Sensory Integration

Theory and Practice

Sensory Integration
Theory and Practice
Second Edition

Anita C. Bundy, ScD, OTR, FAOTA
Professor
Department of Occupational Therapy
Colorado State University
Fort Collins, Colorado

Shelly J. Lane, PhD, OTR/L, FAOTA
Professor and Department Chair
Department of Occupational Therapy
School of Allied Health
Virginia Commonwealth University
Richmond, Virginia

Elizabeth A. Murray, ScD, OTR/L, FAOTA
Senior Instructional Designer
CAST
Peabody, Massachusetts

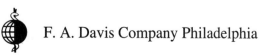 F. A. Davis Company Philadelphia

F. A. Davis Company
1915 Arch Street
Philadelphia, PA 19103
www.fadavis.com

Printed in the United States of America

Last digit indicates print number: 10 9 8 7 6 5 4 3 2

Acquisitions Editor: Margaret Biblis
Developmental Editor: Peg Waltner
Production Editors: Jessica Howie Martin, Nwakaego Fletcher-Perry
Cover Designer: Louis Forgione

As new scientific information becomes available through basic and clinical research, recommended treatments and drug therapies undergo changes. The author(s) and publisher have done everything possible to make this book accurate, up to date, and in accord with accepted standards at the time of publication. The author(s), editors, and publisher are not responsible for errors or omissions or for consequences from application of the book, and make no warranty, expressed or implied, in regard to the contents of the book. Any practice described in this book should be applied by the reader in accordance with professional standards of care used in regard to the unique circumstances that may apply in each situation. The reader is advised always to check product information (package inserts) for changes and new information regarding dose and contraindications before administering any drug. Caution is especially urged when using new or infrequently ordered drugs.

Library of Congress Cataloging-in-Publication Data

Bundy, Anita C.
   Sensory integration : theory and practice / Anita C. Bundy, Shelly J. Lane, Elizabeth A.
Murray.—2nd ed.
     p. cm.
   Previous ed. publisher under: Sensory integration : theory and practice / Fisher, Anne
G., 1991.
   Includes index.
    ISBN 0-8036-0545-5 (alk. paper)
    1. Sensorimotor integration. 2. Occupational therapy for children. I. Lane, Shelly. II. Murray,
Elizabeth A. III. Fisher, Anne G. Sensory integration. IV. Title.

RJ53.O25 F57 2002
616.8′515′083—dc21

           2002019174

This book is dedicated to A. Jean Ayres who changed occupational therapy practice and, in so doing, enhanced the lives of countless individuals. Jean lives on in our hearts and in our work.

To those who live with sensory integrative dysfunction. More than anyone, they understand what it means.

■■ Foreword

"I am so grateful for the occupational therapy my Anna and our family have obtained. My nephew also has severe symptoms of sensory integration dysfunction, dropped out of high school, was unable to complete the job corps, and now, as an adult, is living at home with his parents. He is lost in a body that he cannot understand, and in a world that doesn't understand him."

Anna's Mother

The 21st century has arrived. Untold numbers of children and their families have been supported by the conceptual and pragmatic legacy of Dr. A. Jean Ayres PhD, OTR (July 18, 1920–December 16, 1988), the originator of and first researcher in sensory integrative dysfunction. Parents, families, communities, therapists, and researchers are moving forward together to help children like Anna and her cousin.

Certainly, many thousands of adults and children with sensory integrative dysfunction and their families have received support and services based on the powerful intervention conceived originally by Dr. Ayres and further developed by her students and others. Yet, while progress has occurred within the profession, skepticism arises outside the field. The result is that obtaining services can be a huge burden for parents and other consumers: Reimbursement for evaluation and intervention is often unavailable; large research grants are difficult to obtain; and physicians, psychologists, educators, and others are *still* asking for verification of the existence of the disorder and for substantiation of the effectiveness of intervention

We need a call to action in the 21st century. In this excellent second edition of *Sensory Integration Theory and Practice,* the new editors Bundy, Lane, and Murray, have assembled an erudite volume. With contributions from renowned scholars and practitioners in the field, they explore theory, assessment, intervention, and research related to sensory integrative dysfunction—a massive and significant undertaking.

Theory

The work in this volume has the insight and focus needed to advance the theory. In Chapter 1, Bundy and Murray revisit sensory integrative theory as expounded by its originator, Dr. Ayres, whose first publication in this field was offered in 1966—almost *40* years ago. The meticulous presentation previews the intricate conceptualization in subsequent chapters. Particularly noteworthy are sections on the boundaries of sensory integration intervention, effectiveness studies, and the importance of an occupation-centered intervention model.

Chapters 2 and 4 by Lane, Chapter 3 by Reeves and Cermak, and Chapter 5 by Henderson, Pehoski, and Murray, provide a theoretical review of the proposed neural underpinnings of behavior that create a conceptual basis for sensory integrative dysfunction and for intervention. They discuss recent studies that have described physiologic mechanisms of sensory integrative dysfunction; these mechanisms provide a foundation for further investigation of the neural underpinnings for atypical behaviors observed in individuals with sensory integrative dysfunction. In Chapter 6, Burleigh, McIntosh, and Thompson explore new territory related to sensory integration theory in a discussion of the central auditory nervous system and intervention for individuals with disorders in central auditory processing. In Chapter 17, Parham ties sensory integration to occupation.

Assessment

The second section of this book explores assessment of sensory integration (i.e., Chapters 7 [Bundy] and 8 [Bundy and Fisher]). These chapters and an appendix (Ayres and Marr) detail standardized and clinical methodologies and their interpretation. The chapters are impressive in scope and originality and provide a framework for comprehensive evaluation and clinical reasoning. They emphasize the need to consider the context of daily life.

Intervention

The next chapters focus on intervention and are a tribute to the thousands of occupational therapists and other health professionals who work persistently, making personal sacrifices to provide services to families, children, and adults with sensory integrative dysfunction. One can both learn from, and revel in, the information provided. From our therapeutic experiences, we generate new ideas for successful research. We also learn how to intervene with our next clients; our clients are our professors.

As detailed, the importance of thoughtful, careful intervention is paramount. In these intervention chapters (9–12), Bundy and Koomar draw upon the theory base presented previously to discuss the complex and powerful intervention first characterized by Ayres. Koomar and Bundy explore insight and wisdom, and play in intervention, highlighting the importance of clinical reasoning and emphasizing the complexity of this approach to intervention. They highlight the *respect* and *individuality* that persons receiving intervention must be afforded as clinicians struggle to understand the many facets of dysfunction and daily life. Intervention, they suggest, is based upon the intuition and artfulness of the therapist, perhaps more than the specific activities and modalities used.

In Chapter 14, several authors (Frick, Gjesing, Harkness, Hickman, Kawar, Shellenberger, J. Lawton-Shirley, P. Wilbarger, and Williams) explore new ideas related to intervention for individuals with sensory integrative dysfunction. The education innovator John Dewey (1859–1952) said, "*Every great advance in science has issued from a new audacity of imagination.*" The creative ideas explored in these chapters have generated new energy as well as controversy in the field. Future research will establish the role of these newer methods in intervention. They *may* be shown to be a leap forward when carefully applied within the context of established principles of occupational therapy. Time and research will tell the unfolding story of the validity of these new ideas.

Another section of this volume explores interventions beyond the clinic, discussing supplemental interventions with children and adults with sensory integrative dysfunction. Included are chapters on consultation (13: Bundy) and combining sensory integration intervention with other methods (15: Anzalone and Murray) such as neurodevelopmental treatment, behavior and learning theory, and coping theory.

The field of sensory integrative dysfunction has a legacy of science from its originator, Dr. Ayres. Since her death in 1988, controversy has abounded.

Men [and women] are apt to mistake the
strength of their feeling
for the strength of their argument.
The heated mind resents the chill touch
And relentless scrutiny of logic.

William Gladstone (1809–1898)

Such has been the case in the field of sensory integrative dysfunction for decades. Some *believe* in sensory integrative dysfunction and some publicly decry its validity. Some *believe* that the research base solidly demonstrates the value of sensory integrative dysfunction, while others *feel* that sensory integrative dysfunction is myths and magic. Some practitioners *believe* the newer intervention methods are superior to the more established methods and others *feel* we must remain solidly within the principles and techniques established by Dr. Ayres when providing intervention.

Research

And this brings us to research. In important chapters, Mulligan and others explore the state of research in the field. The lesson is that we need more high-quality research, the type Dr. Ayres herself conducted and advocated. Of course research, "*never solves a problem without creating ten more*" (G.B. Shaw, 1856–1950). And yet, as Dr. Ayres would assert, that is the purpose and beauty of science—growth.

There must be no barriers to freedom of inquiry
... or dogma in science. The scientist is free, and
must be free to ask any questions, to doubt any
assertion, to seek for any evidence, and to correct
any errors.

J. Robert Oppenheimer (1904–1967)

We have learned so much ... and yet we have so much more to learn. Our research agenda in the 21st century includes studying:

- The validity of sensory integrative dysfunction as a distinct syndrome, separate and distinct from other known disorders. What are its phenotypic and genotypic characteristics?

- The effectiveness of intervention. With what specific types of problems and under what specific intervention conditions is treatment useful?
- The underlying neurologic, physiologic, and/or biochemical mechanisms that result in sensory integrative dysfunction.
- The etiologies, incidence, and prevalence of the condition.

The 20th century brought the identification of sensory integrative dysfunction, the development of initial assessment and intervention methodologies, and the birth of research in the field. The 21st century promises a revolution in knowledge created by an intricate and essential research agenda. The complexity of the research is ours to behold and investigate. Only through continued study of what we do not know, can our theories and practice be legitimized.

Some believe that science is a proving ground for theory; I perceive science as a path along which knowledge can be improved. We go forward with uncertainty, and with humility, hoping and worrying and working towards the ultimate truth—truths that in their finality will bring calm and joy to children and adults with sensory integrative dysfunction and their families. This volume will aid us greatly upon that path.

"Truth, like infinity, is to be forever approached, but never reached"

A. Jean Ayres, 1972 p.4

Lucy Jane Miller, PhD, OTR
April 30, 2001

Foreword Bibliography

Ayres, A.J. (1965). Patterns of perceptual-motor dysfunction in children: A factor analytic study. *Perceptual and Motor Skills, 20,* 335–368.

Ayres, A.J. (1972). *Sensory integration and learning disorders.* Los Angeles: Western Psychological Services.

■■ Preface

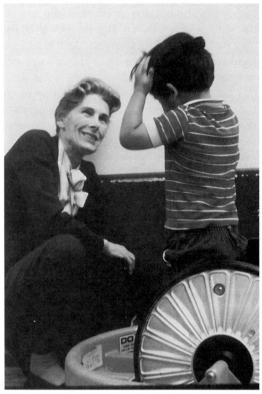

Dr. Jean Ayres with "Roy."

More than 10 years ago, I (AB) first saw a video-tape of an intervention session that Jean Ayres conducted with an almost-4-year-old-boy I'll call "Roy." I was so "taken" by the tape that I made a bootleg copy and I have shown it in countless courses in many countries. However, most often I used it in courses about play. In fact, until very recently, I did not know the actual story of that session.

The tape began with Roy sitting inside a tire tube atop a platform swing, pulling on handles to make it move. Within a few moments, Roy held his arms out to Jean using the age-old gesture that means, "pick me up." The overall impression is of a very young child. Jean, however, did not pick Roy up. Instead, she showed him where to place his leg and facilitated his active movement. In effect, she nonverbally said, "You do it yourself. I'm here to help."

Jean and Roy moved from one activity to another. Each time, he tried to get her to "rescue him" and each time she gently, firmly, and nonverbally insisted that he take control. Roy got on a "horse swing" suspended from the ceiling by two points, but it was too great a challenge to his poorly developed postural mechanism and he tried to throw himself off onto the mat below. Jean gently placed his hands back on the horse and held it to make it more stable. "Give it a good try," she seemed to be saying. After a few moments, she helped him get off by facilitating his movements again.

Within 20 minutes, Roy had gotten on and off no less than six pieces of equipment. He seemed unable to get really involved with any of the equipment for more than a few moments. Jean followed his lead—always facilitating rather than doing for him. At one point, Roy stood on a vibrating platform and Jean offered to brush him but Roy said, "No." And something about the way he said it suggested that he was taking control. Although it had once seemed that the session might never get underway (which I, as an experienced practitioner, found oddly comforting), that was no longer the case. A remarkable transformation was taking place: Roy shed his babyish ways before my eyes.

Roy's growth began surreptitiously but accelerated. He got involved in a game in which he drove a pretend truck along a makeshift road to deliver packages to "Teresa," the therapist assisting Jean. In his actions and limited words, Roy *became* a deliveryman. And the game continued for 15 minutes or more with Roy becoming more and more assertive. At one point, when Teresa told Roy that he had room for only two packages, Roy screeched, "No, no, no, no!" at the top of his lungs. A sturdy truck driver had replaced the passive child who began the session.

Although Roy's mother undoubtedly would not have been amused, I cannot stifle a grin whenever I see the tape. "You go, Roy!" This almost-4-year-old, who should long ago have outgrown the "terrible twos," suddenly seemed to have come into his own.

Jane Koomar, who, with Elise Holloway, was

responsible for the taping of this wonderful session, gave the following account:

> Jean was addressing Roy's vestibular and postural problems, reinforcing language as opportunities arose and addressing his dyspraxia by allowing him to have a lot of control, initiating things on his own, and expanding on themes in which he showed interest. At this point he rarely imitated the therapist, but Jean tried that strategy when she could. He loved Jean and really worked hard for her. He was one of many children who seemed to know that Jean understood him. He could be his best self with Jean and knew that she would appreciate everything he tried to do. Although Jean was not his primary therapist, he was very bonded to her and would look for her and go over and give her a big hug whenever he saw her in the clinic. (Jane Koomar, personal communication, March 10, 2001.

A. Jean Ayres was both a master theoretician and a master clinician. One of the most incredible things about her work is that we can view it through a number of lenses. When I see the tape of Roy, I cannot resist imposing my play theory lenses on it. Jane Koomar saw it as an exquisite example of sensory integration theory.

When we were writing the first edition, Jean cautioned us about equating intervention with play. She feared that an association between play and sensory integration theory would denigrate the science of the theory. But the power of the play that occurs between Roy and Jean is undeniable. The play reflects the *art* of practice. Sensory integration theory, as much as any theory in occupational therapy, depends on a partnership of art and science. Science gives sensory integration credibility; art gives it meaning. Toward a partnership of art and science, we offer these works from a number of outstanding theorists, researchers, clinicians, and artists. Jean Ayres touched us all. We carry the torch that she passed to us at her death, fueling it with new perspectives and new knowledge.

Anita C. Bundy
Shelly J. Lane
Elizabeth A. Murray

■■ Acknowledgments

This book has been a long time in the making. It definitely reflects the efforts and support of countless individuals to whom we owe a tremendous debt of gratitude.

Many people at F. A. Davis were particularly helpful. Lynn Borders Caldwell, Margaret Biblis, and Christa Fratantoro enabled us to spend time together, which made all the difference. They also answered our unending questions. When we thought we had corrected all the errors and inconsistencies, Peg Waltner found more. Jean François Vilain cheered us on from the sidelines: We needed that. We will miss him a great deal in his retirement.

The authors represent some of the greatest minds in their respective fields. Each has made a significant contribution to sensory integration theory. In addition, some authors whose work was critical to the first edition, notably Anne Fisher, Gary Kielhofner, and Ken Ottenbacher, have made more important contributions to this edition than may be readily apparent.

Our reviewers guided us to clarify, rethink, and reorganize. The end product reflects their collective wisdom. We thank: Lila Bartmann, Patti Davies, Ginny Deal, Lynne Harkness, Marge Luthman, Nancy Payjak, Andrew Potts, Sharon Ray, Becky Robler, Eva Rodriquez, Pat Sample, Gretchen Stone, Brenda Wilson, Louise White, and the Colorado State University students in the OT 421 class in Spring, 2000 and the OT 480 classes in Fall, 2000 and Fall, 2001. We are particularly grateful to Sharon Ray, Margaret Short, and Brenda Wilson, who reviewed large chunks of this manuscript—sometimes more than once!

Linda McDowell, Cindy Weaver, Barbara Ball, Wendi Wetherell, and Nancy Hughes provided significant technical assistance. David Greene drew draft after draft of the major schematic that appears throughout the text. Shay McAtee shot a substantial number of the photographs, including the one that appears on the cover.

Finally, those who are closest to us offered unending support, including, but not limited to, waiting on us while we worked and setting aside many of their own needs: Ginny Deal; Rick, Hannah, and Lucas Thornton; and Jackie Dalton. We truly could not have done it without them.

We have heard that Aldous Huxley once said, "If you want to write, keep cats." Dogs are pretty good too—especially golden retrievers. PJ, Morgan, Amy, Shadey, and Smokey (our cats), and Cody, Socks, and Moffat (our dogs) offered comic relief and a sympathetic ear whenever we needed them. PJ stood on the keyboard a number of times, and is no doubt responsible for any errors.

A.C.B.
S.J.L.
E.A.M.

■■ Contributors

MARIE ANZALONE, ScD, OTR, FAOTA
Assistant Professor of Clinical Occupational
  Therapy
College of Physicians and Surgeons
Columbia University
New York, New York

A. JEAN AYRES, PHD, OTR, FAOTA
(deceased)
Emeritus Adjunct Associate Professor
Department of Occupational Therapy
University of Southern California
Los Angeles, California

ANITA C. BUNDY, ScD, OTR, FAOTA
Professor
Department of Occupational Therapy
Colorado State University
Ft. Collins, Colorado

JOAN M. BURLEIGH, PhD
Director
Center for Central Auditory Research
Research Scientist
Department of Electrical and Computer
  Engineering
Colorado State University
Ft. Collins, Colorado

SHARON A. CERMAK, EdD, OTR, FAOTA
Professor and Program Director
Boston University MCH Center for Leadership
  in Pediatric OT
Department of Occupational Therapy
Boston University
Boston, Massachusetts

ANNE G. FISHER, ScD, OTR, FAOTA
Professor
Department of Occupational Therapy
Colorado State University
Ft. Collins, Colorado

SHEILA M. FRICK, OTR
Director, Therapeutic Resources
Madison, Wisconsin

GUDRUN GJESING
O.T. in Children's Health
Swimming instructor and recognized Halliwick
  Lecturer
Pedagogic Psychological Counseling
Haderslev, Denmark

LYNNE HARKNESS MS, OTR
Occupational Therapist
Brighton Public Schools 27J
Brighton, Colorado

ANNE HENDERSON, PhD, OTR/L, FAOTA
Professor Emeritus
Department of Occupational Therapy
Boston University
Boston, Massachusetts

LOIS HICKMAN, MA, OTR, FAOTA
Director, Jen-Lo Therapy Farm
Lyons, Colorado

MARY KAWAR, MS, OTR
Director, Mary Kawar & Associates
San Diego, California

JANE A. KOOMAR, PhD, OTR, FAOTA
Executive Director
Occupational Therapy Associates–Watertown,
  P.C.
Watertown, Massachusetts

SHELLY J. LANE, PhD, OTR/L, FAOTA
Professor and Department Chair
Department of Occupational Therapy
School of Allied Health
Virginia Commonwealth University
Richmond, Virginia

NANCY LAWTON-SHIRLEY, OTR
Occupational Therapist
Special Children Center
Hudson, Wisconsin

DIANA MARR, PhD
Measurement Statistician
Educational Testing Services
Princeton, New Jersey

KATHLEEN W. MCINTOSH, PhD
Speech and Language Pathologist
Ft. Collins, Colorado

LUCY J. MILLER, PhD, OTR
Associate Professor of Pediatrics and
    Rehabilitation Medicine
University of Colorado Health Sciences Center,
    Denver CO.
Director
Sensory Integration Dysfunction Treatment and
    Research Center (STAR)
The Children's Hospital
Denver, Colorado
Executive Director
KID Foundation
Littleton, Colorado

SHELLEY MULLIGAN, PhD, OTR
Associate Professor
Department of Occupational Therapy
School of Health and Human Services
University of New Hampshire
Durham, New Hampshire

ELIZABETH A. MURRAY, ScD, OTR/L, FAOTA
Senior Instructional Designer
CAST, Inc.
Peabody, Massachusetts

L. DIANE PARHAM, PhD, OTR, FAOTA
Associate Professor
Department of Occupational Science and
    Occupational Therapy
University of Southern California
Los Angeles, California

CHARLANE PEHOSKI, ScD, OTR/L, FAOTA
Assistant Professor
Worcester State College
Worcester, Massachusetts

GRETCHEN DAHL REEVES, PhD, OT/L, FAOTA
Associate Professor
Eastern Michigan University
Occupational Therapy Program
School of Associated Health Professions
Ypsilanti, Michigan

SHERRY SHELLENBERGER, OTR/L
Co-owner
TherapyWorks Inc.
Albuquerque, New Mexico

TRACY MURNAN STACKHOUSE, MA, OTR
Director of Occupational Therapy and Research
    Associate
UC Davis Medical Center
M.I.N.D. Institute
Davis, California

MICHAEL W. THOMPSON, PhD
Associate Professor
Department of Engineering
Baylor University
Waco, Texas

SHAREN TRUNNELL, OTR
Occupational Therapist
Department of Rehabilitation
The Children's Hospital
Denver, Colorado

JULIA L. WILBARGER, MA, MS, OTR
Doctoral Candidate
University of Denver
Denver, Colorado

PATRICIA L. WILBARGER, MEd, OTR, FAOTA
Private Practice
Santa Barbara, California

MARY SUE WILLIAMS, OTR/L
Co-owner
TherapyWorks Inc.
Albuquerque, New Mexico

■■ Contents

2. Structure and Function of the Sensory Systems   35

Shelly J. Lane, PhD, OTR/L, FAOTA

5. Visual-Spatial Abilities

*Anne Henderson, PhD, OTR/L, FAOTA, Charlane Pehoski, ScD, OTR/L, FAOTA, and
Elizabeth Murray, ScD, OTR/L, FAOTA*

6. Central Auditory Processing Disorders   141

Joan M. Burleigh, PhD, Kathleen W. McIntosh, PhD, and Michael W. Thompson, PhD

PART II Assessment and Intervention

7. Assessing Sensory Integrative Dysfunction   169

Anita C. Bundy, ScD, OTR, FAOTA

8. Interpreting Test Scores and Observations: A Case Example

Anita C. Bundy, ScD, OTR, FAOTA and Anne G. Fisher, ScD, OTR, FAOTA

9. The Process of Planning and Implementing Intervention

Anita C. Bundy, ScD, OTR, FAOTA

10. Play Theory and Sensory Integration

Anita C. Bundy, ScD, OTR, FAOTA

11. Orchestrating Intervention: The Art of Practice

Anita C. Bundy, ScD, OTR, FAOTA and Jane A. Koomar, PhD, OTR, FAOTA

12. Creating Direct Intervention from Theory

Jane A. Koomar, PhD, OTR, FAOTA and Anita C. Bundy, ScD, OTR, FAOTA

13. Using Sensory Integration Theory in Schools: Sensory Integration and Consultation

Anita C. Bundy, ScD, OTR, FAOTA

14. Alternative and Complementary Programs for Intervention   333

15. Integrating Sensory Integration with Other Approaches to Intervention   371

Marie E. Anzalone, ScD, OTR, FAOTA and Elizabeth A. Murray, ScD, OTR/L, FAOTA

PART III   Focus on Research and Occupation

16. Advances in Sensory Integration Research   397

Shelley Mulligan, PhD, OTR

17. Sensory Integration and Occupation   413

L. Diane Parham, PhD, OTR, FAOTA

Appendix A. Use of Clinical Reasoning in Occupational Therapy: The STEP-SI Model of Intervention of Sensory Modulation Dysfunction   435

Lucy J. Miller, PhD, OTR, Julia Wilbarger, MA, MS, OTR, Tracy Stackhouse, OTR, and Sharon Trunnell, OTR

Appendix B. Sensory Integration and Praxis Tests   453

A. Jean Ayres, PhD, OTR, FAOTA and Diana B. Marr, PhD

PART I

Theoretical Constructs

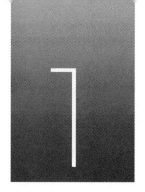

Sensory Integration: A. Jean Ayres' Theory Revisited

Anita C. Bundy, ScD, OTR, FAOTA
Elizabeth A. Murray, ScD, OTR, FAOTA

> *Just as the continued production of research results in constantly changing neurological concepts, so also will [sensory integration] theory need to undergo frequent revision.*
>
> —A. Jean Ayres (1972a, p. ix)

A. Jean Ayres' theory of sensory integration has sparked more research, generated more controversy, and had a more marked effect on occupational therapy practice than any other theory developed by an occupational therapist. Originally, Ayres, an occupational therapist with advanced training in neuroscience and educational psychology, developed the sensory integration theory to explain the relationship between deficits in interpreting sensation from the body and the environment and difficulties with academic or motor learning. Specifically, she hypothesized that a subgroup existed among individuals with learning disorders, whose members displayed deficits in interpreting sensation (Ayres, 1972a). Poor sensory integration without other apparent cause (e.g., peripheral sensory loss, neurological damage) contributed to learning difficulties.

Sensory integration theory has a long history.

As in a novel that begins with an event and then traces the steps leading to it, we will begin with an example and a current view of sensory integration theory and then recount its evolution.

AN EXAMPLE

Sensory integration cannot be observed. We hypothesize that it occurs on the basis of evidence from neuroscience. However, although we *observe* deficits in behavior, we only *hypothesize* that these deficits are the result of poor sensory integration. Furthermore, we observe whether intervention affects a change in behavior, but when behavioral changes do occur, we can only hypothesize that they are caused by improved sensory integration or enhanced neural functioning.

For example, Mark had diminished tactile discrimination, as indicated by his low scores on standardized tests. He also had poor posture, as evidenced by low extensor muscle tone, poor proximal stability, and poor equilibrium reactions. However, Mark had no evidence of frank peripheral or central nervous system (CNS) damage, and he was of average intelligence. Therefore we hypothesized that he had difficulty processing and integrating tactile, vestibular, and proprioceptive sensations within the CNS.

Mark was also clumsy. Although other children his age were playing baseball, Mark could not catch, throw, or bat nearly as well as his peers. Although Mark could tie his shoes and ride a bicycle, learning took more effort for him than for others. Mark's ability to hop, skip, and jump were not as good as expected for a child of his age. On standardized testing, he had difficulty imitating postures and reproducing movement sequences that involved coordinated use of both sides of the body.

Because Mark showed no evidence of frank cognitive or neurological deficits that could account for his motor incoordination, we hypothesized that these problems were related to poor motor planning (i.e., praxis). Furthermore, because empirical evidence has consistently linked diminished ability to discriminate tactile, vestibular, and proprioceptive sensations with problems in motor planning, we speculated that Mark's motor planning problems were related to, and possibly caused by, poor tactile, vestibular, and proprioceptive processing.

We concluded that intervention providing enhanced tactile, vestibular, and proprioceptive sensations in the context of meaningful activities would improve Mark's ability to integrate sensation and plan movement. Although we could not observe improvements in his CNS processing after intervention, we did observe that Mark's coordination improved.

INTRODUCTION TO SENSORY INTEGRATION THEORY

Ayres (1972a) defined sensory integration as "the neurological process that organizes sensation from one's own body and from the environment and makes it possible to use the body effectively within the environment" (p. 11).

Although she believed that visual processing was central to learning, Ayres focused her theory on the vestibular, proprioceptive, and tactile systems. In 1981, she wrote to Kay Sieg, "If you just look at children from a behavioral standpoint and do behavioral type research, and modeling, you'll never really discover that a main foundation to visual perception is the vestibular system with proprioception and other senses also contributing" (Sieg, 1988, pp. 99–100). Ironically, until very recently, the role of vision in sensory integration theory was reduced primarily to form and space perception, construction, and visual-motor coordination (i.e., paper and pencil tasks). In Chapter 5, Henderson and colleagues propose a new conceptualization of visual-spatial ability and relate it more clearly to sensory integration.

Recognizing the provisional nature of sensory integration theory, Ayres nonetheless hoped to be able to identify patterns of dysfunction among children with sensorimotor and learning problems and tailor specific intervention strategies to different subgroups. In fact, Ayres' primary objective in developing sensory integration theory was to explain the underlying cause of these problems in order to determine the optimal mode of intervention (Ayres, 1972a, 1975a, 1979).

Over time, sensory integration theory and its evaluation and intervention technology have undergone numerous revisions. Ayres (1972a) anticipated the need for the theory to evolve, indicating that:

> . . . in many instances, [sensory integration] theory falls short of its goals, but a useful purpose will have been served if a new focus on the problem of learning disorders stimulates further search for an even more effective and comprehensive theory that will yield procedures that may enhance CNS integration and, consequently, ameliorate associated learning and behavior problems. Truth, like infinity, is to be forever approached but never reached (p. 4).

SENSORY INTEGRATION THEORY

Sensory integration is a *theory* of brain–behavior relationships. Theories are not facts; rather, theories represent provisional statements based on assumptions. The value of a theory is that it helps to explain, plan, and predict. Sensory integration theory is used to:

- *Explain* why individuals behave in particular ways.
- *Plan* intervention to ameliorate particular difficulties.
- *Predict* how behavior will change as a result of intervention.

Sensory integration theory has three components. The first pertains to development and describes typical sensory integrative functioning; the second defines sensory integrative dysfunction; and the third guides intervention programs. Each component, in turn, has a major, overarching postulate. The three major postulates of sensory integration theory are:

1. Learning is dependent on the ability to take in and process sensation from movement and the environment and use it to plan and organize behavior.
2. Individuals who have a decreased ability to process sensation also may have difficulty producing appropriate actions, which, in turn, may interfere with learning and behavior.
3. Enhanced sensation, as a part of mean-

ingful activity that yields an adaptive interaction, improves the ability to process sensation, thereby enhancing learning and behavior.

Because sensory integration theory has components that pertain to dysfunction and intervention, it has evaluation and intervention technology. Thus, when we speak of sensory integration, we refer to three interrelated elements of practice:

1. The theory itself
2. Evaluation methods (i.e., the Sensory Integration and Praxis Tests [SIPT] [Ayres, 1989]), measures of sensory modulation (e.g., the Sensory Profile [Dunn, 1999]), and related clinical assessments of neuromotor behavior
3. A specific approach to intervention

The relationships of the three elements of practice to processes associated with sensory integration are shown schematically in Figure 1–1.

A Schematic Representation of Sensory Integration Theory

Schematic representations reflect the relationships among a parsimonious set of constructs drawn

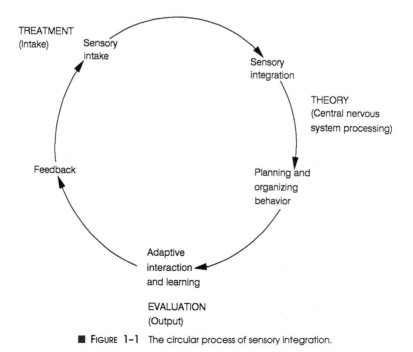

■ FIGURE 1–1   The circular process of sensory integration.

from the theory. For simplicity, theories are often depicted schematically. The creator of the schematic selects the specific constructs. Thus, a theory may be represented schematically in numerous ways by numerous authors.

As shown schematically in Figure 1–2, sensory integrative dysfunction manifests itself in two major ways: poor modulation and poor praxis. Individuals can have evidence of one or both types of dysfunction.

Although Figure 1–2 provides a useful overview of sensory integrative dysfunction, it does not convey the complexity of the theory. Based partly on Ayres' (1979) representation, we have created a schematic that reflects hypothesized relationships among sensory systems and behavior (Fig. 1–3). Although this representation refers to relationships germane to all three postulates (i.e., development, dysfunction, and intervention), for simplicity we have depicted only the dysfunction postulate.

Central nervous system processing of vestibular, proprioceptive, and tactile sensation, including processing in the limbic and reticular systems, is represented in a central column. Expressions of modulation dysfunction emanate from the left side of the central column. Expressions of dyspraxia are to the right of sensory processing. The closer a construct is to the column representing sensory processing, the clearer the neurophysiological relationship. Poor processing of vestibular and proprioceptive information have been related to deficits in practic dysfunction, and two modulation disorders, gravitational insecurity and aversive responses to movement. The tactile system has been related to somatodyspraxia and sensory defensiveness. As shown by the overlapping circles in Figure 1–2, an individual can have practic deficits, modulation deficits, or both. Although we discuss each of the difficulties associated with sensory integrative dysfunction (see Fig. 1–3) in detail in subsequent chapters, we have also described each briefly here.

Practic Dysfunction

In sensory integration theory, praxis refers to the ability to plan new movements. We have identified two levels of motor planning dysfunction: BIS and somatodyspraxia.

Patterns of test scores associated with somatodyspraxia and BIS have appeared consistently in research related to sensory integrative testing (Ayres, 1965, 1966a, 1966b, 1969, 1972b, 1977, 1989; Ayres et al., 1987; Mulligan, 1998, 2000).

To have sensory integrative–based dyspraxia, individuals must have deficits in processing one or more types of sensation. Different types of praxis are associated with dysfunction in different sensory systems. Specifically, whereas deficits in BIS are associated with vestibular and proprioceptive processing, somatodyspraxia is associated with processing tactile, vestibular, and proprioceptive sensations.

Fisher and Bundy (1991b) suggested that somatodyspraxia is a more severe form of practic disorder than is BIS. Lai et al. (1996) supported this speculation by showing that the SIPT praxis tests associated with BIS were more difficult than those typically associated with somatodyspraxia. In fact, one might consider practic ability to represent a spectrum from hyper-normal, evidenced by super-athletes such as Michael Jordan, to very severely impaired, as seen in some individuals with significant brain damage. The practic ability of individu-

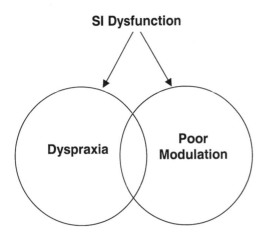

■ FIGURE 1–2 Simplified representation of manifestations of SI dysfunction.

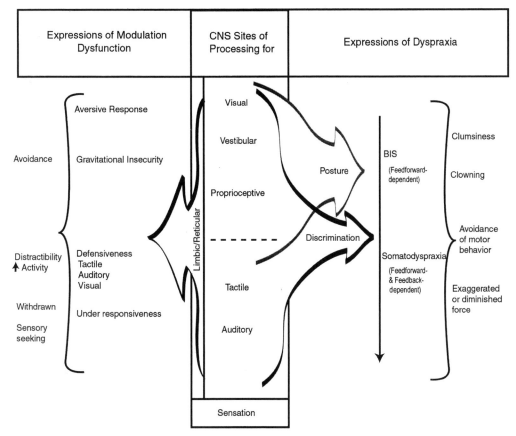

■ FIGURE 1-3 Schematic representation of SI theory (Revised by Bundy, Lane, and Murray from Fisher and Bundy (1991) and Sass (1995), with permission. Graphic courtesy of David Greene.)

als with the two types of sensory integrative–based practic deficits (i.e., BIS and somatodyspraxia) likely fall somewhere in the middle. This hypothesized spectrum of practic ability is illustrated in Figure 1–4.

Postural Deficits

Posture is assumed to be the outward manifestation of vestibular and proprioceptive processing. Thus, although it is not a type of practic disorder, postural deficits are thought to reflect the basis for deficits in BIS in particular, and sometimes for somatodyspraxia. A diagnosis of postural deficits is based on the presence of a meaningful cluster of indicators (see Chapter 8 for a discussion of meaningful clusters). Relevant postural indicators include:

• Extensor muscle tone (assessed by examining posture in standing)

• Prone extension
• Proximal stability
• Ability to move the neck into flexion against gravity (part of supine flexion)
• Equilibrium

Postrotary nystagmus is also often a part of this grouping, in which case the cluster may be called "postural-ocular."

Deficits in Tactile Discrimination

Deficits in tactile discrimination are assumed to be an outward manifestation of tactile processing. They are thought to be one basis for somatodyspraxia. A diagnosis of deficits in tactile discrimination is based on the presence of a meaningful cluster of standardized test scores indicating that an individual has difficulty identifying the characteristics of touch. Generally, these tests are drawn from the SIPT.

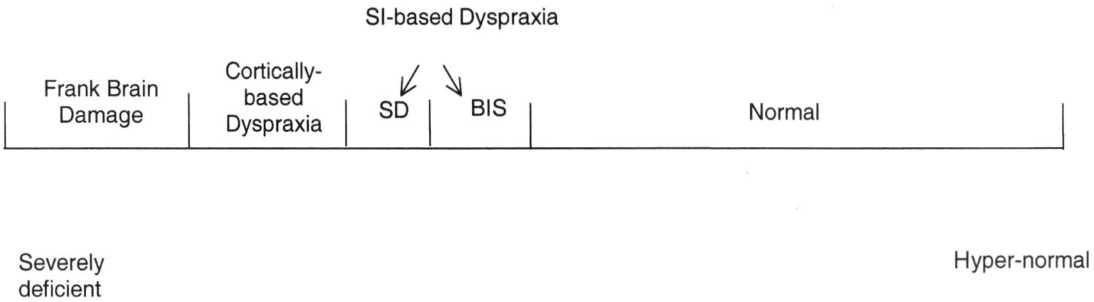

SI-based Dyspraxia

Frank Brain Damage	Cortically-based Dyspraxia	SD ↙ ↘ BIS	Normal

Severely
deficient

Hyper-normal

■ FIGURE 1–4 Spectrum of practice ability.

Deficits in Bilateral Integration and Sequencing

As the name suggests, individuals with BIS have difficulty using the two sides of their body in a co-ordinated fashion and sequencing motor actions. Fisher (1991) indicated that "sequencing" referred specifically to anticipatory projected movement sequences (i.e., the feedforward-dependent sequence of movements necessary to get one's limbs to a particular place in time to act). For example, to catch a ball, one must project the hands to the precise location where the ball will be in time to receive it. Fisher indicated that many projected action sequences are bilateral. BIS is presumed to have its basis in poor vestibular and proprioceptive processing. Additionally, the visual system plays a major role in anticipating the location of moving objects and in guiding our movements to these locations (see Chapters 3 and 5).

Somatodyspraxia

Individuals with somatodyspraxia have difficulty with both feedback- (simple) and feedforward-dependent (difficult) motor tasks. That is, they have difficulty with the whole range of gross motor tasks. Often they have difficulty with fine motor tasks as well. Keogh and Sugden (1985) and Henderson and Sugden (1992) offered a simple model for gauging the degree to which an activity is feedback or feedforward dependent. This model is shown in Figure 1–5. The more movement by the client or target on which the client is acting, the greater the feedforward demand of the task.

To have somatodyspraxia, an individual must have deficits in somatosensory (usually tactile) processing. However, the individual usually also has poor vestibular and proprioceptive processing.

Sensory Modulation Disorders

Although therapists (e.g., Dunn, 1997; Kinneally et al., 1995; Wilbarger & Wilbarger, 1991) have frequently referred to sensory modulation disorders, statistical evidence of their occurrence has been more elusive. Until very recently, no formal tests related to sensory modulation existed. Rather, such diagnoses were made based on observation or history alone. Thus, Ayres rarely included evidence of sensory modulation disorders in her analyses, and then only of tactile defensiveness. Recently, Dunn and colleagues (Dunn, 1994; Dunn & Brown, 1997; Dunn & Westman, 1997) and Miller and colleagues (McIntosh et al., 1999; McIntosh et al., 1999; Miller et al., 1999) conducted a series of studies that have provided preliminary information about the nature of sensory modulation disorders. Dunn's work has included a series of factor analytic studies using a tool called the *Sensory Profile* (Dunn, 1999). Miller (McIntosh et al., 1999) used both physiological measures and a shortened version of the *Sensory Profile* to examine sensory modulation disorders.

Although the term "modulation" is familiar to many therapists, its precise meaning is elusive. Ayres (1979), who first applied the concept to sensory integration theory, defined modulation as the CNS's regulation of its own activity. Engineers liken modulation to tuning a radio to the amplitude and frequency of the sound waves emitted by a particular station. When the amplitude and frequency detected by the radio tuner match those of the station's sound waves, the station comes in clearly. However, when the tuner is not properly modulated, the radio is rendered ineffective. Individuals who have difficulty modulating sensation behave as though the amplitude of their response is consistently greater or less than that of most in-

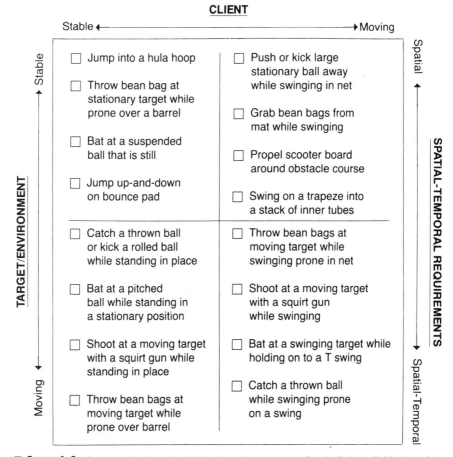

CLIENT

Stable ←——————————————————————————→ Moving

TARGET/ENVIRONMENT Stable	
☐ Jump into a hula hoop	☐ Push or kick large stationary ball away while swinging in net
☐ Throw bean bag at stationary target while prone over a barrel	☐ Grab bean bags from mat while swinging
☐ Bat at a suspended ball that is still	☐ Propel scooter board around obstacle course
☐ Jump up-and-down on bounce pad	☐ Swing on a trapeze into a stack of inner tubes
☐ Catch a thrown ball or kick a rolled ball while standing in place	☐ Throw bean bags at moving target while swinging prone in net
☐ Bat at a pitched ball while standing in a stationary position	☐ Shoot at a moving target with a squirt gun while swinging
☐ Shoot at a moving target with a squirt gun while standing in place	☐ Bat at a swinging target while holding on to a T swing
☐ Throw bean bags at moving target while prone over barrel	☐ Catch a thrown ball while swinging prone on a swing

(Left axis label: TARGET/ENVIRONMENT, Stable ↑ / Moving ↓)
(Right axis label: SPATIAL-TEMPORAL REQUIREMENTS, Spatial ↑ / Spatial-Temporal ↓)

■ FIGURE 1–5 Common treatment activities by category, according to their spatial-temporal requirements. (Adapted from Keogh and Sugden, 1985.)

dividuals, decreasing the effectiveness of their performance. This is illustrated in Figure 1–6.

Depending on the sensory system (or systems) most affected and whether individuals tend to underreact or overreact to sensation, deficits in sensory modulation can be manifest in several different ways. Commonly, four types of modulation disorders include:

1. Sensory (including tactile) defensiveness
2. Gravitational insecurity
3. Aversive responses to movement
4. Underresponsiveness

Sensory Defensiveness

Sensory defensiveness is a fight-or-flight reaction to sensation that others would consider nonnoxious. Although tactile defensiveness was the first to be described, defensiveness is widely believed to occur in all sensory systems, with the possible exception of the vestibular and proprioceptive systems. Sensory defensiveness is often linked to poor limbic or reticular system processing (see Chapter 4).

Gravitational Insecurity

Gravitational insecurity is manifested as fear of movement, being out of the upright position, or having one's feet off the ground. As with sensory defensiveness, reactions reflecting gravitational insecurity are out of proportion to any danger and also to any postural deficits the individual has. Gravitational insecurity is associated with poor otolithic vestibular processing (Fisher, 1991).

Aversive Responses to Movement

Aversive responses to movement occur in response to movements that most individuals would consider non-noxious; they are characterized by

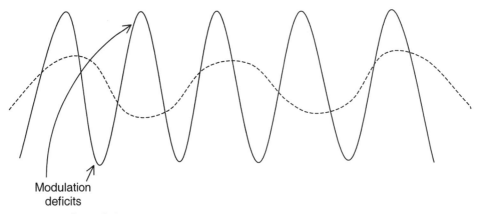

Modulation
deficits

■ Figure 1–6   Schematic representation of modulation and modulation deficits.

autonomic nervous system reactions. Similar to gravitational insecurity, aversive responses to movement are associated with poor processing of vestibular information. However, rather than otolithic processing, aversive responses are thought to reflect poor processing of semicircular canal-mediated information (Fisher, 1991).

Underresponsiveness to Sensation

Although each of the mentioned sensory modulation disorders involves individuals *overreacting* to sensation, some individuals are *underresponsive* to sensation. They react in a way that suggests they do not notice sensation, or their responses are far less than expected. There is some clinical indication that certain individuals with this disorder also may have a delayed reaction to sensation. An example of delayed reaction to pain occurs when an individual does not respond immediately to—or seems unaware that—a painful event has occurred. Of course, underresponsivity or delayed reactions can also occur in other sensory systems (see Chapter 4).

Assumptions of Sensory Integration Theory

As with all theories, several assumptions underlie sensory integration theory. These assumptions relate to the neural or behavioral bases of sensory integration.

Assumption 1: The Central Nervous System Is Plastic

Plasticity refers to the ability of brain structures to change. Intervention derived from sen-

sory integration theory is hypothesized to effect changes in the brain because of plasticity. Ayres (1989) indicated that:

> . . . the brain, especially the young brain, is naturally malleable; structure and function become more firm and set with age. The formative capacity allows person-environment interaction to promote and enhance neurointegrative efficiency. A deficiency in the individual's ability to engage effectively in this transaction at critical periods interferes with optimal brain development and consequent overall ability. Identifying the deficient areas at a young age and addressing them therapeutically can enhance the individual's opportunity for normal development (p. 12).

Ayres consistently stressed the structural and behavioral plasticity of the young brain. In earlier writings, she assumed that age 3 to 7 years was a critical period for development of sensory integration (Ayres, 1979). Unfortunately, this has been incorrectly interpreted to mean that individuals older than age 8 years could no longer benefit from intervention based in sensory integration theory. Our experience in treating older children and adult clients clearly indicates that these individuals have the potential for significant change. Furthermore, experimental brain research has indicated that plasticity persists into adulthood and possibly throughout life. There is little evidence that younger children benefit more or change faster than do older children or adults who participate in intervention programs based on the principles of sensory integration theory. Law et al. (1991) are among very few researchers to have demonstrated such a relationship.

In their critique of sensory integration theory, Ottenbacher and Short (1985) noted that "recent environmental enrichment studies now indicate that brain alterations do occur in mature organisms and even in geriatric organisms" (p. 302). However, they also differentiated between plasticity (i.e., structural or morphological change) and learning (i.e., functional or "adaptive change in behavior as a result of experience") (p. 300). Behavioral change does not necessarily indicate a specific change in neural structure, and future research may lead to modification of the theory.

Assumption 2: Sensory Integration Develops

Behaviors present at each stage in the developmental sequence provide the basis for the development of more complex behaviors. Parham and Mailloux (2001) described adaptive interactions typical of young children from the prenatal period through about age 7 years.

When sensory integrative dysfunction occurs, normal development is disrupted. As Short-DeGraff (1988) indicated that:

> . . . sensory integration theory assumes that the brain is immature at birth and also is immature [or dysfunctional] in some individuals with learning problems. The goal of sensory integration therapy is to provide stimulation that will address certain brain levels (primarily subcortical), enabling them to mature [or function more normally], and thereby assisting the brain to work as an integrated whole (p. 200).

Assumption 3: The Brain Functions as an Integrated Whole

Ayres consistently stressed the idea that the brain functioned as a whole. Nonetheless, she believed that higher-order integrative functions evolved from, and were dependent on, the integrity of "lower-order" structures and on sensorimotor experience. She viewed higher-order (cortical) centers of the brain as responsible for abstraction, perception, reasoning, language, and learning. In contrast, she viewed sensory integration as occurring mainly within lower (subcortical) centers. Furthermore, she conceptualized lower parts of the brain as developing and maturing before higher-level structures. She believed

that development and optimal functioning of higher-order structures were dependent, in part, on the development and optimal functioning of lower-order structures (Ayres, 1972a, 1974a, 1974b, 1975a, 1979, 1989).

Sensory integration theory has been criticized because of the inclusion of hierarchical concepts (Ottenbacher & Short, 1985; Short-DeGraff, 1988). However, as Short-DeGraff (1988) pointed out, Ayres incorporated both holistic and hierarchical concepts into her theory. Ayres used hierarchical concepts to facilitate communication of difficult ideas and as a guide for intervention; however, she never lost sight of the holistic or systems view of the brain. Unfortunately, the use of hierarchical concepts has led to an overemphasis on linear or reductionistic thinking when describing sensory integration theory and practice.

Thus, in this text, we have emphasized a systems view of the nervous system. In this view, Ayres' concept of an interactive, holistic hierarchy is retained. According to Pribram (1986), "the essence of biological . . . hierarchies is that higher levels of organization take control over, as well as being controlled by, lower levels. Such reciprocal causation" (p. 507) exists throughout brain structures. When clients demonstrate evidence of inadequate processing of sensation, it seems most appropriate to think in terms of one or more systems not functioning optimally. Systems interact, and both cortical and subcortical structures contribute to sensory integration. Furthermore, both the person and the CNS are open systems. Through interaction with the environment, an open system is capable of self-regulating, self-organizing, and changing (Kielhofner, 1985, 1995).

Assumption 4: Adaptive Interactions Are Critical to Sensory Integration

An adaptive interaction represents give and take with the environment in which an individual meets a challenge or learns something new (Ayres, 1972a, 1979, 1985) and the environment changes. An assumption of sensory integration theory is that adaptive interactions *promote* sensory integration and the ability to contribute to an adaptive interaction also *reflects* sensory integration. Although this assumption may appear to reflect circular logic, we believe that sensory integration is a spiraling process characteristic of an open system.

Humans learn from past experience only when we recognize our actions as successful. Knowledge of success is provided by feedback. For example, active movement produces vestibular and proprioceptive sensations (production feedback) that form the basis for memories (neuronal models) of "how it felt" to move. Similarly, knowledge of the outcome of a transaction forms the basis for memories of "what was achieved" (outcome feedback) (Brooks, 1986). Neuronal models, derived from production and outcome feedback, form the basis for planning more complex transactions. Active participation is critical. "Learning from previous experience . . . depends on sensing and moving, not just on sensing" (Brooks, 1986, p. 14). The performance of increasingly complex movements indicates that new neuronal models have developed.

Assumption 5: People Have an Inner Drive to Develop Sensory Integration Through Participation in Sensorimotor Activities

Ayres (1972a, 1975b, 1979, 1989) linked inner drive and motivation to self-direction and self-actualization. She indicated that children with sensory integrative dysfunction often showed little motivation (or inner drive) to be active participants, try new experiences, or meet new challenges. Improvement from intervention often appears first in clients' improved beliefs in their own abilities and in satisfaction derived from mastery of elements within the environment. According to Ayres, inner drive can be seen in the excitement, confidence, and effort that a child brings to an activity. Intervention leads to a stronger inner drive to seek out self-actualizing or growth-promoting activities that, in turn, enhance sensory integration (Ayres, 1972a).

BOUNDARIES OF SENSORY INTEGRATION THEORY AND PRACTICE

Sensory integration theory was designed to describe the difficulties of a particular group of individuals. Similarly, when intervention is based on sensory integration theory, certain principles apply. As sensory integration theory has grown in popularity, it has been applied in ways that exceed the boundaries of the theory. Furthermore, the term *sensory integration* has been used inappropriately

to describe intervention that does not meet the criteria of the theory. When planning and reporting on progress, occupational therapy practitioners should be explicit about the approaches they have used in intervention. When therapists apply testing or intervention outside the circumstances for which it was developed, they must proceed with caution because the boundaries of the theory have been exceeded.

Boundaries and the Population

Sensory integration theory is intended to explain mild to moderate problems in learning and behavior, especially problems associated with motor incoordination and poor sensory modulation that cannot be attributed to frank CNS damage or abnormalities. Ayres hypothesized that sensory integrative dysfunction was related to central processing of sensation. The theory is not intended to explain the neuromotor deficits associated with such problems as cerebral palsy (e.g., spasticity), Down syndrome (e.g., hypotonicity), or cerebrovascular accident (CVA) (e.g., decreased tactile perception). A diagnosis of sensory integrative dysfunction requires evidence of deficits in the central processing of vestibular, proprioceptive, or tactile sensation that are not attributable to frank peripheral or CNS damage or associated with cognitive deficits.

Although the major focus of sensory integration theory has been on children, it also applies to adults who continue to demonstrate dysfunction that was present during childhood. However, the theory is not meant to explain adult-onset deficits. A person with an adult-onset learning, behavior, or neurological problem (e.g., dementia, CVA, schizophrenia) would not have sensory integrative dysfunction unless he or she had it as a child.

Children with mental retardation, cerebral palsy, or other developmental disorders caused by frank CNS damage or abnormality *may* have *concomitant* deficits in sensory integration (i.e., poor modulation, dyspraxia). However, one always must consider the possibility that observed impairments could be attributed to the CNS. For example, children with Down syndrome often have depressed postrotary nystagmus, hypotonicity, poor proximal joint stability, poor equilibrium, and difficulty extending against gravity to assume the prone extension posture. Although this cluster of symptoms may be suggestive of deficits in vestibular and proprioceptive processing, in children with Down syndrome, the problem can be attributed to abnormalities of the cerebellum (Nommensen & Maas, 1993).

Similarly, children with hearing loss may also show a cluster of depressed postrotary nystagmus, low muscle tone, poor proximal joint stability, poor equilibrium, and difficulty extending against gravity to assume the prone extension posture. However, in these cases, the problem may be attributed to a peripheral problem (i.e., damage to the eighth cranial nerve.) The problems in children with hearing loss and children with Down syndrome are *not* likely to be caused by sensory integrative dysfunction.

Although Ayres (1972a, 1975a, 1979) clearly articulated the boundaries of sensory integration theory, many researchers and theorists seem to have exceeded those boundaries (cf. Arendt et al., 1988; Bonder & Fisher, 1989; Densem et al., 1989; Mason & Iwata, 1990; Reisman, 1993; Robichaud et al., 1994; Soper & Thorley, 1996). By using data from children with known CNS disorders (e.g., cerebral palsy) to demonstrate that the SIPT were valid assessments of sensorimotor behavior, Ayres (1989) may have contributed to this problem. She seemed to imply that some of the sensorimotor deficits seen in the children with known CNS dysfunction reflected poor sensory integration. In referring to 10 children with cerebral palsy, Ayres stated that:

> . . . the scores on Standing and Walking Balance (SWB), Motor Accuracy (MAc), and possibly Design Copying (DC) must be considered depressed by the neuromotor incoordination typical of cerebral palsy. This group as a whole has trouble with both visuopraxis and somatopraxis. Poor tactile perception is associated with the dyspraxia (p. 210).

Unfortunately, Ayres (1989) did not explicitly state that the praxis and tactile perception deficits were most likely attributed to the higher-order brain damage characteristic of children with cerebral palsy rather than indicative of impaired sensory integration (see Chapter 15).

Children with Pervasive Developmental Disorders: A Brief Note

A special note about children with autism and other forms of pervasive developmental disorder

(PDD) is in order. Children with PDD are frequently thought to have abnormal processing of sensory information. Several individuals (e.g., Ayres, 1979; Ayres & Tickle, 1980; Baranek et al., 1997; Grandin & Scariano, 1986) have related poor sensory processing to PDD. Others (e.g., Edelson et al., 1999; Linderman & Stewart, 1999; McClure & Holtz-Yotz, 1991; Zissermann, 1992) have examined the effectiveness of sensory stimulation or sensory integration procedures on function in children with PDD or autism. In general, although most studies reflected single case research or case reports and thus may have limited generalizability, the findings have been relatively positive. These findings ranged from decreases in tension and anxiety (Edelson et al., 1999) or self-stimulatory behavior (McClure & Holtz-Yotz, 1991; Zissermann, 1992) to increases in social interaction, approach to new activities, and responsiveness to holding or hugging and movement (Linderman & Stewart, 1999).

Boundaries and Intervention

The boundaries of sensory integration theory also apply to intervention. Direct intervention based on the principles of sensory integration theory involves enhanced sensation in the context of meaningful, self-directed, adaptive interactions. The emphasis is on the integration of vestibular, proprioceptive, and tactile sensations and not just on the motor response. Thus, "the availability of suspended equipment is a hallmark of this treatment approach" (Parham & Mailloux, 2001, p. 364).

Many direct intervention programs referred to as sensory integration probably are more appropriately referred to as sensorimotor or sensory stimulation.

Sensorimotor approaches emphasize specific motor responses (e.g., altered muscle tone, movement). Although sensory is an important part of sensorimotor programs, it is secondary to motor. Generally, suspended equipment is not used. Sensorimotor approaches may be applied to individuals or groups.

In *sensory stimulation* programs, sensation (i.e., olfactory, touch-pressure, vestibular, visual, auditory) is applied *to*, rather than sought *by*, the individual. Sensory stimulation programs are relatively passive. Generally, their purpose is to elicit a generalized response (e.g., increased attention, calming). Sensory stimulation is a component of both sensorimotor and sensory integration approaches but, by itself, cannot be considered to be either (see Chapter 15 for a more detailed discussion of sensorimotor approaches and sensory stimulation).

Service Delivery Models: A Special Note

We have one final note regarding intervention that pertains to service delivery models (i.e., direct intervention, consultation). In many settings, intervention is most appropriately delivered through *consultation*. In consultation, the therapist works with caregivers (or occasionally with a client) to enable them to understand the difficulties of the client in a new way (reframing) and develop strategies to interact more effectively with the client.

In consultation, sensory integration theory provides a new framework for the client's behavior. Strategies may or may not involve the provision of enhanced sensation and require an adaptive response from the client. When the strategies involve altering elements of the human and nonhuman environment but do not include enhanced sensation and an adaptive response, the therapist is likely to be using a rehabilitative frame of reference (Trombly, 1995). We discuss consultation in more detail in Chapter 13.

THE SPIRALING PROCESS OF SELF-ACTUALIZATION

Although Ayres (1972a) emphasized the neurobiological basis of sensory integration and indicated that intervention could "be carried out by educators, psychologists, or health related professionals" (p. ix), occupational therapy practitioners have been the primary professionals to adopt the theory into practice. Seeing a need to bring sensory integration theory more explicitly in line with occupation, Fisher and Murray (1991) proposed a model of sensory integration that emphasized self-actualization (Fig. 1–7.) Their model illustrated the merging of two spiraling processes, one (depicted by the medium gray spiral) reflecting sensory integration theory, and the second (depicted by the white spiral) drawn largely from the Model of Human Occupation (Kielhofner, 1985, 1995). Fisher and Murray named their model "the spiral process of self-actualization."

Fisher and Murray (1991) began with inner drive and a relatively traditional depiction of sen-

sory integration theory. Inner drive provided the impetus to become involved in meaningful activities that were the source of sensation. Participation in meaningful activity was central to Fisher and Murray's model. They defined "meaningful" as having significance, value, or purpose. For an activity to be meaningful, a client must be in control of and able to make sense of the experience.

Taking in sensation (*sensory intake*) is an early step in the sensory integrative process. There are many sources of sensation, including the physical and social environments (represented by arrows labeled *environment*) and *production* and *outcome feedback*. Production feedback arises from the body and informs us about how it felt to move; outcome feedback arises from actions that produce a change in the environment.

Sensation is *integrated* and gives rise to the planning and production of *adaptive interactions* with the environment. *Adaptive* implies that an individual has met the demands of a desired task. Ayres emphasized the need for a client's actions to be just a little better than they had ever been before. *Interaction* implies give and take with environmental elements. Interactions are behaviors that we can observe, evaluate, and change. Adaptive interactions give rise to production and outcome feedback.

Planning an adaptive interaction means knowing "what to do" and organizing "how to do it." Planning depends, in part, on body scheme developed as a result of feedback from previous plans, active participation (production), and outcomes of previous adaptive interactions.

Thus, production and outcome feedback are important to learning. After a neuronal model of an action is developed, it can be used to plan new, more complex interactions. Thus, Fisher and Murray added a third loop (dark lines) to their spirals to depict neuronal models (see Fig. 1–7).

The white loop of the spiral reflects the core assumption of occupational therapy: that humans have an occupational nature and, according to Fisher and Murray (1991), places sensory integration within the greater context of occupational science. Adaptive interactions are basic to occupational behavior. Two core assumptions of occupational science are that humans have an innate need to participate in occupation and that occupation is intrinsically motivating. In turn, humans develop meaning, satisfaction, confidence, self-control, and a sense of mastery from participation

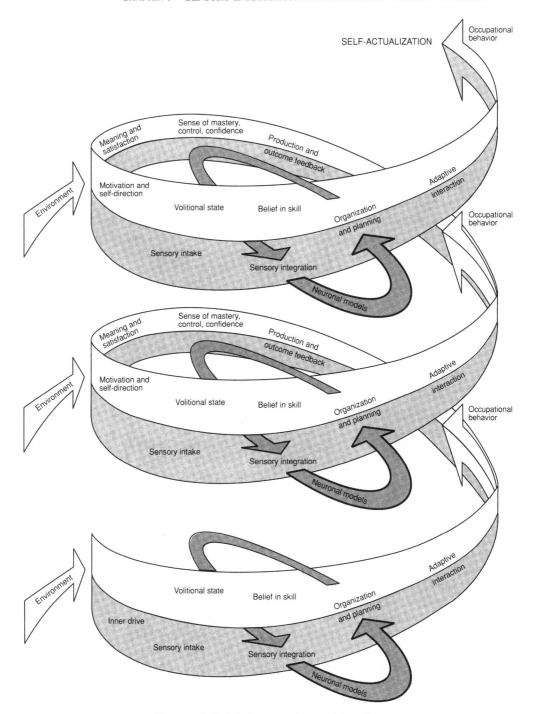

■ FIGURE 1–7 Spiral process of sensory integration.

in occupation (White, 1959). Thus, the impetus for planning and organizing adaptive interactions includes both sensation and volitional factors (e.g., motivation, self-direction).

Adaptive interactions imply that individuals feel a certain amount of control over the environment. People who develop a *sense of mastery* also develop belief in their own abilities (i.e., *belief in skill*). Belief in their abilities enables individuals to become self-directing. They become motivated to explore their capacity through the *planning and production of adaptive interactions* and participation in meaningful occupation.

In summary, Fisher and Murray (1991) hypothesized that through the spiraling process of self-actualization, sensory integration, and adaptive interactions led to organized and effective occupational behavior (e.g., self-care, self-management, play, academic performance). Furthermore, volition is an important prerequisite for adaptive interactions. As individuals develop control over the environment and belief in their own skills, interactions with the environment become more meaningful and satisfying.

THE MIND–BRAIN–BODY PROCESS

Fisher and Murray's (1991) model grew out of criticism leveled against sensory integration theory by Kielhofner and Fisher (1991). They believed that, although Ayres clearly cared about children's self-esteem and self-actualization (i.e., mental phenomena), she portrayed sensory integration very much as a brain–body theory. Recognizing that sensory integration and sensory integrative dysfunction involved a mind–brain–body process, Kielhofner and Fisher (1991) believed it was necessary to couple sensory integration theory with another theoretical framework that operationalized the mind.

> It is not enough to have a general, or vague, reference to the nature of the mind. That is, while recognition of a relationship between sensory integrative dysfunction, clumsiness, and self-esteem is an important beginning, it does not [describe] how the child's view of self emerges, nor does it explain how self-perception influences choices of behavior. If we consider that mental events are at least as complex as is the process of sensory integration, then we can readily see the requirement for a comparably sophisticated view of the mind (Kielhofner & Fisher, 1991, p. 35).

Kielhofner and Fisher (1991) illustrated their concern with separating brain–body from mind with the story of Joe, a 9-year-old boy with sensory integrative dysfunction who was up to bat in a Little League practice session.

> Joe's brain lacked the ability to integrate sensation from his body and the environment. Joe's in-

ability to integrate sensory information seemed to be related to the difficulty he experienced in planning and producing motor action sequences. As a result, his motor behavior was clumsy and his timing was off. But what does this tell us about how or what Joe felt? Joe deeply wanted to be able to play baseball well, but he felt extremely frightened as the pitcher got ready to throw the ball. Joe knew the challenge was to meet the pitched ball with the swing of his bat, but he did not know how to do it. He had little awareness of how it should feel to swing the bat and hit the ball. What he could feel was the eyes of his peers bearing down on him as the ball raced in his direction. Joe became increasingly aware of an aching feeling in the pit of his stomach; his anxiety was acute and physically distressing. Joe had a deep and pervasive feeling that he was "no good."

> This emotional state manifested itself in Joe's brain as overarousal. As the ball approached, Joe was unable to really watch it. The ball seemed to disappear from his visual consciousness and he did not have an awareness of his relationship to it in time and space. He swung the bat almost in self-defense and in the vain hope that somehow it would connect with the ball. But he missed widely and the whole performance had a tragicomic appearance. A chorus of jeers and laughter from his peers painfully drove home his error. And this was not a new experience for Joe. His discomfort with using his body for many of the coordinated actions required in sports was familiar to him. The harder he tried, the more difficult it seemed to be to get things right. For Joe, not being able to physically execute the motor actions he wished, and feeling uncomfortable around peers as his performance missed the mark, was a familiar and uncomfortable experience.

> In Joe's case, we may speculate that inefficient brain processing was responsible for the quality of his motor performance. But we can hardly argue that the inability of Joe's brain to process sensory information, and nothing else, caused the performance. Clearly, Joe's psychological state had something to do with how he performed. What went on as Joe performed badly was much more than just a case of poor sensory integration and uncoordinated motor behavior. Neither Joe's behavior nor his experience could be captured adequately by explanations grounded only in neuroscience. Rather, the important dimension of men-

tal experience was also a critical part of what Joe did and felt (pp. 28–29).

Kielhofner and Fisher (1991) pointed out that fragmentation in the knowledge base concerning mind–brain–body relationships had more than intellectual consequences. When therapists focused on one component of the dysfunctional complex (e.g., the state of the nervous system or neurobehavior) with relative inattention to mental phenomena—or vice versa—intervention became disjointed and incomplete (DiJoseph, 1982). A therapeutic approach that considered both the brain–body and the mind and appreciated how they were interrelated, had obvious advantages over a more narrow or fragmented approach. Thus, in an attempt to address the very real concerns discussed by Kielhofner and Fisher, Fisher and Murray (1991), created the spiraling process of self-actualization, just discussed, as a model that blended sensory integration theory with the model of human occupation.

DEVELOPMENT OF SENSORY INTEGRATION THEORY: HISTORY AND RESEARCH

Fisher and Murray's spiraling process was the result of an evolution that began 25 years before. A. Jean Ayres, the creator of sensory integration theory, continued to work together with numerous students and colleagues until her death in 1988. Since then, a number of researchers and theorists have followed in Ayres' footsteps and continued to shape sensory integration theory. Critics, too, have played a role in its development. All of this work has been crucial to the face that sensory integration theory wears today.

Factor-Analytic and Related Studies

To analyze patterns of dysfunction among children with learning disabilities, Ayres used three statistical procedures: principal components, factor analysis, and cluster analyses. The studies that served as a basis for sensory integration theory were based on principal components and factor analyses. Principal components and factor analysis are conceptually similar in that both can be used to determine whether some small number of underly-

ing constructs accounts for the variability in test scores of a large group of people (Stevens, 1986).

For example, we might administer motor-free tests of visual perception and tests of motor proficiency to a group of children. We expect some to be better at visual perception and some to be more coordinated. We expect that some well-coordinated children will have poor visual-perceptual abilities, and some poorly coordinated children will have good visual-perceptual skills. We expect children who are more skilled at visual perception to obtain higher scores on tests of visual perception and children who are less skilled to obtain lower scores. Similarly, we expect coordinated children to obtain high scores on motor tests and children who are poorly coordinated to obtain low scores. Finally, we expect that some children who obtain high scores on tests of visual perception will attain high scores on motor tests and vice versa. In other words, we expect the tests of visual perception to statistically correlate, and we expect the tests of motor behavior to correlate. However, we do not expect the tests of visual perception to correlate with the tests of motor proficiency or, at least, we do not expect the strength of the correlation to be as strong. Principal components and factor analysis enable researchers to identify correlations among test scores. In our example, we expected two factors, one that included the visual-perceptual tests and another that included the motor tests.

Between 1965 and 1977, Ayres completed six factor-analytic studies of the Southern California Sensory Integration Tests (SCSIT) (Ayres, 1972c) and related measures, using data from children with and without perceptual-motor or learning disabilities (Ayres, 1965, 1966a, 1966b, 1969, 1972b, 1977). Sensory integration theory evolved, in large part, on the basis of Ayres' interpretations of these analyses. Although the factors emerging in the studies were not identical and the labels that Ayres attached to them varied over time, careful analysis revealed certain similarities that suggested the presence of several different—but relatively consistent—patterns of dysfunction. The patterns of dysfunction that appeared most consistently included:

- Dyspraxia (i.e., poor motor planning) associated with poor tactile discrimination (commonly referred to as somatosensory-based dyspraxia)
- Poor bilateral integration associated with postural deficits, thought to reflect poor

processing of vestibular and proprioceptive sensation and commonly called vestibular bilateral integration disorder

- Tactile defensiveness (i.e., an aversive reaction to being touched) was sometimes associated with increased activity level and distractibility
- Poor form and space perception (visual and tactile)
- Auditory-language dysfunction
- Poor eye-hand coordination

Ayres' goal was the identification of discrete patterns of dysfunction (i.e., typologies). Although Ayres found domains of dysfunction using factor analysis, they were not discrete typologies. A child's test scores could reflect more than one pattern, and some children were more correctly described as having generalized sensory integrative dysfunction (Ayres, 1972b). In 1987, Ayres et al. published the results of a seventh factor-analytic study based on the SCSIT, preliminary versions of the SIPT, and clinical observations. Two consistent factors emerged. Ayres named one of them *visuo- and somatodyspraxia*. The second reflected *poor bilateral motor and sequencing abilities*. Other, more unstable, factors appeared to reflect sensory processing deficits. A comparison of this factor analysis and the more recent of the earlier factor analyses is shown in Table 1–1.

Later, in analyzing data from the SIPT, Ayres (1989) used cluster analysis in addition to principal components and factor analysis. Cluster analysis is similar conceptually to principal components or factor analysis, except that the researcher is interested in identifying groups (clusters) of participants whose scores are similar to those of others in one cluster but different from those in any other cluster. In the example we described, we would expect exploratory cluster analysis to identify four clusters of children. One group should be composed of children who obtained high scores on both motor and visual-perceptual tests; another group would be composed of children who attained low scores on both types of tests. We would expect the other two groups to be a high visual-perceptual: low motor group and a low visual-perceptual-high motor group.

The patterns that emerged from the factor and cluster analyses of the SIPT data included:

- Somatosensory processing deficits
- Poor BIS
- Impaired somatopraxis
- Poor praxis on verbal command
- Visuopraxis factor, more appropriately considered poor form and space perception, and visual construction deficits, visual-motor coordination deficits
- Generalized sensory integrative dysfunction

Ayres' factor-analytic and related studies have been appropriately criticized for limitations in design and interpretation (Cummins, 1991; Hoehn & Baumeister, 1994). Because Ayres was constantly exploring new ideas, she used a different battery of assessments in each study. Thus, none

■ TABLE 1–1 SUMMARY OF AYRES' FACTOR ANALYTIC STUDIES, 1972 TO 1989

1972	1976	1977	1987	1989
Apraxia	Praxis-somatosensory	Praxis	Somatodyspraxia	Somatodyspraxia
Form and space	Form and space	Form and space	Visuopraxis	Visuomotor, form and space, visual construction
Hyperactivity, distractibility, tactile disorder		Tactile defensiveness		
Postural-ocular, bilateral integration	Postural-ocular, integration of two body sides	Postural-ocular, integration of two body sides	Bilateral motor and sequencing abilities	Bilateral integration and sequencing
Auditory-language	Auditory-language	Auditory-language	Auditory-memory	Praxis on verbal command
	Duration of postrotary nystagmus	Duration of postrotary nystagmus	Prolonged nystagmus	Postrotary nystagmus
	Eye–hand coordination	Eye–hand coordination		Visuomotor coordination

of the studies was ever a true replication of a preceding one. Furthermore, her sample sizes were consistently small relative to the number of tests administered. When sample sizes are small, there is a great risk that individual tests will "load" on (i.e., correlate with) a given factor purely by chance. Had Ayres replicated any of her studies, it is very likely that the resultant factor loadings would have varied considerably.

A preferable approach would have been to use confirmatory factor analysis (as Mulligan [1998] later did) to "confirm" the existence of hypothesized constructs (factors) rather than exploratory factor analysis to "explore" unknown underlying constructs. However, these limitations did not lessen the impact Ayres' studies had on the development of sensory integration theory; even conservative interpretation of the results revealed reasonably consistent patterns of dysfunction that were represented by somewhat different individual test scores over time.

The initial factor and cluster analyses of the SIPT marked a major milestone in sensory integration theory. Although many of the pattern labels differed from those Ayres labeled earlier, the initial SIPT data expanded on—and further clarified—the results of earlier research. For example, in earlier studies, Ayres identified vestibular bilateral integration disorder. The SIPT data indicated that the ability to plan and execute sequenced movements was also associated with bilateral integration. Although the term "vestibular" was dropped from the pattern label, central vestibular and proprioceptive processing deficits continued to be hypothesized as the basis for some disorders in bilateral integration. However, when vestibular and proprioceptive disorders are separated from BIS disorders, it is clearer that each can occur in isolation from the other. Thus, these SIPT analyses added to and built on previous knowledge.

More recently, Mulligan (1998) completed the largest study to date using SIPT data from more than 10,000 children. Mulligan attempted to confirm the five factors that Ayres reported most consistently. Although she found the five-factor model to have a reasonable fit to the data, confirmatory factor analysis revealed a second-order, four-factor model with more satisfactory fit. That is, Mulligan found that the data were best described by a higher-order factor that she labeled "generalized practic dysfunction" and four first-order factors. Mulligan labeled the first-order factors visual perceptual deficit, BIS deficit, dyspraxia, and somatosensory deficit.

Although Mulligan (1998) labeled the higher-order factor "generalized practic dysfunction," she indicated that, "the strong relationship between dyspraxia and the higher-order factor . . . identified in this study raises the question of whether this higher-order factor is merely dyspraxia" (p. 826). Subsequently, Mulligan agreed that the higher-order factor might actually be better named "general sensory integrative dysfunction" or that it may reflect some "very general 'inefficiency' marker of central nervous system functioning particularly in the areas/systems measured by the SIPT" (Mulligan, personal communication, June 1, 1999). "General sensory integrative dysfunction" seems to capture better the essence of the first-order factors because neither visual perceptual deficit nor somatosensory deficit can be described accurately as practic deficits. Mulligan's model, with the higher order renamed "general sensory integrative dysfunction," is shown in Figure 1–8. However, as Praxis on Verbal Command, thought to be a measure of "higher level praxis," loads strongly on "dyspraxia," it is worth considering whether the second-order factor is not actually something bigger than sensory integrative dysfunction.

The significance of Mulligan's (1998) findings is unclear. As with all research, her study has limitations. Most notably, "the modified models tested were derived from the data themselves." Thus, "future research should include replication of this study with a new sample" (p. 827). However, because Mulligan's study is by far the largest study of SIPT data, her findings deserve serious consideration. Two findings seemed particularly notable.

First, three tests (i.e., Postrotary Nystagmus, Kinesthesia, and Standing and Walking Balance) failed to load on any factor. This has raised interesting questions about the ability of the SIPT to measure postural deficits, thought to be the behavioral manifestation of vestibular and proprioceptive processing. Furthermore, it suggested that therapists must always include clinical observations of posture (e.g., prone extension, postural stability, equilibrium) in their assessments of sensory integration (Fisher & Bundy, 1991a; Mulligan, 1998).

Second, unlike Ayres (1966b, 1977, 1989; Ayres et al., 1987), who consistently associated poor praxis with somatosensory deficits, Mulli-

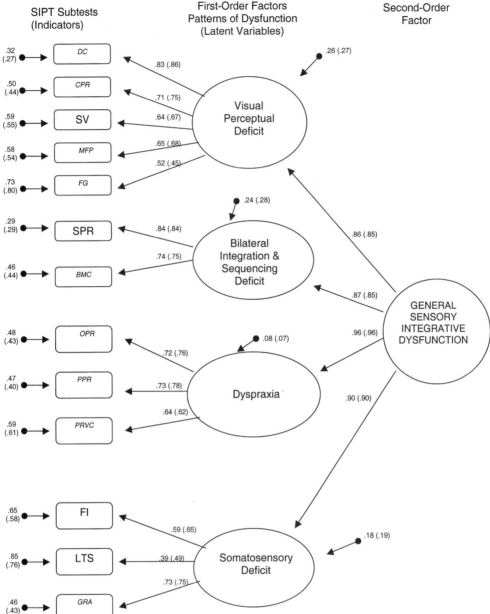

■ FIGURE 1–8 Mulligan's model.

gan (1998) did not find a factor containing tests reflecting both. She explained that there were strong associations among all patterns of dysfunction, including praxis and somatosensory.

Mulligan (2000) also subjected SIPT data to cluster analysis. As with her factor analyses, Mulligan's results were both similar to and dissimilar from Ayres' findings. Although Ayres had identi-

fied six clusters, Mulligan believed that a five-cluster solution best represented the data. Mulligan indicated that her findings supported Ayres' low average BIS and generalized sensory integrative (SI) dysfunction clusters and that a cluster she named "average SI and praxis" represented a merging of Ayres' "high" and "low average SI and praxis" clusters. Furthermore, embedded within a cluster Mulligan named "generalized SI dysfunction and dyspraxia—moderate" was a pattern of very low scores on Praxis on Verbal Command and relatively higher scores on Postrotary Nystagmus, a cluster Ayres also had identified. Mulligan labeled a fifth cluster "dyspraxia," which was characterized by below-average scores on many tests with a motor component as well as some tests potentially representing underlying sensory processing deficits. Mulligan urged practitioners to use caution in interpreting test results suggesting sensory integrative dysfunction.

CURRENT VIEW OF SENSORY INTEGRATION THEORY REVISITED

In synthesizing the results of the many factor and cluster analyses, we find four broad groupings. One group, dyspraxia, includes the patterns we have described earlier under practic functions (i.e., BIS deficits, somatodyspraxia). This group also contains outward manifestations of central sensory processing deficits (i.e., postural deficits and poor tactile discrimination). A second group reflects expressions of sensory modulation dysfunction (i.e., sensory defensiveness, gravitational insecurity, aversive response to movement, underresponsiveness). Sensory modulation dysfunction did not emerge from the SIPT data, and the SIPT data do not provide a basis for evaluating them. However, tactile defensiveness appeared in several factor analyses. Furthermore, modulation disorders, in some form, have been described consistently in conjunction with sensory integrative dysfunction. These first two groupings are shown in Figure 1–3.

A third group includes various measures of visual perception and visual-motor coordination. However, the measures used to identify this grouping had a strong cognitive component, and the link between these tests and an underlying sensory processing deficit is weak at best (see Chapter 5 for a more detailed discussion).

Finally, some of the factor analytic studies included auditory-language measures. Again, many of these measures were strongly dependent on cognition. Chapter 6 discusses deficits in auditory processing and their sequelae.

EFFICACY OF INTERVENTION BASED ON SENSORY INTEGRATION THEORY

A number of researchers, beginning with Ayres (1972d, 1976, 1978), have examined the postulate that intervention can enhance sensory integration. Ayres implemented two intervention studies with children who had learning disabilities. In the first, Ayres (1972d) assessed the effects of intervention on children with sensory integrative dysfunction and children with auditory-language problems. Both experimental groups made significant gains in reading and auditory-language skills. In the second study, Ayres' (1976, 1978) goal was to determine which subgroups of children with learning disabilities were most likely to benefit from intervention based on the principles of sensory integration theory. She found that children who had depressed postrotary nystagmus made greater gains academically than did similar children in the control group.

Ayres believed that the results of these studies provided initial support for her hypothesis that improving sensory integration resulted in enhanced learning. The latter study also led her to conclude that central vestibular processing disorders were a common basis of learning problems and that children with central vestibular processing disorders, including shortened postrotary nystagmus, may respond better to intervention based on the principles of sensory integration theory than children with prolonged nystagmus.

All the studies of the efficacy of intervention that followed in the early years after Ayres published her theory have been criticized, legitimately, for various design-related issues. Nonetheless, Ottenbacher (1982) was able to identify eight studies published between 1972 and 1981 that he judged to be of sufficient rigor for inclusion in a meta-analysis. Furthermore, he found sufficient evidence to suggest that intervention based on the principles of sensory integration theory was effective. In fact, Ottenbacher found a mean effect size of 0.79 across all measures, with the greatest effect (1.03) associated with motor-reflex variables and the smallest effect, although it is relatively large (0.43), associated with language.

Ottenbacher's analysis drew criticism for lack

of rigor of the studies included and for failing to examine data comparing SI with other approaches to intervention (Hoehn & Baumeister, 1994). However, for many years, therapists held out Ottenbacher's analysis as "proof" of the efficacy of intervention based on the principles of sensory integration. Recently, Vargas and Camilli (1999), who also used meta-analysis to examine studies conducted between 1972 and 1982, supported Ottenbacher's results. They found an average effect size of 0.60 (95% confidence interval [CI], 0.33–0.86) for studies conducted during this decade.

Since the early 1980s, a number of researchers (e.g., Carte et al., 1984; Densem et al., 1989; Humphries et al., 1991; Humphries, Wright et al., 1992; Humphries et al., 1993; Kaplan et al., 1993; Polatajko et al., 1991; Wilson & Kaplan, 1994; Wilson et al., 1992) have attempted to validate intervention based on the principles of sensory integration theory with children who have learning disabilities. Unfortunately, these researchers have been somewhat less successful than the earlier researchers. In fact, although they also included studies whose participants were children and adults with mental retardation and other disorders not necessarily reflective of sensory integration theory, Vargas and Camilli (1999) found a very small effect size (0.03; 95% CI, −0.20–0.26) in studies completed between 1983 and 1993 (including many of those already listed).

Some of the studies listed above can be criticized for procedural faults (e.g., using the Southern California Sensory Integration Tests [SCSIT] as an outcome measure). However, most were conducted in a highly rigorous fashion. Furthermore, it seems clear that many of the researchers wanted— and expected—to find that intervention based on sensory integration theory was effective. And children receiving this intervention *did* make gains, even a few that were statistically significantly greater than those of children receiving alternate intervention (i.e., perceptual motor, tutoring) (e.g., Humphries et al., 1991, 1992, 1993; Law et al., 1991; Polatajko et al., 1991; Wilson & Kaplan, 1994; Wilson et al., 1992). Nonetheless, the gains were so few and so unpredictable that, based on a review of seven studies published between 1982 and 1992, Wilson, et al. (1992) concluded:

> . . . this review has failed to find any statistical evidence that SI treatment improves the *aca-*

demic performance of learning disabled children more than a placebo (the positive impact of attention or the therapeutic relationship). With respect to *sensory or motor* performance, the results are not as consistent, but do suggest that, statistically, overall SI treatment may be similar to perceptual-motor training (p. 337).

Efficacy Reconsidered

In recent years, the evidence in support of intervention based on the principles of sensory integration theory is mixed at best and downright negative at worst. Thus, as Kaplan et al. (1993) indicated, "this leaves one wondering why so many therapists and the families of their clients are still strongly devoted to sensory integration treatment [SIT]. What is it about SIT that makes people *think* it is working?" (italics added) (p. 346).

In a desperate attempt to find solutions to difficult problems, do families, therapists, and even teachers (Stonefelt & Stein, 1998) simply *want to think* that intervention based on the principles of sensory integration theory is effective? Is it the research that is misleading, or the theory? Perhaps, in some respects, it is both.

Kaplan et al. (1993) concluded their paper with the following:

> It is possible that sensory integration in the 1990s is in the same developmental stage that psychotherapy research was during the 1950s. In 1952, Eysenck published a widely publicized study that questioned the effectiveness of psychotherapy. That article had a powerful effect in stimulating psychotherapy research. Good empirical research began in the 1960s (Hersen, Michelson et al., 1984). The effectiveness of a wide variety of types of psychotherapeutic approaches is now well established, but only after 40 years of intensive research with increasingly rigorous methodologies. A significant portion of this research literature has investigated process variables, patient characteristics, and therapist characteristics. Although SIT researchers have begun to consider many of these variables, they have a long road to travel before its effectiveness is established or refuted (p. 347).

Kaplan et al. (1993) also offered several other potential answers to their question regarding the popularity of intervention based on the principles of sensory integration theory even in the absence of empirical support for its efficacy. First, the intervention may be effective, not because of the theory on which it is based, but because of the intense bond that often forms between the client and therapist. Furthermore, as a child *does* improve and his or her family has no basis for comparison, they attribute the change to improved sensory integration.

These "answers" are based on the assumption that although individuals' experiences are valid, they lack the perspective gleaned from empirical research. However, Kaplan et al. (1993) offered another answer, one that focuses on a different aspect of sensory integration theory as it pertains to intervention.

The theoretical framework of sensory integration dysfunction enables the clients and families to "reframe" the motor and behavioral problems ("poorly disciplined, immature, destructive, careless, rigid, or overactive") (Bundy, 1991, p. 319) into terms that are based on a theory that integrates mind and body. When the frame for viewing the client's behavior is changed to a more positive one, the parents and teachers are provided with the basis for developing different kinds of strategies for working with the child. The resulting improvements in behavior, skills, and attitudes are often attributed to the actual physical treatment, not necessarily to any attitudinal change resulting from consultation with the therapist (p. 347).

Because consultation with families was not a part of any of the studies examining the efficacy of intervention, it is possible that Kaplan et al. (1993) are correct. That is, changing the perceptions and attitudes of those around the client is more effective than working directly with the client to change his or her ability to process sensory information. However, one interesting twist to these authors' point is that apparently sensory integration theory as a possible explanation for client's behavior and difficulties "rings true" to a lot of parents, therapists, and teachers. Would *any* explanation offered be just as effective as long as it was relatively positive (i.e., did not question a child's basic goodness, integrity, or intelligence or blame the parents or teacher)? We think not, but these questions all remain to be tested.

Invariably, when the efficacy of an intervention seems to be elusive, researchers and supporters of the intervention question the appropriateness and sensitivity of the outcome measures

used. Sensory integration is no exception. In fact, Polatajko et al. (1992) also suggested this as a problem.

Clinicians themselves often experience frustration when a child shows no gains on tests, but the therapist, teacher, and parents detect improvements they consider to be important. The development of tests in occupational therapy has focused on the functions of screening and diagnosis [i.e., descriptive tests] more than that of sensitivity to change [i.e., evaluative measures]. The tests used both in the clinic and in research are not always appropriate for assessing change over time. It may be that clinicians and researchers are trying to detect change with a yardstick while change is occurring in inches (p. 338).

Cohn and Cermak (1998) expressed related concerns about the appropriateness of outcome measures:

The outcome assessments we choose implicitly display our belief systems and the underlying assumptions regarding the behaviors we hope to change. In practice, the assessment tools and the variables measured often become the operational definition for the changes we are attempting to measure (Haley, 1994). . . . Miller and Kinnealey (1993) . . . argued that changes in test scores are meaningful only if "documentation can be supplied that the test scores are indicative of changes in performance in daily life" (pp. 5 and 540).

Cohn and Cermak (1998) continued: "By focusing primarily on the underlying components of performance of children, occupational therapists have neglected to explore how sensory integration affects the everyday occupation of children in the context of their families" (p. 540). Although this is an important point, in fairness to researchers attempting to validate sensory integration theory, *sensory integration is an underlying component of performance.* Furthermore, Ayres relied heavily on such measures. A major postulate of sensory integration theory pertains to the efficacy of intervention based on its principles to change the underlying capacity of the client to process sensory information. Of course, Ayres' main concern was that children act more effectively and efficiently within their environments. Perhaps a more germane question is, "To what extent does performance on standardized measure predict an individual's ability to perform related tasks in daily life?"

This, of course, is a question of validity that is addressed only occasionally. However, it *is* asked (e.g., Burton & Miller, 1998; Coster, 1998). Its answer, elusive as that may be, may lead us to a whole new conceptualization of assessment within occupational therapy (Coster, 1998). Assessment related to intervention based on the principles of sensory integration theory will be only one small part of that conceptualization.

In their recent meta-analysis, Vargas and Camilli (1999) reported two interesting findings that also may help to explain why recent research examining the efficacy of intervention based on the principles of sensory integration theory has generally failed to achieve significant results. They found that studies that use four or fewer outcome measures and those that measure effectiveness in only one dependent category (i.e., psychoeducational, behavior, language, motor, or sensory-perceptual) had significantly greater effect sizes than did studies that included more outcome measures or measures from a greater number of categories. Although increasing the number of outcome measures or categories may be one way of increasing the reliability of a study (Vargas & Camilli, 1999), intervention must be goal directed to be maximally effective. How would a therapist know how to plan intervention directed at improving outcomes in up to five categories? Put another way, what would an intervention look like that was designed to improve simultaneously the psychoeducational, behavioral, language, motor, and sensory-perceptual performance of a client?

Granted, Ayres (1972a, 1989) and others (e.g., Fisher & Murray, 1991; Kimball, 1999; Parham & Mailloux, 2001) have indicated that sensory integration is a neurological process that underlies a number of higher-order functions. Depending on the author, these have included such variables as attention, self-esteem, motor planning, and academic learning. In Ayres' (1972a) words, "The objective is modification of the neurological dysfunction interfering with learning rather than attacking the symptoms of that dysfunction" (p. 2). But however powerful sensory integration may be, it is neither a miracle nor a cure. In fact, Ayres (1972a) went on to say, "This type of therapy . . . does not necessarily eliminate the need for the more symptomatic approach. Therapy is considered a supplement, not a substitute, to formal classroom instruction or tutoring. It reduces the severity of the difficulty and allows specifics . . . to be learned more rapidly"

(p. 2). No doubt, the same could be said about learning to ride a bike or pump a swing as of classroom learning.

Furthermore, the average amount of intervention provided in the studies by Vargas and Camilli (1999) in their meta-analysis was 60 hours when sensory integration was compared with no treatment and 36 when it was compared with an alternate intervention (range, 13 to 180). That amount of intervention may seem like a lot, particularly if it is being reimbursed at $100.00 per hour. However, it would be nothing short of a miracle if, even in 180 hours, a client with learning disabilities who was already significantly behind in school could develop more efficient CNS processing *and* enough ability to score significantly higher on measures of IQ, behavioral function, self-esteem, language, gross and fine motor function, praxis, and visual perception. Have proponents of sensory integration theory developed so much zeal as to suggest this is possible? Or have researchers lost sight of the constraints of reality?

NEW PERSPECTIVES ON INTERVENTION

In developing new perspectives on theory and intervention based on the principles of sensory integration theory, we have been influenced by a number of factors. Among them are:

- The return of occupational therapy to its occupation-based mission
- Developing theories of nervous system function, motor control, and motor learning
- Current reimbursement practices within the educational and health-care systems

The Return of Occupational Therapy to Its Occupation-Based Mission

In recent years, a number of authors (e.g., Coster, 1998; Fisher & Short-DeGraff, 1993; Mathiowetz, 1993; Mathiowetz & Haugen, 1995; Trombly, 1993) have written eloquently about the need for occupational therapists to take a "top-down" perspective in assessment and intervention (Fig. 1–9). The top-down perspective is contrasted with a "bottom-up" approach. Both are based on a hierarchical view of occupation in which performance components (e.g., sensory integration, strength, developmental level) form the bottom level of a hierarchy that includes occupational performance (e.g., self-care, play) and roles as upper levels. In a bottom-up approach, therapists target performance components in assessment and intervention. They then infer a relationship between impairments or improvements in performance components and occupational performance. For example, poor praxis results in difficulty learning to ride a bike.

There are many problems with a bottom-up perspective. For example, difficulty learning to ride a bike may be caused by a number of factors—*in addition to or instead of*—poor praxis. Furthermore, improvements in praxis may not automatically result in the child's ability to ride the bike.

Recently, Coster (1998) proposed an occupation-centered model for the assessment of children, which provides a different perspective on intervention. Coster's model contained four levels. From top to bottom, they included:

1. Participation (in the occupations typically expected of or available to a child of this age and culture)
2. Complex task performance
3. Activity (simpler tasks comprising complex tasks) performance
4. Component processes (performance components)

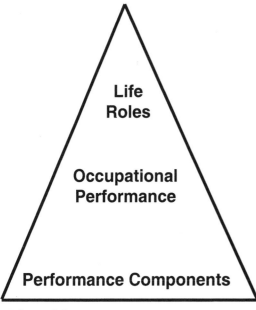

■ FIGURE 1-9 The "top-down" perspective in assessment and intervention. (Adapted from Mathiowetz (1993) and Trombly (1993), with permission.)

To illustrate her model, Coster provided the example of a child with limited participation in playground activities, particularly complex tasks involving group interactions and physical games. Contributing activity limitations might include limited skills to initiate and sustain peer interactions, inability to remember and follow game rules, difficulty with physical tasks (e.g., running, kicking a ball), or limited endurance. In turn, these activity limitations may result from sensory processing difficulties, motor incoordination, or difficulties with emotional regulation (i.e., component processes). Coster acknowledged that therapists have little access to assessments that would tell them about the first three levels of her model. For the most part, we depend on observation and interview. To determine which component processes might be responsible for the difficulties, therapists might use existing standardized tools. However,

> . . . the difference in the present approach [over a more traditional bottom-up approach] is that these [standardized] assessments would be used to determine *how* to intervene, not *what* the goals of intervention would be. . . . The measure of successful outcome of intervention for this child is not whether there has been a change in sensory processing but whether there is a change in his or her occupational engagement to a pattern that is more personally satisfying and more growth supporting (p. 340).

Developing Theories of Nervous System Function, Motor Control, and Motor Learning

Increasing knowledge of CNS function, in conjunction with developments in cognitive psychology, motor learning, kinesiology, and biomechanics, has resulted in the replacement of neuromaturational and reflex-hierarchical theories, widely accepted by Ayres and her contemporaries, with systems approaches to development. Systems approaches view behavior as the end product of activity of a number of internal and external subsystems (e.g., sensorimotor, cognitive, mechanical, and task demands). Many concepts drawn from the systems approach to motor behavior are critical to our developing beliefs regarding intervention incorporating the principles of sensory integration theory. Perhaps most importantly, in the systems approach, motor behavior is viewed as organized by the demands of specific tasks within particular contexts.

(Haugen & Mathiowetz, 1995; Heriza, 1991; Mathiowetz & Haugen, 1995; McEwen & Shelden, 1995).

Haugen and Mathiowetz (1995) and Mathiowetz and Haugen (1995) have applied contemporary theories of motor control and motor learning to a model of practice for occupational therapists. They referred to this model as the Contemporary Task-Oriented Approach. In this approach, assessment and intervention are conducted in the context of activities that clients need and want to do (i.e., occupational performance or activity performance in Coster's model). After those activities have been identified, therapists analyze clients' performance to determine what performance or environmental components are limiting their ability to perform tasks successfully. Intervention involves assisting clients to develop necessary components as much as possible *in the context of* the desired activity. The type of teaching strategy, type of feedback, and optimal forms of practice are critical to success in the Contemporary Task-Oriented Approach. These are selected based on the characteristics of the task to be mastered. Readers are referred to Mathiowetz and Haugen (1995) and Haugen and Mathiowetz (1995) for further discussion of the Contemporary Task-Oriented Approach. Other contemporary approaches to motor learning and motor control are discussed in Chapter 3.

Current Reimbursement Practices Within Educational and Health Care Systems

We once had virtually unlimited time and comparatively greater resources for intervention. But increasingly, occupational therapy practitioners must be accountable for their time and the efficacy of their interventions. Schools, hospitals, and clinics are increasingly strapped for space, money, and time from practitioners. Administrators are demanding that services be provided in the most efficient and effective manner with a minimum of resources. Further, the focus of intervention is no longer at the discretion of the practitioner. All services are becoming increasingly family centered.

Family-centered services mean that families and children must be involved in identifying intervention goals that are meaningful to them and that intervention approaches clearly help to accomplish their desired outcomes. In pediatric therapy we have often assumed that our intervention will

mysteriously result in functional improvement sometime in the future (Gordon, 1987), but the future is now. Palisano said, "In the present climate of health care reform, the extent that consumers identify our services as being responsive to their needs will impact greatly on how well we will be positioned to face the challenges of the 21st century" (Palisano, 1994, p.140). This is true regardless of the service setting and who pays for the services (McEwen & Shelden, 1995, p. 42).

We believe that intervention based on the principles of sensory integration theory can be extremely powerful. Judging by the number of parents requesting it for their children, parents also believe in its power. However, when it is delivered in the traditional fashion, intervention based on the principles of sensory integration theory can be extremely time consuming (i.e., often 6 months to 3 years of weekly sessions) and expensive. Unless families are willing and able to pay out of pocket, few resources exist for such extensive intervention. Thus, if we are to preserve the power of sensory integration, we must be willing to change its face. The reasons for this change, however, are not purely economical. They also rest in current knowledge of CNS function and developing theories of motor control and motor learning and in the mission and philosophy of occupational therapy.

PUTTING IT ALL TOGETHER: A PROPOSED MODEL OF INTERVENTION INCORPORATING THE PRINCIPLES OF SENSORY INTEGRATION THEORY

We propose that when sensory integrative dysfunction, manifested as poor praxis or modulation, limits clients' abilities to perform tasks they need or want to do, intervention can be most effectively and efficiently implemented using the following principles. These principles are drawn from sensory integration theory, theories of motor control and motor learning, and the philosophical base of occupational therapy:

- Objectives (goals) are limited in number (one is optimal) and are relatively short term in nature (four to six sessions expected for mastery).

- Objectives (goals) are explicit and determined by clients and caregivers.
- Helping clients and caregivers reframe behaviors and difficulties is an important part of intervention.
- Clients and caregivers often implement aspects of intervention, particularly when the objectives depend on altering sensory modulation.
- Even when sensory integrative dysfunction is found to limit clients' performance, other factors may also be contributing to the difficulties. When present, these may require intervention of a different type.
- The form of intervention (i.e., what it looks like) is determined through task analysis in which the limiting components of the targeted task (or tasks) are identified.
- As much as possible, the form of intervention "mimics" or incorporates the limiting components of the targeted task.
- When sensory integrative dysfunction limits performance, intervention incorporates enhanced sensation. The type (or types) of sensation depend on the desired outcome.
- Intervention activities demand an adaptive interaction.
- When improved motor performance is a crucial part of the objective, intervention activities incorporate appropriate amounts and types of practice and feedback.
- Intervention concludes when objectives are met and no important needs remain that are appropriate targets for occupational therapy intervention.

Example I: A Child with Poor Praxis

Lars was an 11-year-old client in a 1-week intervention course incorporating the principles of sensory integration theory conducted in Norway. Lars had been referred to occupational therapy because of poor coordination and low endurance that prevented him from engaging in many of the activities his peers enjoyed. The occupational therapist working with Lars had interviewed both him and his parents to determine his level of participation in meaningful activity and his ability to engage in complex tasks and activities. The therapist also had observed Lars as he carried out some of the complex tasks he and his family had identi-

fied as problematic. Because it seemed likely that sensory integrative dysfunction, manifested in poor praxis, contributed significantly to Lars' difficulties, his therapist also evaluated his sensory integrative functioning. The results indicated that Lars had difficulty processing vestibular-proprioceptive information, which seemed to contribute to difficulties with BIS. No difficulties with sensory modulation, including gravitational insecurity, were noted.

The first day of the course, the therapists working with Lars met with his mother and him to determine an objective for intervention. Because it was a course on intervention incorporating the principles of sensory integration theory into intervention, they were asked to select an objective that would respond logically to this type of intervention. After considerable discussion, Lars and his mother settled on "descending a flight of open stairs reciprocally and without hesitation."

Having set the objective, the therapists engaged in a task analysis to attempt to uncover the reasons for Lars' difficulty with the stairs. An important part of that task analysis was to observe Lars descending a flight of stairs. Because we had no open stairwell, we observed him descending a closed stairwell. We videotaped his performance for analysis and comparison at the end of the intervention. Lars descended the stairs slowly and in a step-tap fashion. He looked downward, carefully monitoring his feet and the stairs. He held the railing securely, appearing fearful.

The results of assessment of sensory integrative functioning had indicated that Lars had difficulty processing vestibular and proprioceptive sensations and that this resulted in impaired BIS. Furthermore, Lars' performance on the stairs suggested that he did not have a good sense of where his feet were in space. While Lars was still on the stairs, a therapist placed cuff weights around his ankles to test her hypothesis. However, rather than improving, Lars' performance actually deteriorated. In one last attempt to examine the theory of poor proprioception as the basis for impaired stair climbing, the therapist moved the weights to Lars' shoulders. This time the improvement was dramatic. Although he still held the handrail, Lars walked reciprocally and much more quickly down the stairs.

Lars was seen in intervention for 1 hour each of the next 4 days. Intervention activities provided him with opportunities to take in enhanced vestibular and proprioceptive (i.e., resistance to movement) sensation in the context of activities that demanded bilateral projected action sequences. The therapists concentrated on creating activities that involved Lars' feet. For example, while he was prone or supine in the net, Lars kicked off a mat leaning against a wall. He did the same thing on a scooter board. Lars also kicked large balls while swinging prone in the net. Because stair climbing is an activity done in an upright position, the therapist also created jumping activities for Lars as well as obstacle courses that he moved through as quickly as possible.

At the end of four intervention sessions, the therapists took Lars back to the stairwell and once again videotaped his descent of the stairs, this time with no weights on Lars' shoulders. Just as Lars began the descent, someone handed him a cap, which he placed on his head. Then he ran quickly down the stairs, his hands in his pockets, looking toward his mother, who stood at the bottom.

Discussion

Lars made significant gains in just 4 hours of intervention that occurred over the course of 1 week. The activities in which Lars engaged during intervention looked very similar to those one would see in any clinic that uses the principles of sensory integration theory. The differences lay in the emphasis during assessment and planning of the intervention activities. Rather than addressing the larger goal of improving sensory integration, the therapists were guided jointly by the demands of stair climbing and their belief that what interfered with Lars' mastery of stair climbing was poor processing of vestibular and proprioceptive sensations and impaired BIS. Because stair climbing is an activity done primarily with the feet and legs, the therapists concentrated on the lower extremities as they planned activities that would provide enhanced vestibular and proprioceptive sensations and demand bilateral projected action sequences. They did not include stair climbing as an activity.

Several things remain unknown about the effects of Lars' intervention. First, because no open stairwell was available, it is not known whether Lars actually met the goal. The logistics of the course prevented us from learning that. Second, although it is unlikely, it is possible that Lars secretly spent a portion of each day practicing stair climbing and that this, in fact, was responsible for his gains. Finally, and perhaps most importantly,

nothing is known about whether Lars' sensory integrative abilities actually improved. However, given current theories about CNS functioning, it seems quite possible that they did.

If Lars had been seen in a more typical situation rather than as part of a course, the therapists working with him would have met again with Lars and his mother to set another goal. They would continue this process until no more concerns appropriate for occupational therapy intervention seemed imminent.

Example 2: A Child with Poor Sensory Modulation

Sam was a 5-year-old kindergarten student whose occupational therapy evaluation suggested that, although he was generally overly active, he seemed actually to have low arousal and to use activity to "keep alert." He found it difficult to get motivated to move but became irritable when he remained still for long periods of time. At times, he actually did become overly active and unfocused in response to activity. Thus, his behavior could be confusing to those around him.

Sam received intensive occupational therapy, including direct intervention (both one to one and in a group) and consultation with his teacher. The common goal for all these services was that Sam participate constructively in classroom activities, including completing assignments. His family and therapist believed that poor self-regulation prevented him from meeting the goal. In each type of service delivery, the therapist approached the problem in a slightly different way.

In *one-to-one direct service,* Sam received traditional intervention based on the principles of sensory integration theory. Because of the available equipment and space, Sam had opportunities to take in "large doses" of enhanced tactile, vestibular, and proprioceptive sensations and produce adaptive environmental interactions. Although this form of intervention seemed to have a powerful short-term effect, it did not produce a lasting effect. After a short period, Sam was back to his typical low state of alertness.

The *group intervention* in which Sam was involved was based on the principles of the Alert program (Williams & Shellenberger, 1996). Here Sam learned to focus on indicators of his level of alertness and to liken his arousal level to an engine running at different speeds. He learned that when "his engine was running low," he needed to engage in particular types of activity to "rev" it to a more optimal level. This intervention seemed to provide Sam with a positive frame for his difficulties. Furthermore, it provided an avenue for "shots" of enhanced sensation when he needed them most—during daily life events—and provided him with control over what might otherwise have seemed like a chaotic existence.

Through *consultation,* Sam's teacher learned about Sam's difficulties with self-regulation. She learned "engine concepts" and ways to adapt activities, demands, and the environment to enable Sam to regulate his level of arousal and thus meet his goal of participating constructively in classroom activity and completing assignments. Among other things, Sam's teacher learned that Sam needed to move a lot, so she sent him on errands or let him walk around the classroom. She also learned that manipulating objects seemed to help Sam focus his attention and that, at times, Sam needed to be able to sit apart from the group, go to a quiet place, or even leave an activity to "adjust his engine level."

Many of the strategies developed during consultation were counterintuitive to Sam's teacher because she, like many adults, viewed sitting quietly as an indicator of paying attention. However, Sam's teacher came to realize that Sam could *either* pay attention *or* sit quietly. This intervention enabled an important caregiver, Sam's teacher, to understand and interact with Sam in more positive ways. Consultation also enabled the teacher to adapt the nonhuman environment in ways that facilitated Sam's accomplishing his goal. (Other children in the classroom probably also benefitted from the therapist's consulting with the teacher regarding Sam's needs.)

This three-pronged approach to intervention was incredibly successful. In fact, it enabled Sam to participate so constructively that he completed his kindergarten year successfully, a goal that once seemed beyond his grasp.

Discussion

As a whole, Sam's intervention enabled him to alter his level of arousal in order to participate more constructively in kindergarten. Each interrelated form of service delivery served a different—but equally essential—purpose. Much of Sam's intervention focused on giving him and his teacher a better understanding of the challenges he faced.

Based on that understanding, the teacher and therapist developed strategies that could be used to address those challenges *in context.* The teacher and therapist both had a clear idea of the goal, how to reach it, and what it would look like when it was met. Sam also developed a better understanding of his body and feelings of increased control over the demands of his environment. If Sam had been older, he would have probably developed even more feelings of control and a wider repertoire of strategies for matching his needs with the demands of the environment.

SUMMARY AND CONCLUSIONS

In this chapter, we have presented an overview of the history of the development of sensory integration theory and practice and our current perspectives of sensory integration theory. In this process, we have attempted to place sensory integration within the greater context of occupational therapy. Members of all helping professions share a common concern for functional independence. What makes occupational therapy practitioners unique is our emphasis on the process of "doing" occupational behavior. The term *praxis,* derived from the Greek, is more than motor planning; praxis means doing. Thus, it can serve to remind us that our primary concern is not sensory integration but whether our clients are able to *do* what they need and want to do.

We also initiated a critical analysis of sensory integration theory. Theory is provisional. As the results of additional research are disseminated and new perspectives are formulated, each must be evaluated in relation to existing theory. Thus, critical analysis of sensory integration theory and practice will remain an ongoing process.

References

Arendt, R. E., MacLean, W. E., & Baumeister, A. A. (1988). Critique of sensory integration therapy and its application in mental retardation. *American Journal on Mental Retardation, 92,* 401–411.

Ayres, A. J. (1965). Patterns of perceptual-motor dysfunction in children: A factor analytic study. *Perceptual and Motor Skills, 20,* 335–368.

Ayres, A. J. (1966a). Interrelations among perceptual-motor abilities in a group of normal children. *American Journal of Occupational Therapy, 20,* 288–292.

Ayres, A. J. (1966b). Interrelationships among perceptual-motor functions in children. *American Journal of Occupational Therapy, 20,* 288–292.

Ayres, A. J. (1969). Deficits in sensory integration in educationally handicapped children. *Journal of Learning Disabilities, 2,* 160–168.

Ayres, A. J. (1972a). *Sensory integration and learning disorders.* Los Angeles: Western Psychological Services.

Ayres, A. J. (1972b). Types of sensory integrative dysfunction among disabled learners. *American Journal of Occupational Therapy, 26,* 13–18.

Ayres, A. J. (1972c). *Southern California Sensory Integration Tests Manual.* Los Angeles: Western Psychological Services.

Ayres, A. J. (1972d). Improving academic scores through sensory integration. *Journal of Learning Disabilities, 5,* 338–343.

Ayres, A. J. (1974a). Reading: A product of sensory integrative processes. In A. Henderson, L. Llorens, E. Gilfoyle, C. Myers, & S. Prevel (Eds.), *The development of sensory integrative theory and practice: A collection of the work of A. Jean Ayres* (pp. 167–175). Dubuque, IA: Kendall/Hunt. (Original work published 1968).

Ayres, A. J. (1974b). Sensory integrative processes in neuropsychological learning disability. In A. Henderson, L. Llorens, E. Gilfoyle, C. Myers, & S. Prevel, (Eds.), *The development of sensory integrative theory and practice: A collection of the work of A. Jean Ayres* (pp. 96–113). Dubuque, IA: Kendall/Hunt. (Original work published 1968).

Ayres, A. J. (1975a). Sensorimotor foundations of academic ability. In W. M. Cruickshank & D. P. Hallahan, *Perceptual and learning disabilities in children,* vol. 2 (pp. 301–358). Syracuse, NY: Syracuse University.

Ayres, A. J. (1975b). *Southern California Postrotary Nystagmus Test Manual.* Los Angeles: Western Psychological Services.

Ayres, A. J. (1976). *The effect of sensory integrative therapy on learning disabled children: The final report of a research project.* Los Angeles: University of Southern California.

Ayres, A. J. (1977). Cluster analyses of measures of sensory integration. *American Journal of Occupational Therapy, 31,* 362–366.

Ayres, A. J. (1978). Learning disabilities and the vestibular system. *Journal of Learning Disabilities, 11,* 18–29.

Ayres, A. J. (1979). *Sensory integration and the child.* Los Angeles: Western Psychological Services.

Ayres, A. J. (1985). *Developmental dyspraxia and adult-onset apraxia.* Torrance, CA: Sensory Integration International.

Ayres, A. J. (1989). *Sensory Integration and Praxis Tests manual.* Los Angeles: Western Psychological Services.

Ayres, A. J., Mailloux, Z. K., & Wendler, C. L. W. (1987). Developmental dyspraxia: Is it a unitary function? *Occupational Therapy Journal of Research, 7,* 93–110.

Ayres, A. J., & Tickle, L. (1980). Hyper-responsivity to touch and vestibular stimulation as a predictor of responsivity to sensory integrative procedures in autistic children. *American Journal of Occupational Therapy, 34,* 375–381.

Baranek, G. T., Foster, L. G., & Berkson, G. (1997). Tactile defensiveness and stereotyped behaviors. *American Journal of Occupational Therapy, 51,* 91–95.

Bonder, B. R., & Fisher, A. G. (1989). Sensory integration and treatment of the elderly. *Gerontology Special Interest Section Newsletter,* Rockville, MD: American Occupational Therapy Association, *12*(1), 2–4.

Brooks, V. B. (1986). *The neural basis of motor control.* New York: Oxford University.

Bundy, A. C. (1991). Consultation and sensory integration theory. In A. G. Fisher, E. A. Murray, & A. C. Bundy (Eds.). Sensory integration: Theory and practice (pp. 318–332). Philadelphia: F. A. Davis.

Burton, A. W., & Miller, D. E. (1998). *Movement skill assessment.* Champaign, IL: Human Kinetics.

Carte, E., Morrison, D., Sublett, J., Uemora, A., & Setrakian, W. (1984). Sensory integration therapy: A trial of a specific neurodevelopmental therapy for the remediation of learning disabilities. *Journal of Developmental and Behavioral Pediatrics, 5,* 189–194.

Cohn, E. S., & Cermak, S. A. (1998). Including the family perspective in sensory integration outcomes research. *American Journal of Occupational Therapy, 52,* 540–546.

Coster, W. (1998). Occupation-centered assessment of children. *American Journal of Occupational Therapy, 52,* 337–344.

Cummins, R. A. (1991). Sensory integration and learning disabilities: Ayres' factor analyses reappraised. *Journal of Learning Disabilities, 24,* 160–168.

Densem, J. F., Nuthall, G. A., Bushnell, J., & Horn, J. (1989). Effectiveness of a sensory integrative therapy program for children with perceptual-motor deficits. *Journal of Learning Disabilities, 22,* 221–229.

DiJoseph, L. M. (1982). Independence through activity: Mind, body, and environment interaction in therapy. *American Journal of Occupational Therapy, 36,* 740–744.

Dunn, W. (1994). Performance of typical children on the sensory profile. *American Journal of Occupational Therapy, 48,* 967–974.

Dunn, W. (1997). The impact of sensory processing abilities on the daily lives of young children and their families: A conceptual model. *Infants and Young Children, 9,* 23–35.

Dunn, W. (1999). *Sensory profile: User's manual.* San Antonio: Psychological Corporation.

Dunn, W., & Brown, C. (1997). Factor analysis on the Sensory Profile from a national sample of children without disabilities. *American Journal of Occupational Therapy, 51,* 490–495.

Dunn, W., & Westman, K. (1997). The Sensory Profile: The performance of a national sample of children without disabilities. *American Journal of Occupational Therapy, 51,* 25–34.

Edelson, S. M., Edelson, M. G., Kerr, D. C. R., & Grandin, T. (1999). Behavioral and physiological effects of deep pressure on children with autism: A pilot study evaluating the efficacy of Grandin's hug machine. *American Journal of Occupational Therapy, 53,* 145–152.

Fisher, A. G. (1991). Vestibular-proprioceptive processing and bilateral integration and sequencing deficits. In A. G. Fisher, E. A. Murray, & A. C. Bundy (Eds.), *Sensory integration: Theory and practice* (pp. 71–107). Philadelphia: F. A. Davis.

Fisher, A. G., & Bundy, A. C. (1991a). The interpretation process. In A. G. Fisher, E. A. Murray, & A. C. Bundy (Eds.), *Sensory integration: Theory and practice* (pp. 234–250). Philadelphia: F. A. Davis.

Fisher, A. G., & Bundy, A. C. (1991b). *Sensory integration theory.* In H. Forssberg & H. Hirschfeld (Eds.), *Movement disorders in children* (pp. 16–20). New York: Karger.

Fisher, A. G., & Murray, E. A. (1991). Introduction to sensory integration theory. In A. G. Fisher, E. A. Murray, & A. C. Bundy (Eds.), *Sensory integration: Theory and practice* (pp. 3–29). Philadelphia: F. A. Davis.

Fisher, A. G., & Short-DeGraff, M. A. (1993). Improving functional assessment in occupational therapy. Recommendations and philosophy for change. *American Journal of Occupational Therapy, 47,* 199–201.

Gordon, J. (1987). Assumptions underlying physical therapy intervention: Theoretical and historical perspectives. In J. H. Carr & R. B. Shepherd (Eds.), *Movement science: Foundations for physical therapy in rehabilitation* (pp. 1–30). Rockville, MD: Aspen.

Grandin, T., & Scariano, M. M. (1986). *Emergence: Labeled autistic.* Novato, CA: Atena.

Haley, S. M. (1994). Our measures reflect our practice and beliefs: A perspective on clinical measurement in pediatric physical therapy. *Pediatric Physical Therapy, 6,* 142–143.

Haugen, J. B., & Mathiowetz, V. (1995). Contemporary task-oriented approach. In C. A. Trombly (Ed.), *Occupational therapy for physical dysfunction* (pp. 510–527). Baltimore: Williams & Wilkins.

Henderson, S. E., & Sugden, D. A. (1992). *Movement assessment battery for children manual.* London: Psychological Corporation.

Heriza, C. (1991). Motor development: Traditional and contemporary theories. In M. J. Lister (Ed.), *Contemporary management of motor control problems: Proceedings of the II Step Conference* (pp. 88–126). Alexandria, VA: Foundation for Physical Therapy.

Herson, M., Michelson, L., & Bellack, A. S. (1984). *Issues in psychotherapy research.* New York: Plenum.

Hoehn, T. P., & Baumeister, A. A. (1994). A critique of the application of sensory integration therapy to children with learning disabilities. *Journal of Learning Disabilities, 27,* 338–350.

Humphries, T. W., Snider, L., & McDougall, B. (1993). Clinical evaluation of the effectiveness of sensory integrative and perceptual motor therapy in improving sensory integrative function in children with learning disabilities. *Occupational Therapy Journal of Research, 13,* 163–182.

Humphries, T. W., Wright, M., McDougall, B., & Vertez, J. (1991). The efficacy of sensory integration therapy for children with learning disability. *Physical and Occupational Therapy in Pediatrics, 10,* 1–17.

Humphries, T. W., Wright, M., Snider, L., & McDougall, B. (1992). A comparison of the effectiveness of sensory integrative therapy and perceptual-motor training in treating children with learning disabilities. *Journal of Developmental and Behavioral Pediatrics, 13,* 31–40.

Kaplan, B. J., Polatajko, H. J., Wilson, B. N., & Faris, P. D. (1993). Reexamination of sensory integration treatment: A combination of two efficacy studies. *Journal of Learning Disabilities, 26,* 342–347.

Keogh, J., & Sugden, D. (1985). *Movement skill development.* New York: MacMillan.

Kielhofner, G. (1985). *A model of human occupation: Theory and application.* Baltimore: Williams & Wilkins.

Kielhofner, G. (1995). *A model of human occupation: Theory and application* (2nd ed.). Baltimore: Lippincott, Williams, & Wilkins.

Kielhofner, G. (1997). *Conceptual foundations of occupational therapy.* Philadelphia: F. A. Davis.

Kielhofner, G., & Fisher, A. G. (1991). Mind-brain-body relationships. In A. G. Fisher, E. A. Murray, & A. C. Bundy (Eds.), *Sensory integration; Theory and practice* (pp. 30–45). Philadelphia: F. A. Davis.

Kimball, J. G. (1999). Sensory integration frame of reference: Postulates regarding change and application to practice. In P. Kramer & J. Hinojosa (Eds.), *Frames of reference for pediatric occupational therapy,* 2nd ed (pp. 169–204). Baltimore: Lippincott, Williams, & Wilkins.

Kinnealey, M., Oliver, B., & Wilbarger, P. (1995). A phenomenological study of sensory defensiveness in adults. *American Journal of Occupational Therapy, 49,* 444–451.

Lai, J. S., Fisher, A. G., Magalhaes, L. C., & Bundy, A. C. (1996). Construct validity of the Sensory Integration and Praxis Tests. *Occupational Therapy Journal of Research, 16,* 75–97.

Law, M., Polatajko, H. J., Schaffer, R., Miller, J., & Macnab, J. (1991). The impact of heterogeneity in a clinical trial: Motor outcomes after sensory integration therapy. *Occupational Therapy Journal of Research, 11,* 177–189.

Linderman, T. M., & Stewart, K. B. (1999). Sensory integrative-based occupational therapy and functional outcomes in young children with pervasive developmental disorders: A single-subject study. *American Journal of Occupational Therapy, 53,* 207–213.

Mason, S. A., & Iwata, B. A. (1990). Artifactual effects of sensory-integrative therapy on self-injurious behavior. *Journal of Applied Behavior Analysis, 23,* 361–370.

Mathiowetz, V. (1993). Role of physical performance component evaluations in occupational therapy functional assessment. *American Journal of Occupational Therapy, 47,* 225–230.

Mathiowetz, V., & Haugen, J. B. (1995). Evaluation of motor behavior: Traditional and contemporary views. In C. A. Trombly (Ed.), *Occupational therapy for physical dysfunction* (pp. 157–185). Baltimore: Williams & Wilkins.

McClure, M., & Holtz-Yotz, M. (1991). Case report—The effects of sensory stimulatory treatment on an autistic child. *American Journal of Occupational Therapy, 45,* 1138–1142.

McEwen, I. R., & Shelden, M. L. (1995). Pediatric therapy in the 1990's: The demise of the educational versus medical dichotomy. *Physical and Occupational Therapy in Pediatrics, 15,* 33–46.

McIntosh, D. N., Miller, L. J., Shyu, V., & Dunn, W. (1999). Overview of the short sensory profile (SSP) (pp. 59–73). In W. Dunn (Ed.), *Sensory profile: User's manual.* San Antonio, TX: Psychological Corporation.

McIntosh, D. N., Miller, L. J., Shyu, V., & Hagerman, R. (1999). Sensory modulation disruption, electrodermal responses, and functional behaviors. *Developmental Medicine and Child Neurology, 41,* 608–615.

Miller, L. J., & Kinnealey, M. (1993). Researching the effectiveness of sensory integration. *Sensory Integration Quarterly Newsletter, 21,* 1–7.

Miller, L. J., McIntosh, D. N., McGrath, J., Shyu, V., Lampe, M., Taylor, A. K., Tassone, F., Neitzel, K., Stackhouse, K., & Hagerman, R. (1999). Electrodermal responses to sensory stimuli in individuals with fragile X syndrome: A preliminary report. *American Journal of Medical Genetics, 83,* 268–279.

Mulligan, S. (1998). Patterns of sensory integration dysfunction: A confirmatory factor analysis. *American Journal of Occupational Therapy, 52,* 819–828.

Mulligan, S. (2000). Cluster analysis of scores of children on the Sensory Integration and Praxis Tests. *Occupational Therapy Journal of Research, 20,* 256–270.

Nommensen, A., & Maas, F. (1993). Sensory integration and Down's syndrome. *British Journal of Occupational Therapy, 56,* 451–454.

Ottenbacher, K. (1982). Sensory integration therapy: Affect or effect? *American Journal of Occupational Therapy, 36,* 571–578.

Ottenbacher, K., & Short M. A. (1985). Sensory integrative dysfunction in children: A review of theory and treatment. In D. Routh & M. Wolrich (Eds.), *Advances in developmental and behavioral pediatrics* (vol. 6, pp. 287–329). Greenwich, CT: JAI.

Palisano, R. J. (1994). Pediatric physical therapy: An individual perspective. *Pediatric Physical Therapy, 6,* 140–141

Parham, L. D. & Mailloux, Z. (2001). Sensory integration. In J. Case-Smith, A. S. Allen, & P. N. Pratt (Eds.), *Occupational therapy for children* (4th ed., pp. 329–351). St. Louis: Mosby.

Polatajko, H. J., Kaplan, B. J., & Wilson, B. N. (1992). Sensory integration treatment for children with learning disabilities: Its status 20 years later. *Occupational Therapy Journal of Research, 12,* 323–341.

Polatajko, H. J., Law, M., Miller, J., Schaffer, R, & Macnab, J. (1991). The effect of a sensory integration program on academic achievement, motor performance, and self-esteem in children identified as learning disabled: Results of a clinical trial. *Occupational Therapy Journal of Research, 11,* 155–175.

Pribram, K. H. (1986). The cognitive revolution and mind/brain issues. *American Psychologist, 41,* 507–520.

Reisman, J. (1993). Using a sensory integrative approach to treat self-injurious behavior in an adult with profound mental retardation. *American Journal of Occupational Therapy, 47,* 403–411.

Robichaud, L., Hébert, R., & Desrosiers, J. (1994). Efficacy of a sensory integration program on behaviors of inpatients with dementia. *American Journal of Occupational Therapy, 48,* 355–360.

Short-DeGraff, M. A. (1988). *Human development for occupational and physical therapists.* Baltimore: Williams & Wilkins.

Sieg, K. W. (1988). A. Jean Ayres. In B. R. J. Miller, K. W. Sieg, F. M. Ludwig, S. D. Shortridge, & J. Van Deusen (Eds.), *Six perspectives on theory for practice of occupational therapy* (pp. 95–142). Rockville, MD: Aspen.

Soper, G., & Thorley, C. R. (1996). Effectiveness of an occupational therapy programme based on sensory integration theory for adults with severe learning disabilities. *British Journal of Occupational Therapy, 59,* 476–483.

Stevens, J. (1986). *Applied multivariate statistics for the social sciences.* Hillsdale, NJ: Lawrence Erlbaum.

Stonefelt, L., & Stein F. (1998). Sensory integrative techniques applied to children with learning disabilities: An outcome study. *Occupational Therapy International, 5,* 252–272.

Trombly, C. (1993). Anticipating the future: Assessment of occupational function. *American Journal of Occupational Therapy, 47,* 253–257.

Trombly , C. A. (Ed.). (1995). *Occupational therapy for physical dysfunction.* Baltimore: Williams & Wilkins.

Vargas, S., & Camilli, G. (1999). A meta-analysis of research on sensory integration treatment. *American Journal of Occupational Therapy, 53,* 189–198.

White, R. (1959). Motivation reconsidered: The concept of competence. *Psychological Review, 66,* 297–333.

Wilbarger, P., & Wilbarger, J. (1991). *Sensory defensiveness in children aged 2–12.* Santa Barbara, CA: Avanti Educational Programs.

William, M. S., & Shellenberger, S. (1996). *How does your engine run?* Albuquerque: TherapyWorks.

Wilson, B. N., & Kaplan, B. J. (1994). Follow-up assessment of children receiving sensory integration treatment. *Occupational Therapy Journal of Research, 14,* 244–267.

Wilson, B. N., Kaplan, B. J., Fellowes, S., Gruchy, C., & Faris, P. (1992). The efficacy of sensory integration treatment compared to tutoring. *Physical and Occupational Therapy in Pediatrics, 12,* 1–36.

Zissermann, L. (1992). The effects of deep pressure on self-stimulating behaviors in a child with autism and other disabilities. *American Journal of Occupational Therapy, 46,* 547–551.

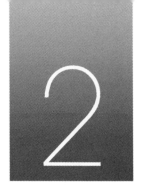

Structure and Function of the Sensory Systems

Shelly J. Lane, Ph.D, OTR/L, FAOTA

> *The task of neural science is to provide explanations of behavior in terms of activities of the brain, to explain how millions of individual nerve cells in the brain operate to produce behavior and how, in turn, these cells are influenced by the environment, including the behavior of other people.*
>
> —*Kandel et al., 1995, p. 5.*

> *... the structure/function duality is merely a didactic convenience. In reality, structure allows function and function gives meaning to structure.*
>
> —*Cohen, 1999, p. 3.*

PURPOSE AND SCOPE

Students faced with their first neuroanatomy class commonly feel a sense of foreboding. There is seemingly endless detail within the central nervous system (CNS), and developing a thorough understanding not only of structure and function but also of interrelationships between and among structures seems a daunting undertaking. Our task in this chapter is a little less daunting: we will examine a small piece of the neuroscience pie to gain an understanding of the essentials of sensory processing and how this relates to the theory and practice of sensory integration. We present an overview of the sensory systems most closely aligned with sensory integration theory. This means that the tactile, vestibular, auditory, and visual systems will be covered, but the olfactory and gustatory systems will not be discussed. A single chapter on even these four senses can hardly do justice to the complex nature of processing within each sensory system. However, we have attempted to provide integrative information that combines structure and function. For more detailed information, readers are referred to the books listed in the reference list and to the other chapters of this book.

We begin by offering brief definitions and descriptions of central and peripheral CNS components. The general functions to be considered are the mechanisms of action that underlie processing in most or all sensory systems:

- Reception
- Transduction and encoding of the sensory stimulus
- Receptor fields and adaptation
- Lateral inhibition
- Convergence and divergence
- Distributed processing and control
- Serial and parallel processing

With this foundation, we will address structure and function within individual sensory systems. We have highlighted the main points relative to each sensory system in an appendix at the end of the chapter. These points paint the big picture for each system and allow readers to absorb the interesting details over the course of time.

We will link function and dysfunction within each sensory system discussion and make reference to other chapters in this book. Within each sensory system presented, readers will find a discussion of the receptors subserving this system, their structure and mechanisms of action, pathways to the CNS, and a brief discussion of function. Function as it relates to sensory integration theory and practice is presented in much greater detail in other chapters of this book.

Neuroscience tends toward discussions of systems within systems. We have attempted to avoid this potentially confusing terminology, but at times it has not been possible. Thus, we have the CNS and within it the somatosensory systems, among which are the anterolateral systems subserving touch. Likewise, we find such redundancy of terminology in other sensory systems. When it has not been possible to avoid embedding discussions of one system within another, we have attempted to be clear on exactly which system is under discussion.

REFERENCE MATERIALS

In developing the material below, we used many sources because no single neuroscience text does it all. Some emphasize function, some emphasize structure, others take a systems approach, and still others take a geographic approach. All have their place and all answer different questions. Cohen (1999), Kandel et al. (1995; 2000), Kingsley (2000), Lundy-Ekman (1998), and Gilman and Newman (1992) approach the topic from a systems perspective. Gilman and Newman (1992) also in-

clude chapters on specific structures (e.g., the thalamus). Lundy-Ekman (1998) focuses on the anatomy of the CNS. Cohen (1992) and Lundy-Ekman (1998) combine a good deal of functional information with neuroanatomy, and both wrote for occupational and physical therapy professionals. Lundy-Ekman (1998) has less text but very useful and plentiful color diagrams and figures. Cohen's book (1999) is more densely packed with information and includes line drawings. Kandel et al. (1995; 2000) and Zigmond et al. (1999) use a systems approach, but their emphasis is on function, and the neuroanatomy is embedded within the functional aspects. The books by Kandel et al. (2000) and Zigmond et al. (1999) are "tombs of knowledge" full of information. Both are excellent resources but neither can be considered an entry-level book. The book by Kandel et al. (1995) is a smaller version of the 2000 book that covers, as the title suggests, the essentials. Rather than reference each statement below, we credit these works in advance as they provided essential background, detail, and guidance to the structural and functional material in this chapter. At appropriate points within this chapter, we reference sources that offer more limited input.

A QUICK REVIEW OF THE BASIC STRUCTURE AND FUNCTION

The CNS is one of three components of the human nervous system. The peripheral nervous system (PNS) and the autonomic nervous system (ANS) are the other two. The human nervous system can be likened to a communications network, with the ANS and PNS transmitting messages into and out of the central core (i.e., the CNS). We will continue to use this analogy in the following descriptions.

The PNS is composed of receptors and neurons, which collect and conduct information to the CNS. The PNS connects the outside world and peripheral structures (e.g., skeletal muscles and glands) to the brain and spinal cord. In a computer system, the PNS would be the equivalent of the keyboard, mouse, and the cables that connect these "peripherals" to the guts of the computer.

Specific receptors for each sensory system are particularly sensitive to one form of physical energy, just as the keyboard and mouse respond to different forms of activation. In the tactile and olfactory systems, the receptors are themselves primary sensory neurons, and information is transmitted along their axons to secondary sensory neurons located within the CNS. In the other sensory systems, the receptors are specialized cells that, after activation, transfer their information to the primary sensory neuron through a process of synaptic transmission. Specifics on receptors are found in subsequent discussions of sensory systems.

The CNS is made up of neurons, pathways, and glia. As can be seen in Figure 2–1, the neuron consists of a cell body, axons, and dendrites. The cell body is the metabolic center of the neuron. Extending from the cell body are two types of processes, axons and dendrites. Typically, there is only one axon, which carries information from the cell body to the target. Although generally only a single axon exits a cell body, it may split into many branches, thereby allowing a single neuron to influence many targets. Axon diameter varies from 0.2 to 20 μm, a feature that will help determine the speed with which information is transmitted; the larger the axons, the more rapid the transmission. Axons may be myelinated, or surrounded by a nodular sheath of fatty substance. Myelin offers insulation to the nerve process and increases transmission speed along the axon. Thus, the axons act like cables in the communication network. Bigger cables, with more insulation, transmit information more quickly and with less loss of signal strength than do the small, uninsulated cables.

Dendrites are responsible for bringing information into the cell body. Thus, the dendrites are cables in the communication network as well. The fibers of the PNS, which carry information from the receptor to the CNS, are dendrites. Dendrites are often extensively branched, allowing communication with many other neurons. They bring information into the central core from an array of sources.

Dendrites and axons combine to form the path-

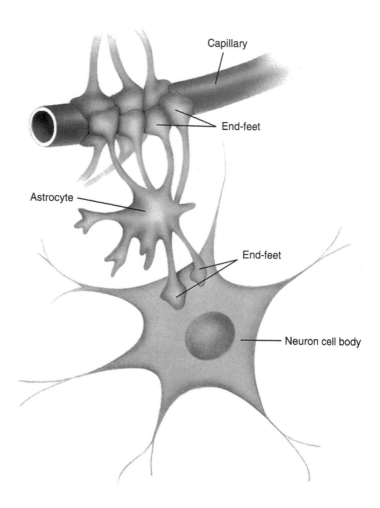

■ FIGURE 2-1 Neuron with astrocytes forming a connection with a capillary. (Reprinted with permission from Lundy-Ekman, L: Neuroscience: Fundamentals for Rehabilitation, p. 22. Philadelphia, WB Saunders Co. 1998.)

Capillary

End-feet

Astrocyte

End-feet

Neuron cell body

ways of the CNS. Fiber bundles and pathways travel varying distances within the CNS and carry information from the CNS to the effector organs and muscles in the body.

Glial cells surround and greatly outnumber neurons. One form of glia, the astrocyte, is shown in Figure 2–1. They do not have the same electrical transmission properties of neurons, but instead, they:

- Provide structural support to the nervous system
- Insulate groups of neurons from each other
- Remove debris after injury or cell death
- Buffer the electrochemical environment in which neurons exist
- Nourish neurons

The ANS is a component of the PNS, and it consists of receptors that respond to pressure and stretch, changes in body chemistry, pain, and temperature. The use of the label "autonomic" suggests that this component of the nervous system functions without conscious control in maintaining the body's physiological homeostasis. Information received is transmitted to the CNS through peripheral and cranial nerves. Within the CNS, the hypothalamus, thalamus, and limbic system, along with areas within the medulla and pons, are responsible for mediating autonomic functions. The efferent fibers of this system innervate smooth muscle, cardiac muscle, and glandular epithelium.

The efferent component of the ANS is composed of two divisions, sympathetic and parasympathetic. The sympathetic division functions to prepare the body for fight or flight; it is active during periods of stress and serves to increase the body's use of energy. The parasympathetic division has a "rest and digest" function, restoring the energy stores in the body by promoting digestion of food and absorption of nutrients. The two divisions of the ANS may innervate the same organ and act in concert to regulate activity in that organ.

We will not further address the specifics of ANS structure or function in this text. However, the way in which sensory processing takes place within the nervous system is often interpreted as a reflection of ANS activity. For instance, when a child with tactile defensiveness overreacts to a nudge from a classmate, the sympathetic component of the ANS may have been activated. Similarly, when we suggest the use of deep pressure or heavy work to act as a calming or focusing agent

for a child, we are considering the potential ability of this input to increase activity in the parasympathetic division of the ANS. Thus, as you read, consider how the behaviors identified in children or the impact of interventions recommended by practitioners potentially reflect activity within the ANS. We have pointed out when systems project to components of the ANS.

Basic Central Nervous System Geography

The CNS can be grossly divided into the brain and the spinal cord. The spinal cord contains both afferent and efferent fibers carrying information to and from the brain and cell bodies located in the PNS. In addition, there are numerous local interneurons (small neurons that reside entirely within the cord) that are responsible for information processing and integration. Using the computer analogy again, the spinal cord is roughly equivalent to a large housing through which several cables run from peripherals to the computer tower. However, because processing does occur in the spinal cord, this analogy falls somewhat short.

The brain (the central processing center in the communication network) has four main components, most of which can also be seen in Figure 2–2:

- The cerebrum or hemispheres
- The diencephalon
- The cerebellum
- The brainstem

The cerebrum includes four lobes with which you are likely familiar (i.e., frontal, parietal, occipital, temporal) and two others, the limbic lobe (visible on the medial surface of the brain) and the insular lobe (forming the floor of the lateral fissure). The diencephalon is composed of the thalamus, epithalamus, and hypothalamus. The brainstem is made up of the pons, medulla, and midbrain.

The midbrain is, at times, referred to as the mesencephalon, a reflection of terminology used in describing embryological brain development. Within the midbrain are the inferior and superior colliculi, associated with the auditory and visual systems, respectively; together they are referred to as the tectum, forming a tent over the cerebral aqueduct. As an aside, the superior colliculus is also considered an important integration center for sensory input because it receives input from

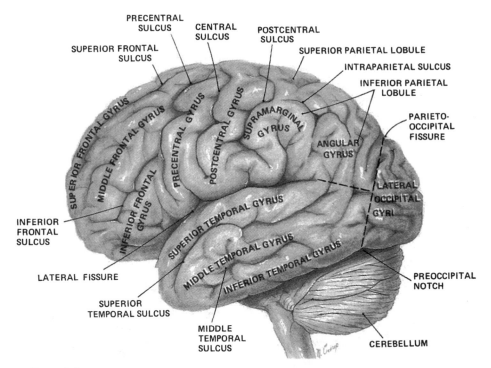

■ FIGURE 2-2 Lateral view of the left cerebral hemisphere or cerebrum. The frontal lobe ends posteriorly at the *central sulcus*. The parietal lobe is bounded by the *central sulcus* and the *parieto-occipital fissure*. The temporal lobe lies below the *lateral fissure*. The occipital lobe lies just posterior to the *parieto-occipital fissure*. The *cerebellum* can be seen below the temporal and occipital lobes; it has a striated appearance in this diagram. Just anterior to the cerebellum is the *brainstem* region, of which the *medulla* and the *pons* are visible here. The *diencephalon* lies deep and cannot be seen in this diagram. (Reprinted with permission from Gilman, S, and Newman, SW: Essentials of Clinical Neuroanatomy and Neurophysiology, 9th edition, p. 7. Philadelphia, FA Davis Co, 1996.)

multiple sensory systems. Another midbrain region, the periaqueductal gray, surrounds the region of the cerebral aqueduct and thus is located adjacent to the tectum. In the subsequent sections of the chapter, we discuss each of these CNS components as they relate to the sensory systems.

Brodmann's areas are also referred to throughout this chapter. Brodmann's areas represent a numbering system of brain regions developed by Brodmann in 1909. He thought that each of the 52 numbered regions defined a discrete histological unit within the brain. Subsequent work has shown that only some of these areas have clear functions. However, the numbering that has survived is a useful reference point for identifying cortical regions. Brodmann's areas are shown in Figure 2–3.

Basic Central Nervous System Function

Organization of function within the CNS was once thought to be strictly hierarchical, with increasing complexity in the interpretation of input and planning of output as information moved from the spinal cord to the cerebral cortex. According to Zigmond et al. (1999), this hierarchical organization does exist and is very apparent in the motor system. In addition, there is a hierarchy in processing sensory input such that at each level within the CNS greater specificity in interpretation of input is attained. However, the complexity of interactions within and between CNS levels indicates that a heterarchical organization also exists. Sensory information reaches all levels within the motor systems, and motor system output is influenced not only by sensory input but also by cognitive processing, other intrinsic activity (e.g., sleep–wake cycles, behavioral state, arousal level, motivation), and sensory feedback from ongoing motor activity. Thus, the CNS is functionally organized both hierarchically and heterarchically. Zigmond et al. (1999) suggested that the relationship between the structure and function of the CNS is "an unsolved problem" (p. 37).

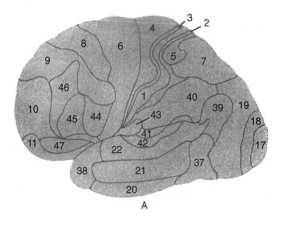

A

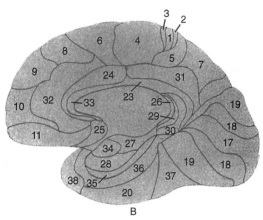

B

■ FIGURE 2-3 Brodmann's areas. (Reprinted with permission from Lundy-Ekman, L: Neuroscience: Fundamentals for Rehabilitation, p. 323. Philadelphia, W. B. Saunders Co., 1998.)

Terminology

Some functional considerations become important as we begin to study the CNS. Because they are all at work in all sensory systems, we define them here and refer to them within each system as appropriate.

Stimulus Reception and Transduction

"In each sensory system the initial contact with the external world occurs through specialized cells called sensory receptors" (Kandel et al., 1995, p. 372). Receptors within each system respond optimally to specific types of sensory input. Thus, specific tactile pressure receptors respond best to touch or pressure, and photoreceptors in the eye respond best to light. However, functional specificity is not absolute, and with a sufficiently intense stim-

ulus, receptors respond to alternative forms of energy. This can be demonstrated by putting pressure on your eye and "seeing stars." The photoreceptors, typically light detectors, respond, in this instance, to pressure. Interestingly, the interpretation of the phenomenon continues to fall along the lines of visual functions—seeing stars. This later phenomenon is related to encoding.

Although the receptors are different for each system, the process of changing the input from physical to electrochemical has some similarities. Using the tactile system as an example, deep pressure activates a receptor, such as the Pacinian corpuscle. The pressure changes membrane characteristics in the receptor, and this process leads to transduction of the mechanical (pressure) input into an electrical signal. From physiology class, you may recall that all cells have an "electrical potential" established by the distribution of charged ions on the inside and outside of the cell membrane. Tactile pressure leads to changes in the distribution of these ions, which changes the charge distribution across the membrane and results in a local depolarization of the immediately surrounding membrane. The term applied to this local depolarization is a "receptor potential." At times, when the stimulus is very weak, the electrical changes are minimal and the receptor potentials are not strong enough to lead to transmission beyond this level, so the input never reaches the CNS. The message "peters out" a short distance from where it began, similar to a whisper spoken to a large group of people. Those close by may hear it, but unless they pass it on, those on the far side of the group will not, and the message will die a short distance from where it began.

If the stimulus is of sufficient intensity or applied for a long enough period of time, receptor potentials can be added together, and the result is the production of an action potential in the sensory neuron. An action potential is also a change in the distribution of charge on the membrane, but it is strong enough to depolarize neighboring areas on the neuron, and a wave of depolarization is generated that carries the information to its first synapse on the way to the CNS.

Stimulus Encoding

One action potential, in any system, generated by any input, is the same as another. How then does the CNS discriminate between bright light and firm touch? Discrimination relies on specificity of receptors for a type of sensory input and requires interpretation within the CNS, based on pathways and connections of the sensory neurons. Receptors convey the information that a touch was firm instead of soft by encoding the stimulus characteristics into a pattern of action potentials that represents intensity, duration, and movement of the stimulus. A stronger stimulus results in an increase in the frequency of action potentials sent to the CNS and is likely to activate more receptors when applied. Thus, strong inputs are read as such in the CNS because they generate more action potentials within one neuron and because the input is detected by multiple receptors so that action potentials are transmitted by a large number of neighboring neurons. This process of specificity in receptors has parallels in computer systems as well. The electrical wires that connect both the keyboard and mouse to your computer are essentially the same; they transmit electrical current in the same manner after the current is generated. The specificity comes from the receptors—the keys and mouse pad. We can change the intensity and duration of input over these "receptors" manually by changing the characteristics of the type (e.g., typing in bold or in all capitals), and this, too, is a characteristic defined by the peripheral receptor.

Receptor Fields

The term *receptor* or *receptive field* refers to the area around a receptor from which input can be transduced into an electrical signal. This concept is applied to mechanical receptors of the tactile system where the receptor field is that area of skin surrounding a single receptor, which activates the receptor. In the visual system, the receptor field of a photoreceptor is that area of the retina in which it is found. Small receptor fields are associated with fine discriminative function because they contribute to a precise representation of input at the CNS. Returning to the computer analogy, this is similar to the receptive area available on a keyboard with very small keys (e.g., a hand-held organizer) versus one with very large keys (e.g., keys on a child-size keyboard).

Receptor Adaptation

Receptors adapt to continued input, and depolarization of the receptor membrane ceases, even with continued input. Some receptors are considered rapidly adapting, responding only at the onset and offset of input. Others are slowly adapting, responding in a more continual manner to ongoing input, but eventually even these will cease to produce action potentials. The adaptation of receptors becomes critical in the function of the sensory systems, and this function plays a role in providing ongoing information about what is happening (slowly adapting receptors), along with information on changes in the internal or external environment (rapidly adapting receptors).

Lateral Inhibition

Lateral inhibition is another phenomenon important to understanding how we receive and interpret neural signals. As shown in Figure 2–4, lateral inhibition is the mechanism used by the CNS to focus input from the receptors and thereby sharpen its interpretation.

Lateral inhibition relies on the presence of inhibitory interneurons. It happens like this: a stimulus—for example, a touch—is applied to the hand. Receptors in the skin are activated, and those with their receptive fields centered under the stimulus respond with greater strength (more action potentials and more rapid firing). This is analogous to speaking softly to a group of people; those directly in front of the speaker will hear the bulk of the message, but those on the edges will capture less of the information. Receptor neurons contact more than one sensory neuron as they transmit information to the CNS, much as the people in this group talk with their neighbors. In the absence of lateral inhibition, the activation pattern spreads widely, with increasing numbers of sensory neurons activated, and the result at the CNS is some general awareness that a large region of the skin was touched. In the speaking example here, it would be as though each person who heard the message spoke it again to a neighbor, and the neighbor shared it with another neighbor so that soon the whole room would be buzzing with sound. However, the specifics of that sound would be rather vague. Lateral inhibition is used to focus the input, rather than allow it to be diffused over many neurons. In sensory systems, using this focusing mechanism, the neurons at the center of the receptor field (i.e., those most intensely activated by the input) activate inhibitory interneurons at

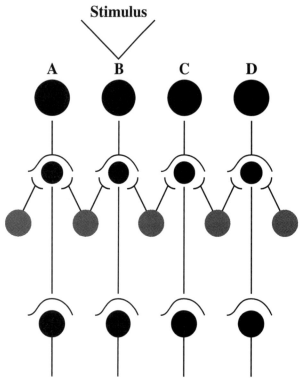

Stimulus

A   B   C   D

**Receptors:
receive stimulus at
strength related to
location**

**Inhibitory Interneurons
Each inhibits strength of
signal by 20%**

■ **FIGURE 2–4** Schematic of lateral inhibition. In this diagram the stimulus is applied as shown, and the receptors directly under it will respond with full strength, whereas those located laterally will respond with less strength. Thus receptor B will respond at 100%, A and C at 80%, and D at 60%. The small inhibitory interneurons reduce the stimulus by 20%. Thus stimulus strength in each neuron is reduced by 40% at this level, and neurons A and C now transmit at only 40%, B at 60%, and D at 20. This information transmitted from this point forth then is more focused; little information is transmitted over neuron A and none over neuron D. This process can occur at all synapses along the route of transmission, and will serve to sharpen the initial input received by the receptor. (The values associated with stimulus strength and interneuron inhibition are arbitrary.)

their first synapse within the CNS. These inhibitory interneurons connect with sensory neurons farther from the center of the receptive field (i.e., less active neurons) and inhibit transmission at the periphery of the receptive field. Other terms used to define this process include *surround inhibition* and *inhibitory surround*. The process is the equivalent of the people in the center of the room gently putting their hands over the mouths of their neighbors to prevent them from speaking. This cuts down on the background noise in the room, making the original message more clearly delivered, at least to the people permitted to hear it. In the CNS, lateral inhibition serves to focus the input at each relay station, reducing background noise. This results in the ability to discriminate and localize the input we receive. Sensory systems with well-developed discriminatory functions rely on this mechanism.

Convergence and Divergence

Convergence and divergence (Fig. 2–5) are concepts that need to be understood in order to appreciate the accuracy with which information is conveyed from the PNS to the CNS. With convergence, many cell processes synapse at one site. Thus, many axons may synapse on the same neuronal cell body or dendrite. When this happens, a great deal of information is condensed. This can be useful for increasing the intensity of the information in the CNS and for promoting integration, but the tradeoff is that the specificity of the original input is decreased, similar to several members of an audience offering input to the speaker in rapid succession. The speaker can listen and integrate the information, but the specifics of where each bit of information came from, exactly what was said and by whom, are likely to be lost.

Divergence, on the other hand, occurs when one

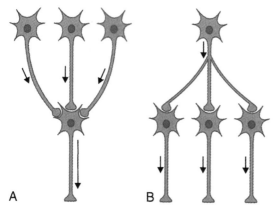

A   B

■ FIGURE 2–5   A schematic depicting convergence (A) and divergence (B) in the CNS. (Reprinted with permission from Lundy-Ekman, L: Neuroscience: Fundamentals for Rehabilitation, p. 37. Philadelphia, WB Saunders Co., 1998.)

process synapses with many different cells in the CNS. Earlier in this chapter, we mentioned that axons can divide and influence many other cells; divergence is such an example. An axon leaves a cell body and subsequently makes contact with cell bodies or dendritic branches in several other areas of the CNS. The functional association here is that the same information is represented at many places, repeated over and over. Thus, the potential impact of this information can be widespread.

Distributed Processing and Control

The CNS can be masterful in its capacity to "multitask." You read this chapter while you maintain your posture, shift weight to relieve uncomfortable pressure, possibly eat and drink, and digest whatever it is you are drinking or eating. All activities are organized and directed by the CNS. You are engaging sensory and motor systems, cognitive processes, and autonomic functions simultaneously via distributed processing within the CNS. When it works well, distributed processing allows for efficient and effective interactions with the world because the load is distributed among different centers of control.

Serial and Parallel Processing

Underlying distributed control of activities are two processing methods: serial and parallel. In serial processing, things occur in sequence, one after another, in a hierarchical manner. Transmitting information from a touch receptor to the CNS oc-

curs this way as the information is mechanically received, transduced into an electrical signal, summed to form an action potential, and transmitted to the CNS. Parallel processing involves the work of more than one pathway at the same time, working simultaneously. Visual, vestibular, and proprioceptive systems often use parallel processing to orient us to our position in space. Each system processes different bits of information about our bodies and the space around us with the integrated endpoint being maintenance of upright posture.

Parallel processing is a term also applied to the parallel processing of the same information in two pathways that have some redundancy. Thus, for instance, pain input is processed via both the dorsal column medial lemniscal and the spinothalamic pathways. This functional overlap can be very useful in the face of disease or dysfunction that interrupts the flow of information in one system. The fact that the same information can be processed in a parallel system can be capitalized upon in intervention.

There are other processes and mechanisms that could be discussed in this background section, but the ones offered provide a very basic anatomic and functional baseline. We now focus on the individual sensory systems and integration among sensory systems as a basis for understanding their contributions to sensory integration and occupational performance.

THE SOMATOSENSORY SYSTEM

We begin our discussion of the somatosensory system with the receptors for the entire system. After gathered by the receptors, processing of somatosensory inputs takes place over the dorsal column medial lemniscal (DCML) and the pathways of the anterolateral system (AL). We present each separately. We also discuss the trigeminothalamic pathway, responsible for the transmission of somatosensory information from the face. A brief description of the functional overlap between the somatosensory pathways completes this section.

Receptors and Transduction

Receptors in the tactile system are, by and large, mechanoreceptors. This means that when a mechanical force (e.g., light touch, deep pressure, stretch, or vibration) is applied to the receptors, the process of neural transmission begins. Proprioceptive input from joints and muscles is certainly a mechanical input, and proprioceptive input is carried along somatosensory pathways. Although we discuss proprioception briefly here, readers will also find proprioception covered in conjunction with the vestibular system in other chapters of this book. The tactile system also includes thermoreceptors, and is thus responsible for the interpretation of temperature input. Table 2–1 lists the receptors within this system and their various characteristics.

Mechanoreceptors within the skin subserve different types of sensory activation. Some respond to the initiation and cessation of input (Meissner's corpuscle, Pacinian corpuscle, some hair follicles) but not to sustained input. These receptors are considered fast adapting because they stop responding to maintained stimuli. They are sensitive to changes in tactile input. Slowly adapting receptors include Merkel's discs, Ruffini endings, and some hair follicle receptors. In contrast to the fast-adapting receptors, this second group of receptors provides the CNS with information regarding the intensity, duration, and speed of input.

Our tactile discrimination ability depends, in part, on the density of receptors and the associated size of the receptor field. In areas of fine tactile discrimination (e.g., finger tips, palms, around the mouth), receptor density is high and the receptor field is small. Areas of high receptor density are more skilled. On the other hand, in areas where less specific information is needed about tactile input (e.g., abdomen and back), receptor density is low

and receptor fields are larger. Researchers (e.g., Heller & Schiff, 1991) examining discrimination abilities have shown that, although some things can be distinguished using either active or passive touch, the use of active touch allows finer and more accurate discrimination. The tactile system also capitalizes on lateral inhibition to focus input and refine discrimination.

The somatosensory system, which carries information from the body to the CNS, has two main subdivisions: the DCML and the AL. Together they provide us with the ability to interpret our tactile world and respond appropriately to touch. Because of the pervasive nature of these two somatosensory subdivisions, they are critical to our interactions with the world. Likewise, the pervasive nature of the somatosensory system means that when problems exist, the impact can be widespread.

Dorsal Column Medial Lemniscal Pathway

Receptors associated with the DCML respond to mechanical stimuli, transmitting primarily tactile, vibratory, touch-pressure, and proprioceptive information. The DCML is consistently associated with functions inherent to tactile discrimination or perception: detection of size, form, and contour; texture; and movement across the skin. Because it carries proprioceptive information, the DCML also transmits information relative to the position of body and limbs in space.

Inputs are transduced into a set of action potentials and transmitted over the axon to the cell

---

■ Table 2–1. **Locations, Modalities of Sensation, Adaptation Rates, and Fiber Types Associated with Skin Receptors**

Type	Location	Stimulus	Fiber Type	Adaptation
Free nerve ending	Dermis, joint capsules, tendons, ligaments	Pain, temperature	A-delta, C	Slow
Hair follicle plexus	Deep dermis	Hair displacement; pain	A-beta	Fast
Meissner's corpuscles (tactile corpuscles)	Papillae of skin, mucous membranes of tongue tip	Touch	A-beta	Fast
Pacinian corpuscles	Subcutaneous tissue	Pressure, vibration	A-beta	Fast
Krause's end bulb	Papillae of hairless skin; near hair follicle plexus	Cold?	A-delta, C	Below 20°C; no adaptation
Merkel's disc	Epidermis of hairless skin; hair follicles	Deformation of skin	A-beta	Slow
Ruffini ending	Joint capsules; connective tissue	Touch; skin stretch; joint movement	A-beta	Slow

body, which, in this case, is in the dorsal root ganglion. There is no synapse here, and the information is passed from the dorsal root ganglion cell body to dendrites that enter the spinal cord and travel to the brain via the dorsal columns of the spinal cord. The DCML is shown in Figure 2–6. The first synapse of the DCML is in the medulla, in the gracile and cuneate nuclei.

From the medulla, fiber tracks cross and form the medial lemniscal fibers, traveling through the brainstem reticular formation and ascending to the ventral posterior lateral (VPL) nucleus of the thalamus. The fact that fiber tracks cross in the brain rather than in the spinal cord has functional implications in the face of an injury or dysfunction. If there is a problem with this pathway at or above the medulla, the functional loss will be on the opposite side of the body. If there is a loss of function within this pathway below the medulla, it will be reflected on the same side of the body.

Fibers enter the thalamus, synapse, and send third-order neurons to the cortex. Cortical reception areas for the DCML include the primary and secondary somatic sensory cortex (S-I and S-II, respectively), as well as areas 5 and 7 of the posterior parietal lobe. The processing up to this point has been an example of hierarchical processing, with more refined information processed at each level. Within the cortex, the hierarchy is less obvious.

In S-I, the somatosensory receptor density and location are precisely represented in a somewhat distorted image of the body known as the *sensory homunculus* (Fig. 2–7). Interestingly, it has been shown that this representation of the body at the cortical level is flexible. Areas representing specific body parts can be increased in size with intense use, and, likewise, representation is decreased with disuse and concomitant diminished skill (Cohen, 1999; Mogliner et al., 1993). This finding is important to occupational therapy intervention in general and sensory integrative intervention specifically.

Processing throughout the DCML promotes its discriminative functions. The somatotopic organization of the fibers is precise, with fibers from the leg and foot taking a medial position. As fibers representing upper leg, trunk, and upper extremity enter the cord, they are added to the pathway laterally. The relationship of the fibers to each other is maintained with high integrity as they travel through the CNS. The somatotopic organization of the fiber pathways is also maintained in the medullary nuclei and in the pathway

as it ascends. However, the pathway twists as it approaches the thalamus so that fibers from the arm come to lie medial to those from the leg.

Precise somatotopic organization is only one reason information in the DCML is transmitted with great accuracy. Others include:

- A minimal number of relays where the signal must be processed
- Little convergence of input en route to the CNS
- Heavy reliance on lateral inhibition to maintain the integrity of a stimulus from the periphery to the CNS

These features allow the brain to interpret the temporal and spatial aspects of DCML inputs, yielding a great deal of information about location and type of somatosensory information received (Haines, 1997; Kandel et al., 2000; Vierck et al., 1985).

Proprioception

Sherrington (1906) defined proprioception as perception of joint and body movements as well as position of the body, or body segments, in space. A more recent description of proprioception includes sensing the direction and velocity of movement, as well as determining the effort needed to grasp and lift objects (Zigmond et al., 1999). Proprioception informs us about the spatial orientation of the body or body parts, the rate and timing of movements, the amount of force our muscles are exerting, and how much and how fast a muscle is being stretched (Kalaska, 1988; Matthews, 1988; McCloskey, 1985). Although Sherrington (1906) identified muscle afferents, joint receptors, *and* the vestibular labyrinth as proprioceptors, we will confine the discussion in this section to the nonvestibular proprioceptors.

Before the early 1970s, researchers distinguished between *conscious* joint proprioception (kinesthesia), thought to arise primarily from joint receptors, and *unconscious* proprioception, thought to arise from the muscle spindle and tendon receptors. More recently, researchers have begun to use the terms *proprioception* and *kinesthesia* synonymously. Although controversy regarding this issue continues to exist, experimental evidence now indicates that all proprioceptive inputs can contribute to conscious proprioception (Matthews, 1988; McCloskey, 1985; McCloskey et al., 1983; Moberg, 1983; Tracey, 1985).

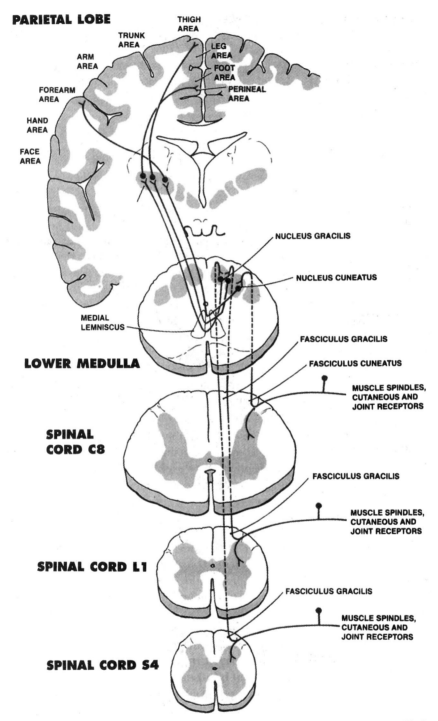

PARIETAL LOBE

TRUNK AREA

THIGH AREA

ARM AREA

LEG AREA

FOOT AREA

FOREARM AREA

PERINEAL AREA

HAND AREA

FACE AREA

NUCLEUS GRACILIS

NUCLEUS CUNEATUS

MEDIAL LEMNISCUS

FASCICULUS GRACILIS

LOWER MEDULLA

FASCICULUS CUNEATUS

MUSCLE SPINDLES, CUTANEOUS AND JOINT RECEPTORS

SPINAL CORD C8

FASCICULUS GRACILIS

MUSCLE SPINDLES, CUTANEOUS AND JOINT RECEPTORS

SPINAL CORD L1

FASCICULUS GRACILIS

MUSCLE SPINDLES, CUTANEOUS AND JOINT RECEPTORS

SPINAL CORD S4

■ Figure 2–6 Dorsal column medial lemniscal system. Note that the information transmitted over this pathway comes from muscle spindles, skin, and joint receptors. That from the lower extremity is transmitted to the *nucleus gracilis* and that from the upper extremity to the *nucleus cuneatus*. (Reprinted with permission from Gilman, S, and Newman, SW: Essentials of Clinical Neuroanatomy and Neurophysiology, 9th edition, p. 62. Philadelphia, FA Davis Co., 1996.)

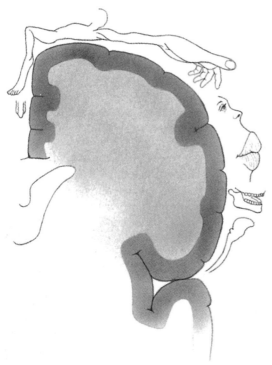

■ FIGURE 2-7 Sensory homunculus located in the primary sensory cortex. (Reprinted with permission from Lundy-Ekman, L: Neuroscience: Fundamentals for Rehabilitation, p. 98. Philadelphia, W. B. Saunders Co., 1998.)

For purposes of studying sensory integration theory, it is more important to understand the distinction between proprioceptors (i.e., proprioceptive receptors) and proprioception (i.e., proprioceptive feedback and perception of joint and body movement). Not all proprioception is derived from peripheral proprioceptive receptors. Internal correlates of motor signals that are sent to the muscles after an action is planned (i.e., corollary discharge) are also an important source of proprioception. Corollary discharge is important for differentiating between active (internally generated) and passive movement generated by an external stimulus, identifying if we have programmed an appropriate level of motor activity, the development of body scheme, and perception of force (Jones, 1988). Knowledge of the body and its movements is important in motor planning, and is also addressed in Chapter 3.

Sources of Proprioceptive Input

Proprioceptive feedback arises primarily from muscle spindles, mechanoreceptors of the skin,

and centrally generated motor commands. Joint receptors, once thought to be a major source of proprioception, are now considered much less important. Joint receptors fire primarily at the extremes of range (flexion or extension) and are probably most important for preventing hyperextension and hyperflexion.

The effective stimulus for the primary and secondary endings of the muscle spindle is stretch. These receptors are mechanoreceptors. Muscle spindles detect both dynamic and static stretch. Primary fibers transmit information regarding the velocity of change in muscle length, as well as amount of change, and secondary fibers transmit information on static positions and sustained stretch and contraction. Both types of fibers are critical for determining the location of body and limbs in space.

Active stretch occurs when higher-level motor commands descend to produce alpha-gamma coactivation and when a muscle contracts against resistance. For example, when we extend the head and upper trunk against gravity from the prone-lying position, extend weight-bearing limbs to jump on a trampoline, or flex our arms while swinging on a suspended trapeze, we are contracting against the resistance of gravity. When a weak muscle contracts against gravity, stretch of the muscle results in recruitment of more motor units so that the muscle can contract harder and become stronger. Therefore, evincing an adaptive behavior against resistance may be the most effective means available for generating proprioceptive feedback. Furthermore, joint compression and traction probably are less effective sources of proprioception than is active muscle contraction against resistance.

Stimulation of cutaneous or skin mechanoreceptors and joint receptors by active joint movement is believed to be particularly important in perception of movement in some, but not all, body areas. For instance, loss of cutaneous input during movement of the knee has not been shown to impair the ability to determine joint position. However, similar loss of input from around the mouth, the hands, or the feet results in significant difficulty with detecting passive movement (Matthews, 1988; McCloskey et al., 1983; Moberg, 1983; Zigmond, et al., 1999).

Although tactile and proprioceptive information travel in the same pathway, it is important not to confuse cutaneous-generated proprioception with tactile sensation. *Proprioception* refers to sensations of movement or position that arise as a result of an individual's own movement. *Tactile sensation* pertains to awareness or perception of the location, or change in position, of an external stimulus applied to the skin. Tactile sensation provides an individual with information about the external environment. Often, tactile information is gathered from movement of joints. However, by definition, deep touch pressure and other tactile sensations are not sources of proprioception.

Centrally generated motor commands and efference copy are also sources of proprioceptive feedback. They are thought to be responsible for the sense of effort or conscious awareness that proprioception is happening (Brooks, 1986; Jones, 1988; Matthews, 1988; McCloskey, 1985).

> We have all experienced the sensation of increasing heaviness of a suitcase which we carry with progressively fatiguing muscles. Ultimately we put down such a load and rest when it has "become too heavy." But the load has not really become heavier: the pressure and tensions in the supporting limbs have not increased, and there is no reason to assume that the discharges from sensory receptors signaling pressures or tensions will have increased either. What makes the load seem heavier is that one perceives the greater effort, the greater efferent barrage of voluntarily-generated command signals, which has been necessary to maintain a contraction with progressively fatiguing and so less responsive muscles. Similar sensations of heaviness or increased muscular force accompany all other states of muscular weakness whether caused experimentally . . . or by disease (McCloskey, 1985, p. 152).

Centrally generated motor commands and efference copy from motor centers are speculated to be necessary for accurate interpretation of sensation (Schmidt, 1999). Centrally generated motor commands and efference copy are also important in motor control, that is, in the planning and producing of an adaptive motor behavior. We present more information on these concepts in Chapter 3.

Interpreting Somatosensory Input

Although we generally consider interpretation of sensation to be a function of the cortex, or at least higher levels of the CNS, some processing begins within the gracile and cuneate nuclei in the medulla for the DCML. In addition to somatosensation, these nuclei receive input from the primary sensory cortex and the reticular formation. This convergence of input means that activity in the primary sensory cortex, as well as the reticular formation, influences the interpretation of tactile input, even before it reaches a cortical level.

Thalamic interpretation of DCML inputs is thought to permit vague conscious discrimination of tactile input. There exist inhibitory interneurons in the VPL that are activated by fibers from the cortex, as well as inhibited by fibers from other thalamic nuclei. Cortical activation of inhibitory interneurons interferes with further transmission of DCML inputs beyond the thalamus. On the other hand, if the inhibitory interneurons are themselves inhibited by other thalamic projections, information can be processed and sent onto cortical areas. Thus, there is some processing at this level that influences transmission beyond the thalamus.

The primary somatosensory cortex (S-I, Brodmann's areas 3,1,2) is subdivided into different processing areas associated with differing types of sensation. The majority of thalamic projections terminate in areas 3a and 3b. Areas 2 and 3a receive information primarily from muscle spindles and Golgi tendon organs, giving these two areas an important role in proprioception and kinesthesia. Areas 3b and 1 receive information from the slow- and fast-adapting tactile receptors in the skin. Loss of texture discrimination has been associated with area 1, and loss of stereognosis has been associated with damage to area 2. Area 3b has been associated with losses of both of these functional skills, and 3b may therefore process information before passing it on the areas 1 and 2. This means that areas 1 and 2 likely elaborate sensory input and are, therefore, associated with higher level interpretation of information. However, there are extensive interconnections within this region of the brain, allowing for both serial and parallel processing of somatosensory inputs (Kandell et al., 2000).

The secondary sensory cortex (S-II, Brodmann's area 43) receives input from the VPL as well as from S-I. However, without a functioning primary sensory cortex, neurons within the secondary cortex do not fire. Thus the secondary cortex depends on the primary cortex for input. Within the S-II, new sensory discriminations are thought to take place. Projections from the secondary cortex to the insular lobe are believed to be involved in tactile memory (Kandell et al., 2000).

Further interpretation of somatosensory inputs

takes place in areas 5 and 7 of the parietal lobe. These regions not only receive input from the thalamus but also from S-I and S-II, and they are connected bilaterally. Both play sensory integrating roles; area 5 for touch and proprioception, and area 7 for somatosensory and visual inputs. Such processing of inputs from multiple sources makes this a good example of heterarchical organization within the CNS. Because of these connections, lesions in areas 5 and 7 result in deficits in spatial perception, visual-motor integration, and directed attention. Both areas are also associated with the manipulation of objects and are important in discerning their tactile qualities (i.e., haptic perception). Any clinician who has tried to evaluate stereognosis in clients who do not automatically manipulate objects can appreciate the importance of manipulation for tactile perception. Lesions in these areas within the right hemisphere have been associated with agnosia of the contralateral side of the body and body space. Tactile sensation is not impaired, but individuals fail to recognize and attend to this side of the body and the environment around it.

Also within the parietal lobe, aspects of tactile and proprioceptive input converge and subsequently project to anterior motor planning areas of the brain. Thus, output from the DCML could be expected to have an impact on both object manipulation and motor planning. In fact, when outputs from area 2 (a region of S-I) to the primary motor cortex are disrupted, hand use becomes uncoordinated. According to Cohen (1999), the decrease in sensory feedback to the motor cortex that occurs secondary to interruption of the DCML is critical and interferes with the production of coordinated fine motor acts.

The DCML may also have a role in modulating arousal. Clinically, certain types of sensory information have been observed to have a calming effect. Deep touch pressure and proprioceptive information can have this quality (Ayres, 1972; Farber, 1982; Knickerbocker, 1980), and both are carried to the CNS via the dorsal columns.

Clinicians and researchers have hypothesized that poor tactile perception may be related to difficulties in manipulative hand skills (Haron & Henderson, 1985; Nathan et al., 1986). Furthermore, difficulty in perceiving the size and form of an object during the process of active manipulation results in difficulty handling the object. We may also speculate that difficulty in perceiving the boundaries of the hand and the relationship of the fingers to one another interferes with manipulation skills.

Anterolateral System

The AL (Fig. 2–8) is composed of separate pathways that function primarily to mediate pain, crude touch (the detection of an object's position but not its movement across the skin), and temperature. Mediation of both neutral warmth and the "tickle" sensation are also related to transmission within these anterolateral pathways. The pathways are spinothalamic, spinoreticular, spinobulbar, spinomesencephalic, and spinohypothalamic.

The term *anterolateral system* is sometimes used interchangeably with *spinothalamic pathway* because the thalamus is a major projection point for many fibers traveling in the anterolateral fasciculus. In fact, some texts have indicated that the AL is but one pathway, the spinothalamic pathway, with intermediate projections to the reticular formation, cranial nerve nuclei, parts of the mesencephalon and hypothalamus on the way to the thalamus, and do not identify the separate projections as separate pathways. Determining which nomenclature is correct is beyond the scope of this text. For clarity in identifying the beginning and end of the projections, we will use the individual pathway designations.

Receptors for the AL system include those that respond to rough stimuli (e.g., rubbing, squeezing, pinching) that do not result in tissue damage; and those that respond when tissue is damaged. These latter receptors are mechanonociceptors. When tissue is damaged, release of chemical substances activate a third class of receptors, called chemonociceptors. There are also receptors for cold and hot sensations. None of these receptors localize inputs well when compared with receptors associated with the DCML.

As with the DCML, cell bodies for neurons associated with the AL are in the dorsal root ganglion. Projections from dorsal root ganglion cells enter the spinal cord, and the fibers ascend or descend one or two spinal segments before synapsing in the dorsal horn. The interconnections of these fibers can be complex. After synapsing, the majority of second-order neurons cross to the other side of the cord and project to the brainstem reticular formation and the thalamus. The crossing pattern defines a different picture for injury or

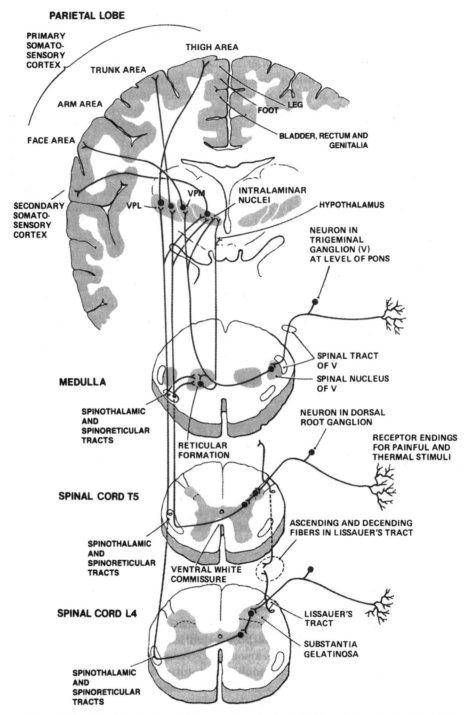

■ Figure 2–8 Anterolateral systems. *Spinoreticular* and *spinothalamic* pathways are both depicted in this figure, and projections to the *somatosensory cortex* indicate regions of the *sensory homunculus,* to which they contribute. Projections to note also include those to the *reticular* formation and the *hypothalamus.* The *trigeminothalamic pathway* is also indicated in this diagram, although it is seen in greater detail in Figure 2–9. (Reprinted with permission from Gilman, S, and Newman, SW: Essentials of Clinical Neuroanatomy and Neurophysiology, 9th edition, p. 51. Philadelphia, FA Davis Co., 1996.)

dysfunction than that seen for the DCML. Any injury to this system above the level of fiber entry into the spinal cord results in deficits on the opposite side of the body.

As suggested by the pathway names, information carried within the AL system projects to the reticular system (spinoreticular), thalamus (spinothalamic), periaqueductal gray and the tectum (spinomesencephalic), and hypothalamic (spinohypothalmic) areas. Interestingly, a large portion of fibers within the AL terminate within the reticular formation. The transmission of both diffuse and chronic pain is thought to be projected to this area of the brain, where arousal is associated with pain. Spinothalamic projections carrying nonspecific touch, temperature, and pain go to the VPL as well as other thalamic nuclei. The thalamus also receives tactile projections from the reticular formation. Fibers sent to midbrain regions (periaqueductal gray and tectum) and the hypothalamus permit pain information to become available to the limbic system and the autonomic nervous system, generating emotional, neuroendocrine, and cardiovascular responses to pain. Interestingly, the emotional components of pain can be separated from pain perception, probably because of the variety of projections within the AL. Medications in the benzodiazepine class (e.g., Valium), when used for pain, do not mask pain perception. Instead, they make the sensation of pain less distressing through their action on the limbic system. Projections to the tectum may be associated with the visual (superior colliculus) and auditory (inferior colliculus) systems; however, the tectum is also an important pain reception center.

Perception of pain relies on projections to the VPL of the thalamus, where it may be interpreted as paresthesia or dull pain and pressure. Because the DCML also projects to the VPL and there is some degree of convergence of AL and DCML inputs, this nucleus is thought to be an important area for interaction of information from these two sources of somatosensory input. DCML input is thought to inhibit transmission in the AL pathways, and the thalamus may be one site for this interaction (Peele, 1977). Interaction in the VPL may partially explain why deep touch-pressure and proprioception have been observed to diminish the sensation of pain and tactile defensiveness (Fisher & Dunn, 1983). Projections from the VPL go to the somatosensory cortices (both S-I and S-II), which, therefore, are also potential anatomi-cal sites for interaction between DCML and AL inputs. Precise localization of pain is thought to take place at the cortical level.

Trigeminothalamic Pathway

The trigeminothalamic pathway (Fig. 2–9) transmits somatosensory input from the face. The cell bodies for the fibers in the peripheral aspect of this pathway are located in the trigeminal ganglion. From there, fibers project to the pons and the spinal cord, where they both ascend and descend before synapsing. Synapses for these fibers take place in the pons, in a column of cells called the principal sensory nucleus, and in the spinal track of the trigeminal nerve. Input to the spinal track of the trigeminal nerve carries primarily pain, temperature, and nondiscriminative touch from the face and mouth to the CNS. Input to the principal sensory nucleus conveys discriminative tactile information from the face and mouth to the thalamus, at the ventral posterior lateral (VPL) nucleus. From there, fibers project to the primary sensory cortex, where the regions around the mouth have a wide representation. The sensory homunculus reflects this wide representation.

Functional Considerations

In sensory integration theory, the tactile system is thought to be of the utmost importance in determining behavior. Touch is our first language; it is the first system to function *in utero,* and it mediates our first experiences in this world. We are nourished, we are calmed, and we first become attached to others (i.e., bonding) through touch (Montagu, 1978). The sensation of touch is, in fact, the "oldest and most primitive expressive channel" (Collier, 1985, p. 29), and it is a primary system for making contact with the external world. We are extremely dependent on touch until language, motor skills, and cognitive processes develop and can guide our experiences and interactions (Collier, 1985; Diamond & Hopson, 1998).

In a recent review of literature, Blackwell (2000) summarized the power of the tactile sensory system:

> There remains little doubt that tactile stimulation is
> an important factor in the social, emotional, physi-
> ological, and neurological development of infants
> and young children. Consequently, it is one of the

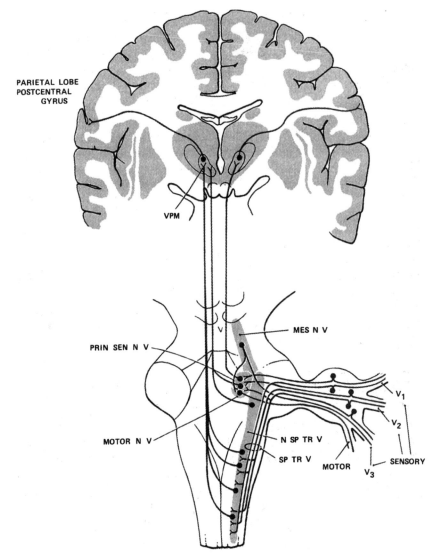

▪ FIGURE 2-9 Trigeminothalamic system. *MES N V:* mesencephalic nucleus of CN V; *N SP TR V:* nucleus of the spinal tract of CN V; *PRIN SEN N V:* principal sensory nucleus of CN V; *SP TR V:* spinal tract of CN V; *V₁:* ophthalmic division of CN V; *V₂:* maxillary division of CN V; *V₃:* mandibular division of CN V; *VPM:* ventral posterior medial nucleus of the thalamus. (Reprinted with permission from Gilman, S, and Newman, SW: Essentials of Clinical Neuroanatomy and Neurophysiology. 9th ed, p. 128. Philadelphia, FA Davis Co., 1996.)

most essential elements in the nurturing and healing environment of the infant and child (p. 37).

All occupational roles can be disrupted by inadequacies in processing tactile input. For example, a difficult time with performance of activities of daily living (ADLs) may be related to inadequate integration of input from tactile receptors responsible for discrimination. Poor student performance may result from difficulty manipulating writing and cutting tools in the classroom. Poor peer inter-

actions may result from inadequate modulation of tactile sensation. The somatosensory system is an incredibly pervasive system from both a receptor and an interactive perspective.

Many aspects of touch associated with tactile defensiveness are hypothetically associated with transmission through the AL pathways and with the central interpretation of the input (Ayres, 1972). Given that the AL pathways project to the regions of the brain responsible for arousal (reticular system), emotional tone (limbic structures), and autonomic regulation (hypothalamus), we postulate that tactile defensive behaviors may be related to the connections among these systems and brain regions. Tactile defensiveness is discussed in more detail in Chapter 4.

Although previous researchers hypothesized that the DCML and the AL were separate and discrete, present understanding delineates considerable functional overlap (Kandell et al., 2000; Melzack & Wall, 1973; Zigmond, et al., 1999). For example, the DCML plays an important role in the localization of pain. Furthermore, clients with lesions in the DCML retain some skill in tactile discrimination. Thus, some aspects of pain are transmitted through the DCML, and some aspects of tactile discrimination must be carried in the AL. Many authors have discussed this redundancy of function in terms of parallel pathways and serial processing. Parallel pathways are advantageous because they add to the depth and flavor of a perceptual experience by allowing the same information to be handled in different ways, and they offer a measure of insurance. If one pathway is damaged, the other can provide residual perceptual capability. Such functional redundancy in the organization of the nervous system may play a role in the efficacy of intervention.

THE VESTIBULAR SYSTEM

We approach the vestibular system in the same manner as the somatosensory system, beginning with receptor structure and function and then examining vestibular projections within the CNS. Subsequently, we discuss proprioception from a functional perspective and briefly look at the interaction between vestibular and proprioceptive sensation as they relate to the control of posture and movement.

Receptors and Transduction

The vestibular apparatus includes the semicircular canals and the otolith organs, the utricle and the saccule (Fig. 2–10). Receptors for the vestibular system are located within these structures in the inner ear, in close proximity to those of the auditory system. In fact, the endolymph that bathes the receptors for the auditory system moves freely between the auditory and vestibular systems.

Vestibular receptors are hair cells located in the otolith organs and in swellings at the base of the three semicircular canals (i.e., anterior, lateral, pos-

terior). The otolith organs are primarily responsible for static functions. The information processed by these receptors is used to detect position of the head and body in space and control of posture. The semicircular canals are the dynamic component of the vestibular system. These structures respond to movement of the head in space.

Vestibular receptors are chalice shaped with hairlike processes extending from their apices. At the base of each cell lies the afferent process of the vestibular nerve. Each cell has a single kinocilium and several stereocilia. Although movement of the kinocilium in one direction leads to depolarization of the hair cell, movement in the opposite direction leads to hyperpolarization. When the cells depolarize, a neurotransmitter (likely aspartate or glutamate, both excitatory) is released into the synaptic cleft. The transmitter interacts with the afferent fiber of the vestibular nerve, sending information about movement to the CNS. We discuss the specifics of depolarization within the semicircular canals and otolith organs below.

In addition to the afferent fibers at the base of each hair cell, there are also efferent fibers that originate in the vestibular nuclei. These efferent fibers provide inhibitory control of the transmission of information from the hair cell and can prevent information from traveling beyond the receptor site.

Utricle and Saccule

The otoliths are saclike organs oriented in horizontal and vertical planes. In the receptor region of the otolith organs, the macula, hair cells synapse with processes from the vestibular ganglion cells. Hair cell processes extend into an overlying substance with gelatinlike qualities, the otolith membrane, in which are embedded otoconia (calcium carbonate crystals). In the upright position, the hair cells in the macula of the utricle are oriented in a horizontal plane, with the otoconia resting on top of them. When the head tilts or moves linearly, there is displacement of the otoconia and the embedded hair cell stereocilia, beginning the process of stimulus detection and transduction. Movement of the stereocilia creates electrical discharges within the hair cell. This electrical energy is changed to chemical energy at the synapse between the macular hair cells and the vestibular ganglion projections. The hair cells in each quadrant of the utricle are systematically oriented in a

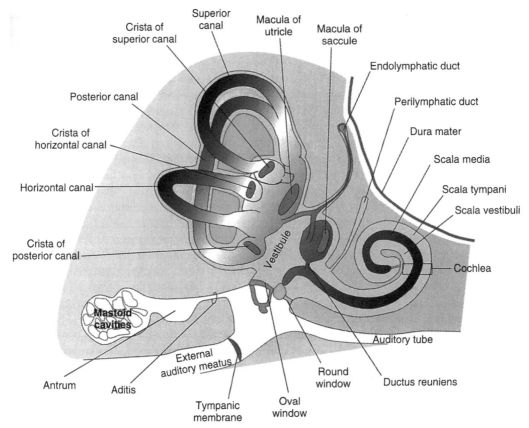

■ Figure 2-10 Vestibular and auditory structures. Simple view of the vestibular and auditory structures as they lie within the body labyrinth. Depicted in this drawing are the receptor regions of the vestibular system, the *cristae* of the semicircular canals, and the *maculae* of the otolith organs. The connectivity between the membranous portions of vestibular and auditory systems can be seen. (Reprinted with permission from Kingsley, RE: Concise Text of Neuroscience, p. 347. Philadelphia, Lippincott Williams & Wilkins, 2000.)

different direction. Thus, systematic variation in the orientation of the utricular hair cells results in the utricle detecting head movement or position (e.g., tilt) in the three orthogonal planes of space. The utricle responds to linear, sustained, and low-frequency stimuli (i.e., stationary head position or slow head movements less than 2 degrees per second) (Fisher & Bundy, 1989; Roberts, 1978; Wilson & Melvill Jones, 1979).

Although the saccule seems to have mechanical properties similar to those described for the utricle, the function of this structure is less well understood. Despite much speculation concerning the possible roles of the saccule (e.g., vertical accelerometer, vibratory receptor), its precise function remains unclear. Kandell et al. (2000) attributed the detection of vertical acceleration to the saccule, noting that gravity is the most "ubiquitous and the most important" (p. 805) of vertical inputs. In addition, these authors associated the detection

of anterior-posterior movement with the saccule. One confirmed function of the saccule, identified in animals, is in acousticoneural transduction; however, the significance of saccular acoustic reception remains unclear (Cazals & Aurousseau, 1987).

Together, the utricle and saccule respond to head tilt in any direction and to linear movement. They constitute slowly adapting receptors and provide tonic input to the CNS pertaining to head position and movement. These structures are critical to the maintenance of upright posture and equilibrium.

Semicircular Canals

The semicircular canals, which are actually closed tubes, detect changes in the direction and rate of angular acceleration or deceleration of the head (Fig. 2–11). Angular acceleration results in rotary head movements–that is, head movements

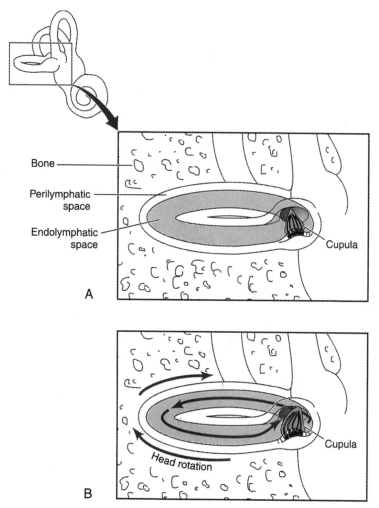

Bone

Perilymphatic space

Endolymphatic space

Cupula

A

Cupula

Head rotation

B

▪ Figure 2-11 Movement of the cupula during head rotation. (A) In the absence of circular movement the *cupula* is positioned upright and mechanical distortion of the embedded hair cells is minimal. (B) With rotary movement the *cupula* is displaced in a direction opposite to that of head movement, bending the hair cells and information about the movement is sent to the CNS. (Reprinted with permission from Kingsley, RE. Concise Text of Neuroscience, p. 354. Philadelphia, Lippincott Williams & Wilkins, 2000.)

that, if continued long enough, would result in the head turning in a circle (e.g., spinning, head nodding). Within each vestibular apparatus, the three semicircular canals are oriented at right angles so that they represent all three planes in space. When the head is tilted forward 30 degrees, the horizontal canal is oriented in the horizontal plane, and the anterior and posterior canals are vertical and oriented at right angles to each other. The semicircular canals have an enlarged ending called the ampulla. Within the ampulla is the receptor apparatus for the semicircular canals, the crista ampullaris, which contains the hair cell receptors.

The receptors are embedded in the cupula, a substance with gelatinlike characteristics similar to the macula. There are no otoconia in the crista ampullaris. Instead, the cupula extends nearly to the top of the ampulla, and its edges are, for the most part, anchored to the epithelium that lines the canal. The canals are filled with endolymph. When the head moves (accelerates), inertia causes the endolymph to lag behind head movement. The result is pressure on the cupula, and its displacement in a direction opposite to that of head movement. Displacement of the cupula leads to bending of the hairs, and this mechanical distortion begins the process of transduction. As head movement continues, the speed of the endolymph catches up with that of the head; the cupula returns to its resting position; and the hair cells are no longer mechanically distorted. With continued movement of the head at a relatively constant velocity, the semicircular canal receptors return to a basal firing rate. When head movement stops or decelerates, the inertia again acts on the endolymph, and it continues to move in the canals, this time in the direction of head movement. Pressure is again placed on the cupula, bending the hairs in the same direction in which the head had been moving. This then changes transmission and activity in the vestibular nerve. Several seconds after the head stops moving, the cupula and hairs return to their normal resting positions.

Afferent fibers carrying information to the vestibular nuclei and efferent fibers from the vestibular nuclei meet the hair cells at their base. Afferent fibers carry information from the receptors to the vestibular ganglion and from there to the vestibular nuclei. Efferent input from the nuclei forms part of an early feedback mechanism within the system. Investigation continues to be warranted on the precise function of these efferent fibers; however, it has been shown that output from these fibers decreases activity in some hair cells and increases it in others.

Canals are paired structures. Movement of the head in one direction leads to movement of the endolymph (and associated distortion of the cupula) in one direction in one ear and in the opposite direction in the other ear. Bending of the hair cells in one direction leads to depolarization; in the other direction, it leads to hyperpolarization. Thus, information sent to the CNS from the two ears is different. Depolarization excites the afferent axon with which the hair cells synapse, increasing activity. Hyperpolarization in the opposite ear leads to a decrease in firing from the hair cells. This is one of the features of this system that allows us to detect direction of movement.

Because the hair cells in each pair of canals are maximally stimulated by head rotation in the same plane, they are able to detect movement of the head in the three orthogonal (right-angle) planes of three-dimensional space. The most efficient stimuli for the semicircular canals are angular, transient (short-term), and fast (high-frequency) head movements of at least 2 degrees per second. When the head moves at slower speeds, the endolymph, cup-

ula, and hair cells all move at the same speed as the head (Fisher & Bundy, 1989; Roberts, 1978; Wilson & Melvill Jones, 1979). Afferent fibers in the vestibular nerve transmit both tonic and phasic information from the receptors, which is critical to function within this system.

Central Projections

There is always some activity within the vestibular nerve, primarily because of tonic activation of otolith organs by gravity (Kandel et al., 2000). Activation of the receptor organs either increases or decreases this baseline activity, depending on the direction of movement. Because the vestibular nerves project both ipsilaterally and contralaterally, the vestibular nuclei can determine direction of movement by comparing the frequency of impulse flow between left and right canals and otolith organs.

The cell bodies for the vestibular nerve are located in Scarpa's ganglion. From these cell bodies, the vestibular nerve carries information to the vestibular nuclei in the brainstem. There are four nuclei on each side: lateral, medial, superior, and inferior. A great deal takes place at this level within the vestibular system. Each nucleus receives direct ipsilateral input as well as contralateral input via fibers crossing from the opposite nuclei. These nuclei receive inputs from the spinal cord, cerebellum, and visual system. The organization of these inputs allows detection of direction and speed of head movement and position of the head relative to gravity.

Vestibular nuclei receive input from other sensory systems, notably the visual system. Visual inputs are relayed through the inferior olive and cerebellum, and the interaction of these inputs is thought to be important in generating eye movements.

From the vestibular nuclei come many fiber pathways that connect the vestibular system extensively within the CNS. Direct connections are found between vestibular nuclei and the cerebellum, oculomotor nuclei, and spinal cord. Projections have also been described to parts of the reticular system, the thalamus (VPL and ventral lateral nuclei), and the cortex (frontal lobe or anterior portion of the parietal lobe). This organization within the vestibular system is an example of heterarchical processing rather than hierarchical; each connection has a unique function.

The vestibular system is the only sensory system with direct connections to the cerebellum. Projections come from the vestibular nerve directly and from vestibular nuclei. In turn, there are direct connections from the cerebellum to the vestibular nuclei. These interconnections are important for ongoing control of eye and head movements as well as posture.

The vestibular nuclei have direct connections with oculomotor nuclei for cranial nerves III (oculomotor), IV (trochlear), and VI (abducens) via the medial longitudinal fasciculus. Fibers are both crossed and uncrossed as they reach these nuclei. These connections serve to fix the eyes as head and body move, providing us with an ongoing stable visual image. The eye movements are termed "compensatory" because they are "equal in direction and opposite in direction to the head movement perceived by the vestibular system" (Haines, 1997, p. 315). When the head is not moving, the eyes remain still. However, with head movement the vestibular-ocular reflex is initiated to enable the visual field to remain stable, even as the head and body move. This constitutes the vestibulo-ocular reflex.

Nystagmus is a specialized compensatory vestibulo-ocular movement. As the head moves in an angular fashion, interactions between the oculomotor nuclei and the vestibular system allow the eyes to remain fixed on an object in space. With continued angular movement of the head, the eyes reach the end of their range of motion. When this occurs, the eyes spring back to a central position, and the process begins again. The initial phase of this process becomes the slow phase of nystagmus. The fast phase occurs when the eyes snap back to a central location. *Nystagmus* is named for the direction of the fast phase, which is the same as the direction of head movement. When nystagmus occurs during head movement, it is termed *per-rotary nystagmus* (i.e., nystagmus that takes place during movement). The nystagmic eye movements are tied to the movement of endolymph in the canals, and they begin with the onset of movement. As movement continues at a steady pace, the endolymph catches up with the movement of the head, the cupula regains an upright position, and input to the CNS returns to baseline. Per-rotary nystagmus declines and eventually stops. When the head stops, endolymph in the canals continues to move in the direction of head turn. This activates the cupula again, in the opposite direction, and triggers the same sequence of events described above but in the opposite direction, this time leading to postrotary nystagmus.

Measurement of postrotary nystagmus is a tool that has been used to examine one aspect of the integrity of the vestibular system. When using this measurement, it is important to have a more complete understanding of the processes underlying nystagmus. These processes were well described by Fisher (1989); we summarize them briefly here. Movement of endolymph in the semicircular canal and displacement of the cupula initiate nystagmus. However, the cupula returns to a resting position and stops activating the vestibular receptors several seconds before nystagmus ceases. This phenomenon is related to *velocity storage,* a mechanism associated with the vestibular nuclei in which velocity information generated by movement is collected and stored, then released slowly, generating nystagmus (Cohen, 1999). Fisher et al. (1986) suggested that this mechanism was impaired in individuals with a vestibular-based dysfunction in sensory integration, resulting in shortened postrotary nystagmus duration. Further investigation is needed to confirm this possibility.

The vestibular nuclei send projections to the spinal cord via lateral and medial vestibulospinal pathways (LVST and MVST, respectively). These pathways are responsible for influences on muscle tone as well as for ongoing postural adjustments. The LVST receives input from semicircular canal pairs, otolith organs, vestibulocerebellum, and spinal cord. Fibers from the LVST terminate directly on alpha and gamma motor neurons in the spinal cord at cervical, lumbar, and sacral levels. Alpha motor neurons supply muscle fibers, and gamma motor neurons project to the muscle spindle; thus, the vestibular system has a strong influence on postural muscles, postural control, and stability. The MVST receives input from the cerebellum and from skin and joint proprioceptors. The fibers in this pathway project to flexor and extensor motor neurons in the cervical region of the cord. This input assists with the maintenance of a consistent position of the head in space. Thus, with descending vestibular projections, we see the interaction of vestibular and proprioceptive inputs.

Responses elicited as a result of utricular or semicircular canal stimulation "act on antigravity extensor muscles so as to elicit compensatory head, trunk, and limb movements, which serve to oppose head perturbations, postural sway, or tilt" (Fisher & Bundy, 1989, p. 240). However, as might be expected, there are differences between the kinds of postural responses ultimately elicited by stimulation to the different receptors. Utricular inputs, conveyed primarily via the LVST to limb and upper-trunk alpha and gamma motoneurons, result in ipsilateral facilitation of extensor muscles and inhibition of flexor muscles. Semicircular canal inputs are conveyed primarily via the medial vestibulospinal pathway to axial alpha and gamma motoneurons and result in bilateral facilitation of neck and upper-trunk muscles. Although utricular inputs elicit more sustained postural responses (i.e., tonic postural extension and support reactions), semicircular canal inputs elicit more phasic equilibrium responses (Fisher & Bundy, 1989; Roberts, 1978; Wilson & Melvill Jones, 1979). More specifically, transient or angular head movements that stimulate the semicircular canals result in phasic (i.e., rapid, transient):

- Stabilization of the head and upper trunk in the upright position
- Extension of the weight-bearing limbs on the side toward which the individual is rotating or tilting (downhill side)
- Flexion of the weight-bearing limbs on the contralateral (uphill) side
- Compensatory abduction and extension of non–weight-bearing limbs

Sustained head tilt or linear head movements that stimulate the utricle result in tonic (maintained):

- Extension of the downhill weight-bearing limbs (support reactions)
- Flexion of the uphill weight-bearing limbs
- Compensatory abduction and extension of the non–weight-bearing limbs
- Stabilization of the head and upper trunk in the upright position (Fisher, 1989; Roberts, 1978; Wilson & Melvill Jones, 1979)

The functional implication is that if the goal is to facilitate tonic postural or support reactions, activities that provide utricular stimulation may be more appropriate. If the goal is to encourage the use of more phasic or transient postural reactions, then activities that provide semicircular canal stimulation may be indicated.

Vestibular connections project bilaterally to the VPL of the thalamus, as well as to the lateral nu-

clear group of the thalamus. The VPL receives somatosensory input and is one anatomical region where interaction of somatosensory and vestibular inputs takes place. Both the VPL and the lateral nuclei project fibers to the cortex, to the base of the precentral gyrus (area 3a) and to the base of intraparietal sulcus (area 2V). Area 2V neurons respond to head movements, and activation of this region leads to sensations of dizziness or movement. Neurons here receive not only vestibular input but also visual and proprioceptive inputs, and this area is likely involved with the perception of motion and spatial orientation. A lesion here leads to confusion in spatial orientation. Area 3a receives vestibular and somatosensory inputs and projects to area 4 of the motor cortex. These connections likely serve to integrate motor control of the head and body.

Vestibular and Proprioception Interactions

Vestibular and proprioceptive processing are hypothesized to jointly contribute to the perception of active movement; the development of body scheme; and the development and use of postural responses, especially those involving extensor muscles (e.g., extensor muscle tone, equilibrium). Matthews (1988) reviewed existing evidence of the contribution of proprioception to body scheme and to our awareness of our relationship to the external environment. He concluded that, under typical circumstances, the role of proprioception was to provide the motor system with a clear and unambiguous map of the external environment and of the body. Goldberg (1985) also suggested that proprioception played a role in programming and planning of bilateral projected action sequences. Nashner (1982) had already proposed that inputs from the vestibular system could be used to resolve vestibular-visual-somatosensory (proprioceptive) conflicts and, as such, the two systems worked together to provide a stable frame of reference against which other sensory inputs were interpreted. Thus, vestibular and proprioceptive inputs, together with vision, provide:

- Subjective awareness and coordination of movement of the head in space
- Postural tone and equilibrium
- Coordination of the eyes, head, and body, and stabilization of the eyes in space during head movements (compensatory eye movements)

THE AUDITORY SYSTEM

Activation of the auditory system is a complex process because sound waves are received by the external ear, transmitted via the middle ear, and finally transduced into action potentials within the inner ear. The structure of the auditory system can be seen in Figure 2–10, adjacent to the vestibular system. Receptors for the auditory system are located in the inner ear, in a membranous structure called the cochlea. The receptors are hair cells, which are components of the organ of Corti. Hair cells are also the receptors in the vestibular system, and the mechanism of transduction from hair cell receptors in the auditory system are similar to that described for the vestibular system.

Receptors and Transduction

Sound begins as sound waves, corralled by the external ear, and transmitted through the external auditory meatus to the tympanic membrane. Attached to the tympanic membrane are the ossicles of the middle ear. The ossicles act to optimize the transfer of sound energy from air to the fluid-filled inner ear, where the organ of Corti lies. Because of this relationship, diseases that impede movement of the ossicles decrease energy transfer and interfere with hearing. This is what happens with inner ear infections (i.e., otitis media).

The transduction of sound into a neurochemical signal begins with movement of the tympanic membrane, which, in turn, creates movement of the ossicles in the middle ear. One of the ossicles fits into the oval window, the opening to the inner ear. Movement of the ossicles creates movement of the fluid in the inner ear (perilymph). This then moves the basilar membrane, upon which sits the organ of Corti, which contains hair cells. Hair cells in the auditory system have projections into the membrane that sits atop them, the tectorial membrane. The basilar membrane changes thickness throughout its length, being thinner at the base than at the apex. This makes it sensitive to different frequencies (i.e., pitches) along its length. As the basilar membrane moves, with different areas moving in response to different sound pitch, the hair cells move, and the projections in the tectorial membrane are bent. This physical movement of these projections initiates transduction in the hair cell. The process from this point parallels that in the vestibular system. Depolarization of the hair cell releases a neurotransmitter (glutamate) that interacts with receptor sites on the afferent component of the auditory nerve, and information is carried to the CNS.

Within the auditory system, the first synapse is very close to the point of transduction. Activation of the hair cells turns physical energy into electrical energy and, almost immediately, chemical energy, as the impulse is transferred to the dendrites of the spiral ganglion, which synapse with the hair cells. Within the organ of Corti are two types of hair cells, those thought to control the sensitivity of the receptor apparatus, the outer cells, and those thought to be primarily responsible for actual hearing, the inner hair cells. A single spiral ganglion cell may innervate as many as 50 outer hair cells. In contrast, the inner hair cells may *receive* dendritic connections from as many as 10 spiral ganglion cells. Thus, whereas outer hair cells converge, inner hair cells diverge at the first synapse in the pathway. The organ of Corti is tonotopically organized; whereas high sounds activate cells on the basilar membrane near its narrow end, low sounds activate cells at the wide end of the membrane. In addition, inner hair cells and the spiral ganglion cells synapsing with them show a "tuning curve," where there is a relationship between the amplitude of sound needed to induce a barely detectable neuronal discharge and the sound frequency. These characteristics of the receptive apparatus account for the accuracy with which sound information is transmitted to the brain.

As in the vestibular system, the auditory nerve has both afferent and efferent components. The afferent components form the cochlear portion of the vestibulo-cochlear nerve (cranial nerve VIII). The efferents come from the superior olivary complex and innervate the outer hair cells directly and the inner hair cells indirectly. When active, the efferent fibers inhibit transmission of information to the CNS and may play a role in the discrimination of specific sounds in the presence of background noise.

Central Connections

The auditory system has two primary pathways to the CNS: the *core pathway,* which maintains tonotopic organization of input and transmits sound frequency with speed and great accuracy, and the *belt pathway,* which is less well organized and transmits information relative to the timing and intensity of input. This latter pathway contributes to bilateral interaction of sound input. Information on both are integrated into the information described below.

Axons from the spiral ganglion cells form the cochlear nerve, which travels from the ear to the brainstem where it synapses with ventral and dorsal cochlear nuclei, ipsilaterally. All fibers have synapses in both nuclei. The tonotopic organization of these connections is maintained at this level. From this point, three routes carry acoustic information onward. From the dorsal cochlear nucleus come fibers that cross to become part of the lateral lemniscus. From the ventral nucleus, one group of fibers follows those of the dorsal nucleus. Another group passes to the ipsilateral and contralateral nuclei of the trapezoid body and the superior olivary nuclei and, from there, joins the lateral lemniscus. Thus, the lateral lemniscus has both ipsilateral and contralateral representation of acoustic information, although contralateral fibers predominate. The superior olive is the first place information from both ears converges. This convergence occurs with accurate representation of the timing of auditory input to the two ears, which is continued onto the cortex. Stimulus localization depends on the accurate rendition of the temporal aspects of sound reception.

Fibers within the lateral lemniscus travel to the inferior colliculus and the medial geniculate body. The inferior colliculus receives essentially all auditory input, both core and belt pathway input, as well as input from the contralateral auditory cortex. As such, it is a major integrating center for the auditory system. Nonetheless, neither the organization nor the function of this structure is well understood. The main nucleus of the inferior colliculus is the central nucleus, where cells are sensitive to both timing and intensity differences in the sound transmissions received. Another site for auditory input in the inferior colliculus is the paracentral nucleus. This structure receives not only auditory input but also inputs from the spinal cord, dorsal column, and superior colliculus. This nucleus is thought to play a role in multisensory integration and auditory attention.

The inferior colliculus sends fibers on to the medial geniculate body, a specialized nucleus within the thalamus. From there, information travels to the transverse temporal gyrus, also called Heschl's gyrus, Brodmann's areas 41 and 42. This region is composed of the primary auditory cortex. It receives core pathway input and is tonotopically organized. The belt area surrounds the area of core pathway input; it is both less organized and less well understood. When information reaches the primary auditory cortex, a sound is heard. This cortical region is critical for the perception of speech.

Brodmann's area 22 corresponds to the secondary auditory cortex, where discriminations for location and direction of sound take place. The planum temporale is a part of this area, and, as noted in Chapter 6, it is an area implicated in dyslexia. Area 22 also receives input from the visual and somatosensory pathways. The specifics of function within this area remain uncertain. According to Kingsley (1999):

> Although it is generally assumed that the secondary auditory cortex on the planum temporale processes one or more specific dimensions of auditory information that are critical for encoding representations of phonemes, syllables and words, there is little experimental evidence to support this localization (p. 355).

The secondary auditory cortex receives input from the paracentral nucleus. As noted, this projection is likely responsible for detecting and directing attention to novel or moving auditory input.

Auditory association cortex encompasses areas 39 and 40 (see Fig. 2–3 to find these regions), the angular gyrus and supramarginal gyrus, respectively. These areas are associated with reading and writing. Damage to area 39 leads to an inability to recognize speech. Projections from the primary auditory cortex are also found in other cortical regions associated with speech. Areas 44 and 45 have been called Broca's area; damage there results in speech that is nonfluent. Speech recognition is not impaired by such damage. The association area of the auditory cortex also receives input from other systems, such as the vestibular and somatosensory systems. Thus, there is multisensory interaction here, and this may play a role in arousal or attention.

Efferent Processes and Feedback Loops

Within the auditory pathways are numerous efferent processes thought to act as feedback loops. Functionally, they may contribute to selective auditory attention. Reticulospinal pathways "sample" activity in the lateral lemniscus and play a role in auditory startle responses. In addition, the inferior colliculus and the auditory cortex project to the superior colliculus, where they are integrated with somatosensory inputs. These pathways are likely responsible for controlling orientation of the head, eyes, and body to sound.

THE VISUAL SYSTEM

Despite the pervasive nature of the tactile system and the importance of the vestibular system, we rely most heavily for day-to-day function on visual input. "It is vision that helps us to navigate in the world to judge the speed and distance of objects; to identify food, members of other species, and familiar or unfamiliar members of our own species" (Zigmond et al., 1999, p. 821). The visual system functions primarily as an edge, contrast, and movement detector. We perceive visual images best when they are still; therefore, our visual abilities depend, in part, on the vestibular-ocular reflex, which contributes to a stabilized visual field. The visual system itself can adjust to movement within the environment with the optokinetic reflex, which works with the vestibulo-ocular reflex to maintain a stable image on the retina. When disparity exists between visual and other sensory inputs (e.g., when we sit in a still car while the car-wash apparatus moves forward and backward over the surface, giving the appearance that the car is moving), we believe the visual system. In this example, we may press on the brake pedal.

Visual processing is complex, with at least three parallel pathways carrying information that must be integrated. We present a greatly simplified examination of structures and mechanisms underlying vision, beginning with a description of receptors, transduction, and visual pathways. We close with a brief consideration of function. Keep in mind that, within the visual system, more than any other sensory system, the whole is much greater than a mere summing of the parts.

Receptors and Transduction

Vision receptors are specialized cells located in the neural retina at the back of the eye. These *photoreceptors,* the rods and cones, transduce light energy into electrical energy that can be transmitted to the CNS. Cones are responsible for day vision and rods for night vision. Cones mediate color vision and provide higher acuity than do rods, which are highly light sensitive and able to amplify light signals to enable vision in dim light. Although cone pathways are not convergent, maintaining a high degree of spatial resolution, rod pathways converge extensively, which further increases the ability to see in dim light by summing light input but decreases the resolution capability of these receptors. In addition, rod cells respond slowly, which adds to their ability to sum dim light, allowing us to see in low light conditions. On the other hand, cones respond rapidly, which allows us to see quick flashes of light.

Cone cells are of three types, each responding to a different spectrum of color: red, green, and blue. Differentiation of other colors depends on differential transmission of information from these three receptors. In contrast, rod cells are achromatic–that is, they respond to all wavelengths of light, but do not allow for discrimination of color. In the center of the retina is an area called the fovea. In this region, light more readily reaches the receptor cells, and acuity is enhanced. There are no rods in the fovea, only a dense concentration of cones.

Transduction of light energy into the electrical signal needed to get information from receptor cells into the CNS is a complicated process. However, a brief look at this process helps us compare activity in this sensory system with that in others. The process of changing light energy into a neural signal begins with the rod and cone cells. These cells maintain tonic activity and transmit information to the CNS in an ongoing manner through neurotransmitter release. With a change in light or the detection of an edge or movement, a change in tonic activity occurs, either increasing or decreasing the amount of neurotransmitter released, and subsequently altering the ongoing signal to the CNS. Because of the complexity of the retina, a great deal of processing occurs in this neural structure before the time when information is transmitted over the optic nerve to the CNS.

Retina

The retina (Fig. 2–12) has 10 layers. The outer layer consists of the pigment epithelium. The neural retina forms the remaining nine layers. Light must travel through the outermost eight layers of the retina before falling on the receptor cells. Light hits the layers in this order: inner limiting membrane, ganglion cell layer, inner plexiform (synapses between ganglion, bipolar, and amacrine cells), inner nuclear layer (bipolar, amacrine, and horizontal cell bodies), outer plex-

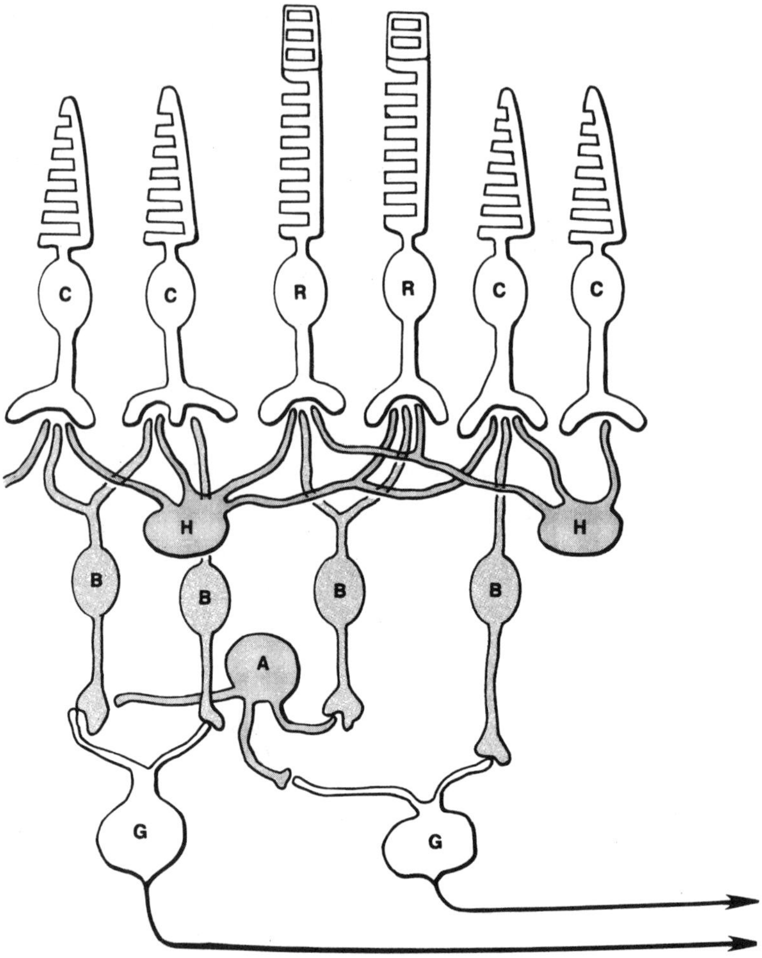

■ Figure 2-12 Simplified diagram of the retina showing five basic retinal cells: A = amacrine; B = bipolar cell; C = cone cell; G = ganglion cell; H = horizontal cell; R = rod cell. The cell bodies of rods and cones form the *outer nuclear layer* and their projections the *receptor layer*. The region where receptor cells are shown synapsing with horizontal and bipolar cells forms the *outer plexiform layer*. The *inner nuclear layer* consists of the cell bodies for bipolar, horizontal, and amacrine cells. Synapses between amacrine, bipolar, and ganglion cells form the *inner plexiform layer* and ganglion cell bodies form the *ganglion cell layer*. Inner and outer limiting membranes are not shown. The processes from the ganglion cells become the optic nerve. (Reprinted with permission from Gilman, S, and Newman, SW: Essentials of Clinical Neuroanatomy and Neurophysiology, 9th ed, p. 182. Philadelphia, FA Davis Co., 1996.)

iform layer (synapses between bipolar, horizontal, and receptor cells), outer nuclear layer (cell bodies for receptor cells), outer limiting membrane, receptor layers (light sensitive receptor cell processes), and pigment epithelium.

Receptor cells synapse onto bipolar cells found in the inner nuclear layer and from there connect with ganglion cells, the axons of which form the optic nerve and project to the lateral geniculate nucleus of the thalamus and the superior colliculus. Intervening in this process are interneurons known as horizontal and amacrine cells, also found in the inner nuclear layer. Although the receptor cells activate bipolar cells, the horizontal and amacrine cells exert an inhibitory influence on receptor, bipolar, and ganglion cells. The inhibition from horizontal cells is an example of lateral inhibition and serves to sharpen the edges of receptive fields, allowing for great accuracy in the information that travels to the CNS. Although bipolar cells work in a different manner, they also serve to sharpen the edges of visual images.

Ganglion cells fall into two categories based on the receptive field associated with the receptor cells. One class of ganglion cell is activated by light directed at the center of its receptor field (on center); another is turned off by light directed at the center of its receptor field (off center). Forming two parallel routes to the CNS, the on-center and off-center information affords the ability to detect contrast in the visual image. We are, therefore, not dependent on the absolute amount of light available in our visual world to detect shape, movement, and color but instead use light and dark contrast for much of this information. The bottom line with this highly complex circuitry is that a great deal of information about contrast, color, form, and

movement in the visual environment is processed before information reaches the CNS.

Central Connections

Gangliar projections form the optic nerve. As can be traced in Figure 2–13, fibers from the nasal region of the retina cross at the optic chiasm and join with fibers from the temporal retina of the opposite eye to form the optic tract, which projects primarily to the lateral geniculate nucleus (LGN) of the thalamus. This is the first of the three processing pathways for visual information that we will discuss. The arrangement of fibers projecting to the LGN allows each hemisphere to

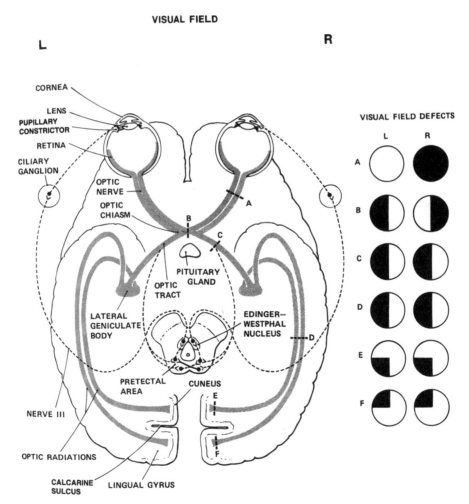

■ FIGURE 2–13 The visual pathways. Lesions to the system (indicated on the right side of the diagram) are reflected in the functional deficits noted in the far right drawing, labeled A–F. (Reprinted with permission from Gilman, S, and Newman, SW: Essentials of Clinical Neuroanatomy and Neurophysiology, 9th ed, p. 183. Philadelphia, FA Davis Co., 1996.)

receive visual information from the contralateral half of the visual world.

A detailed organization of fibers within the optic nerve continues into the optic tract and is then projected into the LGN. As with the tactile system, the representation within the LGN reflects the size of receptor field in the periphery. Thus, the fovea, which has the greatest number of receptor cells and the smallest receptor fields, has the greatest area of representation in the LGN.

Ganglion cells are subdivided into two groups based on both size and function. The magnocellular cells have large receptive fields and respond only briefly to sustained light. These large cells with large receptive fields are thought to be concerned with the general features of objects and object movement. Parvocellular cells are smaller; greater in number; have small receptive fields; and, consequently, convey information about the finer details of vision, with information pertaining to form and color. Magnocellular and parvocellular cells project to different cell layers in the LGN, forming pathways with different functions. The magnocellular pathway contributes to our understanding of *where* an object is in our visual environment; the parvocellular pathway contributes to our understanding of the *what* of an object.

Information from the LGN is projected to the ipsilateral primary visual cortex, or area 17. Here magnocellular and parvocellular pathways maintain their integrity, giving information about the "what" and "where" of visual images. Simple and complex cells are present in the primary visual cortex; these are sensitive to the outline of an object but not its interior. They respond to the specific position of an object as well as its axis or orientation. This is why the visual system is sometimes referred to as a contrast or edge detector.

The organization of the visual cortex is highly complex. Cells there form columns; neurons within a single column respond to a single axis or orientation. The columns are interrupted by what have been called *blob regions* of cells that are sensitive to color rather than axis. A third level of organization within this cortical region is a system of ocular dominance columns. These columns receive input from either the left or right eye, and they alternate at regular intervals, leading to binocular vision.

Visual perception depends on projections beyond area 17. Parvocellular pathway projections run from area 17 to area 19 and then to the inferior temporal region, where form and color are perceived. Projections to the inferior temporal cortex result in interpretations of the "what" of a visual image. This area of the brain is also associated with face and shape recognition.

Perception of motion has its origins in the responsivity of magnocellular ganglion cells in the retina and their projections to the LGN, area 17, area 18, and the middle or superior temporal area. Visual signals, then, project to the visual-motor area of the parietal lobe. This pathway carries information pertaining to the interpretation of speed and direction of object motion and assists in determining where objects are.

The second visual pathway begins with fibers from the optic tract projecting to the superior colliculus (SC). Cells here have large receptive fields and, as such, do not interpret the specifics of the visual world. Instead, these cells respond to horizontal movement within the visual field. Other inputs to the SC come from the visual cortex and the spinotectal pathway, the latter of which carries somatosensory information from both the spinal cord and the medulla. Projections from the SC include those to the thalamus and others to the spinal cord via the tectospinal pathway. Other fibers are sent to the oculomotor nuclei. Thus, the SC plays a role in the visual coordination of posture and the control of eye movements.

The smallest visual pathway is called the *accessory optic tract*. Projections from the optic tract are sent to small (i.e., accessory) nuclei around the oculomotor nucleus, the medial vestibular nucleus, the LGN, and other regions of the thalamus. The efferent processes from these regions project largely to the inferior olive, which sends projections to the vestibular component of the cerebellum. With these connections, the accessory optic tract plays a role in oculomotor adaptation.

Light Reflex

Although not of major concern to the theory of sensory integration, the light reflex is mediated by a pathway that also begins with the rods and cones in the retina. Information forming the foundation for this reflex travels with other light information via the optic nerve, chiasm, and tract but is directed toward the superior colliculus, not the LGN, ending in the pretectal area. From there, fibers are sent to the Edinger-Westphal nucleus, where the motor component of the light reflex begins. Axons travel to the ciliary ganglion and the

Pathway	Organization	Function	Fibers cross . . .	First synapse	Second synapse	Third-order synapse	And beyond . . .
DCML	Precise somatotopic organization throughout Little convergence Few relays	Transmit size, form, texture information Detect movement of touch on skin Convey spatial and temporal aspects of touch	Gracile and cuneate nuclei of medulla	Gracile and cuneate nuclei	VPL of thalamus Reticular formation	Primary and secondary somatic cortex Areas 5 and 7 of parietal lobe	
Anterolateral	Somatotopic, but less specific More convergence	Pain, crude touch, temperature, tickle, neutral warmth	Dorsal horn of the spinal cord	Dorsal horn of the spinal cord	VPL of the thalamus Reticular formation Periaqueductal gray Tectum Hypothalamus	Primary and secondary somatosensory cortex Other thalamic nuclei	
Trigeminothalamic	Somatotopic	Discriminative touch from face and mouth Pain, temperature, nondiscriminative touch	After synapsing in the pons and brainstem	Principal sensory nucleus of the trigeminal nerve Spinal nucleus of the trigeminal nerve	Ventral posterior medial nucleus of the thalamus	Primary somatosensory cortex	
Vestibular		Position and movement of the head in space Maintenance of balance Coordination of the eyes Fixation of the eyes as the body moves through space Detection of speed and direction of movement	After synapsing in the vestibular nuclei in the medulla and pons	Vestibular ganglion	Cerebellum Oculomotor nuclei Alpha and gamma motor neurons VPL of the thalamus	Areas 3 and 2v of the cortex	

(continued)

■ TABLE 2–2. SENSORY SYSTEMS AND PROJECTIONS (*CONTINUED*)

Pathway	Organization	Function	Fibers cross . . .	First synapse	Second synapse	Third-order synapse	And beyond . . .
Auditory	Tonotypic Amplitude tuning curve	Sound detection and localization	Spiral ganglion in ear	Ventral and dorsal cochlear nuclei	Superior olive Trapezoid body	Inferior colliculus Medical geniculate nucleus of thalamus	Auditory cortex Precentral gyrus
Visual	Cones: little convergence, high degree of spatial resolution Rods: significant convergence; high light sensitivity; low resolution Detailed organization of information carried throughout this system	Cones: day vision, color Rods: night vision	At optic chiasm	Bipolar cells in retina	Ganglion cells in retina	Superior colliculus Lateral geniculate nucleus of thalamus	Primary visual cortex

reveal about proprioception? *Psychological Bulletin, 103,* 72–86.

Kalaska, J. F. (1988). The representation of arm movements in postcentral and parietal cortex. *Canadian Journal of Physiology and Pharmacology, 66,* 455–463.

Kandel, E. R., Schwartz, J. H., & Jessell, T. M. (1995). *Essentials of neural science and behavior.* Norwalk, CT: Appleton & Lange.

Kandel, E. R., Schwartz, J. H., & Jessell, T. M. (2000). *Principles of neural science,* (4th ed.)New York: McGraw-Hill.

Kingsley, R. E. (2000). *Concise text of neuroscience.* Philadelphia: Lippincott, Williams & Wilkins.

Knickerbocker, B. M. (1980). *A holistic approach to learning disabilities.* Thorofare, NJ: C.B. Slack.

Lundy-Ekman, L. (1998). *Neuroscience fundamentals for rehabilitation.* Philadelphia: W.B. Saunders Co.

Matthews, P. B. C. (1988). Proprioceptors and their contribution to somatosensory mapping: Complex messages require complex processing. *Canadian Journal of Physiology and Pharmacology, 66,* 430–438.

McCloskey, D. I. (1985). Knowledge about muscular contractions. In E. V. Evarts, S. P. Wise, & B. Bousfield (Eds.), *The motor system in neurobiology* (pp. 149–153). New York: Elsevier.

McCloskey, D. I., Cross, M. J., Honner, R., & Potter, E. K. (1983). Sensory effects of pulling and vibrating exposed tendons in man. *Brain, 106,* 21–37.

Melzack, R., & Wall, P. D. (1973). *The challenge of pain.* New York: Basic Books.

Moberg, E. (1983). The role of cutaneous afferents in position sense, kinaesthesia, and motor function of the hand. *Brain, 106,* 1–19.

Mogliner, A., Grossmann, J. A., Ribary, U., Joliot, M., Volkmann, J., Rapaport, D., Beasley, R. W., Llinas, R. R. (1993). Somatosensory cortical plasticity in adult humans revealed by magnetoence-phalography. *Proceedings of the National Academy of Sciences, USA, 90,* 3593–3597.

Montagu, A. (1978). *Touching: The human significance of the skin.* New York: Harper and Row.

Nashner, L. M. (1982). Adaptation of human movement to altered environments. *Trends in Neuroscience, 5,* 351–361.

Nathan, P. W., Smith, M. C., & Cook, A. W. (1986). Sensory effects in man of lesions of the posterior columns and of some other afferent pathways. *Brain, 109(pt. 5),* 1003–1041.

Peele, T. L. (1977). *The neuroanatomic basis for clinical neurology, (*3rd ed.) New York: McGraw-Hill.

Robb, R. M., Mayer, D. L., & Moore, B. D. (1987). Results of early treatment of unilateral congenital cataracts. *Journal of Pediatric Opthalmology and Strabismus, 24,* 178–181.

Roberts, T. D. M. (1978). *Neurophysiology of postural mechanisms,* (2nd ed.) Boston: Butterworths.

Schmidt, R. A. (1999). *Motor control and learning: A behavioral approach.* Champaign, IL: Human Kinetics Publishers, Inc.

Sherrington, C. S. (1906). *The integrative action of the nervous system.* New Haven: Yale University Press.

Tracey, D. J. (1985). Joint receptors and the control movement. In E. V. Evarts, S. P. Wise, & B. Bousfield (Eds.), *The motor system in neurobiology* (pp. 178–182). New York: Elsevier.

Vierck, C. J., Cohen, R. H., & Cooper, B. Y. (1985). Effects of spinal lesions on temporal resolution of cutaneous sensations. *Somatosensory Research, 3,* 45–46.

Wilson, V. J., & Melvill Jones, G. (1979). *Mammalian vestibular physiology.* New York: Plenum.

Zigmond, M. J., Bloom, F. E., Landic, S. C., Roberts, J. L., & Squire, L. R. (1999). *Fundamental neuroscience.* Boston: Academic Press.

sphincter muscles of the eye. When light is shone in one eye, the eye undergoes pupillary constriction via this pathway. Because of the crossing of fibers, the other eye also constricts.

Visual Experience Counts

Development of skills within the visual system is dependent on experiences, both prenatally and postnatally. Cooperation and competition of axons from the same and opposite eye, respectively, are critical to the postnatal formation of ocular dominance columns, and thus depth perception and binocular vision. Several studies have shown that early deprivation during critical postnatal periods of development results in compromises in visual perception. For instance, when congenital cataracts are present, it is critical to remove them very early. Robb et al. (1987) reported that the critical period to reverse deprivation amblyopia, and achieve adequate acuity, involved removing cataracts before the age of 17 months. Kandel et al. (2000) conclude that cataracts not removed until 10 or more years of age lead to a permanent impairment of form perception, although color perception remains intact. Other incidences and studies of vision deprivation support this finding. Because of its impact on the connections among cortical cells, experience is critical to the development of normal visual perception. We present more detailed information on visual-spatial components of visual perception in Chapter 6.

SUMMARY AND CONCLUSION

The major sensory systems subserving sensory integration theory are complex, and we have only scratched the surface in explaining their structure and function. Each system relies on receptors that respond to one primary form of input and on the transformation of this input into an electrochemical form that can be read by the CNS. Because all input to the CNS eventually takes the form of electrochemical signals, interpretation of specific input depends on the receptors; the specific pathways over which the information is sent; and characteristics of the input, including frequency and intensity of transmission. Integration of inputs takes place in a multitude of CNS locations. In Table 2–2 and the appendix that follows, we

provide key points regarding the stru... tion, and interaction among these syst...

References

Ayres, A. J. (1972). *Sensory integration and disorders*. Los Angeles: Western Psychol Services.

Blackwell, P. L. (2000). The influence of tou... child development: Implications for interv... *Infants and Young Children, 13*(1): 25–39.

Brooks, V. B. (1986). *The neural basis of mot... control*. New York: Oxford University.

Cazals, Y., & Aurousseau, C. (1987). Saccular acoustic responses in the guinea pig involve... rior olive but not inferior colliculus. In M. D. Graham & J. L. Kemnick (Eds.), *The vestibul... system: Neurophysiologic and clinical resear...* (pp. 601–606). New York: Raven.

Cohen, H. (1999). *Neuroscience for rehabilitatio...* (2nd ed.) Baltimore: Lippincott, Williams & Wilkins.

Collier, C. (1985). *Emotional expression*. Hillsdale NJ: Lawrence Erlbaum Associates.

Diamond, M. C., & Hopson, J. (1998). *Magic trees... the mind*. New York: Dutton.

Farber, S. D. (1982). *Neurorehabilitation: A multise... sory approach*. Philadelphia: W. B. Saunders.

Fisher, A. G. (1989). Objective assessment of the quality of response during two equilibrium tests. *Physical and Occupational Therapy in Pediatrics, 9*(3), 57–78.

Fisher, A. G., & Bundy A. C. (1989). Vestibular stimulation in the treatment of postural and related disorders. In O. D. Payton, R. P. DiFabio, S. V. Paris, E. J. Prostas, & A. F. VanSant (Eds.), *Manual of physical therapy techniques* (pp. 239–258). New York: Churchill Livingstone.

Fisher, A. F., & Dunn, W. (1983). Tactile defensiveness: Historical perspectives, new research: A theory grows. *Sensory Integration Special Interest Section Newsletter, 6*(2), 1–2.

Fisher, A. G., Mixon, J., & Herman, R. (1986). The validity of the clinical diagnosis of vestibular dysfunction. *Occupational Therapy Journal of Research, 6*, 3–20.

Gilman, S., & Newman, S. W. (1992). *Essentials of clinical neuroanatomy and neurophysiology*, (9th ed.) Philadelphia: F.A. Davis.

Goldberg, G. (1985). Supplementary motor area structure and function: Review and hypotheses. *Behavioral and Brain Sciences, 8*, 567–616.

Haines, D. E. (1997). *Fundamental neuroscience*. New York: Churchill Livingstone.

Haron, M., & Henderson, A. (1985). Active and passive touch in developmentally dyspraxic and normal boys. *Occupational Therapy Journal of Research, 5*, 102–112.

Heller, M. A., & Schiff, W. (1991). *The psychology of touch*. Hillsdale, NJ: Erlbaum Associates.

Jones, L. A. (1988). Motor illusions: What do they

■■ Appendix 2–1
System Highlights

Somatosensory System

- Receptors are in the skin and around the joints, making this system very pervasive.
- Interpretation of input depends on the combination of receptors activated, receptor density, and receptor field size.
- Two major subdivisions carry information from the body to the CNS: the DCML and the antero-lateral system.
- DCML:
  - Tactile discrimination, vibration, touch-pressure, proprioception, temporal and spatial aspects of a stimulus
  - Main projections: thalamus, S-I, S-II, Areas 5,7
- Proprioception:
  - Information travels within the DCML
  - Perception of joint and body movement, and position of body and body segments in space
  - Main sources: muscle spindles, skin mechanoreceptors, centrally generated motor commands
  - Proprioceptive and vestibular inputs are closely connected functionally, contributing to development of body scheme and postural responses, postural tone and equilibrium, and stabilization of head and eyes during movement
- AL:
  - Pain, temperature, light touch, tickle
  - Includes the following pathways: spinothalamic, spinoreticular, spinomesencephalic, spinohypothalamic
  - Main projections: thalamus, S-I, S-II; reticular formation, periaqueductal gray and midbrain tectum; hypothalamus (as suggested by pathway names)
- Trigeminothalamic pathway:
  - Carries all forms of somatosensory information from the face to the CNS
  - Main projections: thalamus, S-I
- Somatosensation has a pervasive influence on occupational performance because of the wide distribution of receptors and widespread projections within the CNS.
- There is considerable overlap among projections of two major subdivisions with many potential points of interaction.

Vestibular System

- Receptors are hair cells in two structures within inner ear:
  - Otolith organs: respond to linear movement and gravity, head tilt in any direction
  - Semicircular canals: respond to angular movement of the head; respond best to transient, quick movements
- Activity of receptors provides tonic input to the CNS about movement and position of head in space
- Project to vestibular nuclei in the brainstem, and from there to:
  - Cerebellum: reciprocal connections for ongoing control of eye and head movements and posture
  - Oculomotor nuclei: serving to fix the eyes as head and body move
    - Source of vestibular-ocular reflex and nystagmus
  - Spinal cord: influences on muscle tone and ongoing postural adjustments
  - Thalamus and cortex: integration with somatosensory inputs; play a role in perception of motion

and spatial orientation
■ Connections with cerebellum are reciprocal

Visual System

■ Receptors are rods and cones, responding to night and day vision, respectively.
■ Rods are slow responding receptors, with the capacity to sum dim light.
■ Cones rapidly respond to changes in light and provide color vision.
■ Retina is a complex multilayer structure, and a great deal of processing goes on here before it is transmitted to the CNS.
■ Three pathways to the CNS:
  • Lateral geniculate pathway
    > Has parvocellular (P) and magnocellular (M) divisions processing information related to the *what* and *where* of an object, respectively
    > Projects to visual cortex (areas 17 and 19) and on to inferior and superior temporal cortex for additional processing and recognition of faces, shape, and motion
  • Superior colliculus pathway
    > Responses to horizontal movement in visual field
    > Integration with somatosensory input from thalamus
    > Projects to thalamus, spinal cord, and oculomotor nuclei to play a role in coordination of posture and eye movements
  • Accessory optic tract pathway
    > Optic tract projections to accessory nuclei around the oculomotor nucleus, medial vestibular nucleus, and thalamus
    > Projects to inferior olive and on to cerebellum
    > Plays a role in oculomotor adaptation

Auditory System

■ Hair cell receptors function similar to those in the vestibular system.
■ Sound energy must be changed to vibration and to fluid movement energy to activate receptors.
■ Two major auditory pathways:
  • Core pathway
    > Fastest and most direct
    > Maintains precise organization throughout course
    > Transmits sound frequency
  • Belt pathway:
    > Less well organized
    > Surrounds core pathway
    > Transmits information relative to timing and intensity of sound input
    > Important in bilateral interaction of sound
■ Main auditory projections of both core and belt pathways from Cochlear nuclei:
  • Most direct route: axons form the lateral lemniscus project to inferior colliculus
  • Ipsilateral and contralateral projections to the superior olivary complex and onto the inferior colliculus
  • Fibers forming the trapezoid body project to the superior olivary complex
■ From the inferior colliculus, most fibers project to the medial geniculate nucleus (MGN) of the thalamus and from there to the auditory cortex, areas 41 and 42, and auditory association cortex, area 22.
■ Other MGN projections go to the limbic system and temporal and parietal lobes; thought to play a role in arousal and attention.
■ Auditory inputs are integrated with somatosensory inputs in the superior colliculus to play a role in controlling orientation of head, eyes, and body to sound.

3

Disorders of Praxis

Gretchen Dahl Reeves, PhD, OT/L, FAOTA
Sharon A. Cermak, EdD, OTR, FAOTA

> *[The] etiology of developmental dyspraxia clearly is not understood, perhaps because there is little agreement as to what it is and how it can be assessed.*
> —Sugden & Keogh, 1990, p. 133

Praxis means "action based on will" and comes from the Greek word for "doing, acting, deed, practice" (Safire, 1989, p. F18). Although praxis may be observed when individuals interact with the physical environment, it entails more than the observed physical act. Praxis pertains primarily to the *planning* of a motor act; it is a process that requires knowledge of actions and of objects, motivation, and intention on the part of the person.

Researchers' interest in praxis arose from investigations with adults who had sustained traumatic brain injury, primarily to the left frontal or parietal lobes, resulting in the inability to perform voluntary or goal-directed actions (Fredericks & Saladin, 1996). This disorder, known as *apraxia,* interfered with the ability to perform learned actions and impeded the ability to learn new movements or use gesture for communication, in the absence of paralysis, sensory loss, or disturbance of muscle tone.

In contrast with apraxia, the term *dyspraxia* is used to describe motor planning deficits that are developmental rather than acquired. Because we observe clients' difficulties with motor actions, we might assume that dyspraxia is a problem of motor execution. Ayres (1985), however, suggested that dyspraxia was primarily a problem of *organizing the plan* necessary for purposeful behavior. Ayres (1972a, 1979, 1985) believed that the ability to process and integrate sensation formed the basis for the development of body scheme, sometimes referred to as body percept. This, in turn, provided a foundation for the conceptualizations needed for motor planning. Thus, occupational therapists who view praxis from a sensory integrative perspective are concerned with individuals' sensory processing and conceptual abilities (Ayres, 1985; Ayres et al., 1987).

Praxis and dyspraxia are complex concepts, and the terminology associated with them can be confusing. In this chapter:

- *Dyspraxia* is a generic term that refers to developmentally based practic disorders with a variety of etiologies.
- *Sensory integrative–based dyspraxia* refers to practic disorders that have their bases in poor sensory processing.
- *Somatodyspraxia* is a type of sensory integrative–based dyspraxia in which there is

evidence of poor processing of *at least* somatosensory information.

- *Bilateral integration and sequencing (BIS)* disorder is a type of sensory integrative–based dyspraxia in which there is evidence of deficits in vestibular and proprioceptive processing.

The names *somatodyspraxia* and *BIS* are not parallel, but we hypothesize that they reflect a spectrum of practic deficits, as depicted in Figure 1–4. We recognize the difficulty with using these two terms because often they do not fully and accurately reflect the sensory basis of the problem. Adding to confusion, the term *dyspraxia* is sometimes applied to children with developmental coordination disorder and deficits in attention, motor control, and perception (DAMP), suggesting that they may share common characteristics. Nonetheless, until more accurate terms are coined, we will continue to use these terms as defined.

PURPOSE AND SCOPE

In this chapter, we describe sensory integrative–based practic dysfunction manifested, in part, as difficulties in planning and organizing movement. Specifically, we describe the characteristics and relationship of two levels of practic dysfunction: BIS deficits and somatodyspraxia. Sensory integrative–based disorders of praxis generally are determined through the administration of the Sensory Integration and Praxis Tests (SIPT; Ayres, 1989), and this chapter discusses their use. This chapter also presents other diagnoses that commonly include symptoms of dyspraxia. Furthermore, because of its pervasive effect, not only on movement but also on self-esteem and well being, we describe the impact of dyspraxia on development and performance. We discuss sensory integration theory as it pertains to intervention. We describe neuroanatomical mechanisms purported to underlie praxis. Finally, we discuss related literature that may be germane to sensory integrative–based dyspraxia, including contemporary theories of motor behavior.

To illustrate the characteristics of practic disorders, we present the cases of two children, Keisha and David. We use these cases to illustrate important concepts. Although Keisha's and David's difficulties are manifested in different ways, similarities are apparent.

CASE STUDIES

■ KEISHA: A CHILD WITH SOMATODYSPRAXIA

REASON FOR REFERRAL

Keisha was a 6-year, 10-month-old girl in her sixth month of first grade. Keisha's parents requested an occupational therapy evaluation to investigate possible problems in sensory integration and to clarify the difficulties she was having in school with pasting, coloring, cutting with scissors, and printing.

The occupational therapist that evaluated Keisha interviewed Keisha's mother and teacher and observed Keisha in class. She also observed her during a variety of nonstandardized clinical observations of neuromotor performance and administered the SIPT (Ayres, 1989). (See Chapter 7 for a description of the SIPT.)

PARENT INTERVIEW

Keisha was the product of a full-term pregnancy and normal delivery. She weighed 6 lb, 8 oz and did not experience neonatal difficulties. She achieved developmental milestones at expected ages: she sat at age 6 months, crawled at age 8 months, and walked at age 14 months. Her speech also developed normally. Keisha was able to say single words at age 12 months and spoke in sentences at age 18 months, although she had mild articulation problems. Because articulation problems are not uncommon, Keisha's mother was not concerned. When the teacher contacted her about some school difficulties, Keisha's mother was surprised because she always believed Keisha was bright and would do well in school.

Although Keisha could print her name, she was not able to copy simple words, even when the letters were the same as those in her own name. Keisha pressed the pencil so hard on the paper that the point often broke. Although she played with other children in the neighborhood, many of her friends were younger than her. Keisha usually directed the play with her friends toward quiet indoor toys such as puppets, dolls, and toy dishes. When her friends did not want to play her games, Keisha played alone. Her preferred activity was watching television. When her parents bought her toys that required fine motor actions, she created fantasy games instead of using them in more typical ways. Keisha had a vivid imagination and loved to tell stories. She appeared to be highly creative and could explain how things worked in great detail, although she often could not demonstrate the actions she described.

Recalling other features of Keisha's motor development, her mother said that Keisha was not able to pedal a tricycle until she was 5 years old. She was not yet walking down stairs reciprocally, and she only recently had learned to pump a swing. Even though she struggled with new motor tasks, she tried hard to do well. She wanted to be able to keep up with the other children and play the same games they played.

CLASSROOM OBSERVATION

When the occupational therapist observed Keisha in the classroom, many of the problems the teacher had described were apparent and new ones emerged. Compared with the other children, Keisha clearly had difficulty with writing, coloring, and cutting with scissors. When given a four- or five-piece puzzle, Keisha was able to determine the correct location for the pieces but was unable to rotate them into place. In preparing to go outside, Keisha put her coat on upside down. She could not manage the zipper on her coat or fasten the button on her pants. During recess, Keisha spent the entire time alone on a swing. At snack time, she needed assistance to open her milk carton and crackers.

When talking with the teacher, the occupational therapist learned that Keisha had excellent verbal skills and memory, which fit with information provided by her mother and other observations made by the therapist. The teacher also mentioned that Keisha was working on articulation with the speech therapist.

■ DAVID: A CHILD WITH BILATERAL INTEGRATION AND SEQUENCING DEFICITS

REASON FOR REFERRAL

David was a 7 ½-year-old boy attending the second grade at a local public school. He was reported to be very active and loved to move and climb. He was sometimes aggressive with other children and often demanded that games be played in the manner that he designated. Although he was quite bright and most of his work was at grade level, he had to try very hard to keep up with his classmates. His handwriting was difficult to read and, in frustration, he often scribbled carelessly on his papers. David generally preferred his right hand for writing but often used other tools, such as a fork, with his left hand.

PARENT INTERVIEW

David's mother experienced a great deal of nausea during her pregnancy. David was delivered by Cesarean section because he was in a breech position. No postnatal complications were apparent. His mother described him as a happy but active baby who had poor sleep habits. He acquired milestone motor skills at appropriate times and began using language before age 1 year. As a preschooler, David had several ear infections but was otherwise healthy. No particular sensitivities to auditory or tactile stimuli were reported, but David was easily distracted. He was learning to ride his two-wheeled bicycle and tie his shoes. David liked to play soccer, but his mother noted that he frequently tripped on the playing field and could not time his kicking actions appropriately. Often he was observed randomly jumping and running during games. He was initially enthusiastic when trying new tasks, but he quickly lost interest when things did not go well. His mother described David as a "thrill seeker" and noted that he was generally happy. He was seldom daunted by his poor coordination.

CLASSROOM OBSERVATION

David's teacher requested an occupational therapy evaluation primarily to assess David's handwriting difficulties. The therapist was also interested in observing David's behavior. David sat near the front of the classroom and did a great deal of fidgeting and wiggling. He often looked around at classmates and dropped things on the floor. He used all five fingers of his right hand to hold the pencil, stabilizing it against his little finger. David used scissors awkwardly with his left hand and struggled to hold the paper in his right. Associated movements were noted in his right hand that mirrored the actions of his left hand. At times, he transferred the scissors to his right hand. He resorted to tearing the paper when he could not maneuver the scissors well.

Many of the presenting concerns identified in Keisha and David are common in children with sensory integrative–based dyspraxia. Descriptions of children with similar difficulties are reported from many locations around the world (Cermak & Larkin, 2002), suggesting that the phenomena are not restricted by geographic location. However, terminology and diagnoses vary according to the perspective of the researcher, diagnostician, or author reporting the problems.

RELATED DIAGNOSES AND TERMINOLOGY

The term *dyspraxia* is often, but not exclusively, used to describe a sensory integrative–based disorder—that is, not all clients who have dyspraxia have sensory integrative dysfunction. In fact, Ayres (1989) described some children as having dyspraxia even though their difficulties were not based on poor processing of sensation. To further complicate matters, a child diagnosed with sensory integrative–based dyspraxia by an occupational therapist may be diagnosed differently by another professional.

Related diagnoses include clumsiness (Gubbay, 1975), developmental coordination disorder (DCD)

(APA, 1994), and DAMP (Gillberg, 1983; Gillberg et al., 1993; Hellgren et al., 1994). Because these diagnostic terms are included in a number of studies, they are pertinent to the discussion of children with sensory integrative–based dyspraxia. However, although similarities among these conditions exist, we cannot assume they are the same.

Gubbay (1975, 1978) described the problems of "clumsy children" and children with "developmental apraxia," likening them to those of adults with acquired apraxia. He stressed impaired voluntary movements not related to primary sensory, motor, or cognitive deficits. Gubbay believed that clumsy children had difficulty performing skilled, purposeful movements but had no cognitive or physical impairments to explain their difficulties. When he examined their birth histories, Gubbay (1978, 1985) noted that 50 percent had pre-, peri-, or neonatal complications. He reported a 2:1 ratio of boys to girls and a higher percentage of first-born children. He also noted delayed motor development, atypical speech, and late development of bladder control (Gubbay, 1978).

Developmental coordination disorder (DCD) is described in the *Diagnostic and Statistical Manual of Mental Disorders* (*DSM-IV;* APA, 1994). In the *DSM-IV,* under the heading of Motor Skills Disorder, DCD (315.4) is identified as impaired development of motor coordination not due to other medical diagnoses. A diagnosis of DCD is made only if poor coordination interferes with academic performance or activities of daily living. Polatajko et al. (1995) and Wright (1997) indicated that more than 5 percent of the pediatric population had DCD.

The *International Classification of Diseases and Related Health Problems* (*ICD-10;* WHO, 1993) includes a "specific developmental disorder of motor function" in which clumsiness is the key feature with additional difficulties noted in visual-spatial cognitive tasks. The ICD-10 will replace the current diagnostic coding system by October 2003. In the United States, health-care practitioners currently use the *ICD-9-Clincal Modification* (ICD-9-CM, 2001) to determine diagnoses for billing and record keeping. The chapter on Mental Disorders lists "Specific Delays in Development"(315) not caused by a known neurological disorder, with a subheading of "Coordination Disorder" (315.4). The main feature is a serious impairment in motor coordination development that is not explained by intellectual delays (ICD-9-CM, 2001, p. 153). Fur-

thermore, clumsiness is often associated with perceptual difficulties. Subheadings within this diagnostic category include "clumsy child syndrome," "dyspraxia syndrome," and "specific motor developmental disorder."

Although we cannot assume that sensory integrative–based dyspraxia and DCD or any of the seemingly related diagnoses refer to the same condition, Piek and Coleman-Carman (1995) found that children with DCD performed significantly poorer on a kinesthetic perception and movement test than matched control subjects. Evidence such as this suggests that these two conditions may overlap or at least be similar in some important ways. Although discussion of terminology may be considered heuristic, Koomar (1999) found that occupational therapists were reimbursed for services provided to children when they used the code for DCD (315.4) more often than for other codes, including motor apraxia (784.69). They also tended to use the code for DCD more frequently than other codes.

As with sensory integrative–based dyspraxia, descriptions of DCD have been criticized. Sugden and Wright (1998) suggested that both the *DSM-IV* and the *ICD-10* descriptions were inadequate because they implied that DCD is only a problem of gross and fine motor performance and did not account for poor spatial and temporal awareness, sensory processing, or motor planning. Wright (1997) stated that although DCD presents as a physical disorder, its secondary consequences, including a problem with attention, distractibility, and fear of failure, present greater concerns. As Henderson and Barnett (1998) indicated, a consensus on terminology has not been attained, even if the terms used in manuals such as *DSM-IV* and *ICD-10* reflect some of the existing literature.

In Scandinavia, some children with motor coordination difficulties are identified as having DAMP (Gillberg, 1983). Deficits are identified in five areas: attention, fine motor skills, gross motor skills, speech and language, and perception. In addition to the difficulties in motor performance, children with DAMP also have behavior and school achievement problems. Langden et al. (1996) examined the extent to which DAMP and attention deficit hyperactivity disorder (ADHD) overlapped in 589 6-year-old children. They found that up to 75 percent of children with DAMP could also be diagnosed with ADHD. Children with DAMP had more deficits in perception and motor function, but impulsivity represented the most powerful indicator of children with ADHD alone. Because children who are impulsive and distractible may often fall or bump into objects and appear clumsy because they are not paying attention to what they are doing, they may not have motor planning problems. Thus, it is important to sort out the attention component when conducting an evaluation.

DEVELOPMENT AND PERFORMANCE OF CHILDREN WITH PRAXIS DIFFICULTIES

Early Childhood

Children with sensory integrative–based dyspraxia often achieve motor milestones within usual timelines, albeit at the later end of the range. Thus, in its milder forms, dyspraxia may not be detected during the first 3 years of life. Although children with dyspraxia bump into things and need more help than their peers, parents may dismiss these difficulties as "individual variations." However, when the parents of children subsequently identified with dyspraxia look back on their children's early development, they often report that "something was wrong all along."

During the preschool years, problems may become more numerous, but they may continue to go unrecognized. Children often have difficulty with self-care (e.g., fastening buttons, blowing the nose). They may also struggle with toys and play activities (e.g., puzzles, cutting and pasting, coloring, and playground equipment). Keisha had some of these difficulties. Because many preschool programs provide children with choices, children with dyspraxia may avoid difficult activities. Teachers as well as parents may interpret this avoidance as individual preference rather than a sign of difficulty.

School Years

Because previously unrecognized problems become evident, elementary school often marks a turning point for children with dyspraxia. Furthermore, problems that had been identified become even more obvious as the requirements of daily events at home and school increase. Tasks must be completed within specified time limits, and expectations for neatness and organization

are greater. Children may be required to participate in activities they previously avoided. Difficulties in dressing often continue, turning morning routines into battles. The time required for dressing and other self-care activities may be lengthy so that children must receive help, be late for school, or arise very early. The parents are frustrated by the child's inconsistency in performance and may attribute problems to carelessness or laziness (Morris, 1997).

In school, many children experience difficulty with handwriting and art projects that involve cutting, coloring, pasting, and assembling. Play skills such as bike riding, skipping rope, and ball activities may be performed with difficulty. Finally, organized sports and physical education become increasingly important, and children with dyspraxia often experience difficulty in these areas (Szklut et al., 1995). Children with dyspraxia often are described by parents and teachers as uncoordinated. They drop things, bump into objects, and trip and fall (Morris, 1997).

By the third and fourth grades, a dramatic increase in the demand for written output occurs (Levine, 1987). Levine used the term "developmental output failure" to describe the problem of children who could not produce sufficient academic work to meet expectations. Output failure may be caused by poor visual-motor coordination, form and space perception, motor planning or motor memory, fine motor skill, organization or sequencing, or somatosensory processing. Failure to keep up with the amount of work required may result in a decline in grades, motivation, and self-esteem (Levine, 1984, 1987). Problems in these areas are major reasons why school-aged children are referred for occupational therapy (Reisman, 1991).

McHale and Cermak (1992) determined from observations in second, fourth, and sixth grade classrooms, that 30 to 60 percent of the school day was devoted to fine motor tasks. Writing was the predominant fine motor task, used for copying text, taking notes, drawing, writing from dictation, creative writing, and completing work sheets and workbooks. Handwriting problems may be characterized by illegibility that results from disorganized or nonuniform letters, improper spacing, inappropriate slant, or poor stroke quality (Cermak, 1991). As pressure mounts for handwriting to be introduced to children at younger ages, it is likely that difficulties will be identified earlier and more frequently.

Several tests are available for measuring specific aspects of handwriting (Amundson, 1995; Phelps et al., 1984; Reisman, 1999). Information from the SIPT can assist therapists in determining if handwriting difficulties are related to somatosensory processing, form and space perception, or visual-motor coordination. Inadequate somatosensory perception may be manifested as difficulty knowing the boundaries of the fingers or position of the joints. Children with poor somatosensory processing may rely heavily on vision to monitor what their hands are doing (Cermak, 1991).

Deficits in motor planning or motor memory may impede automaticity in writing and prevent the retrieval of neuronal models of letters. As a result, children may make the same letter several different ways (Cermak, 1991). Spontaneous writing depends on memories of letters and words that accumulate with practice. Copying, on the other hand, involves an immediate source of guidance and feedback because a representation of the letters or words is readily available. Although children with BIS deficits may have more difficulty with spontaneous writing, children with somatodyspraxia may struggle with both aspects (Cermak, 1991). Both Keisha and David struggled with the demands of handwriting.

Low muscle tone, inadequate muscle strength, poor postural control, and poor joint stability may also add to problems in handwriting. Kimball (2002) referred to these as functional support capabilities. David's need for a very stable grasp (i.e., all five fingers on the pencil) may fall into this group of problems, relating to his need to compensate for poor postural control. Fatigue, laborious writing, reduced speed, and poor pencil grasp are possible sequelae to these factors.

Adolescence and Adulthood

Studies focusing on sensory integrative–based dyspraxia in adolescents have not been carried out. As such, for information pertinent to this age group, we must look to the literature on DCD, DAMP, and related motor coordination deficits. Here we find that parents are often told that children with coordination difficulties will outgrow them; however, several studies indicate that this may not be the case. For instance, in a 10-year follow-up study of children identified at ages 5 to 7 years as clumsy, Losse et al. (1991) found evidence of poorer motor skills, lower academic achievement, lower IQ scores, and more behavior problems than in a matched sample without evidence of poor coordination. Examining children identified as having DCD at age 5 years, Cantell et al. (1994) identified motor skill deficits persisting into adolescence and found this group to be unlikely to be physically fit or to participate in motor events. Furthermore, in another follow-up study, 16-year-old clients diagnosed with DAMP as children had more speech and language disorders, longer reaction times, greater clumsiness, and higher rates of accidents resulting in bone fractures than adolescents who had no evidence of DAMP (Hellgren et al., 1993). Unfortunately, Losse et al. (1991) had also found that gains made from intervention were not maintained after the intervention was discontinued. These final findings may suggest the need to target intervention on more than motor skills.

In adulthood, dyspraxia may limit career and avocational choices. Knuckey and Gubbay (1983) found that adults who had been identified as very clumsy as children had jobs requiring less manual dexterity than control subjects. Dysfunction in both academic and motor realms is likely to influence future roles and feelings of competence, impeding the ability to explore various available options.

Behavioral and Emotional Characteristics

Individuals with dyspraxia lack skills to interact effectively and efficiently with people and objects, which may lead, in turn, to decreased belief in skill and sense of control. Clients who feel little control or who believe themselves incapable likely feel less self-confident and satisfied with their lives. They may have little drive to perform meaningful occupations (Kielhofner, 1995). For example, children with dyspraxia may be teased by peers and excluded from sports and games, resulting in low self-esteem and increased isolation. Shaw et al. (1982) found that children with learning disabilities and poor motor coordination had more problems with self-esteem than did children with learning disabilities and no motor problems. They named this phenomenon "developmental double jeopardy."

Many children with dyspraxia are aware of the things they cannot do and avoid difficult situations. Even at a young age, children with coordination disorders are more introverted and engage with fewer other children than do their peers (Shoemaker & Kalverboer, 1994). In a longitudinal study, Smyth and Anderson (2000) found that children with DCD spent more time alone or watching others on the playground than children in a control group. In addition, they were less involved in large group play and team games.

Intellectual and Cognitive Factors

Tests of Intelligence

The relationship of intelligence to dyspraxia has been the source of considerable disagreement. Can we consider individuals with cognitive impairments to have dyspraxia? According to Gubbay (1975, 1985), children with dyspraxia have normal intelligence, and this criterion is specified in *ICD-10* (WHO, 1993). Dawdy (1981), however, believed that it was unrealistic to assume normal or near-normal intelligence as a diagnostic criterion. *DSM IV* (American Psychiatric Association, 1994) criteria do not specify that IQ must be normal but state that a diagnosis of DCD should be made only when a child's motor skills are significantly lower than his or her cognitive skills.

We believe individuals with cognitive impairments typically are delayed in all areas, including language and motor planning. When a client's language delays are consistent with delays in other areas, we would not diagnose him or her with aphasia. Similarly, when delays in motor planning are consistent with cognitive and motor development, we would not diagnose the client with dyspraxia. Furthermore, care must be taken to differentiate delays in motor skill development or execution from poor motor planning. *We consider clients with cognitive impairments to have dyspraxia only when their motor deficits are caused by poor motor planning, not simply poor execution, and their motor planning is significantly poorer than their performance in other areas of cognition.*

Gubbay (1975) stated that the single most important diagnostic criterion for dyspraxia was a significantly lower (>1 standard deviation [SD]) performance than verbal IQ score. This pattern characterizes some, but not all, children with dyspraxia (Henderson & Barnett, 1998). For example, poor visual-spatial ability may contribute to lower scores on performance tasks (Henderson & Barnett, 1998). Furthermore, children with both language impairments and dyspraxia may manifest lower verbal than performance IQ scores. Such a scoring pattern is seen in adults with apraxia who typically have left hemisphere damage (Heilman & Rothi, 1993).

Higher Level Processes and Praxis

"As movement assumes meaning, the child learns to motor plan or how to *cortically* direct his movements" (Ayres, 1972a, p. 170, italics added). Although Ayres (1972a, 1979) emphasized the roles of sensory processing and body scheme in motor planning, she also stressed the importance of cortical and diencephalic processing and indicated that the brain required a variety of information to plan actions. First, the brain must have the idea of the intended act—that is, it must be able to conceptualize the goal. Then it must know how the body is designed and how it functions mechanically. That information comes, in part, from the tactile, proprioceptive, and vestibular systems. Furthermore, Ayres (1989) suggested that visual perception and praxis were closely aligned and stated: "A conceptual system common to praxis also appears to serve visual perception" (p. 199).

Thus, Ayres (1989) described two components of praxis: ideation (knowing what to do) and planning of the actions or motor planning. Ideation is a function of cognitive processes; it contributes to our ability to be creative and playful as we interact with the environment (see Chapter 11). We think of ideation as a contributor to imagination and note that difficulties with ideation may be present in some children who struggle to create play scenarios.

Keisha used her imagination to tell stories but struggled with conceptualizing creative ways to act on objects. Her high intelligence may have supported her story making and language abilities, but she could not engage in dynamic physical interactions using her body. She was intelligent enough to know that she did not perform as well as her peers and compensated by seeking younger companions and sedentary play.

DYSFUNCTION IN SENSORY INTEGRATION AND DISORDERS OF PRAXIS

Keisha and David Revisited: Sensory Integration and Praxis Tests and Clinical Observations

Because Keisha's and David's daily life concerns potentially reflected a sensory integrative basis, both children were given the SIPT and clinical observations of neuromotor performance. We present the results of their testing in five categories:

1. Tactile discrimination
2. Vestibular and proprioception processing
3. Praxis
4. Form and space, visual-motor, and construction
5. Sensory modulation

Keisha

Keisha was cooperative with the evaluator throughout the administration of the SIPT. Even on items that were difficult for her, she attempted to do a good job. She especially liked the tests that involved building with blocks and finding hidden pictures.

TACTILE DISCRIMINATION

Keisha's scores were significantly low (<-1.0 SD) on three of four tactile tests. She had difficulty identifying the finger the examiner touched (Finger Identification), replicating designs drawn of the back of her hand (Graphesthesia), and recognizing shapes of objects through manipulation (Manual Form Perception). Only her ability to locate the precise place on her arm where she was touched (Localization of Tactile Stimuli) was in the average range. Keisha's SIPT scores are shown in Table 3–1.

VESTIBULAR AND PROPRIOCEPTIVE PROCESSING

Clinical observation revealed that Keisha had low muscle tone and poor proximal joint stability. Her equilibrium responses were slightly delayed; she tended to hold on to the examiner rather than use equilibrium to maintain balance. Keisha was unable to assume prone extension or maintain head control while in supine flexion. On the SIPT, Keisha's ability to remember the direction and extent of passive arm movements (Kinesthesia) was in the low-average range, but the duration of her postrotary nystagmus was within the average range. In contrast, her static and dynamic balance abilities (Standing and Walking Balance) were below average.

PRAXIS

One of Keisha's lowest scores on the entire SIPT was on Postural Praxis, a test of the ability to reproduce unusual postures assumed by the examiner and an important indicator of dyspraxia. Her ability to copy sequenced arm and finger movements (Sequencing Praxis) was also low. On Bilateral Motor Coordination, a test of smooth, coordinated movements of the arms and legs, Keisha scored below average. Her ability to replicate positions and movements of her tongue, lips, and jaw (Oral Praxis) was also below average. Keisha was able to

■ TABLE 3–1 KEISHA'S SIPT RESULTS

Category	Test	Standard Score
Tactile	Manual Form Perception (MFP)	−1.3
	Localization of Tactile Stimuli (LTS)	0.7
	Finger Identification (FI)	−1.9
	Graphesthesia (GRA)	−1.8
Vestibular and Proprioceptive Processing	Kinesthesia (KIN)	−0.8
	Standing and Walking Balance (SWB)	−2.1
	Postrotary Nystagmus (PRN)	−0.2
Praxis	Postural Praxis (PPr)	−2.3
	Oral Praxis (OPr)	−1.4
	Sequencing Praxis (SPr)	−1.4
	Bilateral Motor Coordination (BMC)	−1.3
	Praxis on Verbal Command (PrVC)	0.1
Form and Space, Visual-motor, Construction	Design Copying (DC)	−1.9
	Motor Accuracy (MAC)	−1.8
	Constructional Praxis (CPr)	0.6
	Space Visualization (SV)	1.2
	Figure-Ground Perception	0.9

carry out movements on verbal command. She achieved an average score on Praxis on Verbal Command, which often is the case for children with somatodyspraxia who have good language skills.

On paper-and-pencil tasks, Keisha showed a right hand preference and used a static tripod grasp. She was unable to assume or maintain prone extension. She was able to perform sequential thumb-to-finger touching with her right or left hand only by visually monitoring her fingers; thus, she could not do it with both hands simultaneously. Keisha's performance was immature, but it was striking that she could perform the action well as long as she could visually monitor her fingers.

FORM AND SPACE, VISUAL-MOTOR, AND CONSTRUCTION

Keisha's ability to trace a line with a pen (Motor Accuracy) and to reproduce two-dimensional forms (Design Copying) was below age expectations, suggesting difficulty with visual-motor control. The rest of Keisha's SIPT scores in this category suggested age-appropriate form and space perception and constructional abilities.

SENSORY MODULATION

Keisha did not demonstrate any avoidance responses to touch, and neither her mother nor her teacher reported any indications of tactile defensiveness. She did not have any evidence of gravitational insecurity or aversive responses to movement. No indication of a drive or craving for increased sensory input was noted.

RELATED TESTING AND SUMMARY

Psychological assessment revealed that Keisha's IQ score was 132, with a higher verbal than performance IQ. Given her competence with language skills compared with her poorer visual-motor and motor planning skills, we were not surprised that her verbal IQ was higher. A significant difference between verbal and performance IQ score, with lower performance scores, fits a common pattern seen in children with dyspraxia.

From the overall pattern of test scores and observations, the occupational therapist identified somatodyspraxia as a major factor that interfered with Keisha's performance. Keisha's dyspraxia appeared to have its basis in poor processing of tactile and vestibular-proprioceptive sensation. Keisha's dyspraxia involved both gross and fine motor (visual-motor) components.

■ TABLE 3–2 DAVID'S LOWEST SIPT SCORES

Test	Standard Score
Kinesthesia (KIN)	−1.2
Graphesthesia (GRA)	−1.0
Postural Praxis (PPr)	−0.9
Bilateral Motor Coordination (BMC)	−1.4
Sequencing Praxis	−1.3
Standing and Walking Balance	−1.1
Motor Accuracy (MAC)	−1.2
Postrotary Nystagmus (PRN)	−1.2

David

David was eager to try many of the tasks requested by the occupational therapist, and, although he was fidgety, he attended well throughout this one-on-one evaluation, exhibiting no distractibility. None of his scores reflected substantial impairments in performance. In fact, many of his scores on the SIPT were within normal limits. However, the pattern of low scores, coupled with a meaningful cluster of clinical observations, is typical of children with BIS deficits. David's lowest scores are reported in Table 3–2.

TACTILE DISCRIMINATION

David did well on most of the tests requiring tactile discrimination. The one exception was Graphesthesia, which required fine motor skill and two-sided body use in addition to tactile discrimination.

VESTIBULAR AND PROPRIOCEPTIVE PROCESSING

David exhibited low proximal muscle tone and hyperextensibility of his elbows, wrists, and fingers. He could not assume prone extension or maintain his head position in supine flexion. David displayed poor postural background movements and equilibrium reactions. These factors, coupled with low scores on Kinesthesia, Standing and Walking Balance, and Postrotary Nystagmus, suggested poor vestibular-proprioceptive processing.

PRAXIS

David's lowest SIPT scores were on the Bilateral Motor Coordination and Sequencing Praxis tests. His performance on the Postural Praxis test was in the low average range. Clinical observation also revealed that tasks requiring bilateral coordination (e.g., jumping jacks, reciprocal stride jumps, and skipping) were poorly coordinated and performed with a great deal of effort. David could not consistently identify his left and right body sides. He carefully monitored isolated movements of his forearms, hands, and fingers with his eyes and moved very slowly when performing simultaneous movements with both hands.

FORM AND SPACE, VISUAL-MOTOR, AND CONSTRUCTION

David had difficulty with the Motor Accuracy test, a pen-and-paper task requiring fine motor control. This score is consistent with his handwriting difficulties.

SENSORY MODULATION

Like Keisha, David did not exhibit aversive reactions to touch or movement. He was, however, distractible and impulsive when observed in unstructured situations and in group activities, such as playing soccer.

Both Keisha and David showed behaviors consistent with sensory integrative–based practic disorders. The behaviors are notable in their reasons for referral, observations made in the classrooms, parental reports of behavior at home, and standardized testing. Interestingly, both children have characteristics consistent with a diagnosis of DCD as well. David's restless behavior and impulsivity may also warrant a diagnosis of ADHD or DAMP.

The Sensory Integration and Praxis Tests and Praxis

As the name suggests, the best use of the SIPT is for the evaluation of praxis and sensory (especially tactile) processing thought to underlie it. Items for the SIPT were selected from sources providing valid measures of sensory processing or praxis. These included the Southern California Sensory Integration Tests (SCSIT) (Ayres, 1972b) as well as procedures used commonly by neuropsychologists to assess acquired apraxia (Ayres, 1989).

Ayres (1965, 1966a, 1966b, 1969, 1972a, 1977) applied a statistical procedure called factor analysis to examine the relationships of measured variables (or test scores) to each other. Factor analysis approaches a set of data by looking at how variables are correlated and creates categories, or factors, that are statistically related (Portney & Watkins, 2000).

Portney and Watkins (2000) described many uses of factor analysis, including the exploration of a large data set to explore relationships, simplification of data, and testing hypotheses. Factor analysis is used to combine many variables into smaller sets or combinations (Royeen, 1989), can provide

insights into the nature of abstract concepts, and can create order from complex data or information.

Over time, using different samples of children and various types of factor analyses, Ayres (1965, 1966a, 1971, 1977, 1987, 1989) found consistent patterns of dysfunction and relationships among variables. For example, she found a link between tactile functions and praxis. In some analyses, she also identified problems in posture, bilateral integration, and motor sequencing linked to vestibular processing.

Ayres (1989) suggested that a good diagnostic assessment should be able to delineate children with typical function from those with dysfunction. In addition, the instrument should help to define differing intervention needs. One method by which this can be accomplished is through a statistical procedure known as cluster analysis (Johnson, 1967). Cluster analysis is a set of statistical procedures that can determine typologies by grouping subjects according to similar characteristics.

Based partly on the results of factor and cluster analyses of SIPT scores, Ayres (1989) identified four major patterns of dysfunction in praxis. She labeled these:

1. Somatodyspraxia
2. BIS deficits
3. Dyspraxia on verbal command
4. Visuodyspraxia

In an attempt to validate Ayres' work, Mulligan (1998) performed factor analyses with data from more than 10,000 SIPT profiles, most of which reflected children evaluated for possible sensory integrative problems. She identified a factor reflecting generalized sensory integrative dysfunction (Mulligan, 1998) and four first-order factors that bear some similarity to Ayres' factors. Mulligan labeled the first-order factors:

1. BIS deficit
2. Dyspraxia (including all praxis tests *except* Bilateral Motor Coordination and Sequencing Praxis, even those reflecting primarily cortical function such as Praxis on Verbal Command)
3. Somatosensory deficit
4. Visuoperceptual deficit

The specific SIPT subtests that contributed to each of Mulligan's factors are shown in Figure 1–8.

Ayres (1989) sought to differentiate among subtypes of dyspraxia as a step toward developing optimal methods for intervention. If she could associate different practic disorders with different types of sensory processing or distinguish among them in some other important way, she also might be able to develop tailored intervention strategies. Although neither Ayres nor Mulligan (1998) entirely accomplished this objective, it seems clear that sensory integrative dysfunction is manifested in a number of different ways in different children. Thus, the clearest interpretation of an individual SIPT profile might be to say, for example, that there is evidence reflecting generalized sensory integrative dysfunction with particular deficits in somatosensation and praxis or BIS and visual perception.

We recognize the many difficulties associated with discussing types of practic deficits. In fact, in keeping with the work of Lai et al. (1996), we believe that, based on research using the SIPT, praxis likely is a unidimensional construct. Nonetheless, we have found it useful to distinguish between *levels* of practic deficit (see Fig. 1–4). Lai et al. (1996) found that SIPT praxis tests associated with BIS were more difficult than those associated with somatodyspraxia, suggesting that BIS represents a less severe form of practic disorder than somatodyspraxia. We have discussed somatodyspraxia and BIS as two levels of the same dysfunction. (See Dewey, 2002 for a discussion of subtypes from a neuropsychological perspective.)

Bilateral Integration and Sequencing Deficits

Bilateral integration and sequencing appears to be a relatively mild form of practic disorder; thus, BIS deficits are generally subtle. They involve poorly coordinated use of the two body sides and deficits in performing sequences of movement. BIS deficits are hypothesized to reflect impaired processing of vestibular and proprioceptive sensations (Fisher, 1991).

During clinical observations of an individual who has BIS deficits, we may observe right–left confusion; poor lateralization of hand function; avoidance of midline crossing; and poor ability to skip, do jumping jacks or stride jumps, and catch and throw a ball. On the SIPT (Ayres, 1989), scores on Bilateral Motor Coordination and Sequencing Praxis generally are low. Ayres also found low scores on Graphesthesia and Oral Praxis to be associated with deficits in BIS. These measures are described more fully in Chapter 7. David's SIPT

scores reflect this pattern. His lowest scores were on Bilateral Motor Coordination (−1.4) and Sequencing Praxis (−1.3), and he also had difficulty with all the clinical observations that reflect BIS.

For deficits in BIS to be considered sensory integrative in nature, they must be accompanied by evidence of poor sensory processing, generally of vestibular and proprioceptive sensation (Fisher, 1991). David and other clients with deficits in BIS generally also have difficulty performing clinical observations associated with vestibular and proprioceptive sensations (e.g., prone extension, proximal stability, equilibrium, postural background movements, and maintenance of neck flexion during supine flexion). On the SIPT, Kinesthesia, Standing and Walking Balance, and Postrotary Nystagmus are most closely associated with vestibular and proprioceptive sensations, although Mulligan (1998) and Fisher and Bundy (1991) believed that clinical observations were better measures of functions related to processing in these sensory systems.

Somatodyspraxia

Somatodyspraxia is characterized by poor planning of both anticipatory, feedforward-dependent movements and actions that depend on sensory feedback. Therefore, clients with somatodyspraxia exhibit difficulties with planning the same kinds of tasks problematic for individuals with deficits in BIS as well as some additional, generally easier, tasks (Cermak, 1991).

Children with somatodyspraxia generally show a characteristic pattern of test scores on the SIPT and clinical observations (Ayres, 1972a, 1975, 1976, 1979, 1989). Low scores commonly are noted on the SIPT in Postural Praxis, Bilateral Motor Coordination, Sequencing Praxis, and Oral Praxis. Keisha had low scores on all of these measures. Constructional Praxis and Praxis on Verbal Command scores may also be low, as may Design Copying and Motor Accuracy. Clinical observations that are difficult for individuals with somatodyspraxia to perform include the ability to assume supine flexion, sequential finger touching, the ability to perform rapid alternating movements (diadokokinesis) (see Chapter 8), and in-hand manipulation skills (Exner, 1992). We noted most of these difficulties in Keisha's case.

Interviews with parents and teachers add information related to daily routine. Delays in the acquisition of self-care skills, poor organization, difficulty manipulating and assembling toys, and strained relationships with siblings or playmates (or a history of these) are commonly reported.

For dyspraxia to have a sensory integrative basis, it must be accompanied by evidence of poor vestibular or proprioceptive or somatosensory processing. Both Ayres (1965, 1966a, 1971, 1977, 1987, 1989) and Mulligan (1998) found relationships between somatosensory processing and praxis. Keisha and many clients with dyspraxia have low scores on tactile tests of the SIPT, including Manual Form Perception, Finger Identification, and Localization of Tactile Stimuli. Because deficits in BIS, based in poor vestibular and proprioceptive processing, seem to represent a higher level of practic dysfunction than somatodyspraxia (Lai et al., 1996), it is reasonable to suspect that most clients with somatodyspraxia will also have difficulty with measures of vestibular and proprioceptive processing.

Ayres' belief in the somatosensory basis for praxis was derived from two sources. First, through case analysis, Ayres found that children with low scores on the praxis tests also often had low scores on the somatosensory tests (A. J. Ayres, personal communication, February 20, 1988). Second, in her early factor analytic studies, Ayres (1965, 1966a, 1969, 1971, 1977) found an association between motor planning deficits and poor tactile discrimination. However, the only somatosensory test that was consistently loaded with practic tests in the factor analyses was Graphesthesia, a test that also involves a degree of motor planning in order to reproduce the geometric shapes.

Unlike Ayres, Mulligan (1998) found somatosensory deficits to form a factor separate from praxis. Although there were reasonably strong correlations between the two factors, suggesting that poor tactile processing may, indeed, play a role in dyspraxia, Mulligan found no evidence of a factor that could be labeled somatodyspraxia.

NEUROANATOMICAL BASES OF PRAXIS AND DYSPRAXIA

The neuroanatomical aspects of the sensory systems are described in Chapter 2. Our purpose here is to examine the neuroanatomical underpinnings specific to praxis. Thus, we have discussed areas of the brain thought to be involved in planning, sequencing, and initiating movement, all important components of praxis.

Although many regions of the brain contribute to praxis, there are no neuroanatomical loci clearly implicated in dyspraxia. Gubbay (1979) defined clumsy children (some of whom may also have dyspraxia) as those "whose ability to perform skilled movement is impaired despite normal intelligence and *normal findings on conventional neurological examination*" (p. 146, italics added). Frank brain damage, therefore, disqualifies clients from his diagnosis of dyspraxia. However, as more sophisticated neurological evaluation procedures (e.g., computed tomography [CT] scans, magnetic resonance imaging [MRI], positron emission tomography [PET] scans, functional magnetic resonance imaging [fMRI], and magnetoencephalography [MEG]) become more accessible, we may acquire greater knowledge of the causes and neurological correlates of developmental dyspraxia.

In one investigation of children with developmental clumsiness using radiologic technology, Knuckey et al. (1983) found that 39 percent of the clients showed abnormal CT scans compared with only 9 percent of control participants. When the group of clumsy children was subdivided into "clumsy" and "very clumsy," the incidence of abnormal CT scans in the very clumsy children was 48 percent. Specific neurological deficits noted included ventricular dilation, peripheral atrophy, and prominent brain regions. There were also several cases with more specific parenchymal abnormalities; however, in these cases, a particular pattern of deficit was not evident. In contrast with individuals who have acquired apraxia, children who were clumsy generally did not have specific left hemisphere involvement. Knuckey et al. (1983) selected their subjects for "clumsiness" based on an eight-item screening test but did not evaluate the clients' sensory integrative status. Thus, it is not possible to know to what extent these results may be applied to children with sensory integrative–based dyspraxia.

Difficulty localizing a specific neurological "substrate" or "locus" for developmental clumsiness supports the viewpoint posited by Luria (1963, 1980) and others (Basso et al., 1980; DeRenzi et al., 1982) that praxis is dependent upon a complex functional system or network involving cortical and subcortical structures. Conrad et al. (1983) suggested a similar belief in their study of children with sensory integrative–based dyspraxia.

Although execution of movement is generally what we observe, praxis primarily entails ideation and planning. In the next section, we examine brain structures purported to be associated with ideation, planning, and execution of action.

Ideation

Ideation, also referred to as knowing what to do (Ayres, 1985) or conceptualizing an action (Rothi & Heilman, 1997), is likely a cortical function. Although ideation cannot be localized to any one area, it is clear that the prefrontal cortex is involved in the process. It plays a major role in setting goals and is active when we perform (or even imagine performing) complex, goal-directed sequences of movements, particularly in novel situations (Fuster, 1997).

Studies with adults who have both ideomotor and ideational apraxia have led researchers to associate ideational deficits with damage to the left hemisphere (Geschwind, 1975; Harrington et al., 2000; Poeck, 1983; Rothi & Heilman, 1997). Adults with ideational apraxia have difficulty establishing the plan of action needed to accomplish an intended goal, resulting in an alteration of the normal sequence (Hecaen, 1981).

Ideation is also thought to be, in part, the result of basal ganglia activity. Although the basal ganglia are clearly associated with motor execution, they have also been linked with cognitive and behavioral aspects of action (Zigmond et al., 1999).

Although the precise location of ideation is not clearly delineated, neither the premotor nor the supplementary motor areas are needed for ideation, nor are these regions associated with motivation to carry out a motor task.

Planning

Both the lateral *premotor* and medial *supplementary motor areas* (SMA) (area 6) play important roles in the planning of movement (Passingham, 1993). These areas are described as being involved in the translation of a movement strategy into movement tactics (the "how to do it") (Deecke, 1996; Kingsley, 2000) or in selection of appropriate movements (Passingham, 1993). The lateral premotor area is polymodal and is active when movement occurs in response to external events. The SMA depends primarily on proprioceptive inputs. It is activated when action is self-initiated (Passingham, 1993). Recent research with monkeys has led Graziano and Gross (1998) to suggest that the process of planning and coordinating movements in response to external stimuli is a function of projections to the premotor area from the parietal lobe. The premotor area has also been shown to play a role in the preparation and anticipation of movement (Decety et al., 1997; Kingsley, 2000) (Table 3–3).

The SMA is proprioceptive dependent and it may be of particular significance in understanding deficits in BIS. The SMA is associated with orientation of the eyes and the head and with planning of bimanual and sequential movements (Lundy-Ekman, 1998). Goldberg (1985) hypothesized that "the medial system operates in 'projectional' action or action that is driven forward by prediction derived from an internal model of the world com-

---

■ TABLE 3–3 A COMPARISON OF FEATURES OF THE MEDIAL AND LATERAL MOTOR PROGRAMMING SYSTEMS

	Medial	Lateral
"Premotor" center	Supplementary motor area	Arcuate premotor area
Sensory dependence	Primarily proprioceptive	Polymodal (including vision)
Control mode	Predictive (feedforward)	Responsive (feedback)
Skilled movement performance	Fluent execution of extended sequences of component actions	Input-dependent, slow, segmented execution
Bimanual control	Simultaneous (parallel or reciprocal)	Alternating (serial or segmental)
Callosal dependence	High	Low
Reaching to target	Trajectory (navigating)	Acquisition (piloting)
Action mode	Projectional (anticipatory)	Responsive (interactive)
Context sensitivity	Internal	External
Subcortical dependence	Basal ganglia	Cerebellum

Source: Adapted from Goldberg (1985).

posed from previous experience which permits the creation of a probabilistic model of the future" (p. 568). In other words, the medial SMA appears to be involved in planning the projected action sequences some children with sensory integrative difficulties find so challenging. The role of the SMA is in contrast with that of the polymodal lateral premotor system that "operates in a responsive mode in which each action is dependent upon explicit external input" (p. 568). The medial system predominates when rapid, well-learned, "skilled" movement sequences are executed using primarily proprioceptive information, independent of the requirements of ongoing visual feedback monitoring.

Area 5 of the parietal cortex is another major site of convergence of bilateral proprioceptive inputs from muscle, cutaneous, and joint receptors of the body with input from other sensory systems (Cohen, 1999). Indirect vestibular signals may also project to area 5. As Jones and Porter (1980) indicated, there is a close association between sensation and motion. Although we do not know if conscious perception is necessarily separate from feedback to higher centers that control movement, there is evidence that cells in area 5 begin firing before movement is initiated (Bear et al., 1996; Snyder et al., 1997), and continue to fire even under conditions of deafferentation and immobilization of joints (Kalaska, 1988). This suggests that some of these cells may play a role in planning active movement (Kandel et al., 2000; Kingsley, 2000). Area 5 has close connections with precentral motor areas, including the SMA, further suggesting a role of proprioceptive inputs to motor planning (Kalaska, 1988; Kandel et al., 2000; Kingsley, 2000).

Execution

The motor cortex provides a mechanism for the execution of the movements that are selected when performing a voluntary action (Passingham, 1993). Neurons in the primary motor cortex receive and encode ongoing input about the speed, direction, and velocity of movement (Kingsley, 2000). This feedback comes from muscles, joints, and skin via the thalamus as well as intracortical projections from the somatic sensory cortex.

Information from the primary motor cortex (area 4) is transmitted to the muscles for execution via the corticospinal and corticobulbar pathways. The corticospinal tract is comprised of fibers from the primary motor cortex, the premotor area, and the primary somatosensory cortex (areas 3, 1, and 2). These fibers synapse in the cord with lateral motor neurons (lateral corticospinal fibers) and medial motor neurons (ventral corticospinal fibers) carrying signals to muscles that will execute the motor command.

Movement depends on information traveling from various areas of the brain to alpha motor neurons in the spinal cord. The motor system relies on a continuous flow of sensory information before and during task performance (Kandel et al., 2000). Information comes in over sensory pathways describing the environment, the position and orientation of the body and extremities, and mechanical information about muscle contraction. In addition, for volitional movement to occur, integration between and among brain structures responsible for all levels of motor output is required.

The cerebellum also has a major role in the execution of coordinated movement (Kiernan, 1998). Because fibers from the cerebellum do not synapse directly with spinal neurons, the role played by the cerebellum in motor planning is less in direct control of movement and more in the integration of movement and feedback (Latash, 1998). The cerebellum serves a highly dynamic function, with high levels of activity as movement is occurring. Specifically, the cerebellum acts as a comparator, offering information to the CNS about movement and improving its accuracy by acting on brainstem and cortical motor areas that, in turn, send information to the spinal cord. The cerebellum also regulates postural control, and guides movements of the eyes, head, body, and limbs (Cohen, 1999).

The cerebellum is also thought to play a role in motor learning because cerebellar circuits are modified through experience. As an act is practiced repeatedly so that it can be done with greater proficiency and less conscious attention, the cerebellum transfers motor tactics from the conscious to the unconscious (Kingsley, 2000).

The basal ganglia receive significant input from the SMA and, via the thalamus, project back to this region. This region of the brain participates in the initiation of movement, but its role may be dependent on context—that is, it may play its role when movements are complex enough to require sequencing (Graybiel & Kimura, 1995). Although basal ganglia neurons are active at the onset of movement, their activity increases after movement initiation. Thus, the basal ganglia are most important in the completion of movement sequences (Zigmond et al., 1999). The ventral system of the basal ganglia receives information primarily from the limbic system. These connections may subserve motivation and emotion important to praxis and may be a part of the evaluator system (Graybiel & Kimura, 1995; Zigmond et al. 1999).

THE ROLE OF SENSATION IN MOVEMENT AND PRAXIS

Knowledge of sensory processing is essential to understanding sensory integrative–based dyspraxia. Use of this knowledge enables practitioners to incorporate enhanced sensation into intervention based on sensory integration theory.

Ayres (1972a) believed that motor planning depended, in part, on the development of a semiconscious body scheme or internal model of the body in action that began with tactile awareness. "Sensory input from the skin and joints, but especially from the skin, helps develop, in the brain, the model or internal scheme of the body's design as a motor instrument" (Ayres, 1972a, p. 168). Ayres further believed that somatic changes arising from movement resulted in memories that guided ensuing movements. Use of the body for action helped integrate the sensory information and develop the body scheme. Thus, "if the information which the body receives from its somatosensory receptors is not precise, the brain has a poor basis on which to build its scheme of the body" (Ayres, 1972a, p. 170).

Although Ayres (1972a, 1975, 1979, 1985) emphasized the contribution of tactile and proprioceptive sensation to the development of body scheme, other investigators have emphasized other contributions to its development. For example, Schilder (1935) and Lackner and DiZio (1988) suggested that vestibular and proprioceptive sensations derived from active movement also contributed to its development. Schilder (1935) also touted the role of vision in body scheme development.

Sirigu et al. (1995) discussed four representations that contribute to "body knowledge processing," a concept broader than body scheme. The first is related to verbal information that gives names to body parts and their purposes. The second is provided by visuospatial information about our own body and bodies in general. Third is a dynamic body image that comes from information about positional aspects of body parts relative to

each other and in relation to the external world. Finally, Sirigu et al. (1995) suggested that motor representations contribute to this knowledge. Heilman and Rothi (1985) suggested that motor planning involves visuokinesthetic engrams that are stored in the left parietal lobe, which can then activate areas of the brain involved in planning and programming movement.

Tactile System

As described in Chapter 2, the tactile system detects qualities and location of external stimuli applied to the skin. Important to the current discussion, the dorsal column medial lemniscal (DCML) system, which conveys information about the spatial and temporal characteristics of touch (Kandel et al., 2000; Morasso, 1981; Mountcastle, 1986), has been linked to behaviors related to praxis (Bear et al., 1996; Caminiti et al., 1990; Vierck, 1978; Wall, 1970). For example, signals that arrive over the system trigger exploratory behavior—that is, they may serve to guide movement for the purpose of gathering sensation. In addition, the DCML system seems to be involved in flexion; programming of complex movement sequences; refined manual dexterity and manipulation, particularly distal to the body; and selective attention, orientation, and anticipation (Snyder et al., 1997). The mechanisms may be through the connections of the DCML with the thalamus (Leonard, 1998). The contributions of the DCML to praxis are summarized in Table 3–4,

Proprioception

Proprioception refers to sensations of movement (i.e., speed, rate, sequencing, timing, and force) and joint position (Kalaska, 1988; Matthews, 1988; McCloskey, 1985; Kandel et al., 2000; Kiernan,

▪ TABLE 3–4 ROLES OF THE DORSAL COLUMN MEDIAL LEMINISCAL SYSTEM	
Motor	**Selective Attention, Orientation, and Anticipation**
Initiation of voluntary movements	Unraveling competing stimuli
Performance of complex movement sequences and refined manual dexterity	Initiating and controlling internal search
Handling objects in space	Anticipatory components of sequential behavior patterns
Flexion of joints	

1998). Matthews (1988) suggested that, under normal conditions, the role of proprioception is to provide the motor system with a clear, unambiguous map of the external environment and of the body. Knowledge of the body and movements that come from proprioception is important for the development of a body scheme, for praxis, and for producing adaptive actions.

Proprioceptive feedback arises primarily from receptors in muscles, with some contributions made by receptors in skin and joints (see Chapter 2 for more information) (Jones, 1999). Primary and secondary endings of the muscle spindle are activated by stretch, including stretch that occurs when muscles contract against resistance. Golgi tendon organs are sensitive to force and the tension of muscles during contraction (Jami, 1992; Jones, 1999). Collectively, Golgi tendon organs and muscle spindle receptors are the primary receptors for muscle proprioception. They provide the central nervous system (CNS) with information about muscle changes during movement, which, in turn, allows generation of the proper amount of force needed to act on objects. The somatosensory cortex, in particular, readily adapts to changing input, modifying the body image and enabling increasingly skilled performance of tasks (Jones, 1999).

Mechanoreceptors of the skin also contribute to proprioception, particularly in the fingers and, to a lesser degree, in the hand. The high density of mechanoreceptors in the skin of the fingers provides feedback regarding movement and may be important for tactile exploration and object manipulation. Stimulation of both cutaneous mechanoreceptors and joint receptors during active joint movement is believed to be particularly important in the perception of movement of the fingers (Fisher, 1991). Receptors on the back of the hand also discharge in response to movement of underlying and adjacent joints and provide information about the direction of the movement (Edin & Abbs, 1991). In contrast, although mechanoreceptors in the palmar surface of the hand respond to flexion and extension, they do not provide a sense of the direction of movement. Signals from joint and cutaneous receptors appear to be more important for detecting proprioception in the hands than the proximal joints (Jones, 1999) because individual finger muscles control several joints.

Proximal joints are more sensitive than distal joints to movement (Hall & McCloskey, 1983, Jakobs et al., 1985) because they move relatively slowly and produce larger displacement of distal limb segments than does an equal amount of movement at a distal joint (Jones, 1999). Furthermore, proprioception (i.e., accuracy in matching joint position) is better for movements in midranges and when individuals move actively rather than passively (Jones, 1999).

Proprioception arising from active movement assists in the development of body scheme and actions used to plan complex movements (Kiernan, 1998; Kingsley, 2000). In contrast, passive movement does not produce the same level of proprioception (Evarts, 1985; Ghez et al., 1990; Kalaska, 1988). Furthermore, passive joint compression and traction may be less effective for providing proprioceptive input than is active muscle contraction against resistance. Thus, within a sensory integration approach, active movement is always preferred over passive movement

Vestibular System

The vestibular system, with receptors in the inner ear, is a source of specialized proprioceptive information. Together with muscle-based proprioception, vestibular input contributes to posture and the maintenance of a stable visual field (Brodal, 1998; Horak et al., 1988; Shumway-Cook et al., 1987). Many of the clinical observations practitioners use to evaluate sensory integration address functions that require proprioception. Although sorting the precise contributions of vestibular- and muscle-based proprioception is neither easy nor necessary, it *is* appropriate to consider the combined impact of vestibular and proprioceptive input on muscle tone, posture, equilibrium, and motor behavior.

Vestibular and proprioceptive feedback contribute to the development of neuronal models of how it feels to perform a given movement (Bear et al., 2001; Evarts, 1985; Kalaska, 1988; Kandel et al., 2000; Kiernan, 1998). According to Brooks (1986), neuronal models of movement are used to regulate ongoing activity and guide the execution of future tasks. Brooks also believed that body scheme, derived at least in part from proprioception, was important for planning anticipatory movements or projected action sequences (i.e., the sequence of movements necessary to project a hand or foot to the place it needs to be at the appropriate time). Playing a game of hopscotch or running forward to catch a bounced ball are examples of activities that involve projected action sequences. Projected action sequences are complex behaviors that require integration of the position of body parts coupled with information about the external environment.

Vision

In combination with the somatic senses (i.e., tactile, vestibular, and proprioceptive) that provide knowledge of the body and its actions, vision also yields much information about the surrounding world. Fox (1999) suggested that vision serves three major purposes: learning about objects, maintaining posture, and informing us about our position in space. Vision also helps us recognize where we are in relation to objects, thus enhancing our ability to approach or avoid those objects. For example, individuals who cannot see their hands before reaching for a visual target direct their hands inaccurately and underestimate the distance to the target. The inaccuracies decrease when individuals can see both their hands and the target in the same workspace (Ghilardi et al., 1995). Thus, when all its functions are considered together, vision influences cognition and plays a significant role in adaptation to the environment (Kosselyn & Koenig, 1992; Zoltan, 1996) and thus influences praxis (see also Chapter 5).

The available research has begun to address the specific relationship of vision to praxis and the various forms of motor incoordination that are discussed in this chapter. Gubbay (1975, 1979) and Henderson and Hall (1982) have found that children classified as clumsy often have visual-perceptual and visual-motor problems. Similarly, in cluster analyses of SIPT data, Ayres (1989) identified a group of children with both visual-perceptual as well as motor planning deficits. Furthermore, Dewey and Kaplan (1994) suggested that visual-perceptual problems disturbed the sensory information these children receive which, in turn, disturbed their performance of planned movement.

Vision is particularly relevant to intervention based on sensory integration theory because of its important contribution to position and movement in space. Although occupational therapy practitioners frequently address deficits related to visual perception, we have much to learn about the relationship between visual perception and praxis. More information on visual-spatial abilities can be found in Chapter 5.

Auditory Processing

Although it is not typically considered when addressing sensory integration theory in understanding praxis, auditory processing may contribute to the organization of movement because it is responsible for providing information regarding the spatial location of objects and events. Research linking the auditory system to *praxis* is virtually nonexistent, but there are some studies that suggest that the auditory system may be an avenue for enhancing movement.

Readers interested in information pertaining to the effect of auditory stimulation on motor and spatial performance in adults with neurological deficits should investigate the work of Thaut et al. (McIntosh et al., 1997, 1995; Thaut et al., 1995, 1996, 1998). In addition, Rauscher et al. (1993, 1995, 1998) have reported improvements in spatial reasoning in college students and more skilled maze negotiation in rats after exposure to classical music. However, other investigations (Newman et al., 1995, Stough et al., 1994; Kenealy & Monseth, 1994) have failed to support these findings.

The investigations referred to involved both subjects and experimental paradigms very unlike those encountered in intervention based on sensory integration theory. However, they contain components that may bear some relationship to praxis; as such, they provide food for thought as we consider the influence of this system on praxis and motor production. Because problems in the timing and sequencing of movement are often noted in children with dyspraxia, it may be useful to examine the role of auditory enrichment, pacing, or cueing to enhance the timing and sequencing of movement. More information on the auditory system can be found in Chapter 6.

THE INTERVENTION PROCESS

The evaluation process—observations in context, interview, clinical observations, and the results of the SIPT—provides critical evidence for determining if sensory integration dysfunction is impairing a client's everyday performance. After evaluation, practitioners, in collaboration with clients and caregivers, can develop plan for interventions. In this section, we provide general comments about the use of sensory integration theory and then examine other contemporary theories that offer additional insight into intervention to facilitate the development of praxis. In Chapter 12, we provide considerable detail about using sensory integration theory to address specific aspects of dysfunction.

Sensory Integration Theory Revisited

Some of the principles and ideas that Ayres promoted are especially important when intervening with individuals who have sensory integrative–based dyspraxia. First, Ayres (1972a) described the adaptive response as central to intervention. Adaptive responses are purposeful actions directed toward a goal that is successfully achieved. Adaptive responses are inherently organizing for the brain. (Please note that throughout this text we have referred to *adaptive responses* as *adaptive interactions*.) Ayres was a proponent of the active participation of the client and made it clear that "doing" had to be initiated by the client.

Second, Ayres (1972a, 1979, 1985) emphasized intervention as a transaction between a client, the task, and the environment. Although praxis enables effective transactions (Ayres, 1985), the environment guides performance by determining its parameters (Connolly & Dalgleish, 1989; Gibson, 1988; Jeannerod, 1988). As the environment changes, so must the client's actions. Ayres (1972a, 1979, 1985) emphasized that an important role of the therapist was to set up environments so that they provided a challenge that was just right.

Sensory integration is not a method by which practitioners *do something to* clients. Rather, practitioners observe how clients respond to cues, interact with significant persons and objects, and adapt to changing environmental demands. They then create environments that entice clients to attempt new skills, adapt in new ways, and master appropriate challenges. Intervention involves challenges that lead to improved organization of brain and behavior. Intervention extends into daily life as clients are enabled to participate more effectively in the family, the classroom, the workspace, and the social environment.

Although many of Ayres' ideas remain contemporary, she was also influenced by early hierarchical models of motor control such as those developed from the work of Hughlings Jackson (Jackson & Taylor, 1932). In such models, successively higher levels of the nervous system control skilled movements. Development was thought to occur in a particular sequence and each level of performance provided a foundation for the more advanced behaviors that would follow. Hierarchical models influenced the development of many therapeutic approaches including proprioceptive neuromuscular facilitation (PNF), neurodevelopmental treatment (NDT), the sensorimotor approach of Margaret Rood (Stokmeyer, 1967), as well as sensory integration. More recently, theorists have disputed some of the basic tenets of the hierarchical models of motor development, making some aspects of Ayres' early beliefs outdated and casting others in new light. New knowledge has influenced—and will continue to influence—the development of sensory integration theory and intervention.

Contemporary Theories of Motor Behavior

A number of theories of motor behavior have emerged in the past 30 years. These theories have been used to guide intervention to address movement dysfunction with a variety of causes; they may well apply to intervention for clients with sensory integrative–based dyspraxia. These theories can be divided into two categories: 1) motor learning and motor control and 2) contextual.

Motor Learning and Motor Control

Motor learning and *motor control* are broad terms that encompass a variety of theories. Whereas motor learning refers to the acquisition or modification of movement, motor control is concerned with the regulation and refinement of movement that has already been acquired (Shumway-Cook & Woollacott, 1995). Some motor learning theories have challenged concepts regarding the order of motor development, supporting instead a notion of flexible, changing behavior in response to the demands of the situation (Thelen, 1995). These are reminiscent of the adaptive transaction, which is an integral part of intervention based on sensory integration theory.

Some motor learning and motor control theorists have categorized movement into two basic systems: a closed-loop system, which relies on sensory feedback for accuracy, and an open-loop system, in which learned actions occur through feedforward (Adams, 1971; Guiliani, 1991; Schmidt, 1988).

Closed-loop processes are based on feedback from discrepancies in motor performance, which are used to refine motor programs. The extent of error in the response is determined, and corrections are made during the action. Sensory feedback is important throughout the action and is produced through sensations associated with the motor response; it is generated during and at the completion of a response. Schmidt and Lee (1988) indicated that closed-loop systems depend heavily on sensory information from the environment and the body. They suggested that exteroceptive information provided by the visual system was the richest source of information for closed-loop control. Vestibular and proprioceptive sensations were also thought to be important. Schmidt (1988) described three types of response-produced feedback. These include feedback that arises from muscles as they contract, movement of the body or body parts in space, and from the environment.

The first two types of feedback arise from the response itself (production feedback). The last arises from changes that occur in the environment as a result of the response (outcome feedback). In closed-loop movements, response-produced feedback is compared with expected feedback. If there is a discrepancy between the actual and expected feedback, an error is detected, and the need for a correction is signaled. Knowledge of results occurs through a comparison of outcome feedback with the intended goal (Mathiowetz & Haugen, 1995). Knowledge of results can occur through the recognition that success has been achieved and can even be verbally described. A child who successfully throws a beanbag at a stack of blocks realizes her success by seeing and hearing blocks fly everywhere. A cheering therapist reinforces the success!

Gentile (1972) described a form of feedback known as knowledge of performance, which is knowledge about the action performed to achieve the goal. This is similar to production feedback. Schmidt (1991) referred to this as kinematic feedback, which depends on information received from the body. Throwing the beanbag was likely achieved through a rapid movement of the upper extremity, with shoulder flexion, elbow extension, and opening of the hand. To describe all of these elements to a child would be overwhelming, but the therapist might say, "You let that beanbag go at the right time!" providing knowledge of performance for the child.

In open-loop control, muscle commands exist before a movement sequence begins and, after they are triggered, run their course without the possibility of correction from sensory feedback (Kelso, 1982; Schmidt, 1988; Stelmach, 1976). An open-loop system uses anticipatory (or feedforward) control, when there is insufficient time to use feedback information to monitor and correct movement (Mathiowetz & Haugen, 1995).

Feedforward processes do not detect errors during movement. Instead, corrections are made based on previous experience, knowledge of one's body and the physical world, and predictions about the anticipated change in the status of movement (Lee, 1988). With feedforward, signals are sent ahead of the movement to prepare for an upcoming motor command or to ready the system for the receipt of some kind of feedback information (Schmidt & Lee, 1999).

Kelso and Stelmach (1976) suggested that internal feedback derived from information processed before the action began (feedforward), was a special form of feedback used in open-loop movements. The internal feedback loops provide a copy of a centrally generated motor command. Other terms for internal feedback are *corollary discharge* and *efference copy*. A "copy" of the motor command to the muscles is sent to other areas of the brain and used to evaluate additional incoming messages. The information can be compared with a reference of correctness, used to correct errors that are detected before the actual production of the action. Therefore, feedforward appears to be particularly important for actions that involve anticipation (Schmidt, 1988). Feedforward, or internal feedback, is differentiated from the response-produced feedback that comes from the movement. The originating stimulus sets a response chain into motion, with the remainder of events determined by associations learned between feedback and the next act in the sequence. After the response chain has been activated, the program is not modified (Schmidt & Lee, 1999).

Most theorists have recognized that neither the closed-loop or the open-loop views is entirely satisfactory and instead have adopted a hybrid view of human motor control, acknowledging various forms of response-produced feedback as well as open-loop conditions, in which no feedback occurs (Schmidt, 1988). What can eventually become open-loop movements are initially learned through a closed-loop system in which attention focuses on the sensory feedback obtained during the movement. Feedback control appears to be particularly important in learning new skills. After the skill is learned, increased reliance on feed-forward becomes possible (Brooks, 1986; Kelso & Stelmach, 1976). Thus, feedforward control appears to represent higher-level ability or skill development in which less conscious control of movement is required (see Figure 3–1).

Application of these motor control theories to sensory integrative–based dyspraxia suggests that children with BIS deficits are less involved than are children with other types of practic disorders because their primary deficits are in proprioceptive-dependent feedforward motor control rather than in actions that require both feedback and feedforward control (Fisher, 1991). Ayres (1978, 1989) found that children with vestibular- and proprioceptive-based bilateral integration disorders are among the least severely affected of children with sensory integrative–based practic disorders. Learning to move or learning to accommodate to new demands appears to be dependent on sensory processing and sensory integration (Wolpert et al., 1995). Acquiring skills and developing motor programs, rather

than using those already learned, seems to be a more difficult process than using skills that have been mastered. This is often the very concern that occupational therapists have in working with children with sensory integrative–based dyspraxia.

Contextual Perspectives

Many newer models of motor behavior emphasize that actions reflect the person, task, and environment. A person's multiple systems (i.e., perceptual, cognitive, and motor) interact with unique tasks in the contexts in which they occur, requiring both feedforward and feedback control to achieve a goal (Shumway-Cook & Woollacott, 1995). Considerable emphasis has been placed on both the environment and the individual's interest for engaging with that environment.

Contextual approaches seem particularly relevant to occupational therapy because active participation in meaningful occupation and the planning and production of adaptive transactions are central

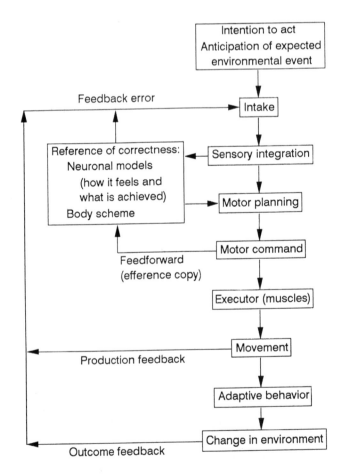

■ FIGURE 3–1 Schematic interweaving of motor control and sensory integration theories.

to the profession and its theories and approaches, including sensory integration theory. For example, Fidler and Fidler (1978) asserted that purposeful activity provided the action–learning experience essential for skill acquisition. Gliner (1985) emphasized the interaction between the individual and the environment (i.e., object and task), rather than the movement itself, and suggested that the environment provided meaning and support to the person performing the action. Similarly, King (1978) maintained that adaptive behavior was organized best through active involvement in occupations. She suggested that in doing purposeful tasks, attention was directed toward the object or the goal rather than the movement. A meta-analysis by Lin et al. (1997) demonstrated that occupationally embedded exercise increased clients' beneficial performance by 50 percent relative to simple rote exercise. This pattern of attention is typical of motor skill development and fits with the previous discussion regarding knowledge of results.

ACTION SYSTEMS THEORY

Some contemporary theories of motor behavior have examined perceptual control of action. A recent approach has focused on the idea that spatial knowledge of the external world is derived from movement experiences associated with vision and memory (Reed, 1982, 1988). This view, known as *action systems theory,* focuses on the functional specificity and meaning of actions and emphasizes the need to study actions within natural contexts. From a sensory integration perspective, this would mean observing children performing in their typical contexts, such as playing on the school playground. Because practitioners are experiencing an increased need to determine appropriate functional goals, systems theories are particularly relevant.

DYNAMICAL SYSTEMS THEORY

Dynamical systems theory challenges traditional views that human development proceeds in an orderly and consistent way with little variability in the acquisition of skills (Gray et al., 1996; Thelen, 1995; Thelen & Smith, 1994). Thelen and Smith (1994) referred to the older perspective as the "view from above." In contrast, in a "view from below," motor behavior is described as fluid, highly variable, and dependent on context. From this viewpoint, dynamical systems theory attempts to explain the unique features of performance that do

not fit well into a static or hierarchical approach. When motor behavior is viewed as a reflection of a dynamic system, one can account for both the global order seen in groups of individuals and the specific variability exhibited by one individual. This union of global with specific underlies the capacity of the individual to adapt.

Thelen and Smith (1994) suggested that context, represented by the immediate situation, matters in three ways. First, context creates a global order through the accumulated experiences within an environment. That is, repeated here-and-now experiences establish the global order. Second, the context selects the global order and allows us to perform qualitatively different acts. For example, the act of grasping varies, depending on whether we hold a bottle, a mug, or a small drinking glass. Grasping is the global feature, but it can be modified by the circumstances in which it is applied. Third, context adapts the global order, fitting the history of past experiences with the task at hand. Because the global order is created by and manifested in the details of the here and now, it is fundamentally context dependent. The expressed pattern of activity includes the sensory messages received within the moment, the preceding activity, and the history of responses that have occurred up to the moment at hand. Continued interaction with the surrounding world through the exploration of new contexts presents opportunities to form associations about events in the world and select details that will cause a reorganization of existing global structures.

Dynamical systems theory eliminates the nature versus nurture debate and suggests that our focus be directed toward the cooperation of components that produce organization, regulation, and stability or facilitate change that is consistent within the context presented (Thelen, 1995). Similar ideas are presented in the theories of E. J. Gibson (1988) and J. J. Gibson (1979), whose research coupled action and perception. J. J. Gibson (1979) defined "affordances" as reciprocal relationships between an actor and the environment that enabled performance of functional tasks. As a child acquires new motor milestones, new opportunities are offered for perceptual discoveries. Environmental interaction, then, is the key to facilitating and fine tuning perception and motor behavior as a basis for further development.

Dynamical systems theory fits well with the theory of sensory integration as it emphasizes doing or acting within a meaningful context. We are struck by the complexity of both approaches and the complexity of the responses required for action within any context, which can appear to the untrained observer to be quite simple.

Practice Effects

In intervention with clients who have dyspraxia, we look for ways to create interesting and challenging tasks that facilitate improved motor planning and skill acquisition. Although we know that practice is important, the characteristics of practice that make it most effective are not clear. In individuals whose motor planning is not impaired, the more variable the practice, the more effective it seems to be for generalization (Mathiowetz & Haugen, 1995). However, it is not clear whether the needs of clients with dyspraxia are similar. Intervention involves considerable repetition. Clearly, the use of practice with clients who have dyspraxia bears further investigation. Larkin and Parker (2002) provide a comprehensive review of task specific interventions for children with DCD.

Movements are generated from past experiences that are successful and stored as long-term memories (Brooks, 1986). Success occurs when the sensory feedback from the movement matches the sensory outflow as the program was expressed and the outcome achieved (Gentile, 1972). A learned motor skill must be practiced to be stored and retrieved in a way that supports expertise (Brooks, 1986). Practicing movements is essential to skill development. Traditional ideas from motor behavior have suggested that blocked practice, or the repeated reproduction of an action within a concentrated time period, would be most beneficial in learning a skill (Mathiowetz & Haugen, 1995). However, it appears that random practice of an action (i.e., practice of one task followed by practice of a different one [Schmidt & Lee, 1999]) across varied time periods enhances retention and use of the movement at later occasions (Shea & Morgan, 1979; Shea & Titzer, 1993). Random practice promotes more comparative analyses of actions and a more memorable mental representation of the action is reported than when repeating the same actions (Shea & Zimny, 1983).

For most individuals, learning is strengthened when practice involves variations on previously learned tasks or circumstances. Lindner (1986) emphasized that "this influence on the learning of a given task from practicing or learning other tasks should be one of the most important factors in learning" (p. 65). Schmidt (1991) pointed out that a major goal of practice is to retain what is learned for later use. However, conditions that enhance long-term retention, such as random practice, do not increase generalizability.

Random practice may be embedded in more variable and novel conditions to increase the adaptability of the movement (Catalano & Kleiner, 1984). Variability occurs quite naturally as children acquire new skills. For example, the grasp a child needs to hold a spoon or stabilize a sock with two hands can be practiced with toys and other objects. Opportunities for varied practice of developing skills are inherent to a therapeutic sensory integration environment that offers interesting and unique challenges. Therapists monitor the ease and success with which clients use equipment and engage objects to determine when to reduce or increase demands.

After a client has learned a skill in a therapeutic environment, it generally is necessary to transfer that skill to situations such as home or school. The more closely the demands of the practice environment resemble those of a client's real-life environment, the easier the transfer of skills (Mathiowetz & Haugen, 1995). This may be especially true for clients who are dyspraxic and who may have difficulty generalizing to new situations. Here therapists are especially challenged and need to find varied and creative ways to facilitate motor learning while selecting tools and materials that are likely to be encountered by the client on a day-to-day basis.

Because of their hypothesized difficulty developing schemas or neuronal models of action that can be generalized, clients with dyspraxia may have particular difficulty realizing gains made during intervention in their daily lives (Ayres, 1985; Brooks, 1986; Schmidt, 1988). Here practitioners are especially challenged to find varied and creative ways to facilitate motor learning while simultaneously selecting tools and materials that are likely to be those clients encounter on a day-to-day basis.

In one study illustrating the difficulty of planning successful intervention for clients with poor motor performance, Polatajko et al. (1995) compared the effects of two different interventions on kinesthesia, tactile discrimination, visual motor integration, manual dexterity, ball skills, and balance in children with DCD. One intervention included a process-oriented approach that emphasized kinesthetic training, the second group received traditional occupational therapy that emphasized sensory and perceptual motor activities, and the third group received no treatment. The most significant improvements occurred in kinesthetic sensitivity in the group that received the process-oriented intervention. However, increased kinesthetic sensitivity did not translate into improved motor performance or generalization of skills. Thus, the authors suggested that training of specific skills may be beneficial.

Teaching clients to attend to specific perceptual or conceptual features of tasks *may* help them transfer newfound skills to daily life tasks. In addition, manual guidance seems to have a positive effect on skill acquisition, although the effect is reduced for later retention and transfer of performance behavior (Carr & Shepherd, 1987). Light manual guidance should direct an individual's *active* movement (Carr & Shepherd, 1987).

Mental practice of an action also has positive influences on motor learning and performance by activating neural areas that are responsible for programming movements and executing a task (Decety, 1996). The effect of mental practice has been confirmed by Ingvar and Philopson (1977), who found significant increases in regional cerebral blood flow (rCBF) to premotor and frontal cortices during mental practice. Increased cerebral blood flow occurs in areas where increased neuronal activity requires additional oxygen and glucose. Similarly, Roland et al. (1980) used rCBF with adults who had no evidence of impairments to record areas of neural activation during imagined movements of the fingers. Blood flow changes were most significant in the supplementary motor area (SMA), which plays an important role in planning complex movements.

During an imagined or actual writing task with the right or left hand, Decety et al. (1988) found significant activation of bilateral prefrontal cortex, SMA, and cerebellum. The cerebellum enhances the force, timing, and organization of skilled movements. Subjects also showed increased activation of the cerebellum when imagining hitting a softball against a wall with a tennis racket (Ryding et al., 1993). Mental practice of imagined right and left arm movements in subjects with poststroke right hemisphere damage produced electrocardiographic (EEG) changes in parietal and frontal regions contralateral to the movement (Weiss et al., 1994). The EEG changes were comparable to those for sub-

jects who had no neurological damage. The authors suggested that imagining actions produces a form of internal proprioceptive feedback that enhances active movement.

We do not know if mental imaging would work for persons with sensory integrative–based dyspraxia. However, clients like David, with mild practic deficits typical and cognitive abilities, could be asked to imagine that they are doing a particular task before actually performing it. Research in this area would greatly enhance our ability to apply this information to children with sensory integrative–based dyspraxia.

Intervention for Keisha and David

When we evaluated Keisha, we found that she had poor processing of tactile, vestibular, and proprioceptive sensations. She also had marked difficulty on tests that require motor planning and visual-motor coordination. We concluded that she had dyspraxia involving both gross and fine motor planning that was related to poor sensory processing. We believed that motor planning difficulties contributed to her poor visual-motor coordination. This affected her handwriting, self-care skills, and play behavior.

In intervention, we provided Keisha with opportunities to receive enhanced sensation in the context of meaningful activities. Keisha initially delighted in opportunities to be contained in small spaces. Climbing into a large cloth bag that was filled with soft foam blocks provided an opportunity for her to plan and organize her movement in a simple way and receive enhanced tactile input. The bag became a washing machine as we closed it up and moved it rapidly back and forth vigorously on the mat. In doing so, we added more vestibular input to the experience. Keisha also liked to pretend that she was a bird in a nest, created with a large inner tube lying on the floor and filled with pillows and beanbags.

After we had worked with Keisha for several weeks, we wanted to involve her in activities that were more demanding. For example, she might engage in an activity of swinging on a trapeze and letting go to land in a pile of pillows. Although this activity, which involves planning and executing projected action sequences, no doubt would be difficult for Keisha, it could also be graded to reduce the demand if necessary. For example, we could set up the situation so Keisha jumped from the top of three steps positioned 10 feet away from the pillows. Or she could start from a small stool 6 feet away from the pillows. We could also adjust the size of the pile of pillows, making the timing of the landing easier or harder. In any case, the goal would be the same—landing on the pillows. If we offered Keisha the opportunity to try (practice) several variations of the activity and if she reached the intended goal each time, her overall action plan would have had to be flexible to meet the changing demands.

David's motor problems were milder. His sensory processing issues were predominantly in vestibular-proprioceptive domains. We speculated that these deficits were interfering with adequate postural control and coordinated use of his two body sides. In addition, his distractibility and decreased attention, which seemed to be separate from his sensory integrative dysfunction, were preventing him from focusing and interfering with his ability to acquire motor skills. We gave David many opportunities for dynamic and intense movement, particularly through the use of suspended equipment.

David was eager to try different swings. He found that he could control the speed of the glider and used it to crash into towers he had built with soft foam blocks. We created a number of challenges to his postural reactions, and he took great pride in his ability to stay on the swing even when moving through wide excursions. He dubbed the bolster swing "the bucking bronco." As he held onto overhead ropes, we moved the bolster in various directions with increasing vigor, and he adapted his reactions to accommodate to the increased demands. Visual-spatial demands are also inherent in such tasks because they involve movement in relation to objects and the environment.

Many aspects of contemporary motor control theories seem complementary to sensory integration theory. For example, in action systems theory, objects provide guides for action. Ayres (1972a, 1985) emphasized the importance of using equipment to design the "just right" challenge. Viewed from the perspective of action systems theory, equipment commonly used in intervention based on sensory integration theory provides "affordances" to perceive the meaning of the situation (i.e., what to do with the equipment) and act on that meaning. The client's actions are guided, in part, by the nature of the equipment and its perceptual characteristics; the activities and equipment pull for the just right challenge.

As we proceeded, we considered certain issues that reflected a broadened view on the nature of dyspraxia. The first of these issues pertained to the use of an approach to intervention that incorporates "cognitive strategies."

One important cognitive strategy, visual direction, involves reminding clients to look at a particular place or object or demonstrating the activity so as to provide clients with a visual model of how the activity is performed. To promote this strategy, when Keisha wanted to climb to the top of a playground jungle gym, we asked her to look up at the top. We might also have shown her a route.

A second cognitive strategy, verbal mediation and monitoring, includes requesting clients to verbalize what is to be done or what has been done. Keisha's verbal skills were very good, and it was especially helpful to her to build on an existing strength as she engaged in motor challenges. For David, whose distractibility and short attention span were problematic, verbal mediation helped him to focus on a specific goal and consider the appropriate sequence of actions. Moreover, when we asked both children to describe what they wanted to do, they had the opportunity to formulate a cognitive representation of the action of climbing to the top of the jungle gym or kicking the ball into the net (Jeannerod, 1988).

For someone with BIS deficits, like David, whose sensory integrative deficits are relatively mild, imagining actions might be another avenue to pursue in intervention. Before engaging in a task, David could be asked to close his eyes and imagine that he is doing the task. This could be followed by the actual performance of the action. Adding the reinforcement of verbal feedback, with the therapist stating what transpired—or perhaps, even better, having David identify the order and success of events—could be included.

We believed that the incorporation of cognitive components (i.e., visual direction and verbal mediation, focusing on the activity as a whole rather than on the components, visualization of the act), together with enhanced tactile, vestibular, proprioceptive, and visual sensation, would result in improved planning and production of movement. That is, Keisha and David could reap the combined benefits of enhanced sensation and cognitive processes that together enhanced their ability to plan "what to do" and "how to do it" (Brooks, 1986).

CONCLUSION

In this chapter, we have attempted to explain some of the very complex issues that surround praxis. Sensation and movement are intricately intertwined in the CNS, as described in this chapter. A growing interest in disorders of movement has produced a rich body of work around motor behavior. However, praxis involves more than movement; cognitive processes also play an important role. Intervention for practic disorders is challenging and exciting. New theories of motor control and motor learning may offer important supplements to sensory integration theory.

References

Adams, J. A. (1971). A closed-loop theory of motor learning. *Journal of Motor Behavior, 3,* 111–150.

Amundson, S. (1995). *Evaluation tool of children's handwriting.* Homer, AK: O.T. Kids.

Ayres, A. J. (1965). Patterns of perceptual motor dysfunction in children: A factor-analytic study. *Perceptual and Motor Skills, 20,* 335–368.

Ayres, A. J. (1966a). Interrelations among perceptual-motor abilities in a group of normal children. *American Journal of Occupational Therapy, 20,* 288–292.

Ayres, A. J. (1966b). Interrelationships among perceptual-motor functions in children. *American Journal of Occupational Therapy, 20,* 68–71.

Ayres, A. J. (1969). Deficits in sensory integration in educationally handicapped children. *Journal of Learning Disabilities, 2,* 160–168.

Ayres, A. J. (1971). Characteristics of types of sensory integrative dysfunction. *American Journal of Occupational Therapy, 25,* 329–334.

Ayres, A. J. (1972a). Improving academic scores through sensory integration. *Journal of Learning Disabilities, 5,* 338–343.

Ayres, A. J. (1972b). *Southern California Sensory Integration Tests manual.* Los Angeles: Western Psychological Services.

Ayres, A. J. (1975). Sensorimotor foundations of academic ability. In W. M. Cruickshank & D. P. Hallahan (Eds.), *Perceptual and learning disabilities in children, volume 2: Research and theory* (pp. 300–360). New York: Syracuse University Press.

Ayres, A. J. (1976). The *effect of sensory integrative therapy on learning disabled children: The final report of a research project.* Pasadena, CA: Center for the Study of Sensory Integrative Dysfunction.

Ayres, A. J. (1977). Cluster analyses of measures of sensory integration. *American Journal of Occupational Therapy, 31,* 362–366.

Ayres, A. J. (1978). Learning disabilities and the vestibular system. *Journal of Learning Disabilities, 11,* 18–29.

Ayres, A. J. (1979). *Sensory integration and the child.* Los Angeles: Western Psychological Services.

Ayres, A. J. (1985). *Developmental dyspraxia and adult onset apraxia.* Torrance, CA: Sensory Integration International.

Ayres, A. J. (1989). *Sensory Integration and Praxis Tests.* Los Angeles: Western Psychological Services.

Ayres, A. J., Mailloux, Z., & Wendler, C. L. (1987). Developmental dyspraxia: Is it a unitary function? *Occupational Therapy Journal of Research, 7,* 93–110.

Basso, A., Luzzatti, C., & Spinnler, H. (1980). Is ideomotor apraxia the outcome of damage to well-defined regions of the left hemisphere? *Journal of Neurology, Neurosurgery and Psychiatry, 43,* 118–126.

Bear, M. F., Connors, B. W., & Paradiso, M. A. (2001). *Neuroscience: Exploring the brain.* Baltimore: Lippincott Williams & Wilkins.

Bear, M. F., Connors, B. W., & Paradiso, M. A. (1996). The somatic sensory system. In M. F. Bear, B. W. Connors, & M. A. Paradiso (Eds.), *Neuroscience: Exploring the brain.* Baltimore: Williams & Wilkins, pp. 308–345.

Brodal, P. (1998). *The central nervous system.* New York: Oxford University Press.

Brooks, V. B. (1986). How does the limbic system assist motor learning? A limbic comparator hypothesis. *Brain Behavior Evolution, 29,* 29–53.

Caminiti, R., Johnson, P. B., & Urbano, A. (1990). Making arm movements within different parts of space: Dynamic aspects in the primate motor cortex. *Journal of Neuroscience, 10,* 2039–2058.

Cantell, M. H., Smyth, M. M., & Ahonen, T. P. (1994). Clumsiness in adolescence: Educational, motor, and social outcomes of motor delay detected at 5 years. *Adapted Physical Activity Quarterly, 11*(2), 115–129.

Carr, J. H., & Shepherd, R. (1987). *A motor relearning programme for stroke.* Rockville, MD: Aspen.

Catalano, J. F., & Kleiner, B. M. (1984). Distant transfer in coincident timing as a function of variability of practice. *Perceptual and Motor Skills, 58,* 851–856.

Cermak, S. (1991). Somatodyspraxia. In A. G. Fisher, E. A. Murray, & A. C. Bundy (Eds.), *Sensory integration: Theory and practice* (pp. 137–165). Philadelphia: F.A. Davis.

Cermak, S., & Larkin, D. (Eds.) (2002). *Developmental coordination disorder: Theory and practice.* San Diego: Singular.

Cohen, H. (Ed.) (1999). *Neuroscience for rehabilitation, 2nd Edition.* Philadelphia: Lippincott Williams & Wilkins.

Connolly, K., & Dalgleish, M. (1989). The emergence of a tool: Using skill in infancy. *Developmental Psychology, 25,* 894–912.

Conrad, K. E., Cermak, S., & Drake, C. (1983). Differentiation of praxis among children. *American Journal of Occupational Therapy, 37,* 466–473.

Dawdy, S. C. (1981). Pediatric neuropsychology: Caring for the developmentally dyspraxic child. *Clinical Neuropsychology, 3,* 30–37.

Decety, J. (1996). Do imagined and executed actions share the same neural substrate? *Cognitive Brain Research, 3,* 87–93.

Decety, J., Grezes, N., Costes, D., Perani, M., Jeannerod, E., Procyk, F., Grassi, F., & Fazio, E. (1997). Brain activity during observation of actions. *Brain, 120,* 1763–1777.

Decety, J., Philippon, B., & Ingvar, D. H. (1988). rCBF landscapes during motor performance and motor ideation of a graphic gesture. *European Archives of Psychiatric Neurological Science, 238,* 33–38.

Deecke, L. (1996). Planning, preparation, execution, and imagery of volitional action. *Cognitive Brain Research, 3,* 59–64.

DeRenzi, E., Faglioni, P., & Sorgato, P. (1982). Modality-specific and supramodal mechanisms of apraxia. *Brain, 105,* 301–312.

Dewey, D. (2002). Subtypes of developmental coordination disorder. In S. Cermak & D. Larkin (Eds.), *Developmental coordination disorder: Theory and practice* (pp. 40–53). San Diego: Singular.

Dewey, D., & Kaplan, B. J. (1994). Subtyping of developmental motor deficits. *Developmental Neuropsychology, 10:* 265–284.

Edin, B. B., & Abbs, J. H. (1991). Finger movement responses of cutaneous mechanoreceptors in the dorsal skin of the human hand. *Journal of Neurophysiology, 65,* 657–670.

Evarts, E. V. (1985). Sherrington's concept of proprioception. In E. V Evarts, S. P. Wise, & B. Blousfield (Eds.), *The motor system in neurobiology* (pp. 183–186). New York: Elsevier.

Exner, C. E. (1992). In-hand manipulation skills. In J. Case-Smith & C. Pehoski (Eds.), *Development of hand skills in the child.* Rockville, MD: American Occupational Therapy Association.

Fidler, G. S., & Fidler, J. W. (1978). Doing and becoming: Purposeful action and self-actualization. *American Journal of Occupational Therapy, 32,* 305–310.

Fisher, A. G. (1991). Vestibular-proprioceptive processing and bilateral integration and sequencing deficits. In A. G. Fisher, E. A. Murray, & A. C. Bundy (Eds.), *Sensory Integration: Theory and Practice* (pp 71–107). Philadelphia: F.A. Davis.

Fisher, A. G., & Bundy, A. C. (1991). The interpretation process. In A. G. Fisher, E. B. Murray, & A. C. Bundy (Eds.), *Sensory Integration: Theory and Practice* (pp 234–250). Philadelphia: F.A. Davis.

Fox, C. R. (1999). Special senses 3: The visual system. In H. Cohen (Ed.), *Neuroscience for Rehabilitation* (2nd ed., pp. 169–194). Philadelphia: Lippincott Williams & Wilkins.

Fredericks, C. M., & Saladin, L. (1996). *Pathophysiology of motor systems.* Philadelphia: F.A. Davis.

Fuster, J. M. (1997). *The prefrontal cortex: Anatomy, physiology, and neuropsychology of the frontal lobe.* Philadelphia: Lippincott-Raven.

Gentile, A. M. (1972). A working model of skill acquisition with application to teaching. *Quest, 17,* 3–23.

Geschwind, N. (1975). The apraxias: Neural mechanisms of disorders of learned movement. *The American Scientist, 63,* 188–195.

Ghez, C., Gordon, J., & Ghilardi, M. (1990). Roles of proprioceptive input in the programming of arm trajectories. *Cold Spring Harbor Symposium in Quantitative Biology, 55,* 837–847.

Ghilardi, M., Gordon, J., & Ghez, C. (1995). Learning a visuomotor transformation in a local area of workspace produces directional biases in other areas. *Journal of Neurophysiology, 73,* 2535–2539.

Gibson, E. J. (1988). Exploratory behavior in the development of perceiving, acting and the acquiring of knowledge. *Annual Review of Psychology, 39,* 1–41.

Gibson, J. J. (1979) The ecological approach to visual perception. Boston: Houghton-Mifflin.

Gillberg, C. (1983). Perceptual, motor and attentional deficits in Swedish primary school children. Some child psychiatric aspects. *Journal of Child Psychology and Psychiatry, 24,* 377–403.

Gillberg, C., Winnergard, J., & Gillberg, I. C. (1993). Screening methods, epidemiology and evaluation of intervention in DAMP in preschool children. *European Child and Adolescent Psychiatry, 2,* 121–135.

Gliner, J. A. (1985). Purposeful activity in motor learning theory: An event approach to motor skill acquisition. *American Journal of Occupational Therapy, 39,* 28–34.

Goldberg, G. (1985). Supplementary motor area structure and function: Review and hypotheses. *Behavioral and Brain Sciences, 8,* 567–616.

Gray, J. M., Kennedy, B. L., & Zemke, R. (1996). Dynamic systems theory: An overview. In R. Zemke & F. Clark (Eds.), *Occupational science: An evolving discipline* (pp. 297–308). Philadelphia: F.A. Davis.

Graybiel, A. M., & Kimura, M. (1995). Adaptive neural networks in the basal ganglia. In J. C. Houk & J. Davis (Eds.), *Computational neuroscience* (pp. 103–116). Cambridge, MA: The MIT Press.

Graziano, A. S., & Gross, C. G. (1998). Spatial maps for the control of movement. *Current Opinion in Neurobiology, 8,* 195–201.

Gubbay, S. S. (1975). *The clumsy child.* New York: W. B. Saunders.

Gubbay, S. S. (1978). The management of developmental apraxia. *Developmental Medicine and Child Neurology, 20,* 643–646.

Gubbay, S. S. (1979). The clumsy child. In F. C. Rose (Ed.), *Pediatric neurology.* London: Blackwell.

Gubbay, S. S. (1985). Clumsiness. In P. J. Vinken, G. W. Bruyn, & H. L. Klawans (Eds.), *Handbook of clinical neurology* (Rev. series). New York: Elsevier Science.

Guiliani, C. A. (1991). Theories of motor control: New concepts for physical therapy. In *Contemporary Management of Motor Control Problems:*

Proceedings of the II STEP Conference. Alexandria, VA: Foundation for Physical Therapy.

Gunzenhauser, N. (1990). *Advances in touch: New implications in human development.* Skillman, NJ: Johnson & Johnson Consumer Products.

Hall, L. A., & McCloskey, D. I. (1983). Detections of movements imposed on finger, elbow and shoulder joints. *Journal of Physiology, 335,* 519–533.

Harrington, D. L., Rao, S. M., Haaland, K. Y., Bobholz, J. A., Mayer, A. B., Binderix, J. R. (2000). Ideomotor apraxia and cerebral dominance for motor control. *Cognitive Brain Research, 3,* 95–100.

Hecaen, H. (1981). The apraxias. In S. B. Filskov & T. J. Boll (Eds.), *Handbook of clinical neuropsychology* (pp. 257–286). New York: John Wiley & Sons.

Heilman, K. M., & Rothi, L. J. G. (1993). Apraxia. In K. M. Heilman & E. Valenstein (Eds.), *Clinical neuropsychology* (3rd ed., pp. 141–163). New York: Oxford University.

Hellgren, L., Gillberg, C., Gillberg, I. C., & Enerkskog, I. (1993). Children with deficits in attention, motor control, and perception (DAMP) almost grown up: General health at 16 years. *Developmental Medicine and Child Neurology, 35,* 881–892.

Hellgren, L., Gillberg, C., Gillberg, I. C., (1994). Children with deficits in attention, motor control and perception almost grown up. *European Child and Adolescent Psychiatry, 3,* 1–15.

Henderson, S. E. & Barnett, A. L. (1998). The classification of specific motor coordination disorders in children: Some problems to be solved. *Human Movement Science, 17,* 449–469.

Henderson, S. E., & Hall, D. (1982). Concomitants of clumsiness in young schoolchildren. *Developmental Medicine and Child Neurology, 24,* 448–460.

Horak, F. B., Shumway-Cook, A., Crowe, T. K., & Black, F. O. (1988). Vestibular functions and motor proficiency in children with impaired hearing or with learning disability and motor impairments. *Developmental Medicine and Child Neurology, 30,* 64–79.

ICD-9-Clinical Modifications (ICD-9-CM). (2001). Salt Lake City: Medicode.

Ingvar, D. H., & Philopson, L. (1977). Distribution of cerebral blood flow in the dominant hemisphere during motor ideation and motor performance. *Annals of Neurology, 2,* 230–237.

Jackson, J. H. & Taylor, J. (1932). *Selected writings of John B. Hughlings, I and II.* London: Hodder & Stoughter.

Jakobs, T., Miller, J. A. A., & Schultz, A. B. (1985). Trunk position sense in the frontal plane. *Experimental Neurology, 90,* 129–138.

Jami, L. (1992). Golgi tendon organs in mammalian skeletal muscle: Functional properties and central actions. *Physiology Review, 72,* 623–666.

Jeannerod, M. (1988). *The neural and behavioral organization of goal-oriented movements: Oxford psychology series.* Oxford: Clarendon.

Johnson, S. C. (1967). Hierarchical clustering schemes. *Psychometrika, 32,* 241–254.

Jones, E. G., & Porter, R. (1980). What is area 3a? *Brain Research Review, 2,* 1–43.

Jones, L. A. (1999). Somatic senses 3: Proprioception. In H. Cohen (Ed.), *Neuroscience for rehabilitation* (2nd ed., pp. 111–130). Philadelphia: Lippincott, Williams & Wilkins.

Kalaska, J. F. (1988). The representation of arm movements in postcentral and parietal cortex. *Canadian Journal of Physiology and Pharmacology, 66,* 455–463.

Kandel, E. R., Schwartz, J. H., & Jessell, T. M. (2000). *Principles of neural science* (4th ed.). New York: McGraw-Hill.

Kelso, J. A. S. (1982). *Human motor behavior: An introduction.* Hillsdale, NJ: Lawrence Erlbaum Associates.

Kelso, J. A. S., & Stelmach, G. E. (1976). Central and peripheral mechanisms in motor control. In G. Stelmach (Ed.), *Motor control: Issues and trends.* New York: Academic.

Kenealy, P., & Monseth, A. (1994). Music and IQ tests. *The Psychologist, 7,* 346.

Kielhofner, G. (1995). *A model of human occupation: Theory and application* (2nd ed.). Baltimore: Lippincott Williams, & Wilkins.

Kimball, J. (2002). Developmental coordination disorder from a sensory integration perspective. In S. Cermak & D. Larkin (Eds.), *Developmental coordination disorder: Theory and practice* (pp. 210–220). San Diego: Singular.

Kiernan, J. A. (1998). *Barr's the human nervous system: An anatomical viewpoint.* Philadelphia: Lippincott-Raven.

King, L. J. (1978). Toward a science of adaptive responses. *The American Journal of Occupational Therapy, 32,* 429–437.

Kingsley, R. E. (2000). *Concise text of neuroscience.* Philadelphia: Lippincott Williams & Wilkins.

Knuckey, N., & Gubbay, S. S. (1983). Clumsy children: A prognostic study. *Australian Pediatric Journal, 19,* 9–13.

Knuckey, N., Apsimon, T., & Gubbay, S. (1983). Computerized axial tomography in clumsy children with developmental apraxia and agnosia. *Brain and Development, 5,* 14–19.

Kosselyn, S. M., & Koenig, O. (1992). *Wet mind.* New York: Free Press.

Koomar, J. (1999, March) Insurance Reimbursement Survey Results. *Sensory Integration Special Interest Section Quarterly, 22* (1), 1–4.

Lackner, J. R. & DiZio, P. (1988). Gravitational effects on nystagmus and perception of orientation. *Annals of the New York Academy of Sciences, 545,* 93–104.

Lai, J. S., Fisher, A., Magalhaes, L., & Bundy, A. (1996). Construct validity of the sensory integration and praxis tests. *Occupational Therapy Journal of Research, 16,* 75–97.

Landgren, M., Pettersen, R., Kjellman, B., & Gillberg, C. (1996). ADHD, DAMP and other neurodevelopmental disorders in 6-year-old children: Epidemiology and co-morbidity. *Developmental Medicine and Child Neurology, 38,* 891–906.

Larkin, D., & Parker, H. (2002). Task specific interventions for children with DCD: A systems view. In S. Cermak & D. Larkin (Eds.), *Developmental coordination disorder: Theory and practice* (pp. 234–247). San Diego: Singular.

Latash, M. L. (1998). Neurophysiological basis of movement. Champaign, IL: Human Kinetics.

Lee, T. D. (1988). Transfer-appropriate processing: A framework for conceptualizing practice effects in motor learning. In O. G. Meijer & K. Roth (Eds.), *Complex motor behavior: The motor-action controversy* (pp. 201–215). Amsterdam: Elsevier.

Leonard, C. T. (1998). *The neuroscience of human movement.* St. Louis: Mosby.

Levine, M. D. (1984). Cumulative neurodevelopmental debts: Their impact on productivity in late middle childhood. In M. D. Levine & P. Satz (Eds.), *Middle childhood: Development and dysfunction* (pp. 227–243). Baltimore, MD: University Park.

Levine, M. D. (1987). Motor implementation. In M. D. Levine (Ed.), *Developmental variation and learning disorders* (pp. 208–239). Cambridge: Educators Publishing Service.

Lin, K., Wu, C., Tickle-Degen, L., & Coster, W. (1997). Enhancing occupational performance through occupationally embedded exercise: A meta-analytic review. *Occupational Therapy Journal of Research, 17,* 25–47.

Lindner, K. J. (1986). Transfer to motor learning: From formal discipline to action systems theory. In L. D. Zaichkowsky & C. Z. Fuchs (Eds.). *The psychology of motor behavior: Development, control, learning and performance* (pp. 65–87). Ithaca, NY: Movement Publications.

Losse, A., Henderson, S. E., Elliman, D., Hall, D., Knight, E., & Jongmans, M. (1991). Clumsiness in children: Do they grow out of it? A 10-year follow-up study. *Developmental Medicine and Child Neurology, 33,* 55–68.

Lundy-Ekman, L. (1998). *Neuroscience fundamentals for rehabilitation.* Philadelphia: W.B. Saunders.

Luria, A. R. (1963). Restoration of function after brain injury. New York: Pergamon.

Luria, A. R. (1980). *Higher cortical functions in man.* New York: Basic.

Mathiowetz, V., & Haugen, J. B. (1995). Evaluation of motor behavior: Traditional and contemporary views. In C. Trombly (Ed.), *Occupational therapy for physical dysfunction* (4th ed, pp. 510–528). Baltimore: Williams and Wilkins.

Matthews, P. B. C. (1988). Proprioceptors and their contribution to somatosensory mapping: Complex messages require complex processing. *Canadian Journal of Physiology and Pharmacology, 66,* 430–438.

McCloskey, D. I. (1985). Knowledge about muscular contractions. In E. Evarts, S. P. Wise, & B. Blous-

field (Eds.), *The motor system in neurobiology* (pp. 149–153). New York: Elsevier.

McHale, K., & Cermak, S. (1992). Fine motor activities in elementary school: Preliminary findings and provisional implications for children with fine motor problems. *American Journal of Occupational Therapy, 46,* 898–903.

McIntosh, G. C., Brown, S. H., Rice, R. R., & Thaut, M. H. (1997). Rhythmic auditory-motor facilitation of gait patterns in patients with Parkinson's disease. *Journal of Neurology, Neurosurgery and Psychiatry, 62,* 122–126.

McIntosh, G. C., Thaut, M. H., Rice, R. R., Miller, R. A., Rathbun, R. A., & Brault, J. M. (1995). Rhythmic facilitation in gait training of Parkinson's disease. *Annals of Neurology, 38,* 338.

Morasso, P. (1981). Spatial control of arm movements. *Experimental Brain Research, 42,* 223–227.

Morris, M. K. (1997). Developmental dyspraxia. In L. J. G Rothi & K. M. Heilman (Eds.), *Apraxia: The neuropsychology of action* (pp. 245–268). Hove, England: Psychology Press.

Mountcastle, V. B. (1986). The neural mechanisms of cognitive function can now be studied directly. *Trends in Neural Science, 9,* 505–508.

Mulligan, S. (1998). Patterns of sensory integration dysfunction: A confirmatory factor analysis. *American Journal of Occupational Therapy, 52,* 819–828.

Newman, J., Rosenbach, J. H., Burns, K. L., Latimer, B. C., Matocha, H. R., & Vogt, E. R. (1995). An experimental test of "the Mozart effect": Does listening to his music improve spatial ability? *Perceptual and Motor Skills, 81,* 1379–1387.

Passingham, R. (1993). *The frontal lobes and voluntary action.* New York: Oxford University Press.

Phelps, J., Stempel, L., & Speck, G. (1984). The children's handwriting scale: A new diagnostic tool. *Journal of Educational Research, 79,* 46–50.

Piek, J. P., & Coleman-Carman, R. (1995). Kinesthetic sensitivity and motor performance in children with developmental coordination disorder. *Developmental Medicine and Child Neurology, 37,* 976–984.

Poeck, K. (1983). Survey of progress: Ideational apraxia. *Journal of Neurology, 230,* 1–5.

Polatajko, H., Fox, A. M., & Missiuna, C. (1995). An international consensus on children with developmental coordination disorder. *Canadian Journal of Occupational Therapy, 62*(1), 3–6.

Polatajko, H. J., Macnab, J. J., Anstett, B. Malloy-Miller, T., Murphy, K., & Noh, S. (1995). A clinical trial of the process-oriented treatment approach for children with developmental coordination disorder. *Developmental Medicine and Child Neurology, 37,* 310–319.

Portney, L. G., & Watkins, M. P. (2000). *Foundations of clinical research: Applications to practice* (2nd ed.). Upper Saddle River, NJ: Prentice-Hall.

Rauscher, F. H., Robinson, K. D., & Jens, J. J. (1998). Improved maze learning through early music exposure in rats. *Neurological Research, 20,* 427–432.

Rauscher, F. H., Shaw, G. L., & Ky, K. N. (1993).

Music and spatial task performance. *Nature, 365,* 611.

Rauscher, F. H., Shaw, G. L. & Ky, K. N. (1995). Listening to Mozart enhances spatial-temporal task reasoning: Towards a neurophysiological basis. *Neuroscience Letters, 185,* 44–47.

Reed, E. S. (1982). An outline of a theory of action systems. *Journal of Motor Behavior, 14,* 98–134.

Reed, E. (1988). From the motor theory of perception to the perceptual control of action. In E. S. Reed (Ed.), *James J. Gibson and the psychology of perception.* New Haven, CT: Yale University.

Reisman, J. (1991). Poor handwriting: Who is referred? *American Journal of Occupational Therapy, 45,* 849–852.

Reisman, J. (1999). *Minnesota handwriting assessment.* San Antonio: The Psychological Corporation.

Roland, P., Skinhoj, E., Lassen, N. A., & Larsen, B. (1980). Different cortical areas in man in organization of voluntary movements in extracorporeal space. *Journal of Neurophysiology, 43,* 137–150.

Rothi, L. J. G., & Heilman K.M. (Eds.) (1997). *Apraxia: The neuropsychology of action.* Philadelphia: Psychology Press.

Royeen, C. B. (1989). Provisional guidelines for the process of data analysis in clinical research. In C. B. Royeen (Ed.), *Clinical research handbook: An analysis for the service professions.* Thorofare, NJ: Slack.

Ryding, E., Decety, J., Sjoholm, H., Stenberg, G., & Ingvar, D. H. (1993). Motor imagery activates the cerebellum regionally. *Cognitive Brain Research, 2,* 94–99.

Schilder, P. (1935). *The image and appearance of the human body.* London: Routledge & Kegan Paul.

Safire, W. (1989, June 11). On language: Rethinking reclama. *The New York Times,* p. F18.

Schmidt, R. A. (1988). *Motor control and learning: A behavioral emphasis.* Champaign, IL: Human Kinematics.

Schmidt, R. A. (1991). Motor learning principles for physical therapy. In *Contemporary management of motor control problems: Proceedings of the II STEP Conference.* Alexandria, VA: Foundation for Physical Therapy.

Schmidt, R. A. & Lee, T. (1999). *Motor control and learning: A behavioral emphasis.* Champaign, IL: Human Kinematics.

Shaw, L., Levine, M., & Belfer, M. (1982). Developmental double jeopardy: A study of clumsiness and self-esteem in children with learning problems. *Journal of Developmental Behavior Pediatrics, 3,* 191–196.

Shea, J. B. & Morgan, R. (1979). Contextual interference effects on the acquisition, retention, and transfer of a motor skill. *Journal of Experimental Psychology: Human Learning and Memory, 5,* 179–187.

Shea, J. B. & Titzer, R. C. (1993). The influence of reminder trials on contextual interference effects. *Journal of Motor Behavior, 25,* 264–274.

Shea, J. B. & Zimny, S. T. (1983). Context effects in memory and learning movement information. In R. A. Magill (Ed.), *Memory and control of action* (pp. 345–366). Amsterdam: Elsevier.

Shoemaker, M. M. & Kalverboer, A. F. (1994). Social and affective problems of children who are clumsy. How early do they begin? *Adapted Physical Activity Quarterly, 11,* 130–140.

Shumway-Cook, A., Horak, F., & Black, F. O. (1987). A critical examination of vestibular function in motor-impaired learning disabled children. *International Journal of Pediatric Otorhinolaryngology, 14,* 21–30.

Shumway-Cook, A., & Woollacott, M. (1995). *Motor control: Theory and practical applications.* Baltimore: Williams & Wilkins.

Sirigu, A., Cohen, L., Duhamel, J., & Pillon, B. (1995). A selective impairment of hand posture for object utilization in apraxia. *Cortex, 31,* 41–55.

Smyth, M. M., & Anderson, H. I. (2000). Coping with clumsiness in the school playground: Social and physical play in children with coordination impairments. *British Journal of Developmental Psychology, 18,* 389–413.

Snyder, L. H., Batista, A. P., & Andersen, R. A. (1997). Coding of intention in the posterior parietal cortex. *Nature, 386,* 167–170.

Stelmach, G. (Ed.) (1976). *Motor control: Issues and trends.* New York: Academic.

Stockmeyer, S. (1967). An interpretation of the approach of Rood to the treatment of neuromuscular dysfunction. *American Journal of Physical Medicine, 46*(4), 900–956.

Stough, C., Kerkin, B., Bates, T., & Mangan, G. (1994). Music and IQ tests. *The Psychologist, 7,* 253.

Sugden, D. A., & Keogh, J. F. (1990). *Problems in movement skill development.* Columbia, SC: University of South Carolina Press.

Sugden, D. A., & Wright, H. C. (1998). *Motor coordination disorders in children.* Thousand Oaks, CA: Sage.

Szklut, S. E., Cermak, S. A., & Henderson, A. (1995). Learning disabilities. In D. A. Umphred (Ed.), *Neurological rehabilitation* (3rd ed., pp. 312–359). St. Louis: Mosby.

Thaut, M. H., Lange, H., Miltner, R., Hurt, C. P., & Hoemberg, V. (1996). Rhythmic entrainment of gait patterns in Huntington's disease patients. *Society for Neuroscience Abstracts, 6,* 727.

Thaut, M. H., McIntosh, G. C., Rice, R. R., & Prassas, S. G. (1995). Effect of auditory stimulation on gait kinematics in hemiparetic stroke patients. *Journal of Neurological Rehabilitation, 9,* 131.

Thaut, M. H., Miller, R. A., & Schauer, L. M. (1998). Multiple synchronization strategies in rhythmic sensorimotor tasks: Period vs. phase corrections. *Biological Cybernetics, 73,* 241–250.

Thelen, E., & Smith, L. B. (1994). *A dynamic systems approach to the development of cognition and action.* Cambridge, MA: The MIT Press.

Thelen, E. (1995). Motor development: A new synthesis. *American Psychologist, 50:* 79–95.

Vierck, C. J. (1978). Interpretations of the sensory and motor consequences of dorsal column lesions. In G. Gordon (Ed.), *Active touch: The mechanisms of recognition of objects by manipulation: A multidisciplinary approach* (pp.139–160). Oxford: Pergamon.

Wall, P. D. (1970). Sensory role of impulses traveling in the dorsal columns. *Brain, 93,* 505–524.

Weiss, T., Hansen, E., Rost, R., Beyer, L., Merten, F., Nichelmann, C., & Zippel, C . (1994). Mental practice of motor skills used in poststroke rehabilitation has own effects on central nervous activation. *International Journal of Neuroscience, 78,* 157–166.

Wolpert, D. M., Ghahramani, Z., & Jordan, M. I. (1995). An internal model for sensorimotor integration. *Science, 269,* 1880–1882.

World Health Organization (1993). *The ICD-10 classification of mental and behavioral disorders. Diagnostic criteria for research.* New York: Churchill-Livingstone.

Wright, H. C. (1997). Children with developmental co-ordination disorder: A review. *European Journal of Physical Education, 2,* 5–22.

Zoltan, B. (1996). *Vision, perception and cognition.* Thorofare, NJ: Slack.

4

Sensory Modulation

Shelly J. Lane, PhD, OTR/L, FAOTA

> *Only recently has the professional literature begun to describe sensory modulation dysfunction. Practicing clinicians desperately need rigorous study designs to provide empirical data related to this disorder. Only through implementing and reporting well-controlled, rigorous studies will investigators be able to answer questions such as, Is SMD a valid syndrome? Does occupational therapy help ameliorate the condition? What are the underlying mechanisms in the disorder?*
>
> *—Miller, L. J. & Summer, C., 2002.*

Sensory processing . . . sensory registration . . . sensory integration . . . sensory modulation . . . sensory responsiveness . . . We use these terms both academically and clinically, yet from one clinic to another, from one academic institution to another, and even from one profession to another, the intended meaning of the terms may differ. Adding complexity, some of these terms suggest neural functions, some suggest the outward behavioral manifestation of what we assume to be neural functions, and some have been used interchangeably to imply either. To avoid confusion, we begin this chapter with some definitions. Relationships between the terms are depicted in Figure 4–1. After the definitions, we examine modulation, first on a cellular level and then on a systems and behavioral level. Next we explain the concept of sensory modulation dysfunction (SMD). Hypothesized links to the limbic system and a proposed relationship between modulation dysfunction and stress leads to a discussion of these issues as well. We discuss specific types of modulation dysfunction within the tactile and vestibular-proprioceptive

systems. We close with a brief look at defensiveness within the visual, auditory, and taste and smell systems. First however, we look at Michael, a child with an SMD.

MICHAEL

Observed in the classroom, Michael appears to not be paying attention to the lesson at hand. He is very quiet and does not volunteer information that adds to the discussion under way. His teacher questions if he is processing the information at all. Michael is currently classified by the school system as "other health impaired." He has an individualized education program (IEP) and receives both educational assistance and occupational therapy. His IEP states that one of his needs is for the opportunity to get more movement and deep pressure input during the day, in order to improve his ability to attend and process. Incorporating this input throughout the school day is becoming difficult because in, fifth grade, Michael's teachers are not comfortable with the accommodations in the classroom, and

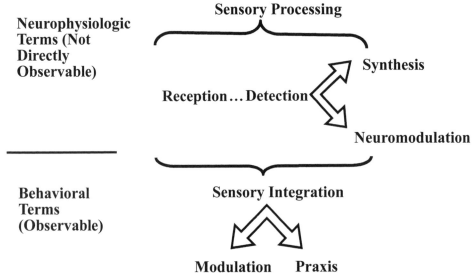

Neurophysiologic Terms (Not Directly Observable)

Sensory Processing

Reception … Detection

Synthesis

Neuromodulation

Behavioral Terms (Observable)

Sensory Integration

Modulation   Praxis

■ FIGURE 4-1 Proposed relationship among neurophysiologic and behavioral terms.

Michael is less comfortable with anything that makes him appear different from his classmates.

A recent Sensory Profile (Dunn, 1999) indicated that Michael underresponds to sensation available in the environment and seeks additional movement and deep touch input throughout his daily routines. Overall, it was determined that Michael has a deficit in sensory modulation, most clearly seen with diminished responsiveness and sensory seeking behavior within the vestibular and proprioceptive systems. These modulation difficulties are linked to both behavioral and emotional regulation problems, presenting as difficulty paying attention to tasks at hand, a tendency to not attend within an active environment, and a high level of emotional reactivity to sensory input. These sensory processing difficulties are very consistent with those over which his mother, Mrs. S., has expressed concern, and are of a nature to impair his ability to work within the classroom.

TERMINOLOGY

Background of Terminology

Terminology associated with sensory integration and sensory modulation falls into at least two categories reflecting neurophysiological processes and behavior. Terms that have neurophysiological definitions include:

- Sensory processing
- Stimulus detection, or detection of sensation

- Integration of sensation or inputs
- Neuromodulation

Other terms suggest something more behavioral than neurophysiological. These include:

- Sensory registration
- Sensory responsiveness
- Some uses of "sensory integration" (as in "He has good sensory integration.")

Being clear on the intent of such terms guides practitioners as they interact with professionals who may not be familiar with the manner in which we use such terms (Miller & Lane, 2000). A diagram is provided in Figure 4–1 to guide readers in understanding the relationship among the definitions provided in this chapter.

Definitions

Processing is the verb form of *process*. A process is defined as "a course or method of operations in the production of something; a series of continuous actions that bring about a particular result" (*Funk & Wagnalls Standard Dictionary,* 1991, p. 633.). As applied to the sensory systems, processing is a broad term that encompasses all that goes on with a sensory signal, including its reception in the periphery, our central detection of this information, its (sometimes multiple) transformations between electrical and chemical signals, and its interaction with other activity within the nervous system. Miller and Lane (2000) defined sensory processing as encompassing "reception, modulation, integration, and organization of sensory stimuli, including behavioral responses to sensory input." (p. 2). *Processing* does not capture the adaptive environmental interaction that we observe; instead, it represents the broader tasks of the nervous system as it deals with incoming information.

Sensory registration is a term that has been used clinically to describe the behavior of noticing sensory stimuli in the environment (Miller & Lane, 2000). To register is to show, record, or document; to make an impression; or to have an effect (*Random House College Dictionary,* 1975). However, *registration* is not a term used in neuroscience literature to reflect the process of taking in and recording sensory information from the environment in such a way as to affect ongoing activity. Used in this way, to include these CNS activities, a better term is *sensory detection.* To *detect* is to discover, manage, or perceive something; to discover the presence, existence, or fact of something (*Random House College Dictionary,* 1975; Webster, 1988). As such, the term *sensory detection* is more consistent with the neurophysiological literature and reflects CNS activity in response to sensory input.

Miller and Lane (2000) defined sensory detection as "the first step that occurs centrally. Incoming sensory information is recorded at multiple levels within the CNS so that it can affect ongoing neural activity . . . by influencing the overall level of activity in the CNS" (p. 3). Thus, in usual situations, sensory detection and the subsequent processing of information are intimately related; sensation makes an impression or has an effect (detection) that is handled in a routine and orderly manner (processed) to allow for adaptive interactions.

Synthesis is a term that represents the neural functions of inter- and intramodal interactions of sensory information that occur at multisensory neurons. Although this could easily be called *integration,* to use this term here leads to confusion. We reserve the phrase *sensory integration* for the bigger, observable sequence of events from reception to the display of an adaptive environmental interaction. Thus, *synthesis* is used to show that after sensory information is received and detected, it must interact with other CNS activities in preparation for the production of observable behavior and adaptive environmental interaction.

Integration is defined as the act of combining into an integral whole behavior in harmony with the environment (*Random House College Dictionary,* 1975). Lane et al. (2000) noted that the term *sensory integration* is used in several contexts and can mean different things, depending on the speaker. As a neurophysiological process, integration within the CNS can be *intrasensory,* in which input from many fiber pathways within one sensory system converges on a single neuron, or group of neurons, to influence ongoing activity. Integration within the CNS can also be *intersensory,* wherein information from multiple sources converges onto a neuron or group of neurons, again influencing ongoing activity. Thus, *sensory integration,* from a neurophysiological perspective, is the process of combining sensation between or within a sensory system (synthesis).

The term *sensory integration* also reflects behavior. Ayres defined it as "the neurological process that organizes sensation from one's own body and from the environment and makes it possible to use the body effectively within the environment" (Ayres, 1979, p. 11). In her early work, Ayres (1972b) defined *sensory integration* as the behavioral manifestation of adequate sensory reception, registration, and synthesis. As deceptively simple as this sounds, integration of sensory information leading to the production of adaptive environmental interactions is a complex central nervous system (CNS) activity.

Sensory integration results in modulation and praxis. To *modulate* is to regulate or adjust to a certain level; to tone down; to adapt to the circumstances (*Random House College Dictionary,* 1975). Neuromodulation, or the modulation of neural activity at the cellular level, is what occurs within the CNS as excitatory and inhibitory inputs from both the external and internal environment are balanced and responses generated. Neuromodulation is a CNS skill. Applied to sensory systems, neuromodulation reflects the balancing of excitatory and inhibitory inputs and adapting to environmental changes.

On a behavioral level, *modulation* refers to responses that match the demands and expectations of the environment. According to McIntosh et al. (1999, p. 1), it is "the ability to regulate and organize reactions to sensory input in a graded and adaptive manner."

Sensory modulation is a dynamic CNS process that is subject to the ebb and flow of continual input over multiple channels. Behaviorally, it is reflected in sensory seeking and sensory avoiding (Dunn, 1999; McIntosh et al., 1999; Parham & Mailloux, 1996). Poor modulation may also be manifested in distractibility, impulsiveness, increased activity level, disorganization, anxiety, and poor self-regulation (Ayres, 1972a; Cohn et al., 1999).

Responsiveness, derived from *respond,* means to react or reply. *Random House College Dictionary* (1975) defined responsive as "reacting readily to influences, appeals, efforts, etc." (p. 1125). Thus, although modulation is a CNS process of balancing inhibitory and excitatory inputs, behaviors such as overresponsiveness or defensiveness and underresponsiveness (which has also been termed *dormancy* [Knickerbocker, 1980; Royeen & Lane, 1991]) have been noted to be reflections of this process; they suggest modulation dysfunction. We observe the *behavioral* response, the over- or underresponsiveness; from these behaviors, we *infer* that neural modulation of sensory information is faulty.

MODULATION

Modulation of sensory input is critical to our ability to engage in daily occupations. Filtering of sensations and attending to those that are relevant, maintaining an optimal level of arousal, and maintaining attention to task all require modulation. When modulation is inadequate, attention may be continually diverted to ongoing changes in the sensory environment. We become distracted and attend to all input; this alters our arousal state such that it is no longer optimal.

Modulation as a Physiological Process at the Cellular Level

The definition of modulation is to adapt or adjust to the circumstances. Within the CNS, modulation is reflected in neuronal activity that is enhanced or dampened in response to various sources of input to meet current demands. At the cellular level, both sensory receptor cells in the periphery and neuronal cells within the CNS may become more or less responsive to input. An incoming sensory signal is received by a receptor specific to that signal. The receptor can be highly responsive to input or, over time, can adapt to continued input and cease to respond. After reception, a stimulus must be transduced into an electrical signal to be carried to the CNS. As noted in Chapter 2, transduction involves

changing the energy of the initial signal (e.g., sound waves for the auditory system or movement for the vestibular system) into electrical and chemical energy. When these changes are of sufficient strength, an electrical signal, known as an *action potential,* is generated and carried to the cell body of the first order neuron. From this initial point of entry, the electrical signal can be propagated to interact with the cell bodies, other axons, or dendrites of other neurons within the CNS.

At the synapse, or point of interaction between neurons, the electrical signal changes to a chemical signal and activates neurotransmission. Neurotransmitters are released and travel across the synaptic cleft to interact with specific receptors on the postsynaptic membrane. Figure 4–2 depicts this process schematically.

For simplicity, we will maintain the perspective that transmitters are strictly excitatory or inhibitory. Because more than one axon makes contact with the same postsynaptic neuron, there will potentially be competing inputs, some excitatory and others inhibitory and some strong and others weak. Thus, no single input is likely to excite the postsynaptic membrane sufficiently to send the message on further. What determines if the signal will be further propagated is, to some extent, the algebraic sum of all inputs. Factors such as the strength and frequency of input and the location of the synapse relative to the cell body influence this sum as well. Thus, modulation at the cellular level comes from activation of specific inputs to a cell; increasing excitatory inputs result in the postsynaptic cell firing and sending the information forward. Increased inhibitory inputs will "block" further transmission of the impulse. In Figure 4–3, this is simplistically diagrammed. Here there is a preponderance of inhibitory inputs; thus, the target cell (shaded) will be *inhibited* from firing.

As an example, consider a very simplified version of the nervous system such as that depicted in Figure 4–3. Neuron A carries sensation from a sharp, quick pinch and releases an excitatory neurotransmitter onto the postsynaptic membrane. Intense or repeated signals activate the postsynaptic cell to further transmission of the signal, say to the thalamus, where the sensation of pain could be identified. However, if the pinched spot is pressed on or rubbed, another set of incoming neurons is activated, (e.g., neuron B), carrying deep pressure. Assume this new input makes a connection with the same central neuron but leads to the release of an

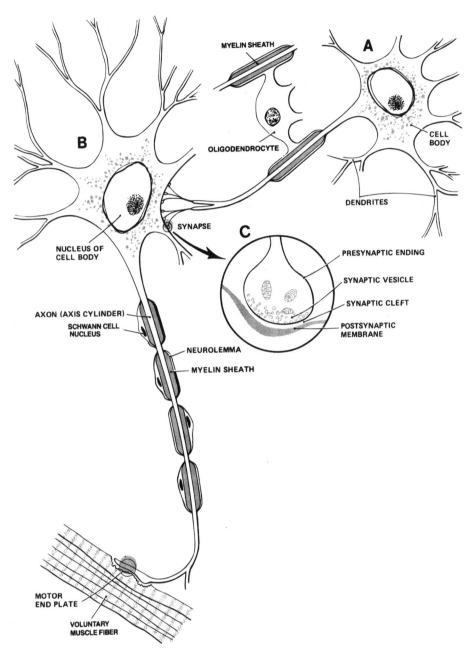

■ FIGURE 4–2 Synapse and synaptic transmission. Neuron A is shown synapsing with neuron B. This synapse is shown in greater detail in C, where the presynaptic visible, synaptic cleft, and postsynaptic membrane are indicated. Neuron A is also shown, surrounded by projections from an oligodendrocyte (a glial cell; see Chap. 2 for more information on neurons and glia). (Adapted from Gilman and Newman, 1992 and reprinted with permission from Gilman, S, and Newman, SW: Essentials of Clinical Neuroanatomy and Neurophysiology, (9th ed) p. 4, Philadelphia, F. A. Davis, 1992.)

inhibitory transmitter. If the signal ratio were one to one (i.e., one pinch activation for one deep pressure rub activation) with similar strength and contact point, then one signal would cancel the other and there would be no propagation of input and no sensation of pain. However, if the pinch is intense or prolonged, an increase in the frequency or intensity of transmission over the deep pressure neuron might be needed to completely cancel the sensation of pain. Even without a complete cancellation, transmission of this painful input is *modulated*, or not as intense as it would have been without the

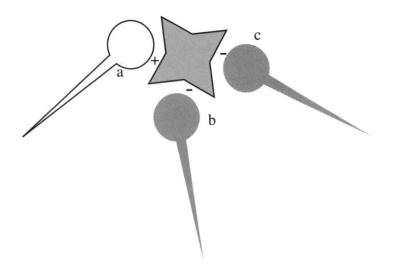

■ Figure 4–3 Balancing excitatory and inhibitory inputs. This neuron (shaded) receives both excitatory (neuron a, white) and inhibitory (neurons b and c, gray) inputs. In this figure the sum of inputs would favor inhibition of further neurotransmission.

deep pressure. In Figure 4–3, neuron c may come from higher level centers in the thalamus. The combination of inhibition from the periphery and the CNS in this case cancel further transmission of pain; it does not reach the level of the CNS required for sensory detection.

Clearly, single cell input to the CNS offers a greatly oversimplified perspective on modulation, but it does provide a useful place to start. The interconnectivity of the CNS is very complex, and many factors influence modulation. Still, the bottom line at the cellular level is that some inputs are excitatory and some are inhibitory; some are strong and some are weak; some are fast and some are slow. The algebraic sum of these factors, along with some essential characteristics of the synapse, determines what the CNS experiences from the periphery and what it does with this information. If we make a cautionary link to the next level, these same concepts can be used to develop a parallel understanding of modulation from a sensory system and behavioral level.

Modulation at the Level of Systems and Behavior

Separating neurophysiological systems from behavior is difficult because we only see systems at work when we observe behavior. Thus, we will look at behavioral and neurophysiological modulation together. However, readers are encouraged to distinguish between descriptions of behavior and those of neurophysiological processes.

If we view the cellular model more realistically,

it becomes clear that many neurons are receiving inputs from many sources simultaneously. CNS structures process incoming input and generate responses that reflect acceptably modulated behavior. Ayres (1979) defined modulation as "the process of increasing or reducing activity to keep the activity in harmony with all functions of the nervous system" (p. 182). Modulation allows a person to respond to relevant input, to not respond to what is irrelevant, and to do so in a manner that promotes adaptive environmental interaction. According to Parham (personal communication, February 1999), modulation facilitates engagement in satisfying and meaningful occupations. Parham maintained that appropriate modulation of sensory input lays a foundation for occupation; this CNS function allows us to engage successfully in self-care, play, and work.

The act of balancing excitatory and inhibitory inputs in the CNS and responding only to those that are relevant (i.e., our work to "maintain harmony") goes on subconsciously. For most, the ability to generate a modulated behavioral response is present, albeit unrefined, at birth. For instance, a fatigued infant begins to cry, finds a thumb, and begins to suck. The clinician may infer that by using somatosensory input (deep pressure to the mouth), the infant has modulated his or her emotional response and has found a way to behave in a socially acceptable manner—to self-calm. Deep pressure and touch within the mouth, transmitted through the somatosensory system, provided sufficient inhibitory input to the cells in the CNS to modulate arousal.

As the nervous system matures, develops more connections, and grows myelin, the ability to modulate one sensory system's activity, via input to another system, becomes refined. This internal growth and development is supplemented by environmental inputs, instilling an understanding of appropriate environmental interactions and how such an interaction is generated.

At some point early in development, the art of modulating behavior through the use of sensation becomes personalized. What works for one does not necessarily work for another. One mother learns early on that close chest-to-chest contact is the only means of quieting her infant. Rocking, bouncing, and patting all seem to increase the infant's agitation rather than help her settle down. In periods of quiet alertness, this baby enjoys these latter inputs, but when she is upset, they only make it worse. Another mother finds that her infant needs to be rocked or jiggled; cuddling alone is insufficient to help this second baby calm down. Different sensations work to help these infants modulate their arousal and anxiety. This was true for Michael; however, he never found tactile input acceptable, and his ability to interpret and modulate tactile input was compromised and he always found it disruptive to his nervous system.

To further illustrate this concept, consider toddlers in a play group using a slide. We see one child, Beth, who is very excited about this opportunity. She has been running in circles from the bottom of the slide to the stairs for several minutes, and this looks like a great way to use up her energy. However, she gets more and more excited each time she gets to slide down the slide. She runs back to the stairs for more but seems to become less coordinated with each turn, finally slipping on the stairs on the way up and screaming in frustration. She requires the intervention of a child care worker before she can calm down and move on to another activity.

Sam, on the other hand, has been sitting and watching, seemingly not looking forward to a turn on the slide or any other activity, for that matter. The care provider guides him to the slide, assists him in the climb, and offers support the first time down. He smiles, walks back to the steps, and looks for assistance to do it again. The next time, Sam climbs alone, checks in with the care provider, and slides alone; another smile emerges. After four or five slides, he is finished and becomes invested in some blocks and cars in another part of the room.

In this instance, the same activity, sliding, increased arousal in both children, but the input had a very different modulatory impact on their behavior. For Beth, the slide was fun but was disorganizing in the long run. Based on her behavior, we infer that the ongoing vestibular and proprioceptive sensations raised her level of arousal beyond the point of adaptive environmental interaction. She needed to pull back and receive another form of input (i.e., comforting from the caregiver) before she was ready for another activity. For Sam, the sliding was activating. His apparently low level of arousal and sensory detection were increased through this activity and, for Sam, this was critical for improving his ability to generate subsequent environmental interactions.

SENSORY MODULATION DYSFUNCTION

A strict definition of modulation includes only toning down, or tempering, CNS responsiveness to input. SMD is more encompassing in that it encompasses modulation dysfunction reflecting both too little and too much "toning down." Hanft et al. (2000) described SMD as:

> a pattern of DSI [dysfunction of sensory integration] in which a person under- or over-responds to sensory input from the body or environment. It is a mismatch between the external contextual demands of a person's world (e.g. culture, environment, tasks, and relationships) and a person's internal characteristics (p. 1).

Over- and underresponsiveness were once thought to represent a continuum (Fisher & Murray, 1991; Knickerbocker, 1980; Koomar & Bundy, 1991; Royeen & Lane, 1991; Williams & Shellenberger, 1994). Although this is a useful simplification, it is no longer an adequate way to depict what we see in children.

A Brief Historical Overview

Knickerbocker (1980) introduced the term *sensory defensiveness* to describe a disorganized response to sensory input resulting from an imbalance between inhibition and excitation within the CNS. The imbalance led to too little inhibition and a consequent flood of input reaching higher CNS structures. Defensive behaviors were the result of this flood. Knickerbocker suggested that such defensiveness could be observed in the olfactory (O), tactile (T), and auditory (A) systems, and called this the "OTA triad." Children with such sensory defensiveness were characterized as overly active, hyperverbal, distractible, and disorganized.

Knickerbocker (1980) also described sensory dormancy that was characterized by disorganized and immature behavior but was thought to result from excessive inhibition of incoming sensory input and a lack of sensory arousal. Dormancy could be observed in the olfactory, tactile, and auditory systems. Knickerbocker described a child experiencing sensory dormancy as being quiet and compliant.

Ayres (1972b) previously had alluded to the concept of a triad of defensiveness, and Knickerbocker's work served as an extension of this. Cermak (1988), Royeen (1989), and Royeen and Lane (1991) further hypothesized that sensory defensiveness and sensory dormancy together formed a continuum, with overresponsiveness at one end and a failure to respond at the other. They suggested that, for at least some children, this continuum was circular, allowing for fluctuations between sensory defensiveness and dormancy in response to environmental sensations. However, Lai et al. (1999) recently examined the relationship between behaviors on the two ends of this proposed continuum and concluded that although defensiveness and dormancy may be related, there is insufficient evidence to conclude that they are signs of the same dysfunction.

Current Conceptualizations

Children who *underrespond* fail to react to the intensity or frequency of a sensory experience in the expected way. Their responses seem dulled or overly modulated. For these children, it takes a lot to get the behavioral system (or systems) activated. Lane et al. (2000) stated that the term *underresponsiveness* suggests a less intense reaction than that seen in most individuals under the same circumstances.

Dunn (1997, 1999) proposed a conceptual model that links the neurological threshold to behavioral responsiveness. In this model, children who underrespond to sensory information are said to have a high neurological threshold that requires a lot of input to reach the threshold and elicit a response. Children who are underresponsive may

seek stronger sensation or be unaware of input as it comes into their CNS. They are prone to danger or injury because of their underresponsiveness and underreactivity. Although practitioners may not consider Sam (presented previously) to have a sensory modulation problem, his environmental interactions reflect underresponsiveness to sensations available in the environment and through activity. He needs a lot of input to get going. Using Dunn's terminology, he has a high threshold to input. Michael would also be considered underresponsive to sensation because he continues to need intense vestibular and proprioceptive sensations to allow for appropriate environmental interactions.

Children who *overrespond* to sensory input react very strongly—and often negatively—to sensory input. In Dunn's model, these children are considered to have a low neurological threshold, meaning it takes very little to activate them. They are often described as having sensory defensiveness because of their strong negative reactions to sensations that most of us do not perceive as negative. Sensations to which they are overly sensitive lead to avoidance and withdrawal behaviors or when this is not possible, they may lash out at the source of the input. According to Lane et al. (2000), these responses to sensation may reflect activation of the sympathetic nervous system.

In the only empirical research on children with SMD, McIntosh et al. (1999) demonstrated differences in electrodermal response (EDR) measures between children with and without SMD when presented with a sensory challenge protocol. The protocol involved presenting 10 trials each of olfactory, auditory, visual, tactile, and vestibular stimuli. Children's EDRs were recorded after each presentation. Two discrete groups of children with SMD were identified: those with hyperresponsive electrodermal activity and those with hyporesponsiveness. Hyperresponsive children showed more responses, responses of greater magnitude, and responses that habituated more slowly than those seen in matched control subjects. Furthermore, these investigators demonstrated that the EDR could predict children's response pattern on the Short Sensory Profile (McIntosh et al., 1999).

Earlier, this same group of investigators had also identified both hyperresponsiveness and hyporesponsiveness in children with fragile X syndrome using the same sensory challenge protocol (Miller et al., 1999). In this work, they found a strong correlation across sensory modalities, suggesting the existence of a generalized dysfunction that crossed all sensory systems, similar to SMD in children without fragile X syndrome. The authors suggested that the response patterns identified in the children with SMD alone "resembles an attenuated form of the pattern in people with fragile X syndrome." They recommended additional research to clarify the similarities and differences between these groups (Miller et al., 1999). Although, as these investigators suggested, this work left many questions unanswered, it has also provided practitioners with the first concrete evidence that there are physiological correlates of the modulation behaviors we have seen clinically.

Clinicians have reported that some children seem to be underresponsive at times but overresponsive at other times. Based on early clinical information, Royeen and Lane (1991) hypothesized a more complex, circular relationship between over- and underresponsiveness. In this model, the shift between under- and overresponsiveness did not require moving from one end of a continuum to the other. Instead, it suggested that a child might exhibit defensive reactions to sensory input until overload led to a shut down in the processing of sensory input. Shutdown then led to the behaviors associated with underresponsiveness. A current conceptualization of this relationship is seen in Figure 4–4, suggesting that there is a group of children who may either over- or underrespond to environmental sensation, but there are also children who fall consistently into one category or the other.

Some support for this conceptualization of over- and underresponsiveness has been found in a recent analysis of data related to sensory processing. Lai et al. (1999) demonstrated a significant relationship between tactile defensiveness (at the overresponsive end of the continuum) and tactile dormancy (at the underresponsive end of the continuum). However, they concluded that the association was not of sufficient strength to warrant the conclusion that over- and underresponsivity to touch are expressions of the same SMD. Further research is needed.

The clinical experiences of other authors (Dunn, 1997; Parham & Mailloux, 1996; Wilbarger, 1993; Wilbarger & Wilbarger, 1991) have led them to suggest that sensory modulation is multidimensional, rather than representing a continuum. The problem, according to these authors, is not so much that children always over- or underrespond to sensation but that their behavior reflects poor modulation and its many ramifications. Responsiveness shifts reflect children's difficulty finding the middle ground where the appropriate level of modulation exists to allow them to interact adaptively with the environment. The resultant behaviors reflect a cascade of events within the CNS that affect attention, arousal, emotional stability, and cognitive processing. This proposal requires further investigation; the work of McIntosh et al. (1999) neither confirmed nor negated this possibility.

In summary, clinicians have identified children with SMD who overrespond to sensory input, those who underrespond, and those who fluctuate between these responsive behaviors. The behavior of

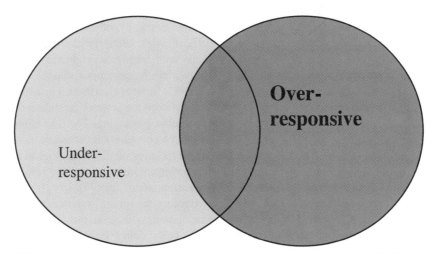

■ FIGURE 4–4 Hypothesized relationship between under- and overresponsiveness in children with modulation disorders. (Note: The proportions in this diagram are not necessarily representative of true proportions; at present they are not known.)

a child who overresponds is characterized by quick, exaggerated reactions to sensation, and at times, withdrawal from such input. They may avoid experiences, thereby limiting the amount of sensation they receive. Children who underrespond may seem to process slowly or they may seek out intense sensory input (Dunn, 1999; Hanft et al., 2000). Such behavioral responses are not necessarily consistent from day to day, and children may sometimes overrespond to sensory input and at other times underrespond to the same input. Such fluctuations make some clinicians believe the two behaviors are part of a unified underlying dysfunction. However, according to Lai et al (1999), although the two are likely related, we lack sufficient information to claim that a single dysfunction exists. Furthermore, although clinicians address subcategories of disorders, including tactile defensiveness; gravitational insecurity; and defensiveness to smell and taste, sound, and light, the work of McIntosh et al. (1999) suggested a more general underlying SMD in which poor modulation in the different systems appears to be related. Much more information is needed to clarify these issues.

Proposed Central Nervous System Links to Sensory Modulation Dysfunction

Aside from the above information that links SMD to electrodermal responsiveness and potentially to the sympathetic nervous system (Miller et al., 1999), our understanding of the mechanisms that underlie sensory modulation deficits remains primarily hypothesis. Ayres (1964) proposed several possible mechanisms for understanding tactile defensiveness, and later, more generally, defensiveness in other systems (Ayres, 1972b, 1979). Ayres' hypotheses have created an interest in seeking more information about modulation disorders. We still have work to do in this area.

Sensory Modulation and the Limbic System

Royeen and Lane (1991) hypothesized that modulation dysfunction may have its roots in regions of the limbic system and hypothalamus. The source of this proposal lies in the functions of these structures. Unfortunately, the functions of the limbic system remain unclear. Called the "mediator of all things emotional" (Restak, 1995, p. 18), the limbic system includes three cortical areas (i.e., the cingulate gyrus, septum, and parahippocampal gyrus) and the gray matter areas of the hippocampus and amygdala. The limbic system receives input from all cerebral lobes and connecting fibers and projects back to these areas as well as extensively within itself. It plays a role in learning and memory; eating and drinking behaviors; aggression; sexual behavior; and, importantly motivation and expression of emotion (Gilman & Newman, 1996; Isaacson, 1982).

Restak said the purpose of limbic function was "[to] integrate and coordinate both our outer- and inner-world experiences into unity" (p. 20). As such, the limbic system is a likely candidate for involvement in SMD.

Royeen and Lane (1991) suggested that involvement of the limbic system:

(a) provides an explanation for the emotional or social difficulties often accompanying tactile and sensory defensiveness, (b) accounts for the presence of defensiveness or dormancy across sensory systems, and (c) allows for extreme shifts or inconsistencies in responsivity (from defensiveness to dormancy) that may be observed in an individual either with regard to a single sensory system or across sensory systems (p. 122).

Miller et al.'s (1999) recent empirical investigation of sensory processing in children with fragile X syndrome supports this suggestion. These investigators demonstrated EDR differences in response to sensory challenge between children with fragile X syndrome and age- and gender-matched controls. The EDR is mediated, in part, by the limbic-hypothalamic system (Edelberg, 1972; Fowles, 1986). Furthermore, studies of patients with fragile X syndrome have implicated the caudate, hippocampus, and thalamus (Reiss et al., 1995; Reiss et al., 1994). Thus, there may be a link between the sensory modulation differences and limbic processing. The link is tentative, and Miller et al. (1999) recommend continued "research focusing on the physiological and anatomical underpinnings of abnormal responses to sensory stimulation" (p. 277).

Because the limbic system may be involved in modulation, a look at the functions associated with its structures is warranted. Studies of the limbic system have largely used animal models. As always, caution must be exercised in making the leap from animal studies to function within the human nervous system. Nonetheless, much can be learned by examining this work.

The septum (septum pellucidum) is one limbic region of great interest. The physiological significance of this structure is only vaguely understood (Kingsley, 2000). Older literature suggested a role in the modulation of pleasure (Isaacson, 1982). Activation has been shown to result in reward-seeking behavior in rats with similar, although much more variable, findings in humans. In humans, activation leads to a significant sense of well being (Kingsley, 2000). The septum is thought to exert an inhibitory influence on the autonomic nervous system (ANS) and to play a role in the use of environmental stimulation; it permits the organism to attend to any stimulus in the environment, even those having low stimulus value (Isaacson, 1982). Thus, in a normal state, this part of the limbic system may be said to contribute to the ability to interact successfully with the environment and, as such, it likely plays a role in sensory modulation.

Lesions of the septal region have been shown to result in transient hyperemotionality in many rodents and humans (Isaacson, 1982). The increased emotionality can be reduced with handling and is less severe when an animal experiences the lesion during its youth. In addition, some animals with lesions appear to demonstrate exaggerated defensive reactions and are hyperresponsive to handling, light touch (air puffs), poking with a stick, temperature changes, light, and sounds (Donovick, 1968; Fried, 1972; Green & Schwartzbaum, 1968; Grossman, 1978; Olton & Gage, 1974). This hyperresponsivity is characterized by increases in motor activity.

Of particular interest is the fact that identical lesions in two different species may not result in the same behavioral outcome. The outcome appears to be related to the genetic background of the animal as well as pre-lesion experiences and the testing environment. This means that we must interpret and apply these findings with great caution. In addition, in considering a possible link to sensory modulation, it is important to look at the child in the context of both family and environment.

The cingulate gyrus has numerous connections; it receives input from the hippocampus and has reciprocal connections with the anterior nucleus of the thalamus and portions of the temporal, parietal, and prefrontal association areas. It also sends input to the dorsal medial nucleus of the thalamus, a connection thought to be important in the affect associated with perception (Kingsley, 2000). As with other limbic structures, the precise physiological function of the cingulate gyrus is unknown, but stimulation of this structure in animals (and, to some extent, in humans) results in behaviors similar to those associated with ablation of the amygdala—that is, diminished aggression. It may play a role in attaching emotional quality or meaning to sensory input, also in concert with the amygdala.

Cohen (1999) defined *affective rage* as the natural response of an animal in the presence of a threatening stimulus. In cats, for example, this might be the presence of another animal within its territory or threat to a litter of kittens. The affective behaviors associated with such rage are strongly inhibited by output from the amygdala and facilitated by connections from the septal area and other regions of the limbic system. This puts the limbic system in a modulatory role for affective rage. Although likening affective rage in animals to sensory modulation deficits is inappropriate, examining this mechanism gives us food for thought because it defines the limbic system as playing a role in the modulation of behavior resulting from environmental input that is perceived to be threatening.

Aside from its role in olfaction, investigators have debated the functions of the amygdala. Pribram (1975) suggested that the amygdala made important contributions to an organism's ability to orient and detect sensory input. Gilman and Newman (1996) indicated that this structure was important in linking "emotional and motivational responses to external stimuli . . . [and] is believed to contribute to the establishment of memories associated with specific constellations of sensory stimuli" (p. 210). Kingsley (2000) echoed this and further stated that this structure played an important role in determining affective perception of sensory input. Both Kingsley and Benarroch et al. (1999) maintain that the basal-lateral region of the amygdala is the site of convergence between sensory input and emotional significance. As such, this region is associated with interpretation of—and attachment of meaning to—a sensory stimulus based on emotional associations.

Information is passed on to another region of the amygdala, the central nucleus, where the emotional response to sensory input is initiated. The amygdala has numerous connections with the hippocampus. This relationship allows amygdalar activity to influence ANS functions. Kingsley (2000) suggested that the connections between the amygdala and components of the temporal lobe, including the hippocampus, were important in linking memories of past events with interpretation of current sensory input. We might consider the possibility that some of the avoidance behaviors associated with SMD may be associated with the attachment of a negative emotional response to that sensory input within the amygdala.

The hippocampus, another limbic structure, has also been hypothesized to play a role in sensory modulation. A large number of fibers link the hippocampus to the cortex. Again, there are holes in our understanding of the precise role of this structure, but it is essential for memory (Kingsley, 2000). Hippocampal lesions result in a wide variety of behavioral alterations that seem to be related to an animal's genetic background and to the conditions under which a behavior was elicited. Here again, extreme caution must be taken in generalizing from animal studies to humans. However, hippocampal lesions result in animals' failing to persist in new tasks; they readily begin a goal-oriented task but will not stay with it to completion. There is also an increase in activity in some situations, especially during "open-field" testing. This increased movement is not associated with increased exploration; the animal seems to move about a great deal but fails to effectively use the environmental information available from this increased movement.

There is also a decreased fear intensity elicited by threatening stimuli and reduced aggression in animals with hippocampal lesions (Isaacson, 1982) as well as sleep disturbances (i.e., the duration of sleep episodes is shortened) (Kim et al., 1971). Again, we have observed certain parallel behaviors in some children who experience sensory modulation deficits.

According to Isaacson (1982), the hippocampus is less closely associated with the ANS, mood, and emotion than are other components of the limbic system, and it is more involved with happenings in the world outside the body. It receives highly processed sensory information from the cortex and uses this to establish our knowledge of position in space and time relative to the external world (Gilman & Newman, 1996). The hippocampus appears to act as "a gatekeeper for both sensory and motor activities" (Isaacson, p. 236).

Finally, a role for the hypothalamus in the process of sensory modulation has been suggested. This structure maintains an important and reciprocal relationship with the limbic structures and is often included in discussions of this system. It integrates information from the cortex (first processed through the amygdala and hippocampus) with input from the spinal cord and brainstem. In this respect, the hypothalamus is a control center for ANS mechanisms (Gilman & Newman, 1996). According to Isaacson (1982), this structure interacts with nearly every other central structure to maintain "suitable conditions for mental actions and for behavior" (p. 108). Cohen (1999) stated that outputs from the amygdala project to the lateral hypothalamus to inhibit affective rage and, as such, it is associated with the expression of this response. Lesions in humans may be responsible for the onset of attack behavior and physically violent outbursts (Kingsley, 2000).

Thus, the purported functions of limbic and hypothalamic structures are consistent with modulation of sensory input. Furthermore, lesions elicit behaviors that, to some extent, parallel those identified by practitioners in children with SMD. However, there are noted differences between humans and animals, and any extrapolations between the two must be hypothetical until further work is done.

Sensory Modulation and Arousal

Arousal is often found in neurophysiology texts to be tied to wakefulness and consciousness. Benarroch et al. (1999) defined consciousness as "an awareness of environment and self. It implies an awake and alert condition in which the person is capable of perceiving his or her internal and external environments and, if the motor system is intact, of responding in an appropriate manner to stimuli" (p. 301). Furthermore, they stated that consciousness is dependent on activity within the reticular activating system, which itself is activated by sensory or cortical inputs. Thus, logic tells us that the modulation of sensory input has a relationship with arousal.

The reticular formation is a diffuse system that runs through the brainstem. In its role of regulating arousal and consciousness, it receives input from every major sensory pathway and projects to the cortex (both directly and via thalamic nuclei) to maintain arousal levels. The presentation of new or novel stimuli increases reticular activation of the cerebral cortex; removal of sensory input decreases reticular activation and leads to a gradual decrease in wakefulness. In response to novel or challenging

stimuli, the cholinergic neurotransmitter pathways to the cortex are responsible for arousal and attention to input and motivation. Histamine plays a role in arousal and motivation, and serotonin acts to produce decreases in arousal and sleep.

With regard to SMD, practitioners have looked to the relationship between optimal arousal levels and the production of an adaptive interaction. Kimball (1999) pointed out that moderate arousal produced an ideal adaptive environmental interaction, but overarousal led to behavioral disorganization, anxiety, and potentially negative responses. The concept of optimal levels of arousal to function has its more "contemporary" roots in the work of Hebb (1949, 1955). Although we now know that the amount of sensory input to the reticular formation regulates arousal, this relationship was less clear years ago when these investigators proposed that stimulus intensity was related to performance and that it was the intensity of input that regulated arousal level. Both of these conceptualizations identified an inverted U curve relationship between arousal and performance and stimulus intensity. Such a relationship is depicted in Figure 4–5. Later work by Berlyne (1960, 1971) expanded on this concept to include

other qualities of sensation as role players in the modulation of arousal. He further suggested that optimum arousal was linked to limbic and ANS functions, and that there may be individual differences in tonic arousal levels and "arousability."

More recently, Kerr (1990) proposed a more complex relationship between arousal and performance that depends on how each individual interprets the positive or negative tone associated with arousal. In Kerr's model, individuals are viewed as arousal seeking or avoiding, depending on whether they find increased arousal to be a pleasant or unpleasant experience. According to Apter's (1984) reversal hypothesis, something that an individual had viewed as pleasant can suddenly reverse to be viewed as unpleasant and anxiety provoking. Such a reversal hypothesis is intriguing to consider for children with SMD who appear to shift from underresponsive and sensory seeking to overresponsive and sensory avoiding. However, these theories continue to require investigation before we can make such a link.

Although it is well accepted that arousal is a function of sensory input, the link to sensory modulation is indirect. Clearly, arousal and modulation are not the same, although practitioners have used

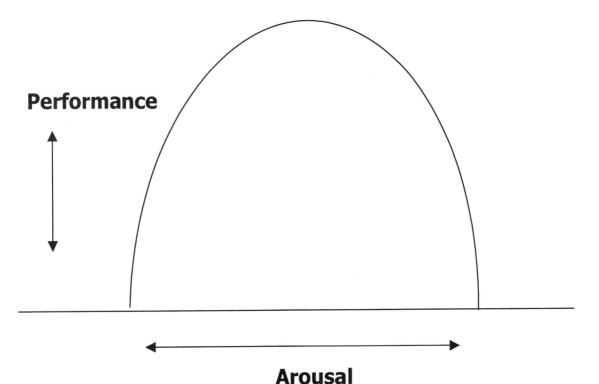

Performance

Arousal

■ FIGURE 4–5   Proposed relationship between arousal and performance.

the terms *overaroused* and *overresponsive* interchangeably. Children who are overly responsive to sensory input but have a limited ability to modulate input often find themselves overaroused. The behaviors seen when this happens can be categorized as disorganized and potentially negative, and some are linked to anxiety (Kimball, 1999).

Alternatively, clinical reports have suggested that, for some children, overresponsiveness to sensory input leads to "shutdown." Kimball related this to ANS changes that include cardiac irregularities, changes in blood pressure, and a nervous system that "cannot respond in normal ways" (Kimball, 1976, 1977), but empirical support for this suggestion is not available. Kimball further suggested that reducing novel stimuli in the environment and decreasing the intensity and variety of input can be used as therapeutic tools to bring arousal back to the optimal range (Kimball, 1999).

Children who display underresponsivity to sensory input appear to be underaroused. For these children, novel, intense stimuli may result in a higher arousal level and more adaptive environmental interaction. As with many of the potential links between CNS function and SMD, this area continues to warrant investigation.

Sensory Modulation Dysfunction and Neurotransmission

Recently, there has been a move to examine the potential role of neurotransmitters in patients with SMD. But we should take caution: if our ability to attach behaviors associated with SMD to specific CNS sites is limited, our ability to do the same with specific neurotransmitter systems is even more limited. As with anatomical structures, the study of transmitters has largely taken place in animals. Studies done in humans are often drug studies, suggesting that the nervous systems under investigation were, in some way, impaired. Understanding central neurotransmitter function through the measurement of peripheral references, such as transmitter metabolites in urine, is complicated by the fact that many transmitters are also present in the periphery, and, as such, metabolites in the urine may reflect peripheral as well as central activity. Nonetheless, alterations in CNS neurotransmitters, notably serotonin (5HT), *may* be tied to defensiveness and, as such, they bear at least a cursory look.

Serotonin is made from the amino acid precursor tryptophan, and dietary intake of tryptophan can influence central levels of the transmitter. According to Cohen (1999), the overall number of central 5HT neurons is limited, but the projections are widespread; virtually all areas of the brain receive 5HT inputs (Zigmond et al., 1999). Such widespread connections suggest that 5HT may be involved in a general way in many CNS functions and the expression of many behaviors and disorders. Cohen noted that 5HT may have either a general CNS inhibitory effect on defensive behaviors in animals or may act to more specifically modulate such behavior. Furthermore, it is important to note that dopamine and norepinephrine are involved in the behavioral response to threat, as are substance P, excitatory amino acid transmitters, gamma amino butyric acid (GABA), and enkephalins (Cohen, 1999). Thus, attributing any behavioral response to sensation to a single neurotransmitter is difficult.

A recent study by Stutzmann et al. (1998) does provide food for thought in regard to a potential role for 5HT in information processing in the rat amygdala. These investigators found that 5HT inhibited excitatory activity in rat lateral amygdala cells and furthermore that corticosterone was needed for this effect to be seen. Thus, the removal of corticosterone prevented 5HT from modulating activity in the amygdala. These authors concluded that both 5HT and corticosterone played a role in the sensitivity of amygdalar neurons to sensory input (this investigation focused on auditory inputs to the amygdala), and that this interaction may be important to the animals ability to respond adaptively to environmental input during times of fear or stress. These investigators also point out that more information is needed before any such conclusions can be confidently made.

In terms of functions, 5HT has been associated with, among other things, the modulation of pain at the level of the spinal cord and control of appetite, sleep, memory and learning, and mood because of connections within the brain. Within the realm of disorders, deficiencies of 5HT (along with norepinephrine) have been associated with depression, obsessive-compulsive disorder (OCD), and migraine headaches, to name just a few. The receptor physiology for the 5HT pathways are complex, with at least four—and as many as seven—populations of receptors, many with subtypes of their own. The physiological function of each receptor has yet to be elucidated. Drugs that produce a depletion of

5HT have been associated with diminished anxiety, and drugs that act as 5HT agonists or those that make more 5HT available have been used to treat patients with depression, OCD, and migraine headaches.

The study of neurotransmitters is an intriguing one. They are, of course, linked with behavior. In fact, it would be safe to say they are all linked to behaviors of some sort. The specificity of this linking, however, presents some difficulty because there are simply too many unknown factors. Thus, further study of 5HT, the behaviors with which it is associated, *and* the relationship of these behaviors to SMD is needed before sound hypotheses can be formulated.

Stress and Modulation

One additional aspect of the relationship between sensory modulation and the limbic system deserves attention. Clinicians have long suspected that anxiety resulting from stress can amplify tactile or sensory defensiveness. Stress is a behavioral response to environmental input that is variable in both its intensity and its triggers. When under stress, we generate responses designed to either reduce or eliminate the stress. In animals, stress responses fluctuate with diurnal rhythm and context. With regard to diurnal rhythm, stress responses are greater during rest than during activity (Zigmond et al., 1999).

The relationship of stress to context is a bit more complex. According to Zigmond et al. (1999), the stress system serves as an active monitoring system that constantly works to compare events in the now with events in the past. Thus, stress responses require past memories and rely on a comparator function that is likely a responsibility of the hippocampus. Relevance of the current event to organism survival dictates the event's importance, which determines which coping mechanisms will be called into action to deal with the situation.

Stress responses begin with release of corticotrophin-releasing factor or hormone (CRF or CRH) from the paraventricular nucleus (PVN) of the thalamus, which, in turn, acts on the ventral hypothalamus to lead to the release of adrenocorticotropin hormone (ACTH). This leads to the release of cortisol from the adrenal gland (Cohen, 1999). Cortisol is often measured as a means of quantifying physiological response to a stressor. Release of ACTH is, in part, regulated by the limbic system and, in part, by enkephalin and endorphin release in the CNS.

The anxiety that results from stress may be associated with unfounded apprehension or fear as well as with concentration difficulties, restlessness, and other symptoms in almost any system of the body (Ashton, 1987). These manifestations of stress and anxiety have been associated with limbic structures and components of the reticular system, hypothalamus, and cortex, as well as with the action of the neurotransmitters norepinephrine, epinephrine, and serotonin, which are associated with these regions (Ashton, 1987). Antianxiety drugs that disrupt the action of these neurotransmitters reduce anxiety-induced behaviors.

Activation of the anxiety system, which Gray (1982) called the behavioral inhibition system, depends on the organism's ability to compare actual input with expected input. Put differently, in any situation, we all have certain expectations of what will occur. We expect a hug from a friend to feel good and a shot to be only slightly painful. If the friendly hug turns into an uncomfortable squeeze or the injection has a burning quality not previously experienced, then our expectation does not match the real situation, and we find ourselves with increased arousal and anxiety. Gray stated that if a match occurred between expected and actual input, the behavioral inhibition system was not activated and general behavior was not altered. If a mismatch occurred, the behavioral inhibition system was activated and took control of behavior, leading to increased arousal and attention to incoming stimuli. This theory of anxiety and stress behavior has been questioned, but it is now fairly well accepted (Gray, 1982).

If one accepts the concept of limbic involvement in sensory modulation, then stress behaviors may play a role in the manifestation of sensory overresponsiveness. When incoming and expected inputs are mismatched, Gray's (1982) behavioral inhibition system takes over, leading to increased arousal and attention to the sensory stimuli, perhaps resulting in a defensive response. These concepts of sensory modulation are extremely hypothetical, however, and require considerably more study.

Tactile Defensiveness

With that background in potential links to CNS structures and functions, we now look at modulation dysfunction that has been associated with specific sensory systems. In this section, we present information on both the *observable behaviors* and the suggested *neurophysiological links*. The most often discussed is tactile defensiveness. In 1964, Ayres proposed a "provisional theory," based in part on earlier observations of Head (1920), to explain a clinical syndrome composed of deficits in tactile defensiveness, distractibility, and increased level of activity. Expanding on these ideas, Ayres (1972b) described the two tactile systems as a continuum rather than a strict dichotomy. They interacted "to provide a continuum of information and response with a need-for-defense interpretation and reaction at one end of the continuum and a discriminative interpretation and discrete response at the other end" (p. 214). Ayres hypothesized that tactile defensiveness was the result of an imbalance between discriminative interpretation and need for defense. She generalized from a protopathic-epicritic continuum to an anterolateral-dorsal column continuum (Ayres, 1964, 1972b). According to Ayres (1972b), tactile defensiveness occurred when the discriminative dorsal column medial lemniscal system failed to exert its normal inhibitory influence over the anterolateral system. As a result, light touch evoked protective, escape-like behavior and strong emotional responses. She hypothesized:

> The tactile defensive response, and other defensive responses to nocioceptive qualities in sensory stimuli, represents an insufficient amount of the inhibitory component in a functional system designed to monitor a certain type of impulse control. Thus, the behavioral response system designed for protection and survival predominated over a system designed to allow the organism to respond to the spatial temporal qualities of the tactile stimuli (Ayres, 1972, p. 215).

Ayres (1964) also suggested that adrenaline (epinephrine), released from the sympathetic nervous system during stress, played a role in the behavioral manifestations of tactile defensiveness, in that the reticular activating system was sensitive to the effects of adrenaline and the dorsal column medial lemniscal pathway was not. Ayres theorized that anxiety was both a cause and an effect of the predominance of the protective system and that the problem was self-perpetuating. Furthermore, a child chronically controlled by the protective system would be offered little opportunity for appropriate environmental exploration, and this might lead to delays in perceptual-motor development.

As early as 1972, Ayres (1972b) recognized that the gate control theory of Melzack and Wall (1965) "unified" various historical perspectives on the duality of the tactile system. She proposed that the gate control theory provided a conceptual model for tactile defensiveness. Briefly stated, this theory suggested that "gate" neurons present in the dorsal horn of the spinal cord controlled the passage of impulses to the CNS. Control of these gate cells was influenced both by incoming tactile inputs and by cortical influences. Tactile inputs carried in large A-beta fibers commonly associated with touch-pressure and other inputs mediated by the dorsal column medial lemniscal pathway, activated the gate cells, which, in turn prevented the transmission of pain to the CNS.

In contrast, inputs mediated by small A-delta and C (pain) fibers inhibited the gate cell. Thus, because the "gate is open" when the gate cell is inhibited, transmission of pain impulses was permitted. Importantly, cortical influences such as anxiety, attention, and anticipation, as well as sensory input over other channels, also mediate gated activity. All of these played a role in determining whether the gate cell was activated (gate closed) or inhibited (gate opened) and, therefore, whether pain transmission could proceed (Melzack & Wall, 1973).

Ayres (1972b) believed that the provision of specific (discriminative) tactile and proprioceptive stimuli would activate the dorsal column medial lemniscal system to "close the gating mechanism" so as to block the protective response to touch and diminish associated increased levels of activity and distractibility. Moreover, she believed that tactile stimuli that elicited a defensive response inhibited the gate cell, thereby permitting transmission of stimuli to the CNS and resulting in a defensive response. Deep touch-pressure and other sensations mediated by the dorsal column seemed to result in gate cell activation, decreasing transmission of defense-eliciting stimuli and, thereby, diminishing the defensive response. These hypotheses also explained the ability of previous stimuli, moods, and so forth, to influence the responses of a child with tactile defensiveness. These factors would be a component of the descending cortical influences on the gate, whereby stressful states, for example, might result in gate cell inhibition and thus permit transmission of defense-eliciting stimuli.

Unfortunately, some aspects of the gate control theory have not been confirmed by research, and others are poorly understood and controversial. For instance, no actual gate neurons have been found in the spinal cord. However, descending central pain controls exist, and stimulation of the dorsal column will lead to pain relief (Kandel & Schwartz, 1985).

In 1983, Fisher and Dunn published a review of pain control theories, including perspectives on the gate control theory of Melzack and Wall (1973) and evidence of inhibitory pain pathways. An important contribution of Fisher and Dunn (1983) was the recognition that the reduction of tactile defensiveness would not lead to improved tactile discrimination. Rather, they stressed that tactile defensiveness and poor tactile discrimination were separate disorders of tactile processing and not two ends of the same continuum; both tactile defensiveness and poor tactile discrimination could, and often did, occur in isolation (Fisher & Dunn, 1983).

One year earlier, Larson (1982) hypothesized that tactile defensiveness was the result of a filtering deficit resulting from too little inhibition. She explained the high arousal, distractibility, and defensiveness observed in children with tactile defensiveness by a lack of inhibition of irrelevant input. Fisher and Dunn (1983) subsequently suggested that the application of the phrase "lack of inhibition" to the child with tactile defensiveness was appropriate in describing the failure of higher CNS structures to modulate incoming tactile stimuli. They pointed out that "clinical descriptions of 'lack of inhibition' in children who display [tactile defensiveness] seem to be compatible with the concept that higher-level influences are not adequately modulating tactile inputs" (p. 2). Thus, they advocated the use of intervention to decrease arousal, including touch-pressure, proprioception, and linear vestibular stimulation.

Although Larson (1982) and Fisher and Dunn (1983) limited themselves to discussions of children with tactile defensiveness, their arguments could readily be applied to children with other manifestations of sensory defensiveness. Although Larson (1982) emphasized a lack of inhibition resulting in tactile defensiveness, she actually described an imbalance in descending mechanisms, resulting in either too little or too much inhibition. "This imbalance decreases the ability to perceive incoming stimuli from tactile and *other sensory modalities* [italics added]" (Larson, 1982, p. 592).

Current hypotheses regarding tactile defensiveness suggest that it is related to a faulty behavioral inhibition system. Input is not only inappropriately modulated, it also fails to generate an adaptive behavioral response. Tactile defensiveness is a problem, in large part, because of inappropriate behaviors that accompany it. A list of behaviors associated with tactile defensiveness is included below. As can be discerned from this list, defensiveness to touch potentially interferes with all occupations and roles. When a child limits food and clothing choices and resists activities such as face and hair washing and nail clipping, basic self-care becomes a trying ordeal. Avoiding sand, refusing to walk barefoot on the grass, or needing to control play activities can negatively affect one's role as a peer or sibling player. These and other behaviors may disrupt classroom behavior, making learning difficult.

Beyond behaviors that are linked easily to defensive responses to touch are those that are secondary to the need to control the sensory environment. Children with defensiveness to touch are often seen as distractible and overly active as they respond to irrelevant incoming sensory input (Ayres, 1965, 1966, 1969; Bauer, 1977). Furthermore, Wilbarger and Royeen (1987) speculated that tactile defensiveness could be a predisposing factor for irregular emotional tone, lability, extreme need for personal space, and disruption in personal care. Scardina (1986) hypothesized that tactile defensiveness interfered with the ability to establish or maintain intimate relationships. Thus, a child or adult with tactile defensiveness may experience a myriad of secondary deficits. Tactile defensiveness may be identified by a meaningful collection of behaviors, such as:

- Avoidance of touch
  - Avoidance of certain styles or textures (e.g., scratchy or rough) of clothing or, conversely, an unusual preference for certain styles or textures of clothing (e.g., soft materials, long pants, or sleeves)
  - Preference for standing at the end of a line to avoid contact with others
  - Tendency to pull away from anticipated touch or from interactions involving touch, including avoidance of touch to the face
  - Avoidance of play activities that involve body contact, sometimes manifested by a tendency to prefer solitary play

- Aversive responses to non-noxious touch
  - Aversion or struggle when picked up, hugged, or cuddled
  - Aversion to certain daily living tasks, including baths or showers, cutting of fingernails, haircuts, and face washing
  - Aversion to dental care
  - Aversion to art materials, including avoidance of finger paints, paste, or sand
- Atypical affective responses to non-noxious tactile stimuli
  - Responding with aggression to light touch to arms, face, or legs
  - Increased stress in response to being physically close to people
- Objection, withdrawal, or negative responses to touch contact, including that encountered in the context of intimate relationships (Royeen & Lane, 1991, p. 112)

Identification of tactile defensiveness is possible by looking for a meaningful *cluster* of behaviors. Many children dislike having their face washed and nails trimmed. These behaviors alone do not constitute tactile defensiveness. As with all disorders of sensory integration, the identification of tactile defensiveness is based on the presence of a consistent pattern (i.e., a sufficient number of aversive or negative reactions to touch) to confirm that it is, indeed, the response to touch that provides the basis of the reaction. This is particularly important when we consider the affective or emotional overlay that may occur with tactile defensiveness. Chapter 7 deals with assessment in greater detail.

Aversive Responses to Vestibular and Proprioceptive Inputs, Gravitational Insecurity, and Vestibular and Proprioceptive Underresponsiveness

Poor modulation within the vestibular system has also been identified. The vestibular system is thought to be a primary organizer of sensory information (Ayres, 1972, 1978, 1979). The vestibular system coordinates movement of the body and eyes in response to environmental demand; it is responsible for awareness of position in space, provides a stable visual field, and contributes to physical and emotional security. According to Ayres, our relationship with gravity is more es-

sential to our well being than is our relationship with our mother (1979).

According to Fisher and Bundy (1989), overresponsivity to vestibular and proprioceptive sensations may be manifested in two ways:

> *Aversive responses* to vestibular-proprioceptive inputs are characterized by nausea, vomiting, dizziness or vertigo, and other feelings of discomfort associated with autonomic (sympathetic) nervous system stimulation. *Gravitational insecurity* is characterized by excessive emotional reactions or fear that is out of proportion to the real threat or actual danger arising from vestibular-proprioceptive stimuli or position of the body in space. Although neither disorder is well understood, both are hypothesized to be a result of hyperresponsiveness or poor modulation of vestibular-proprioceptive inputs (Fisher & Bundy, 1989), and there is some evidence that increased sensitivity to vestibular stimulation or visual-vestibular conflict can result in motion sickness (Baloh & Honrubia, 1979) [italics ours] (p. 92).

Children with gravitational insecurity fear generic, everyday movement experiences, slow or fast, particularly those that involve head movements out of the vertical. Clinicians report that children with gravitational insecurity perceive small movements to be larger than they are. Children with this disorder may avoid activities that require new body or head positions, especially when the feet cannot be in contact with the floor. Fisher (1991) had speculated the source of this dysfunction to be poor modulation of input from the otolith organs, which are responsible for gravity perception. Furthermore, Fisher suggested that gravitational insecurity was related to an inability to resolve sensory conflict and inadequate development of body scheme. Because children with this modulation disorder seem to misjudge the amount of head movement they are experiencing, it may also be that gravitational insecurity is a problem of discrimination within this system. An alternative explanation has been suggested to be inefficient proprioceptive processing because proprioception has been said to modulate vestibular inputs (Ayres, 1979). The fear caused by gravitational insecurity is basic and profound and can affect emotional and behavioral development. Seemingly simple tasks such as getting into and out of a car or stepping down off a curb present anxious moments for individuals with gravitational insecurity. Of particular concern for these individuals is backward space and, as such, they avoid activities such as swinging on swings.

Aversive responses to, or intolerance of, movement is the reaction we feel when we become car-, plane-, or seasick. It is characterized by strong feelings of discomfort, nausea, vomiting, or dizziness after movement that activates the semicircular canals (i.e., angular acceleration). This disorder may result from faulty modulation of semicircular canal inputs. Alternatively, aversive reactions to movement may result from an inability to resolve sensory conflict among visual, vestibular, and proprioceptive inputs (Fisher, 1991).

Aversive responses to movement may not appear during or even directly after an activity. Clients may have difficulty interpreting the sensory input and may respond several hours later with a negative reaction. Fisher and Bundy (1989) and Fisher (unpublished data) described an individual with whom they had carried out an in-depth interview and vestibular testing. She was described as experiencing "sensory overload" or "sensory disorientation" after a period of visual-vestibular stimulation that included visual-vestibular conflict. Fisher (1991) describes this client's response as follows:

> Approximately 3 hours after stimulation, the subject began to experience the feeling that her head, arms, and legs had become detached from her body and were floating in space. When she attempted to walk on a level surface, she felt as if she were walking on an uneven, unpredictable surface. Sometimes the surface would seem to be higher than she expected it to be, and sometimes the ground would be lower than she expected it to be (p. 90).

Thus, an inability to resolve movement, proprioception, and visual input had a strongly disruptive effect on this individual's internal body scheme. Intervention for aversiveness to movement and gravitational insecurity is addressed in Chapter 12. Underresponsivity to movement is seen in children such as Michael, in this case, in conjunction with underresponsivity to proprioception. Michael seeks activities that provide movement and proprioceptive sensations in order to obtain what he considers to be an optimal level of arousal and attention in the classroom and at home.

Presently, clinicians are debating the existence of a SMD related strictly to proprioception that appears to resemble underresponsiveness, in that it is characterized by behaviors designed to obtain a great deal of proprioceptive input (Blanche & Schaff, 2001). Thus, children may hit, bang, bump, or fall on purpose. They may appear very aggressive in their interactions, and their movements may seem clumsy. Whether this is a specific disorder or a reflection of other sensory integrative problems will require further clinical and empirical investigation.

Vestibular modulation deficits have the potential to interfere with occupational performance in many ways. When children are overresponsive to vestibular input, they generally avoid many types of movement. Fearing movement through space, infants and toddlers engage in diminished environmental exploration and gross motor activity. As preschoolers, children with vestibular modulation deficits may become tense and anxious on playground equipment, avoid rough and tumble play, or become easily nauseated when riding in a vehicle. School-age children may avoid amusement parks, camp activities, and sports. Children may also have a very poor sense of where their bodies are in space. The social ramifications of these avoidance behaviors can be profound as they find themselves left out of activities, unable to join in.

Sensory Modulation Dysfunction in Other Sensory Systems

In addition to these somewhat classic examples of specific SMD that have been under study for several years, clinical evidence has suggested that overresponsiveness may be a factor in both the auditory and visual systems as well. This observation would be very consistent with the work of McIntosh et al. (1999) and fits well with the concept of a general SMD. Careful documentation of behaviors that appear to reflect modulation deficits in these sensory systems—and examination of the underlying neuroscience correlates of the behaviors—is needed. Suggestions for intervention with patients who have SMD can be found in Chapter 12, and the STEP SI protocol, developed as an intervention by Miller and colleagues, can be found in Appendix A.

SUMMARY AND CONCLUSION

In summary, SMD is complex and multidimensional. When any sensory input is not modulated in an expected way, the behavior that results is "out of step" with what is needed for an adaptive environmental interaction. Poor modulation has ramifications, both within the nervous system (e.g., affecting attention, arousal, and modulation of other inputs) and in the outside world because it results in the production of behaviors that do not match environmental demand or expectation. Although we are still uncertain of neural links that underlie poor modulation, we are becoming more astute at identifying the problems (see Chapter 7) and intervening (see Chapter 12).

References

Apter, M. J. (1984). Reversal theory and personality: A review. *Journal of Research in Personality, 18,* 265–288.

Ashton, J. (1987). *Brain disorders and psychotropic drugs.* New York: Oxford University.

Ayres, A. J. (1964). Tactile functions: Their relations to hyperactive and perceptual motor behavior. *American Journal of Occupational Therapy, 18,* 6–11.

Ayres, A. J. (1965). Patterns of perceptual-motor dysfunction in children: A factor analytic study. *Perceptual and Motor Skills, 20,* 335–368.

Ayres, A. J. (1966). Interrelationships among perceptual-motor functions in children. *American Journal of Occupational Therapy, 20,* 288–292.

Ayres, A. J. (1969). Deficits in sensory integration in educationally handicapped children. *Journal of Learning Disabilities, 2,* 160–168.

Ayres, A. J. (1972a). Improving academic scores through sensory integration. *Journal of Learning Disabilities, 5,* 336–343.

Ayres, A. J. (1972b). *Sensory integration and learning disorders.* Los Angeles: Western Psychological Services.

Ayres, A. J. (1978). Learning disabilities and the vestibular system. *Journal of Learning Disabilities, 11,* 18–29.

Ayres, A. J. (1979). *Sensory integration and the child.* Los Angeles: Western Psychological Services.

Baloh, R. W., & Honrubia, V. (1979). *Clinical neurophysiology of the vestibular system.* Philadelphia: F.A. Davis.

Bauer, B. (1977). Tactile-sensitive behavior in hyperactive and non-hyperactive children. *American Journal of Occupational Therapy, 31,* 447–450.

Benarroch, E. E., Westmoreland, B. F., Daube, J. R., Reagan, T. J., & Sandok, B. A. (1999). *Medical neurosciences.* Philadelphia: Lippincott, Williams & Wilkins.

Berlyne, D. E. (1960). *Conflict, arousal, & curiosity.* New York: McGraw-Hill.

Berlyne, D. E. (1971). *Aesthetics and psychobiology.* New York: Appleton-Century-Crofts.

Blanche, E. I. & Schaff, R. C. (2001). Proprioception: A cornerstone of sensory integration intervention.

In S. S. Roley, E. I. Blanche & R. C. Schaff (Eds.), *Sensory Integration with Diverse Populations* (pp. 109–124). United States: Therapy Skill Builders.

Cermak, S. (1988). The relationship between attention deficits and sensory integration disorders (Part 1). *Sensory Integration Special Interest Section Newsletter, 11,* 1–4.

Cohen, H. (1999). *Neuroscience for rehabilitation* (2nd ed.). Baltimore: Lippincott, Williams & Wilkins.

Cohn, E., Miller, L. J., & Tickle-Degnen, L. (1999). Parental homes for therapy outcomes: Children with sensory modulation disorders. *American Journal of Occupational Therapy, 56,* 36–43.

Donovick, P. J. (1968). Effects of localized septal lesions on hippocampal EEC activity in behavior in rats. *Journal of Comparative and Physiological Psychology, 66,* 569–578.

Dunn, W. (1997). The impact of sensory processing abilities on the daily lives of young children and their families: A conceptual model. *Infants and Young Children, 9,* 23–25.

Dunn, W. (1999). *Sensory profile.* San Antonio: The Psychological Corporation.

Edelberg, R. (1972). The electrodermal system. In N. S. Greenfield & R. A. Sternbach (Eds.), *Handbook of psychophysiology* (pp. 367–418). New York: Hold, Rinehart, & Watson.

Fisher, A. G. (1991). Vestibular-proprioceptive processing and bilateral integration and sequencing deficits. In A. F. Fisher, E. A. Murray, & A. C. Bundy (Eds.), *Sensory integration theory and practice* (pp. 71–107). Philadelphia: F.A. Davis.

Fisher, A. G., & Bundy, A. C. (1989). Vestibular stimulation in the treatment of postural and related disorders. In O. D. Payton, R. P. DiFabio, S. V. Paris, E. J. Protas, & A. F. VanSant (Eds.), *Manual of physical therapy techniques* (pp. 239–258). New York: Churchill Livingstone.

Fisher, A. G., & Dunn, W. (1983). Tactile defensiveness: Historical perspectives, new research: A theory grows. *Sensory Integration Special Interest Section Newsletter, 6*(2), 1–2.

Fisher, A. F., & Murray, E. A., (1991). Introduction to sensory integration theory. In A. G. Fisher, E. A. Murray, & A.C. Bundy (Eds.), *Sensory integration: theory and practice* (pp. 3–26). Philadelphia: F.A. Davis.

Fowles, D. C. (1986). The eccrine system and electrodermal activity. In M. C. H. Coles, E. Dorchin, & S. W. Porges (Eds.), *Psychophysiology: Systems, processes, and applications* (pp. 51–96). New York: Guilford Press.

Fried, P. A. (1972). The effect of differential hippocampal lesions and pre- and post-operative training on extinction. *Revenue Canadienne de Psychologie, 26,* 61–70.

Funk and Wagnalls Standard Dictionary (1991). New York: Funk and Wagnalls.

Gilman, S., & Newman, S. W. (1992). *Essentials of clinical neuroanatomy and neurophysiology* (Ed. 9). Philadelphia: F.A. Davis.

Gray, J. A. (1982). *The neuropsychology of anxiety.* New York: Claredon.

Green, R. H., & Schwartzbaum, J. S. (1968). Effects of unilateral septal lesions on avoidance behavior, discrimination reversal, and hippocampal EEG. *Journal of Comparative and Physiological Psychology, 65,* 388–396.

Grossman, S. P. (1978). An experimental "dissection" of the septal syndrome. Functions of the septo-hippocampal system (pp. 227–273). *Ciba Foundation Symposium 58 (new series).* New York: Elsevier.

Hanft, B. E., Miller, L. J., & Lane, S. J. (September 2000). Towards a consensus in terminology in sensory integration theory and practice: Part 3: Sensory integration patterns of function and dysfunction: Observable behaviors: Dysfunction in sensory integration. *Sensory Integration Special Interest Section Quarterly, 23,* 1–4.

Head, H. (1920). *Studies in neurology* (Vol. 2). New York: Oxford University.

Hebb, D. O. (1949). *The organization of behavior.* New York: Wiley.

Hebb, D. O. (1955). Drives and the CNS (conceptual nervous system). *Psychological Review, 62,* 243–254.

Isaacson, R. L. (1982). *The limbic system* (2nd ed.). New York: W.B. Saunders.

Kandel E. R., & Schwartz, J. H. (1985). *Principles of neural science.* New York: Elsevier.

Kerr, J. H. (1990). Stress and sport: Reversal theory. In J. G. Jones & L. Hardy (Eds.), *Stress and performance in sport* (pp. 107–131). Chichester: Wiley.

Kim, C., Choi, H., Kim, J. K., Kim, M. S., Huh, M. K., & Moon, Y. B. (1971). General behavioral activity and its component patterns in hippocampectomized rats. *Brain Research, 19,* 379–394.

Kimball, J. G. (1976). Vestibular stimulation and seizure activity. *Center for the Study of Sensory Integrative Dysfunction Newsletter* (now Sensory Integration International), July, 4.

Kimball, J. G. (1977). Case history follow up report. *Center for the Study of Sensory Integrative Dysfunction Newsletter* (now Sensory Integration International), 5.

Kimball, J. G. (1999). Sensory integration frame of reference: Theoretical base, function/dysfunction continua, and guide to evaluation. In P. Kramer & J. Hinojosa (Eds.), *Frames of reference for pediatric occupational therapy* (2nd ed., pp. 119–168). Philadelphia: Lippincott Williams & Wilkins.

Kingsley, R. E. (2000). *Concise text of neuroscience.* Philadelphia: Lippincott Williams & Wilkins.

Knickerbocker B. M. (1980). *A holistic approach to learning disabilities.* Thorofare, NJ: C. B. Slack.

Koomar, J. A. & Bundy, A. C. (1991). The art and science of creating direct intervention from theory. In A. G. Fisher, E. A. Murray, & A. C. Bundy (Eds.), *Sensory integration theory and practice* (pp. 251–317). Philadelphia: F.A. Davis.

Lai, J-S, Parham, D. L., & Johnson-Ecker, C. (1999). Sensory dormancy and sensory defensiveness: Two sides of the same coin? *Sensory Integration Special Interest Section Quarterly, 22,* 1–4.

Lane, S. J., Miller, L. J., & Hanft, B. E. (June 2000). Towards a consensus in terminology in sensory integration theory and practice: Part 2: Sensory integration patterns of function and dysfunction. *Sensory Integration Special Interest Section Quarterly, 23,* 1–3.

Larson, K. A. (1982). The sensory history of developmentally delayed children with and without tactile defensiveness. *American Journal of Occupational Therapy, 36,* 590–596.

McIntosh, D. N., Miller, L. J., Shyu, V., & Dunn, W. (1999). Overview of the Short Sensory Profile (SSP). In W. Dunn (Ed.) *Sensory profile: User's manual* (pp. 59–73). San Antonio, TX: Psychological Corporation.

McIntosh, D. N., Miller, L. J., Shyu, V., & Hager, R. J. (1999). Sensory-modulation disruption, electrodermal responses, and functional behaviors. *Developmental Medicine & Child Neurology, 41,* 608–615.

Melzack, R., & Wall P. D. (1965). Pain mechanisms: A new theory. *Science, 50,* 971–979.

Miller, L. J.,& Lane, S. J. (March 2000). Towards a consensus in terminology in sensory integration theory and practice: Part 1: Taxonomy of neurophysiological processes. *Sensory Integration Special Interest Section Quarterly, 23,* 1–4.

Miller, L. J., McIntosh, D. N., McGrath, J., Shyu, V., Lampe, M., Taylor, A. K., Tassone, F., Neitzel, K., Stackhouse, T., & Hager, R. J. (1999). Electrodermal responses to sensory stimuli in individuals with Fragile X Syndrome. *American Journal of Medical Genetics, 83,* 268–279.

Miller, L. J., & Summers, C. (2001). Clinical applications in sensory modulation dysfunction: Assessment and intervention considerations. In S. S. Roley, E. I. Blanche, & R. C. Schaaf (Eds.), *Understanding the nature of sensory integration with diverse populations.* San Antonio, TX: Therapy Skill Builders.

Olton, D. S., & Gage, F. H. (1974). Role of the fornix in the septal syndrome. *Physiology and Behavior, 13,* 269–279.

Parham, D. L., & Mailloux, Z. (1996). Sensory integration. In J. Case-Smith, A. S. Allen, & P. N. Pratt (Eds.), *Occupational Therapy for Children* (3rd ed., pp. 307–355). St Louis: Mosby.

Pribram, C. (1975). Arousal, activation and effort in the control of attention. *Psychological Review, 82,* 116–149.

Random House College Dictionary (1975). Revised edition. New York: Random House, 1975.

Reiss, A. L., Abrams, M. T., Greenlaw, R., Freund, L., & Denkla, M. B. (1995). Neurodevelopmental effects of the FMR-1 full mutation in humans. *Nature and Medicine, 1:* 159–167.

Reiss, A. L., Lee, J., & Freund, L. (1994). Neuroanatomy of fragile X syndrome: The temporal lobe. *Neurology, 44,* 1317–1324.

Restak, R. (1995). *Brainscapes*. New York: Hyperion.

Royeen, C. B. (August 1989). Tactile defensiveness. An overview of the construct. Paper presented at the International Society for Social Pediatrics, Brixen, Italy.

Royeen, C. B., & Lane, S. J. (1991). Tactile processing and sensory defensiveness. In A. G. Fisher, E. A. Murray, & A. C. Bundy (Eds.) *Sensory integration: Theory and practice* (pp. 108–136). Philadelphia: F.A. Davis.

Scardina, V. (1986). A. Jean Ayres Lectureship. *Sensory Integration Newsletter, 14,* 2–10.

Stutzmann, G. E., McEwen, B. S., & LeDoux, J. E. (1998). Serotonin modulation of sensory input to the lateral amygdala: Dependency on cortricosterone. *The Journal of Neuroscience, 18,* 9529–9538.

Webster's new collegiate dictionary (1988). Springfield, MA: G. &. C. Merriam Co.

Wilbarger, P. (1993). *Sensory defensiveness*. Videotape. Hugo, MN: PDP.

Wilbarger, P., & Royeen, C. B. (May 1987). Tactile defensiveness: Theory, applications and treatment. Annual Interdisciplinary Doctoral Conference, Sargent College, Boston University.

Wilbarger, P., & Wilbarger, J. (1991). *Sensory defensiveness in children aged 2–12: An intervention guide for parents and other caregivers*. Denver, CO: Avanti Educational Programs.

Williams, M. S., & Shellenberger, S. (1994). *How does your engine run?* Albuquerque, NM: TherapyWorks, Inc.

Zigmond, M. J., Bloom, F. E., Landic, S. C., Roberts, J. L., & Squire, L. R. (1999). *Fundamental neuroscience*. Boston: Academic.

5

Visual-Spatial Abilities

Anne Henderson, PhD, OTR, FAOTA
Charlane Pehoski, ScD, OTR, FAOTA
Elizabeth Murray, ScD, OTR, FAOTA

> *Space: the final frontier*
>
> —James T. Kirk

When he was 6 years old, Ricky was referred to an occupational therapist for significant motor clumsiness. He could not walk through his classroom without bumping into desks or tripping over objects in his path. Although he lived only two blocks from school, he was not allowed to walk to school by himself because he could not determine when it was safe to cross the street. On the playground, he misjudged the movement of the swings, resulting in many "near misses" when he walked by children who were swinging.

Ricky had trouble finding his way around the school and did not seem to know how to use landmarks as a guide. Gym class was a disaster; Ricky could not catch a ball unless it hit him in the chest so that he could trap it. When playing dodgeball, he was always the first eliminated.

In his classroom, Ricky was able to read as well as his peers. Printing, however, was a challenge. He could not keep his letters within the lines, and the size and spacing of his letters varied tremendously. Math was also difficult. When using counters to solve a problem, Ricky counted some of them more than once and some not at all.

Ricky still needed help in dressing. He put on shirts backward, and both his legs ended up in the same pants leg. He wore slip-on shoes because he could not tie shoelaces, but sometimes he tried to put one shoe on upside down, with the sole facing up, and he could not figure out what was wrong.

Children like Ricky are familiar to many occupational therapists, and his description fits many children with sensory integrative dysfunction. Undoubtedly, Ricky's problems are partly the result of disorders in processing vestibular and proprioceptive sensations. However, they also most likely reflect poor visual processing, particularly of the aspects of vision that process and interpret spatial information. We can see that he has trouble both in moving himself through space and in understanding the spatial features of objects.

Visual processing has not received the same careful analysis in sensory integration theory that other sensory systems have. Yet children with

Ricky's problems are frequently referred to occupational therapy for evaluation and treatment using sensory integrative procedures. In addition, several tests of the Sensory Integration and Praxis Tests (SIPT) have been described as assessing form and space perception.

PURPOSE AND SCOPE

In this chapter, we present current research on the visual system, with an emphasis on the aspects that contribute to spatial abilities. We first look at how vision is processed in the nervous system. Then we focus on two important roles of the spatial aspects of vision. One is its part in controlling our movements in the environment, and the other is the contribution of visual-spatial abilities to cognition.

DUAL NEURAL PROCESSING OF VISION

Visual processing is commonly divided into two systems. One of these systems recognizes objects (including "living" objects). It is attuned to the features of objects that enable us to identify and remember them. This system is referred to as *object vision,* or the "what" system (Kosslyn & Koenig, 1992; Ungerleider & Haxby, 1994).

The other system is the "where" system, or *spatial vision.* This system determines the locations and positions of objects, relative both to ourselves and to other objects. It processes the features of objects that are needed for actions—for example, to reach for a cup or to avoid bumping into a chair. The spatial processing that occurs in the "where" system is unconscious (Goodale, 2000). It is this contribution of vision to our ability to move in our environment and interact with objects that makes understanding visual-spatial abilities important to sensory integration.

Object vision and spatial vision are differentiated in several places in the human nervous system. We will describe those found in cellular layers and in the cortex. Additional information on the neuroanatomic organization of the visual system can be found in Chapter 2.

Cellular Divisions: Magnocellular and Parvocellular Systems

Evidence that the brain responds differently when recognizing objects and when determining spatial

locations comes from the study of neural cellular layers in the lateral geniculate nucleus (LGN) and its projections to the primary visual cortex (Livingstone, 1993). As described in Chapter 2, two types of ganglion cells are found in the retina: M type and P type. These cells project to the magnocellular and parvocellular layers of the LGN and then to the primary visual cortex, maintaining, for the most part, separate pathways or channels (Kandel et al., 1991). The parvocellular channel projects from the small P type ganglion cells in the retina to the parvocellular layers in the LGN, from there to the visual cortex, and then they terminate mainly in the inferior temporal cortex. This channel is thought to be important for color perception and for analyzing in great detail the shape and surface properties of objects. The magnocellular channel projects from the large M type ganglion cells to the magnocellular layers of the LGN and then to the visual cortex. It terminates primarily in the posterior parietal cortex and serves the sensory-motor function of that area (Mountcastle, 1995). Neurons respond rapidly but transiently, and the system is further associated with motion and depth detection, stereoscopic vision, and interpreting spatial organization (Atkinson, 1993; Hendry & Calkins, 1998; Livingstone, 1993; McCarthy, 1993).

An aside: there is some evidence that the magnocellular system is implicated in some forms of dyslexia. Autopsies of adults with histories of dyslexia have shown magnocellular cells to be fewer than in nondyslexic adults (Livingstone et al., 1991). Some researchers (Barnard et al., 1998; Demb et al., 1998; Livingstone et al., 1991; Vidyasagar & Pammer, 1999) have suggested that a subgroup of children with dyslexia, particularly those with visual disturbances, have a defect in some elementary visual functions served by the magnocellular system. Other researchers have questioned this defect (e.g., Walther-Müller, 1995), and the mechanism by which a deficit in the magnocellular system would result in impaired reading is uncertain (Stein et al., 2000).

Cortical Divisions: The Dorsal and Ventral Streams

In the early 1980s, Mishkin et al. (1982) described two classes of visual function mediated by separate cortical systems. They termed these classes *object vision* and *spatial vision.* According to these researchers, object vision mediates the recognition of objects and the perception of form, color, texture, and size. Its pathway, referred to as the *ventral stream,* projects from the primary visual cortex to the inferior temporal lobe. Spatial vision provides information on the visual location of objects in space. Its pathway, the *dorsal stream,* projects from the primary visual cortex to the posterior parietal lobe (Mishkin et al., 1983; Ungerleider & Mishkin, 1982) (Fig. 5–1). As we have noted, the magnocellular channel is dominant in the dorsal stream, and the parvocellular is dominant in the ventral stream.

These anatomical divisions have been verified repeatedly. However, more recently, researchers (Goodale, 2000; Goodale & Milner, 1992; Milner & Goodale, 1993; Ungerleider & Haxby, 1994) who studied the function of these two pathways or streams have emphasized differences in how these two areas use visual information. In the ventral stream, visual information about object characteristics such as shape, size, and texture permits the formation of long-term perceptual representations that support object identification and visual learning (i.e., what an object is). In the dorsal stream, vision provides information about the location of objects relative to the body and in relationship to each other (i.e., where objects are located). The dorsal stream also mediates the control of visually guided motor actions and processes information about object qualities that is needed to guide actions such as adjusting the hand during reach to the size and orientation of an object (Goodale, 2000). Goodale et al. (Goodale, 2000; Goodale & Milner, 1992; Milner & Goodale, 1993) viewed the role of the dorsal stream as subserving the control of skilled actions directed toward an object. Others (Kosslyn & Koenig, 1992; Shen et al., 1999; Ungerleider & Haxby, 1994) have provided evidence that the motor component is not necessarily the only feature of dorsal stream function because it may also provide information for discriminating spatial properties of objects. All agree, however, that this processing occurs at an unconscious level.

Object vision and spatial vision have been found to be selectively impaired in adults with brain injuries (Milner & Goodale, 1993; Newcombe & Russell, 1969; Newcombe et al., 1987; von Cramon & Kerkhoff, 1993). Clients with more ventral lesions show impairments in visual recognition of objects but no impairment on visual spatial tasks or in navigating through space. Clients with right superior parietal lesions, on the other hand, are impaired on spatial tasks but not on visual recognition.

Neuroimaging studies have also demonstrated differential activation of the ventral and dorsal streams, depending on the task. Cortical regions in the ventral stream are selectively activated when a subject performs an object recognition task, such as matching faces. Spatial tasks, such as shifting attention to different spatial locations, activate regions of the dorsal stream (Chen et al., 2000; Ungerleider & Haxby, 1994).

The two cortical visual areas appear to have dif-

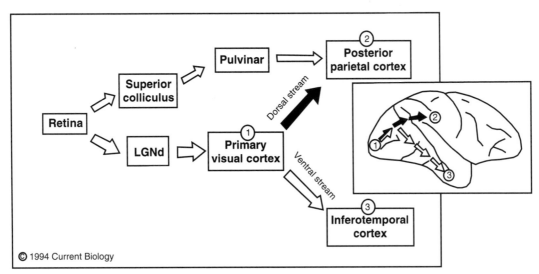

■ FIGURE 5-1 The pathways of the ventral and dorsal streams. (Reprinted from *Current Biology, 4,* Goodale, MA, Meenan, JP, Bulthoff, HH, Nicolle, DA, Murphy, KL, and Racicot, CI: Separate neural pathways for the visual analysis of object shape in perception and prehension, 604–610, 1994, with permission from Elsevier Science.)

ferent reliance on subcortical structures. Girard et al. (1991, 1992) studied the firing of the neurons in the inferior temporal and posterior parietal visual streams in monkeys when the primary visual cortex itself had been cooled or lesioned. (Cooling the primary visual cortex was a way of disrupting neuronal function temporarily. Disruption of the primary visual cortex should thus diminish or abolish any action "downstream" from this area.) The researchers found that whereas visual responses were completely abolished in the inferior temporal cortex after ablation or cooling of the primary visual cortex, some responses could still be recorded from the posterior parietal cortex. The researchers believed that this remaining activity came directly from subcortical structures of the visual system (see Fig. 5–1). This input could be responsible for the fast and unconscious processing of visual information. In contrast, the newer temporal area appeared to be more dependent on primary visual cortex input (Jeannerod, 1997).

Summary of the Neural Processing of Vision

There are parallels between the "what" and "where" functions of the two levels of processing. For example, the high visual acuity and color perception of the parvocellular channel serves form perception and the spatial analysis of object characteristics. Rapid processing and sensitivity to movement in the magnocellular channel foster the perception of direction and location. Although it is tempting to assign the parvocellular system to the ventral stream and the magnocellular system to the dorsal stream, the systems are not that neat. For example, some parvocellular cells are found in the dorsal stream, and quite a few magnocellular cells are found in the ventral stream.

There is, nevertheless, strong support for the contention that the central nervous system (CNS) processes visual information for spatial perception differently than for visual object perception. We should note, however, that the neurophysiology of the two visual systems is far more complex than the simple differentiation described here and that their functions and interactions are far from established. What is known is that the two visual systems are functionally different. This differentiation of the "what" and "where" systems in visual processing has important implications. Using vision to identify a cup and using vision to reach for a cup

are separate skills. In the same vein, although spatial vision contributes to reaching for a cup, other parts of the CNS contribute differentially to different tasks—for example, finding one's way through a department store to buy a cup and mentally rotating an image of a cup to determine if it matches another image. Here we must go beyond the visual system itself and look at how spatial vision is integrated with other parts of the CNS.

VISUAL CONTROL OF MOVEMENT IN SPACE

Vision guides our movements, whether we are simply reaching for an object or moving from one place to another in the environment while avoiding obstacles. To guide movements, vision works in concert with other sensory systems. The auditory system can compensate partially as a spatial sense when vision is lost, and it enhances vision by signaling the direction of noise, which is important in shifting attention to a speaker or warning of an approaching car. Touch confirms the location and characteristics of objects reached for and indicates the qualities of the surfaces we walk on. Vestibular input indicates that we are upright and, along with touch, tells us the direction of gravity. We are not aware of the proprioceptive input from our eyes and neck, but what we perceive is interpreted in the context of our head and eye position and movement.

In discussing the role of vision in guiding motor actions, we first consider the concept of body schema. Accurate visual guidance of the whole body in space or of a limb in space requires that the visual system be integrated with an internal, ever-changing representation of the body. We also need to consider that, as we move, the visual array (i.e., what appears on the retina) changes, and these changes are integrated into movement plans. The posterior parietal cortex is an important area of the brain for integrating vision with other sensory input. Neurons in this area receive somatosensory, proprioceptive, vestibular, auditory, and visual input together with information about eye, head, limb, and locomotor movements (Jakobson & Goodale, 1994).

Vision and the Body Schema

The body schema is an unconscious mechanism underlying spatial motor coordination that provides the CNS with the necessary information about the relationship of the body and its parts to environmental space (Henderson, 1973). The body schema is the proprioceptive-motor-spatial structure of our bodies defined by our orientation to gravity and the position of our head and limbs (Stein, 1991). Body schema is dependent on information about both ongoing and intended patterns of movement that come from tactile, proprioceptive, and vestibular inputs (Lackner & DiZio, 2000). Gibson (1966) wrote that everyday perception occurs in the context of nested motions: eyes within head, head on body, body in an environment filled with objects that may move. In walking toward or reaching for an object, the position of the eyes in the head, the position of the head on the body, and the position of the limbs are registered centrally and integrated with what is seen. Our actions in space are accurate because the visual-spatial coordinates and the body reference coordinates are integrated. For example, when walking and attempting to pass through a narrow opening, vision provides the information about the opening's size, and our knowledge of our body's dimension and position provided by multiple sensory inputs determine if we need to turn to the side or can walk straight through without turning. Warren and Whang (1987) found that adults can make the decision of "passability" unconsciously, based on the width of their shoulders. In stair climbing, adults consistently select as the most comfortable a step height that is one half the length of their lower leg (Warren, 1984). These results for stepping up have been found in 6-, 8-, and 10-year-old children. As they grow, children continually adapt their perception of the critical limits of their leg length.

Vision alone could not adequately direct the body in space without the information in the body schema that is provided through the integration of multiple sensory inputs. Ayres recognized this when she said that ". . . a main foundation to visual perception is the vestibular system with proprioception and other senses also contributing" (Sieg, 1988, pp. 99–100). The posterior parietal lobe and its connections to the premotor area of the frontal lobe are considered major centers for this integration.

Movement and the Visual Array

When we move, as when we walk or turn our head or eyes, the visual array is constantly chang-ing. Several mechanisms help us to accurately interpret these changes. When the changes in visual array are well integrated with the body schema, they provide us with the perception of both our movement and the surroundings. Four of these mechanisms are *optic flow*, by which we differentiate self movement from object movement; *spatial constancy*, which provides stable vision; and *motion parallax* and *optic expansion*, by which we perceive the depth or distance of stationary and moving objects. Two of the mechanisms—optic flow and spatial constancy—appear to have connections to the posterior parietal cortex.

Optic Flow

With every movement of the eyes, head, or body, the optic array, or the pattern of visual stimulation on the retina, changes and "streams" across the retina. When we move forward, the visual pattern flows by us, but when we turn our heads back and forth, the direction of the flow is side to side. This visual stream across the retina is called optic flow. Optic flow is a major source of information for the perception of depth and distance and of movement, both of the self and of objects. For example, when walking through woods or a crowded room, we unconsciously monitor the optic array that is streaming to either side of us as we move forward. This information helps guide our movements so we can navigate the environment without bumping into objects that are in our path. Cells driven by optic flow have been reported in the posterior parietal cortex, and they may play a role in the visual guidance of locomotion through space (Milner & Goodale, 1993; Mountcastle 1995).

Spatial Constancy

Another aspect of vision that is related to moving through space is spatial constancy. Because of spatial constancy, as the term is used in neurophysiology and psychology, the world around us appears to remain stable when our eyes are moving (Mountcastle, 1995). Because the retina registers a visual scene only for an instant, the visual stimulation of an active observer is continually changing. However, this is not what we perceive. Spatial constancy depends on the central registration of eye, head, and body movements coordinated with the central registration of the changes in the retinal pattern caused by those movements. Spatial constancy is a critical mechanism of the human visual system and the foundation of motor and perceptual functions in the physical world. We are not generally aware of the constant changes in the retinal patterns or of our eye and head positions, but a person can experience loss of spatial constancy by looking in a hand mirror and rotating the body while focusing on the reflection of the scene behind him or her. The scene in the mirror will seem to rotate behind the observer because the scene's registration on the retina is not coordinated with body movement. Some clients with parietal lesions may experience a similar problem. O'Conner and Padula (1997) observed that some of these clients reported various problems that appear related to a problem with spatial constancy. Some believed that all visual space moved when they moved their heads. For others, only larger objects moved or words seemed to "jump" on a page when they attempted to read.

Motion Parallax and Optical Expansion

The most powerful mechanisms for perceiving depth and distance involve movement of the self or objects (Kellman & Banks, 1998). When we move, we provide a change in visual information that yields depth and distance cues. As the head is moved back and forth, objects that are nearby appear to "move" more rapidly than far-away objects. You can experience this by closing one eye, holding up your finger, turning your head from side to side and focusing on a distant object. Your finger will seem to move in relation to objects further away. This phenomenon has been termed *motion parallax*.

Another depth cue is *optical expansion*. Optical expansion occurs in relation to the distance of an object from the observer. Objects that are nearby take up more of your field of vision than far-away objects. Consider the difference in what you see when watching a movie sitting directly behind a large person and watching it from six rows behind the same person. Optical expansion is important in judging the movement of objects coming toward you. As they draw closer, the area that they occupy in your field of vision increases. Optical expansion is a critical component in games that require catching, such as baseball, because it provides cues both about the distance and the velocity of the ball.

With these and other depth cues such as stereoscopic vision and linear perspective, the visual system converts two-dimensional retinal images into three dimensions. This perception of depth is as direct as the perception of color. As with optic flow and spatial constancy, visual information is unconsciously integrated with head and eye movement, and we experience depth, distance, and object movement without knowing how we do it. Spatial information on depth is not stored in memory but is processed repeatedly and directly into action or perception (or both).

Visual-Motor Abilities

The unconscious knowledge of the body necessary for visual-motor actions and the changes in the visual array that result from movement of the body are integral to all movement through space and all interactions with objects. Interactions in the environment include kicking a ball and avoiding obstacles, but the most widely studied interaction is the use of vision in reach and grasp.

Visual Guidance for Reach to Grasp

Both reach and preparation for grasp rely on the visual input of the dorsal stream, which transforms visual information into motor commands (Jeannerod, 1997; Milner & Goodale, 1993; Mountcastle, 1995). Reach and the preparation to grasp are highly coordinated, but they are separate and distinct subsystems of visual-motor behavior and depend on different sorts of visual information. The transport of the hand needs information about the distance and direction of the object, but preparation for grasp needs information about the object's size, shape, and orientation (Jeannerod, 1994). As the hand touches the object, tactile input adjusts the hand pressure to qualities such as hardness and texture.

Reaching

The function of reach is to move the hand to a desired location. Reach is coded for direction and distance in relationship to the body schema, and the object's location in relation to a person is important for the action (Jeannerod, 1997). During the transport phase, there is an initial acceleration of the arm toward the target that slows as the hand nears contact. The hand is now in central vision, and a final visual adjustment can be made so that the hand lands exactly on target. The initial movement of the arm to the target is preplanned and not disturbed by the loss of vision after the movement has been initiated. What is disrupted when vision is eliminated during reach is the terminal correction of the movement at the end of the trajectory. This requires visual feedback (Jeannerod, 1981; Jeannerod & Biguer, 1982).

Preparation for Grasp

Reaching for an object not only involves the coordinates for the movement of the arm but also the preparation of the hand for grasp. This involves a complex interplay of the motor system with the visual registration of the object. During the grasp process, the object has been fixated and the intrinsic properties of the object are processed to guide motor control. Size, shape, orientation, and texture influence how the object will be grasped, and all are registered so that as the arm moves, the hand begins to shape to accommodate to the size of the object and the forearm rotates to position the hand to match the orientation of the object. You can try this yourself. Note the automatic change in forearm rotation when using a palmar grasp to reach toward a dowel or small rod held in either a vertical or horizontal direction. When reaching for a horizontally presented rod, the hand is positioned with the thumb facing down. When the rod is in a vertical position, the forearm is rotated so that the thumb faces up. Vision registers the difference in the orientation of the object and, without conscious awareness, the hand accommodates to these two different situations. A similar automatic adjustment of the opening of fingers can be seen when reaching for a small or larger block. Contact with the object is planned so that the grasp points of the fingers are located on regions of the object's boundary that would be expected to yield the most stable grip (Goodale et al., 1994).

Whole Body Movement

Information on the role of neurological structures involved in the movement of the body through space is less precise than that describing movements of the hand in space. (This is probably because the exploration of single neuron responses in monkey is possible when the animal can be confined to a primate chair. Studying total body movements using this method would be extremely diffi-

cult.) Peripheral vision serves optic flow and is important in posture and locomotion. Neurons in the posterior parietal cortex have been described as driven by optic flow and may play a role in the visual guidance of self-movement through space (Mountcastle, 1995). Mechanisms of depth perception, in particular those based on movement, are also critical to negotiating moving objects.

Vision and Balance

The influence of vision on balance is secondary to the integration of the vestibular, proprioceptive, and tactile signals that orient our bodies to the direction of gravity and to the surface of support (Stoffregen & Ricco, 1988). Although the somatic senses are primary in postural control, vision also exerts a powerful influence through the mechanism of optic flow. The effect of a moving visual surround on postural reactions has been demonstrated on adult subjects in a laboratory setting (Nashner, 1985). The postural response to vision, particularly peripheral vision, is very rapid. The importance of vision in balance is seen in the Standing and Walking Balance Test of the SIPT, which involves activities such as standing on one foot and walking heel to toe in a straight line. In typical individuals, performance on these balancing activities is significantly better when the eyes are open than when they are closed.

At age 9 months, children have been shown to lose sitting balance when the side "walls" of an experimental room were moved. The response to movement in the visual surround indicates that infants use optic flow to control their posture (Bertenthal & Clifton, 1998; Lee & Aronson, 1974). Older children were found to inhibit the postural response better; they swayed but did not fall. As balance control and muscle tone develop, older children appear to compensate for the optic flow (Kellman & Banks, 1998). Children with mental retardation show delay in controlling their response (Butterworth & Ciccheti, 1978). Their problem may be the result of inadequate processing of peripheral vision, which may be related to delayed maturation of the nervous system.

Locomotion

Locomotion requires the negotiation of obstacles, apertures, changes of height, and moving objects. Adults perform these actions automatically, without being aware of the information that regulates their performance. These actions require the registration of depth and distance along with the integration of the body schema and the processing of the ever-changing visual array during movement. Gibson (1979) considered vision, proprioception, and vestibular function all to be critical for posture and balance but believed that the sensory information needed for walking was primarily visual (from the optic flow pattern).

Moving through a room without bumping into objects requires accurate perception of the location of the objects as well as a central image of the boundaries of our bodies. Infants have this ability before they can walk. Myklebust (1975) found the difficulty of one child in avoiding obstacles, even when repeatedly warned, to be associated with other problems of depth and movement perception. In the early perceptual-motor literature, the inability to avoid obstacles was attributed to poor body schema (Kephart, 1960). Another hypothesis is that a child who bumps into things may have a problem processing peripheral vision (Titcomb et al., 1997). These suggestions are not necessarily mutually exclusive because poor avoidance of obstacles may have different origins.

Dealing with Moving Objects

The perception of motion includes the motion of the self relative to stable surroundings, the motion of objects relative to the surroundings, the motion of the surroundings relative to self, and the relative motion of moving objects (Owen, 1990). Optic flow specifies the direction, magnitude, path, speed, and acceleration of one's movement (Owen, 1990; Warren, 1990). Mechanisms of depth perception detail the features of the environment as well as the direction, path, speed, and acceleration of moving objects (Lappin, 1990). These perceptual systems are mutually supported and together serve coordinated action between the self and both stationary and moving objects. Figure 12–21 classifies sensory integration activities according to the relative movement of the self and objects (i.e., a target on which the client acts).

Negotiating moving objects requires the monitoring of self-movement as well as the perception of the distance, direction, and speed of the approaching object. Some children may have difficult with this. For example, children with severe spatial problems, such as Ricky, may not be accurate in judging the speed and distance of oncoming cars and thus be unable to cross a street alone (e.g., Myklebust, 1975).

Catching a moving object is primarily a spatial-temporal skill. It requires three-dimensional detail of features of the environment and perception of the direction, path, speed, and acceleration of the object. The motor response must be precise in time and place so perception and motion coincide as to where and when the object arrives. Both the motion of the self and the motion of the object must be monitored.

Assessing the trajectory and timing in ball playing is a learned skill. In ball catching, the time to contact is specified by optic expansion (Bertenthal & Clifton, 1998). However, the motor system, driven by feedforward, must be timed for the hand to be in position at the moment judged for the ball's arrival. The relative importance of these two processes for the accuracy of catching depends on how much experience a person has had with the task.

Summary of Visual Control of Movement in Space

Two of the primary functions of human vision are the guidance of motor actions and the visual identification of the objects in the environment. There are strong indications that different neural networks at subcortical and cortical levels mediate these two functions. Spatial vision is believed to be more related to the processing of vision in the parietal lobe and object vision to processing in the temporal lobe.

Efficient movement requires coordination between visual-spatial processing and proprioceptive and vestibular information. As the body moves, the visual array changes, and vision must adjust to these changes. Mechanisms such as optic flow, spatial constancy, motion parallax, and optical expansion help us to accurately interpret these changes.

As occupational therapy practitioners, we cannot fully define the neurophysiological processes of the people with whom we work. However, the observable behaviors represented in a child like Ricky certainly seem to point to difficulty with visual control of movement in space. Ricky could not negotiate the classroom environment without bumping into objects or tripping. He did not know when it was safe to cross a street by judging the speed of an oncoming car. Each of these tasks required the visual analysis of where objects and the body were in space.

Although critical to basic human actions, efficient control of movement is not the only contribution of spatial vision. In the next section, we look at *spatial cognition.*

VISUAL-SPATIAL ABILITIES AND COGNITION

Up to this point, we have described the unconscious visual spatial processing that guides our movements. However, visual-spatial inputs also contribute to the conscious processing referred to as spatial cognition (Kosslyn & Koenig, 1992). At this level, visual-spatial abilities are a component of many cognitive skills. Higher-order visual-spatial abilities involve the ability to recognize and remember the relationships between features within an object or design, between two or more objects, or between oneself and objects. They also include the ability to mentally manipulate objects or imagine how an object would appear if either the whole object or parts of it were moved. These are the skills we use when understanding relationships between lines, angles, and curves that are needed in geometry or architecture or in visualizing potential chess moves that master chess players do with ease. We also use spatial cognition when finding our way around in a new place or moving through familiar surroundings without getting lost.

Both movement through space and spatial cognition draw on the dorsal stream for the discrimination of spatial properties, such as the position, orientation, and size of objects and their parts. However, aside from this, they differ markedly. Although object recognition, the main function of the ventral stream, does *not* play a role in the movement of our bodies through space, it is an important part of spatial cognition (Kosslyn & Koenig, 1992). Furthermore, spatial cognition draws heavily on the *conscious* analysis that is a function of the prefrontal cortex (Baddeley, 1992; Collette et al., 1999; Frith & Dolan, 1996; Mellet et al., 1998); when describing movement through space, we have specifically focused on movements that are not on a conscious level. Thus, although movement in space requires coordination of vestibular, proprioceptive, and visual systems (primarily through the dorsal stream), spatial cognition depends primarily on both the ventral and dorsal streams of the visual system as well as the

prefrontal cortex (Fig. 5–2.) The common link is the dorsal stream, which tells us where objects are relative to ourselves and to each other. Without this, there is no spatial component.

Spatial cognition can be divided into two major groups. One, *topographical orientation,* has at its basis an individual's relationship to his or her environment. The other group, which we have labeled *object-focused spatial abilities,* relates to objects themselves.

Topographical Orientation

Topographical orientation, or wayfinding, is the ability to go from place to place in familiar surroundings without getting lost and to learn how to find the way in new environments. It has several distinct components that can be used singly or in combination, depending on the demands of the setting or the person's ability. These components draw on both the ventral and dorsal visual streams because both the identification of places and their positions must be processed (Aguirre & D'Esposito, 1999; Aguirre et al., 1998).

Basic to topographical orientation is the knowledge of the location of places with respect to oneself. Objects or landmarks in our environment identify places within the spatial framework and orient us to where and in which direction to turn. As we become familiar with landmarks in our environment, we build mental representations of the locations of and directions toward familiar places. This internal sense of direction, together with our memory of landmarks, is what we use primarily when finding our way around the environment.

The highest level of topographical representation is that of a spatial schema or mental map of the spatial relationship between multiple locations. A spatial schema makes it possible to make spatial inferences and allows the use of shortcuts, perspective taking, and the making of models or maps.

Wayfinding dysfunction may manifest itself primarily in novel places. Brain-injured clients with wayfinding dysfunction complain that it takes them longer to learn their way around new places. This appears to be because they must learn how to use compensatory techniques to find their way (Newcombe & Ratcliff, 1989). Fine et al. (1980) described a man who succeeded in working as a delivery truck driver only because his coworkers provided him daily with a written checklist of landmarks and turnings.

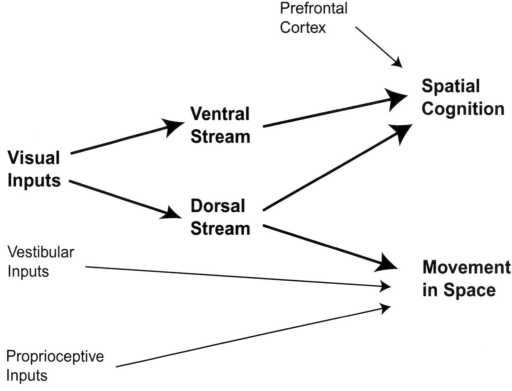

■ FIGURE 5–2 Contributions of the visual system to spatial abilities.

Children who have difficulty with wayfinding are familiar to many occupational therapy practitioners. Ricky is a good example. For 6 months, Ricky came weekly to an outpatient occupational therapy clinic. It took him nearly 3 months to learn the route from the front door to the clinic, which involved making only two turns. Even after that time, if anyone stopped Ricky while he was on his way from the door to the clinic, he became disoriented and could not find his way on his own.

We do not know how common wayfinding problems are in children with spatial dysfunction. Studies of children with learning disabilities are generally limited to the use of standardized psychological tests such as the Wechsler Intelligence Scales for Children (WISC), supplemented by standardized academic measures. Tests such as these would not indicate whether problems in wayfinding exist. Severe disorders of daily life skills may surface, but more subtle problems may not be identified.

Children with problems in wayfinding can be helped to develop compensatory strategies if they have the ability to use visual and verbal cues. Ther-

apists, teachers, and parents can help by understanding the disorienting effect of featureless objects, and being sure that landmarks such as desks or lockers are easily identifiable. Assisted practice in route learning can be provided by pointing out landmarks and by having the child verbalize the way to help with memorizing relevant turns. When needed, written directions or drawings of landmarks with directional arrows can be provided.

Object-Focused Spatial Abilities

Another aspect of spatial cognition focuses on the spatial relations of objects themselves, irrespective of the individual. This aspect, which we refer to as *object-focused spatial abilities,* includes skills tapped by many formal assessments, including several of the performance subtests of the WISC, such as Block Design and Object Assembly. Definitions of spatial abilities that come from cognitive psychology frequently are limited to object-focused spatial abilities (Voyer et al., 1995). Often these abilities have been defined primarily by features of the tests used to assess them, rather than by any functional behavior (Voyer et al., 1995). This is an important point; a deficit in wayfinding can be determined because an individual frequently gets lost, but poor performance on a formal test of object-focused spatial ability may or may not be directly linked to functional behavior. Although a deficit in object-focused spatial abilities is strongly associated with other cognitive deficits (and is often assessed in standard intelligence tests), the actual functional implications of poor performance are not clear.

An additional confounding factor is the complexity of many of the tests themselves. Often they require general cognitive abilities such as attention, memory, or verbal facility. Because of this complexity, it is often not clear what a given test is evaluating, and a child may perform poorly on any given test for reasons other than a spatial disability (Farah, 1990; Kolb & Wishshaw, 1995). A further complication is that spatial dysfunction might not be detected by a test. Some tests can be completed successfully using other cognitive strategies, so success does not rule out disability. We cannot assume that a spatial disorder has been excluded based on the normal performance in one or two tests (Newcombe & Ratcliff, 1989). An analytic approach is needed to look for the reasons for a poor performance on a test (Ratcliff, 1982).

As we stated earlier, the common element between movement in space and spatial cognition is the contribution of the dorsal stream. Knowing the role that the dorsal stream plays in object-focused tasks will help to clarify what aspects of these tasks relate to spatial abilities. Neuroimaging studies have shown that the dorsal stream is active when we judge location and relative distances among objects (Chen et al., 2000) and when we mentally turn or rotate an object (Alvisatos & Petrides, 1997; Carpenter et al., 1999; Tagaris et al., 1996). Clients with damage to the posterior parietal lobe, where the dorsal stream projects, have difficulty making judgments about object location and line orientation (Benton et al., 1983; Benton & Tranel; 1995; DeRenzi, 1985; Warrington & Rabin, 1970). Because the dorsal stream is associated with spatial relationships *and* spatial transformations, it is these aspects of tests that may reflect a common function in visual-spatial abilities (Chen et al., 2000). We will look at two different types of skills requiring visual-spatial abilities, one in which the spatial properties of objects are analyzed (spatial analysis) and one that requires the replication of the spatial aspects of objects (construction).

Spatial Analysis

Many object-focused tasks depend primarily on the ability to analyze the position and relationship of objects. The tasks can be as simple as finding two lines that are in the same orientation. More complex spatial analysis may involve mentally monitoring a series of steps that transform a spatial display and then predict the outcome. Games such as chess rely heavily on this ability. A good chess player visualizes a potential move on the board, the potential responses by an opponent, and the player's possible moves in response. Top chess players can predict several moves in advance. As the tasks become more complex, successful performance depends more and more on the problem-solving functions of the prefrontal cortex.

An example of a complex task that requires spatial analysis is paper folding, in which a person is shown a folded piece of paper in which holes have been punched and must determine what the paper will look like (i.e., where the holes will be) when it is unfolded (Fig. 5–3). The Paper Folding Test (Witkin, 1950) uses this format. Subjects must determine which one among four unfolded pieces of paper is the same as a folded model in which holes were punched. The number of folds increases as the test progresses, requiring the subject to visualize each step of the unfolding.

Although we might assume from its name that the Space Visualization Test of the SIPT requires spatial analysis, this is not true for all of the test items. The earliest items require only matching shapes. This involves ventral stream processing, not dorsal, and it is a measure of form perception, not spatial perception. The next group of items in this test uses the same form. The task is to match the location of the hole to that of the peg in the formboard, which requires analysis of the location of an internal detail. At the highest level, the test requires mental rotation of the forms to determine which one will fit. Thus, it measures two different aspects of spatial abilities at the higher levels. For young children, who complete only the form discrimination items, Space Visualization measures object perception but not spatial perception.

The Figure-Ground Perception Test of the SIPT does not require spatial analysis. Instead, it requires recognition of objects or forms when other objects or forms are used as distracters. The spatial relationship of the objects is not important,

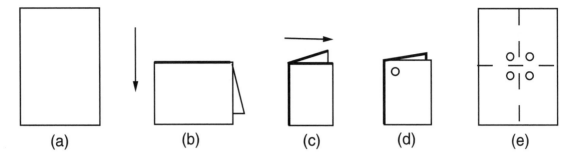

(a) a sheet of paper
(b) paper folded in half
(c) paper folded in half again
(d) hole punched in corner
(e) appearance of paper when unfolded

■ FIGURE 5–3 An example of paper folding.

and the objects do not need to be mentally moved or turned in order to find them.

Constructional Ability

Constructional performance is a perceptual activity with a motor response that includes drawing and assembling. Construction has a strong spatial component, just as accurately reproducing a two-dimensional or three-dimensional design requires grasping the spatial relationships among the parts of a design. Construction requires not only spatial abilities processed by the dorsal system and elementary form perception as processed by the ventral system but also a wide range of cognitive abilities, which may include attention, concentration, or verbal facility, depending on the task. Despite this complexity, clients with parietal lesions (which disrupt dorsal but not ventral stream processing) show a marked inability to demonstrate even a rudimentary understanding of the spatial relationships needed for construction.

Constructional ability is commonly divided into two types, drawing and assembly. Assembly is the use of objects to construct a design.

DRAWING OR COPYING

Drawing and copying are the most common forms of testing constructional performance. Copying tasks include imitation, copying with model present, or copying from memory. The models themselves are two dimensional, but they may represent three-dimensional figures, and they range from replication of simple lines to complex combinations of forms. Drawing in response to verbal command requires visual imagery. Although much is yet unknown about the capacities that underlie the ability to draw and copy drawings, some clues can be found in extensive research in child development and neuropsychology.

Differentiation between some aspects of drawing ability can be found in child development. First, form discrimination and form reproduction are widely separated developmental skills. Infants can discriminate simple forms such as a square and circle at age 6 months but cannot draw a circle until age 3 years or a square until age 4 years. Second, the perceptual nature of copying is demonstrated by the developmental sequence of the skill. Copying a square requires drawing horizontal and vertical lines, something 3-year-old children can do, but it is several years before a child has the perceptual skills needed to analyze and draw a square using these horizontal and vertical lines.

Maccoby and Bee (1965) studied copying in preschool children and concluded that errors stemmed from what they termed "failure to perceive the attributes of a form." Perceptual attributes include curved versus straight lines, open versus closed forms, the number and slant of lines, and the size of angles. Children in the study not only matched forms correctly but also recognized that their own incorrect drawings did not match. Success required perception of attributes.

Children's performance is also influenced by the method of examination. They first are successful in the *imitation of drawing strokes* that place little demand for the perception of attributes or memory. Next, children can *copy models with sticks;* shortly after they are able to *draw the model*. The highest level, *drawing with the model removed*, is a memory task and is not asked of young children.

In addition, the orientation of strokes and figures has been found to be influenced by the background on which children draw (Naeli & Harris, 1976). When preschool-aged children copied triangles and squares onto a triangular sheet of paper, the triangles were more accurate than the squares. This is the reverse of the usual developmental sequence of success in drawing squares preceding success in drawing triangles.

An example of a construction test that uses drawing is the Design Copying test of the SIPT. Part I has children copy designs onto a dot grid. The dot grid provides cues to the spatial relationship of the lines. Part II does not involve a grid. In addition to evaluating the completed designs, the scoring for Design Copying also considers the process children used in their construction, and parts of this analysis look at the spatial relationships among the parts (e.g., reversals, inversions).

HANDWRITING

Handwriting is a particularly important skill in children's daily school activities. Poor execution of the spatial aspects of writing numbers and letters leads to errors in math, illegibility, and messy homework. An accomplished handwriter uses vision only for spot checks to make sure horizontal alignment and proper spacing between words is maintained, but beginning handwriters depend on vision for guidance when learning to write.

Letter formation in manuscript writing requires a spatial analysis similar to that of copying geometric forms, and copying forms at some early level of proficiency generally precedes writing (Ziviani, 1995). When a child with a spatial disability has difficulty with letterforms, the errors may be the poor shaping or closure of individual letters or a lack of uniformity in orientation or size.

Handwriting requires organization in the placement of writing on a page. The external spatial demands for organization include attention to the edges of the paper and to the conventions of going from top to bottom and left to right. A line of writing must be in horizontal alignment, not slanting up or down, and sequential lines must be parallel. Beginning writers are given lined paper, so the task becomes placement of the letters and words on the line and control of size to stay between lines.

The most common spatial errors in handwriting involve incorrect and inconsistent spacing between writing units (Stott et al., 1985; Ziviani & Elkins, 1984). These may include overspacing between letters in a word and underspacing between words (or running words together).

CONSTRUCTION WITH OBJECTS

A second class of constructional abilities requires the manipulation of objects that must be assembled to match a model. Tasks such as these place less demand on memory and imagery; trial-and-error may be possible in finding correct solutions. In other ways, the demands for spatial cognition are similar to those in paper and pencil spatial tests. There is less research to date on construction with objects than on drawing and copying.

A simple assembly task is the copying of models of cubes as used in the testing of young children. Young children are able to stack cubes before they can arrange them in a line (Stiles-Davis, 1988). Cube designs ranging from a three-block bridge through 10 block steps are age graded through age 6 years (Gesell et al., 1940). With older children and adults, the age level of success provides an indication of the severity of constructional disability (Lezak, 1995).

More complex two-dimensional designs include the WISC Block Design and Object Assembly subtests, stick construction, and parquetry blocks. The SIPT Constructional Praxis test requires the assembly of a construction of blocks to replicate a three-dimensional model. Part II analyzes the construction by looking at the spatial relationships among the parts, such as whether blocks are displaced or at an incorrect angle.

CONSTRUCTION AND BRAIN DYSFUNCTION

Constructive disability resulting from right hemisphere damage is associated with a spatial perceptual disorganization not usually seen after damage to the left hemisphere. The spatial errors that may occur include both a loss of the overall configuration of the model and an inability to perceive the spatial relationships of the parts of the drawing. Poor orientation of forms, inappropriate spacing between elements of a model, and difficulty representing three dimensions also occur. The most severe disability results in piecemeal, fragmented drawings (Guerin et al., 1999; Lezak, 1995). The same spatial errors in drawing construction are seen in children with congenital damage to the right hemisphere and in children with spatial problems secondary to other kinds of brain dysfunction (Bellugi et al., 1988; Stiles-Davis, 1988). These children commonly show normal form perception.

Children with learning disabilities may demonstrate one spatial error but not another. For example, one child might show disorganization of the spatial relationships within a figure, and another may have difficulty with orientation or the spatial relationships among figures (Henderson, 1992, 1992–1993). Still others may have more difficulty with the overall contour of a model than with its internal detail (Denkla, 1985).

There is no "drawing center" in the brain (Kosslyn & Koenig, 1992). The studies of constructional disability have shown that many separate component abilities are used. This is illustrated by a report from Ratcliff (1991) that described two clients who showed a striking dissociation between form perception and spatial perception. One client was able to draw exceptionally realistic copies of pictures. They were not exact but captured the essential features of the original. However, his copies of meaningless geometric designs were distorted and incomplete. A second client could not recognize objects or draw even simple objects on command, but he was able to analyze and accurately reproduce the spatial relationships between the parts, edges, and contours of complex geometric designs. He drew these designs line by line with attention to the relative position of the elements to each other. He could copy pictures of objects, but he could not recognize what he had drawn. These clients provide added information about the separability of perception of forms and construction.

A classification of constructional ability needs further research, but, as the components are clarified, greater precision in the design of remedial strategies in constructional disability will be possible. For the present, it is important to observe and record how a child accomplishes constructional tasks (Loikith, 1997).

Summary of Spatial Cognition

Visual-spatial abilities contribute significantly to cognition. Skill in finding our way around our house, school, neighborhood, and city, and in telling others how to do the same, depends to a great degree on these abilities. They also play a major role in solving geometry problems, winning a game of chess, repairing an engine, or designing a skyscraper. Even basic skills, such as handwriting or aligning numbers to solve an addition problem, rely on spatial cognition.

Although we may use formal tests of spatial abilities to assess spatial cognition, the test scores themselves do not tell us how our clients function in everyday life. Low test scores may lead us to hypothesize that a client will have difficulty with handwriting or with mathematics, but this may not be the case. Furthermore, we must analyze the process clients use to complete test items so that we can clarify whether or not a poor performance is caused by poor spatial abilities.

SUMMARY AND CONCLUSION

Vision is the process of discovering from what we see what is present in the visual world and where it is (Marr, 1982). Distinct anatomical neural pathways serve "what" and "where" functions, a ventral pathway for object perception and a dorsal pathway for spatial organization. In this chapter, we have focused on two different aspects of the dorsal pathway, movement in space and spatial cognition. Both spatially guided movement and the discrimination of the spatial characteristics of objects originate in the dorsal pathway, but the visual information for these two aspects is further integrated in different areas within the CNS.

In the processing of movement in space, vision is integrated with the vestibular, proprioceptive, and tactile input to the posterior parietal lobe, and spatial information is relayed directly to the motor system. This visual spatial information is used at an unconscious level for functions that range from reach and grasp to whole body movement to and around objects.

Spatial cognition draws on both the dorsal and the ventral pathways for visual information that is integrated with other areas of the cortex that do not contribute to movement. Spatial cognition requires memory and conscious analysis of the objects perceived and thus depends on increasingly complex interactions of these many areas.

Visual control of movement in space and spatial cognition are related in their mutual dependence on the dorsal system. However, a spatial dysfunction in one is not indicative of a dysfunction in the other. Motor problems or problems in depth perception might be accompanied by problems in spatial cognition, as we have seen with Ricky, but poor performance on cognitive spatial tests in no way indicates a movement disorder. *Spatial cognition is less likely than the visual control of movement to be affected by sensory integrative dysfunction.*

The complexity of tests of spatial cognition makes it difficult to determine what a given test is evaluating in a given child. The form and space tests of the SIPT require many skills of a child in addition to spatial analysis. Some children appear to have a visual-spatial problem based on test scores, but the underlying problem might be in cognition. Alternately, bright children might use other strategies to circumvent a spatial problem when they are actually weak in this area. *Therefore, poor test scores on the form and space tests of the SIPT may not be reflective of sensory integrative dysfunction.* Thus, spatial dysfunction may be expressed in two very different ways, and occupational therapists need to be aware of both aspects.

References

Aguirre, G. K., & D'Esposito, M. (1999). Topographical disorientation: A synthesis and taxonomy. *Brain, 122,* 1613–1628.

Aguirre, G. K., Zarahn, E., & D'Esposito, M. (1998). Neural components of topographical representation. *Proceedings of the National Academy of Science USA, 95,* 839–846.

Alvisatos, B., & Petrides, M. (1997). Functional activation of the human brain during mental rotation. *Neuropsychologia, 35*(2), 111–118.

Atkinson, J. (1993). A neurobiological approach to the development of 'where' and 'what' systems for spatial representation in human infants. In N. Eilan, R. McCarthy, & B. Brewer, (Eds.), *Spatial representation* (pp. 325–339). Cambridge, MA: Blackwell.

Barnard, N., Crewther, S. G., & Crewther, D. P. (1998). Development of a magnocellular function in good and poor primary school-age readers. *Optometric Vision Science, 75,* 162–168.

Baddeley, A. (1992). Working memory. *Science, 255,* 556–559.

Bellugi, U., Sabo, H., & Vaid, J. (1988). Spatial deficits in children with Williams Syndrome. In J. Stiles-Davis, M. Kritchevsky, & U. Bellugi (Eds.), *Spatial cognition: Brain bases for development* (pp. 273–298). Hillsdale, NJ, Erlbaum.

Benton, A., Hamsher, K., Varney, N., & Spreen, O. (1983). *Contributions to neuropsychological assessment.* New York: Oxford University.

Benton, A., & Tranel, D. (1993). Visuoperceptual, visuospatial, and visuoconstructive disorders. In K. M., Heilman, & E. Valenstein, (Eds.), *Clinical neuropsychology* (3rd ed., pp. 165–213). New York: Oxford University.

Bertenthal, B. I., & Clifton, R. K. (1998). Perception and action. In W. Damon, (Ed. in chief), D. Kuhn, & R. Siegler (Vol. Eds.), *Handbook of child psychology,* 5th ed. vol. 2, *Cognition, perception and language* (pp. 51–102). New York: John Wiley & Sons.

Butterworth, G., & Cicchetti, D. (1978). Visual calibration of posture in normal and motor retarded Down's syndrome infants. *Perception: 7,* 513–525.

Carpenter, P. A., Just, M. A., Keller, T. A., Eddy, W., & Thulborn, K. (1999). Graded functional activation in the visuospatial system with the amount of task demand. *Journal of Cognitive Neuroscience, 11,* 9–24.

Chen, J., Myerson, J., Hale, S., & Simon, A. (2000). Behavioral evidence for brain-based ability factors in visuospatial information processing. *Neuropsychologia, 38,* 380–387.

Collette, F., Salmon, E., Linden, M. V. D., Chicherio, C., Belleville, S., Degueldre, C., Delfiore, G., & Franck, G. (1999). Regional brain activity during tasks devoted to the central executive of working memory. *Brain Research: Cognitive Brain Research, 7,* 411–417.

Demb, J. B., Boynton, G. M., Best, M., & Heeger, D. J. (1998). Psychophysical evidence for a magnocellular pathway deficit in dyslexia. *Vision Research, 38,* 1555–1559.

Denkla, M. B. (1985). Motor coordination in dyslexic children: Theoretical and clinical implications. In F. Duffy, & N. Geshwind (Eds), *Dyslexia: Theoretical and clinical implications* (pp. 187–195). Boston: Little Brown.

DeRenzi, E. (1985) Disorders of spatial orientation. In J. Fredricks (Ed.), *Handbook of clinical neurology,* vol. 1, *Clinical neuropsychology* (pp. 405–422). New York: Elsevier Science.

Farah, M. J. (1990). *Visual agnosia: Disorders of object recognition and what they tell us about normal vision.* Cambridge, MA: MIT.

Fine, E., Mellstrom. M., Mani, S., & Timmins, J. (1980). Spatial disorientation and the Dyke-Davidoff-Masson syndrome. *Cortex, 16,* 493–499.

Frith, C., & Dolan, R. (1996). The role of the prefrontal cortex in higher cognitive functions. *Brain Research: Cognitive Brain Research, 5,* 175–181.

Gesell, A., Halverson, H., Thompson, H., Ilg, F., Castner, B., Ames, L., & Amatruda, C. (1940). *The first five years of life.* New York: Harper and Row.

Gibson, J. J. (1966). *The senses considered as perceptual systems.* Boston: Houghton-Mifflin.

Gibson, J. J. (1979). *The ecological approach to visual perception.* Boston: Houghton-Mifflin.

Girard, P., Salin, P., & Bullier, J. (1991). Visual activity in areas V3A and V3 in the macaque monkey. *Journal of Neurophysiology, 66,* 1493–1503.

Girard, P., Salin, D., & Bullier, J. (1992). Response selectivity in neurons in area MT in the macaque monkey during reversible inactivation of area VI. *Journal of Neurophysiology, 67,* 1–10.

Goodale, M. (2000). Perception and action in the human visual system. In M. S. Gazzaniga (Ed.). *The new cognitive neurosciences* (2nd ed., pp. 365–377). Cambridge, MA: MIT.

Goodale, M., & Milner, L. S. (1992). Separate visual pathways for perception and action. *Trends in Neurosciences, 15,* 20–25.

Goodale, M. A., Meenan, J. P., Bulthoff, H. H., Nicolle, D. A., Murphy, K. J., & Racicot, C. I. (1994). Separate neural pathways for the visual analysis of object shape in perception and prehension. *Current Biology, 4,* 604–610.

Guerin, F., Ska, B., & Bellville, S. (1999). Cognitive processing of drawing abilities. *Brain and Cognition, 40,* 464–478.

Henderson, A. (1973). Body schema and the visual guidance of movement. In A. Henderson & J. Coryell (Eds.). *The body senses and perceptual deficit. Proceedings of the Occupational Therapy Symposium, Boston University, March, 1972* (pp. 1–15). Boston: Author.

Henderson, A. (Fall 1992). A functional typology of spatial disabilities and disabilities. Part 1. *Sensory Integration Quarterly, 20,* 1–6.

Henderson, A. (Winter 1992–1993). A functional typology of spatial disabilities and disabilities. Part 1. *Sensory Integration Quarterly, 20,* pp. 1–5.

Hendry, S. H. C., & Calkins, D. J. (1998). Neuronal chemistry and functional organization in the primate visual system. *Trends in Neurosciences, 21,* 344–349.

Jakobson, L. S., & Goodale, M. A. (1994). The neural substrates of visually guided prehension: The effects of focal brain damage. In K. M. B. Bennett & U. Castiello (Series Eds.), G. E.. Stelmach, & P. A. Vioon, (Vol. Eds.). *Advances in psychology,* Vol. 105. *Insights into the reach and grasp movements* (pp. 199–214). North-Holland: Elsevier Science.

Jeannerod, M. (1981). Intersegmental coordination during reaching at natural visual objects. In J. Long & A. Baddeley (Eds.). *Attention and performance IX* (pp. 153–168). Hillsdale, NJ: Erlbaum.

Jeannerod, M. (1994). Object oriented action. In K. M. B. Bennett & U. Castiello (Series Eds.). G. E. Stelmach, & P. A. Vioon, (Vol. Eds.). *Advances in psychology,* Vol. 105. *Insights into the reach and grasp movements* (pp.129–150). North Holland: Elsevier Science.

Jeannerod, M., (1997). *The cognitive neuroscience of action.* Cambridge, MA: Blackwell.

Jeannerod, M., & Biguer, (1982). Visuomotor mechanisms in reaching within extrapersonal space. In D. Ingle, M. A. Goodale, & R. Mansfield (Eds.).

Advances in the analysis of visual behavior (pp. 387–409). Cambridge, MA: MIT.

Kandel, E. R., Schwartz, J. H., & Jessell, T. M. (1991). *Principles of neural science.* New York: Elsevier.

Kellman, P., & Banks, M. (1998). Infant visual perception. In W. Damon (Ed. in Chief), D. Kuhn, & R. Siegler (Vol. Eds.). *Handbook of child psychology,* 5th Ed. Vol. 2. *Cognition, perception and language* (pp. 103–146). New York: John Wiley & Sons.

Kephart, N. C. (1960). *The slow learner in the classroom.* Columbus, Ohio: Merrill.

Kolb, B., & Whishaw, I. (1995). *Fundamentals of human neuropsychology* (4th ed.). New York: W. H. Freeman.

Kosslyn, S. M., & Koenig, O. (1992). *Wet mind.* New York: Free.

Lackner, J. R., & DiZio, P. A. (2000). Aspects of body self-calibration. *Trends in Cognitive Sciences, 4,* 279–288.

Lappin, J. S. (1990). Perceiving the metric structure of environmental objects: form, motion, self-motion, and stereopsis. In R. Warren & A. H. Wertheim (Eds.). *Perception and control of self-motion* (pp. 541–578). Hillsdale, NJ: Erlbaum.

Lee, D. N., & Aronson, E. (1974). Visual proprioceptive control of standing in human infants. *Perception and Psychophysics, 15,* 529–532.

Lezak, M. D. (1995). *Neuropsychological assessments* (3rd ed.). New York, Oxford University.

Livingstone M. (1993). Parallel processing in the visual system and the brain: Is one subsystem selectively affected in dyslexia? In A. M. Galaburda (Ed.). *Dyslexia and development: Neurobiological aspects of development* (pp. 237–257). Cambridge, MA: Harvard University.

Livingstone, M. S., Rosen, G. D., Drielane, F. W., & Galaburda, A. M. (1991). Physiological and anatomical evidence for a magnocellular defect in developmental dyslexia. *Proceedings of the National Academy of Science USA, 88,* 7943–7947.

Loikith, C. C. (1997). Visual Perception: Development, assessment, and intervention. In M. Gentile (Ed.). *Functional visual behavior: A therapist's guide to evaluation and treatment options* (pp. 197–247). Bethesda, MD: American Occupational Therapy Association.

Marr, D. (1982). *Vision: A computational investigation into the human representation and processing of visual information.* San Francisco: Freeman.

McCarthy, R. (1993). Assembling routines and addressing representations: An alternative conceptulization of 'what' and 'where' in the human brain. In N. Eilan, R. McCarthy, & B. Brewer. (Eds). *Spatial representation* (pp. 373–399). Oxford, UK: Blackwell.

Maccoby, E. E., & Bee, H. L. (1965). Some speculations concerning the gap between perceiving and performing. *Child Development, 36,* 367–378.

Mellet, E., Petit, L., Mazoyer, B., Denis, M., & Tzourio, N. (1998). Reopening the mental imagery debate: Lessons from functional anatomy. *Neuroimage, 8,* 129–139.

Milner, A. D., & Goodale, M. A. (1993). Visual pathways to perception and action. In T. P. Hicks, S. Molotchnikoff, & T. Ono (Eds.). *The visually responsive neuron: From basic neurophysiology to behavior* (pp. 317–337). New York: Elsevier Science.

Mishkin, M., Ungerleider, L., & Macko, K. (1983). Object vision and spatial vision: Two cortical pathways. *Trends in Neuroscience, 6,* 414–417.

Mountcastle, V. B. (1995). The parietal system and some higher brain functions. *Cerebral Cortex, 5,* 377–390.

Myklebust, H. R. (1975). Nonverbal learning disabilities: Assessment and intervention. In H. R. Myklebust (Ed.). *Progress in learning disabilities* (pp. 85–121). New York: Grune & Stratton.

Naeli, H., & Harris, P. (1976). Orientation of the diamond and the square. *Perception, 5,* 77–78.

Nashner, L.M. (1985). Strategies for organization of human posture. In M. Igarashi Blac (Ed.). *Vestibular and visual control of posture and locomotion equilibrium.* Basel, Switzerland: Karger.

Newcombe, F., & Russell, W. R. (1969). Dissociated visual perceptual and spatial deficits in focal lesions of the right hemisphere. *Journal of Neurology, Neurosurgery, and Psychiatry, 32,* 73–81.

Newcombe, F., Ratcliff, G., & Damasio, H. (1987). Dissociable visual and spatial impairments following right posterior cerebral lesions: Clinical, neuropsychological, and anatomical evidence. *Neuropsychologia, 25,* 149–161.

Newcombe, F., & Ratcliff, G. (1989). Disorders of visuospatial analysis. In E. Boller & J. Grafman, (Eds.). *Handbook of neuropsychology* (Vol. 2, pp. 333–356). New York: Elsevier.

O'Conner, M., & Padula W. (1997). Visual rehabilitation of the neurologically involved. Gentile, M. (Ed.). *Functional visual behavior: Therapist's guide to evaluation and treatment options* (pp. 295–319). Bethesda, MD: American Occupational Therapy Association.

Owen, D. H. (1990). Lexicon of terms for the perception and control of self-motion and orientation. In R. Warren & A. H. Wertheim (Eds.). *Perception and control of self-motion* (pp. 33–50). Hillsdale, NJ: Erlbaum.

Ratcliff, G. (1982). Disturbances of spatial orientation associated with cerebral lesions. In M. Potegal (Ed.). *Spatial abilities: Development and physiological foundations* (pp. 301–331). New York: Academic.

Ratcliff, G. (1991). Brain and space: Some deductions from clinical evidence. In J. Paillard, (Ed.). *Brain and space* (pp. 237–250). Oxford, UK: Oxford University.

Shen, L., Hu, X., Yacoub, E., & Ugurbil, K. (1999). Neural correlates of visual form and visual spatial processing. *Human Brain Mapping, 8,* 60–71.

Sieg, K. W. (1988). A. Jean Ayres. In B. R. J. Miller,

K. W. Sieg, F. M. Ludwig, S. D. Shortridge, & J. Van Deusen (Eds.). *Six perspectives on theory for practice of occupational therapy* (pp. 95–142). Rockville, MD: Aspen.

Stein, J. P. (1991) Space and the parietal association areas. In J. Paillard (Ed.), *Brain and space* (pp. 185–222). Oxford, UK: Oxford University.

Stein, J., Talcott, J., & Walsh, V. (2000). Controversy about the visual magnocellular deficit in developmental dyslexics. *Trends in Cognitive Sciences, 4,* 209–211.

Stiles-Davis J. (1988). Spatial dysfunctions in young children with right cerebral injury. In J. Stiles-Davis, M. Kritchevsky, & U. Bellugi (Eds.), *Spatial cognition: Brain bases for development* (pp. 251–272). Hillsdale, NJ: Erlbaum.

Stoffregen, T. A., & Ricco, G. E. (1988). An ecological theory of orientation and the vestibular system. *Psychological Review, 95,* 3–14.

Stott, D. H., Moyes, F. A., & Henderson, S. E. (1985). *Diagnosis and remediation of handwriting problems.* Guelph, Ontario: Brook Educational.

Tagaris, G. A., Kim, S. G., Strupp, J. P., Andersen, P., Ugurbil, K., & Georgopoulos, A. P. (1996). Quantitative relations between parietal activation and performance in mental rotation. *Neuroreport, 7,* 773–776.

Titcombe, R. E., Okoya, R., & Schiff, S. (1997). Introduction to the dynamic process of vision. In M. Gentile (Ed.). *Functional visual behavior: A therapist's guide to evaluation and treatment options* (pp. 3–39). Bethesda, MD: American Occupational Therapy Association,

Ungerleider, L. G., & Haxby, J. V. (1994). 'What' and 'where' in the human brain. *Current Opinion in Neurobiology, 10,* 157–165.

Ungerleider, L., & Mishkin, M. (1982) Two cortical visual systems. In D. J. Ingle, M. A. Goodale, & R. J. Mansfield (Eds). *Analysis of visual behavior* (pp. 549–585). Cambridge, MA: MIT.

Vidyasagar, T. R., & Pammer, K. (1999). Impaired visual search in dyslexia relates to the role of the magnocellular pathway in attention. *Neuroreport, 10,* 61283–61287.

von Cramon, D., & Kerkhoff, G. (1993). On the cerebral organization of elementary visuo-spatial perception. In B. Gulyas, D. Ottoson, & P. E. Roland (Eds.). *Functional organisation of the human visual cortex* (pp. 211–231). Oxford, UK: Pergamon.

Voyer, D., Voyer, S., & Bryden, M. P. (1995). Magnitude of sex differences in spatial abilities: A meta-analysis and consideration of critical variables. *Psychological Bulletin, 117,* 250–270.

Walther-Müller, P. U. (1995). Is there a deficit of early vision in dyslexia? *Perception, 24,* 8919–8936.

Warren. W. H. (1984). Perceiving affordances:Visual guidance of stair climbing. *Journal of Experimental Psychology, Human Perception and Performance, 10,* 683–703.

Warren, R. (1990). Phenomena, problems, and terms.

In R. Warren, & A. H. Wertheim (Eds.). *Perception & control of self-motion* (pp. 1–32). Hillsdale, NJ: Erlbaum.

Warren, W., & Whang, S. (1987). Visual guidance of walking through apertures. *Journal Experimental Psychology: Human Perception and Performance, 13,* 371–383.

Warrington, E. K., & Rabin, P. (1970). Perceptual matching in patients with cerebral lesions. *Neuropsychologia, 8,* 475–487.

Witkin, H. A. (1950). Individual differences in ease of perception of embedded figures. *Journal of Personality, 19,* 1–15

Ziviani, J. (1995). The development of graphomotor skills. In A. Henderson & C. Pehoski (Eds.). *Hand function in the child: Foundations for remediation* (pp. 184–193). St. Louis: Mosby.

Ziviani, J., & Elkins, J. (1984). An evaluation of handwriting performance. *Educational Review, 36,* 251–261.

Central Auditory Processing Disorders

Joan M. Burleigh, PhD
Kathleen W. McIntosh, PhD
Michael W. Thompson, PhD

> *John has perfect hearing but has significant difficulty understanding speech when other noises are present.*
>
> —*The parent of a child diagnosed with central auditory processing deficits*

The study of central auditory processing disorders (CAPD) in children and adults has received increasing attention over the past 30 years. Although a host of information has been available pertaining to visual processing, central auditory processing (CAP) has received less attention. Nevertheless, over the years, the central auditory nervous system (CANS) has intrigued a variety of professionals, including audiologists, speech and language pathologists, educators, occupational therapists, and psychologists.

Ayres' (1972a, 1972b) early work in sensory integration reflected a belief in the importance of the auditory system to learning. However, over the years, sensory integration theory has become dominated by examination of three particular sensory systems: vestibular, tactile, and proprioceptive (Fisher et al., 1991). Thirty-five years after its inception, sensory integration theorists, researchers, and clinicians are again beginning to recognize the need to situate the auditory system

in the study of sensory integration theory (Dunn, 1999; see also Chapter 14). We contend that, because the auditory system is an essential element in human performance, the study of sensory integration theory and practice must also include an examination of CANS function.

PURPOSE AND SCOPE

The purpose of this chapter is to provide broad-based information regarding the complex nature of CANS function in children and adults. We explore behavioral manifestations of dysfunction, incidence of CAPD and auditory maturation, CANS function, CAP tests, and management of dysfunction.

We work from a functional description of CAPD relating to integrity of function along the CANS pathways (i.e., auditory channel capacity). Because of this focus, we provide a detailed description of the CANS and describe various tests used by audiologists. We also address management, with special attention to accommodating inefficiencies in CANS processing.

DEFINITIONS

The American Speech-Language-Hearing Association (ASHA) (1996) described CAP as a functional entity:

> Central auditory processes are the auditory system mechanisms and processes responsible for the following behavioral phenomena: sound localization and lateralization; auditory discrimination; auditory pattern recognition; temporal aspects of audition including, temporal resolution, temporal masking, temporal integration, and temporal ordering; auditory performance with competing acoustic signals; and auditory performance with degraded acoustic signals (ASHA, 1996, p. 41).

Audiologists have entertained a variety of definitions for CAPD over the past 20 years (ASHA, 1996; Katz, 1992; Keith, 1986). As with any complex area of study, differences exist among professionals as to the best ways to describe CAPD.

A functional description of CAPD may include the following: a condition in which one has problems processing or interpreting auditory information when it is presented in a less than optimal listening environment. Typically, individuals with CAPD have normal hearing on traditional pure tone and speech tests but are unable to perform well on a CAP test battery that evaluates the integrity of the CANS. The most baffling aspect of this difficulty is that the vast majority of children and adults with CAPD can hear even the faintest speech signals, but when listening to speech input in a dynamic auditory environment, they have difficulty understanding the speech message. This is possibly caused by an internal distortion of the signal or an "overloaded" auditory system.

One problem with defining CAPD probably results from the complexity of CANS function and its diverse impact on many aspects of human function. Willeford and Burleigh (1985) indicated that professionals do not easily recognize CAPD for a number of reasons:

- Knowledge of the CANS is limited.
- Traditional hearing tests are not designed to evaluate the complexity of the CANS.

- CAPD often is viewed too simplistically.
- Terminology describing CAPD is often nonspecific and misleading.
- Auditory stimuli are very transient in nature and cannot be held in time.

Another source of confusion in defining CAPD has arisen from descriptions of auditory processing difficulties associated with learning disabilities, attention deficit disorders (ADD), or attention deficit with hyperactivity disorder (ADHD), or specific auditory language impairment. It is often inferred that the determination of auditory perceptual difficulties associated with these diagnoses implies the presence of CAPDs. A *distinction between the processing of information presented auditorily and CAP* is often overlooked. It is our contention that when difficulties processing auditory language content or remembering auditory sequential information are identified, it is impossible to know, from that testing alone, if impairments arise from primary CAP inefficiencies, from primary linguistic or cognitive deficits, or from all three. A CAPD, as it is discussed in this chapter, refers specifically to primary auditory dysfunction or inefficiency in function at any level along the CANS pathways and structures. Therefore, CAPDs will be defined only by impairments quantified on the basis of a specific battery of tests designed to evaluate responses to specific acoustic variations in auditory stimuli while holding constant cognitive or linguistic context.

BEHAVIORAL MANIFESTATIONS

Although identification of CAPD relies on a specific battery of tests, certain behaviors can enable recognition of at-risk children and adults. The following section reviews behaviors commonly observed in children with confirmed CAPD. These behavioral manifestations of CAPD were drawn, in part, from case histories of children with both typical and atypical CANS function. The children were selected either from our clinical population or participated in a study conducted by researchers at the Center for Central Auditory Research at Colorado State University in conjunction with staff at a local school district. Case history information was obtained from parents.

Fifty students with atypical CAP (60 percent boys; 40 percent girls; mean age, 9.46 years) were referred to the Center for Central Auditory Research for a variety of reasons. Each of these students had low scores on at least one measure of a CAP test battery. A total of 41 students with normal CAP (43 percent boys; 57 percent girls; mean age, 10.48 years) from a local school district, pre-identified by teachers as having adequate listening ability in their classrooms, served as a control group. These students performed within normal limits on the same comprehensive CAP battery. The results appear in Tables 6–1 through 6–4.

The majority of students with atypical CANS function were reported by their parents to have difficulty following directions. They were often distractible and easily flustered or confused, had short attention spans, and were sensitive to loud sounds.

Eighty percent of children with CAPD had difficulty following directions compared with only 12 percent of children with normal CANS function. Furthermore, large differences in reports of distractibility, confusion in noisy places, and attention span were also recorded. A total of 36 percent of children with atypical CANS function were overly sensitive to loud noises compared with only 7 percent of children with normal CANS function (see Table 6–1).

Children with CAPD may appear to be inconsistently aware of sound; they are not always alerted by new auditory information in the same way as other children (Willeford & Billger, 1978; Willeford & Burleigh, 1985). They may be classified as poor listeners because of a tendency to ignore important auditory information. Apparently inconsistent auditory attention is related to being distracted by extraneous auditory stimuli. Although these listeners appear to be inconsistent, they are actually consistent. It is their auditory environment that is constantly changing, therein placing demands on their inefficient CANS and resulting in variable performance.

Children with CAPD may also demonstrate delayed responses to verbal stimuli in an effort to "buy time" to process incomplete information. Much of the auditory input they receive may be degraded enough that they need more time to integrate incomplete information into a meaningful message.

Classroom Behaviors

Behaviors especially notable for children with CAPD are listed in Table 6–2 and include:

- Daydreaming
- Forgetfulness
- Problems sitting still
- Difficulty with time concepts
- Problems completing assignments
- Dislike of school
- Excessive talking in the classroom

Parents classified children with CAPD as underachievers far more frequently than did parents of children without CAPD. A number of referrals for CAP evaluation have come from psychologists who have noted discrepancies between children's achievement and performance on intelligence tests.

Social-Emotional Behaviors

Children with CAPD may also exhibit atypical social behaviors such as (see Table 6–3):

- Increased anxiety and tension
- Low self-confidence
- Increased frustration
- Attention seeking
- Temper tantrums
- Being easily upset in new situations

Parents of children with CAPD often reported that their children preferred to play with younger

---

■ ☐ TABLE 6–1   **PERCENTAGE OF ABERRANT AUDITORY BEHAVIORS REPORTED IN SCHOOL-AGE CHILDREN WITH CONFIRMED CENTRAL AUDITORY PROCESSING DISORDERS AND NORMAL CENTRAL AUDITORY PROCESSING FUNCTION**

	Clients with CAPD, %	Normal Subjects, %
Problems following directions	80	12
Easily distracted	72	22
Easily flustered or confused	66	10
Appears confused in noisy places	42	0
Has short attention span	72	10
Is sensitive to loud noises	36	7

■ Table 6–2 **Percentage of Aberrant Classroom Behaviors Reported in School-Age Children with Confirmed Central Auditory Processing Disorders and Normal Central Auditory Processing Function**

	Clients with CAPD, %	Normal Subjects, %
Daydreams	64	22
Forgetful	74	24
Restless, has problems sitting still	58	10
Has difficulties with time concepts	46	0
Does not complete assignments	52	7
Dislikes school	28	10
Talks excessively	48	12
Is an underachiever	46	5

children. Based on differences in traits between the two groups, we developed the behavioral checklist found in Figure 6–1. This checklist may be helpful for identifying children with potential CAPD.

Disinhibition Behaviors

Behaviors commonly associated with disinhibition and noted in some children with confirmed CAPD are shown in Table 6–4. These include:

- Irritability
- Hyperactivity
- Impulsivity
- Disobedience
- Rowdiness
- Oppositional behaviors

Children with CAPD may also be described as disruptive, uncooperative, and destructive. Interestingly, these disinhibition behaviors are also very commonly noted in children identified as having ADD or ADHD. Riccio et al. (1994) found that teachers and parents described disinhibition behaviors in children with CAPD significantly more frequently than in typically developing children. However, only 50 percent of the children with CAPD met the diagnostic criteria for ADHD. Although disinhibition behaviors may be observed in children with either CAPD or ADHD, disinhibition symptoms appear as primary and persist for longer than 6 months in children with ADHD (American Psychiatric Association, 1994). In children with CAPD, these symptoms appear secondary to auditory overload and vary over time.

INCIDENCE AND MATURATION

The incidence of CAPD is not known; however, some demographic information is available. In a study of 307 children with confirmed CAPD by Burleigh et al. (1982), the incidence of difficulty on the Willeford Central Auditory Processing Battery was similar for boys and girls; however, referral rates were three times higher for boys. These authors also reported that left-handed children or children who had not developed a hand

■ Table 6–3 **Percentage of Aberrant Social Emotional Behaviors Reported in School-Age Children with Confirmed Central Auditory Processing Disorders and Normal Central Auditory Processing Function**

	Clients with CAPD, %	Normal Subjects, %
Exhibits anxiety or tension	48	10
Lacks self-confidence	54	17
Is easily frustrated	70	20
Seeks attention	58	27
Has temper tantrums	38	7
Prefers playing with younger children	54	12
Is easily upset in new situations	40	5

Source: J. M. Burleigh, 1991.

■ TABLE 6–4 **PERCENTAGE OF DISINHIBITION BEHAVIORS REPORTED IN SCHOOL-AGE CHILDREN WITH CONFIRMED CENTRAL AUDITORY PROCESSING DISORDERS AND NORMAL CENTRAL AUDITORY PROCESSING FUNCTION**

	Clients with CAPD, %	Normal Subjects, %
Irritability	34	5
Hyperactivity	34	7
Impulsivity	32	15
Disobedience	28	7
Rowdiness	16	10
Doing opposite of what is requested	26	7
Disruptive	28	7
Uncooperative	28	7
Destructive	20	2

preference tended to show more difficulty on this CAP test battery, specifically the tests that were associated with cortical processing of auditory information. Burleigh et al. (1995) observed similar distributions of CAPD across genders.

One challenge to defining the incidence of CAPD is that CAP dysfunction may appear as a distinct impairment or may co-occur with other heterogeneous conditions such as attention deficit disorders, learning disabilities, developmental language disorders, or sensory integrative dysfunction. Because CAPD is observed in so many clinical populations (Katz, 1992; Keller, 1992; Riccio et al., 1994), data regarding its incidence are not currently available.

Another obstacle to determining the incidence of CAPD in children is the maturation of the CANS. Normative data strongly suggest that adult level functioning occurs between approximately age 9 and 12 years (Chermak, 1996; Willeford, 1977; Willeford & Burleigh, 1985). Because of this maturation effect, it is important to use age-appropriate tests and age-normed data for identification and determination of potential CAPD.

Although there has been criticism regarding the identification of CAPD in children younger than 9 years, we believe that the use of age-normed tests allows for the identification of performance deficits in children whose CANS maturation is not yet completed. Some children do "outgrow" apparent auditory processing difficulties. However, we do not know when or which children will eventually develop a mature CANS. The risk of not identifying children before age 9 years is that early learning experiences may be altered in a way that prevents affected children from attaining maximum performance.

AUDITORY SYSTEM

Efficient processing of auditory information relies on intricate sequencing of neural events that are dependent on the combined function of the peripheral hearing mechanism (Fig. 6–2) and the CANS (Fig. 6–3). After adequate sensory reception of the auditory stimulus in the peripheral hearing mechanism, auditory input must then be processed through a series of neurological events and specialized cellular structures and nerve fibers. Faulty function at any point in the network may result in inaccurate processing. The following review focuses on events that occur beyond the peripheral hearing mechanism.

Central Auditory Nervous System

The CANS begins functionally at the point where the auditory nerve synapses in the cochlear nucleus and where all cochlear nerve fibers have been determined to terminate.

Cochlear Nuclei

Much has yet to be learned concerning the function of structures within the cochlear nuclei, but there is general agreement that they are intricate structures. Auditory nerves entering the cochlear nuclei are arranged in an orderly fashion in each of three divisions to maintain the tonotopic organization of the cochlea (Webster, 1971). The cochlear nuclei maintain ipsilateral afferent transmission of auditory information from the cochlea and auditory nerve. Because of this factor, an insult to this structure may result in decreased pure tone thresholds (Dublin, 1985). Pure tone thresh-

CENTRAL AUDITORY PROCESSING DISORDERS BEHAVIOR CHECKLIST

NAME _____ AGE ____ GRADE _____ DATE _____ SEX _____

SCHOOL _____**RATED BY**

_____

(*name*)   (*position*)

Please circle the number that best describes how this child usually functions.

5 = always, 4 = usually, 3 = sometimes, 2 = seldom, 1 = never

1.	Can follow directions when presented to the class	5 4 3 2 1
2.	Can sit and listen for 20 minutes	5 4 3 2 1
3.	Can concentrate on a task	5 4 3 2 1
4.	Is not easily frustrated	5 4 3 2 1
5.	Does not become flustered or easily confused	5 4 3 2 1
6.	Can attend for 20 minutes without fidgeting	5 4 3 2 1
7.	Can remember assignments and new duties	5 4 3 2 1
8.	Can concentrate in a noisy environment	5 4 3 2 1
9.	Completes assignments within time limit	5 4 3 2 1
10.	Understands time concept	5 4 3 2 1
11.	Works up to his/her potential	5 4 3 2 1
12.	Possesses good self-confidence	5 4 3 2 1
13.	Makes good use of classroom time	5 4 3 2 1
14.	Prefers playing with children his/her own age	5 4 3 2 1
15.	Is calm and not anxious	5 4 3 2 1
16.	Routinely possesses a good disposition	5 4 3 2 1
17.	Easily motivated to begin new tasks	5 4 3 2 1
18.	Readily adapts to new situations	5 4 3 2 1
19.	Can tolerate loud sounds	5 4 3 2 1
20.	Prefers to listen and take turns talking	5 4 3 2 1

(J. M. Burleigh, 1991)

■ FIGURE 6-1 Central auditory processing disorders behavior checklist.

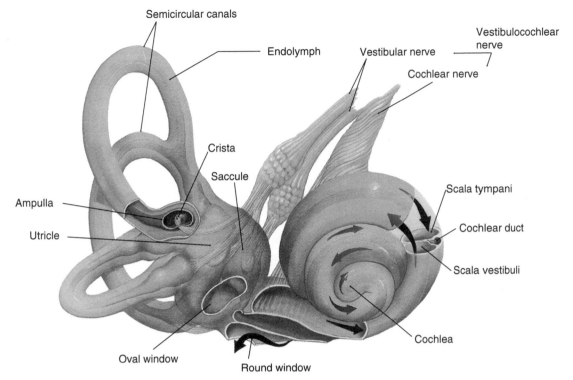

Figure 6-2 Schematic of the peripheral auditory and vestibular system. (Reprinted with permission from Scanlon, VC, and Sanders, T: Essentials of Anatomy and Physiology, 3rd edition, p. 199. Philadelphia, F.A. Davis Company, 1999.)

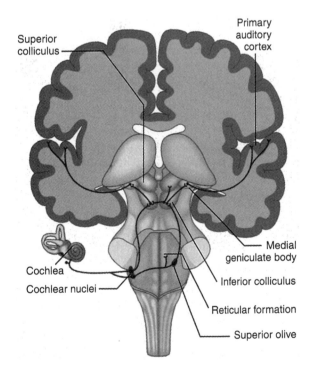

Figure 6-3 Schematic of central auditory nervous system. (Reprinted with permission from Lundy-Ekman, L: Neuroscience: Fundamentals for Rehabilitation, p. 300. Philadelphia, W.B. Saunders Company, 1998.)

olds are the levels at which pure tone stimuli are barely perceptible. Operationally, a threshold is the level at which an individual detects the presence of sound 50 percent of the time.)

The cochlear nuclei have been shown to be highly multifarious and consist of several different cell types that respond with a variety of different discharge patterns (Kiang, 1975; Oertel, 1997). Various cells within the cochlear nuclei may provide the first mechanism for CAP and the coding of various characteristics of sound (Musiek & Lamb, 1992). Thus, the cochlear nuclei are important in the accurate processing of auditory information.

From the cochlear nuclei, CANS complexity increases and the speech message is transmitted to the auditory cortex via various routes. Because of the complexity of transmission and redundancies in speech, inefficiencies in the CANS do not manifest themselves on conventional audiometric evaluation, a phenomenon termed the "subtlety principle" (Jerger, 1960). As explained by Bocca and Calearo (1963), this principle suggests that, because of the general redundancies of speech, information can be transmitted and interpreted in the auditory cortex even if the CANS is inefficient. However, if redundancies of speech are reduced, as in even a minimally noisy listening environment, intact transmission of auditory input will be reduced.

Decussation of Neural Fibers

Before arriving at the next structure, the superior olivary complex, the majority of nerve fibers cross over (i.e., decussate) via the trapezoid body to the opposite side of the brainstem. A minority (25 to 30 percent) of the fibers continue on the ipsilateral side. Therefore the right side of the brainstem and brain processes auditory stimuli received primarily from the left ear. The contralateral fibers represent the dominant pathways, and the ipsilateral pathways are secondary. These structures are all located in the lower pons region (Noback, 1985).

Superior Olivary Complex

The superior olivary complex is an important relay center in the brainstem for binaural integration, which is critical for accurate interpretation of auditory signals presented to both ears. Through binaural listening capabilities, we are able to attend to important auditory information while ignoring extraneous information. For adequate binaural listen-

ing to occur, signals from both ears must arrive simultaneously (Kiang, 1975). Certain audiological tests (e.g., binaural fusion and rapidly alternating speech) are dependent on binaural integration at the level of the superior olivary complex (Tobin, 1985).

Lateral Lemniscus

From the superior olivary complex, auditory information travels through the lateral lemnisci, the primary auditory pathways for ascending and descending pathways in the brainstem. Goldstein (1967) theorized that the auditory cortex was alerted to incoming stimuli by the "rapid transmission" lines of the lateral lemnisci.

Inferior Colliculus

The majority of fibers ascend from the lateral lemnisci to the inferior colliculi. Little is known about the inferior colliculus; however, it is well accepted that it is an important relay center for transmitting auditory information to the thalamus (Carpenter, 1972; Noback, 1985). The inferior colliculus consists of an elaborate network of neurons and axons, subdivisions, and banding patterns that may each contribute to different aspects of auditory processing (Oliver & Morest, 1984). Rose et al. (1966) demonstrated that the inferior colliculus facilitated binaural localization of both high and low frequencies and provided further crossover between contralateral and ipsilateral pathways (Whitfield, 1967), which implies a role in sound localization (Musiek & Baran, 1986).

Medial Geniculate Body

Even though the medial geniculate body is located in the thalamus and the inferior colliculus in the midbrain, they are separated by approximately 1 cm (Musiek & Lamb, 1992). The medial geniculate body represents the final subcortical level of the CANS. Its structure and organization are intricate, and little is known concerning its function. Galaburda (1994a) and Galaburda et al. (1994) have shown fundamental changes in the medial geniculate body in individuals with dyslexia. Galaburda (1994b) speculated that structural anomalies in the brainstem could make it difficult for individuals with dyslexia to interpret the rapidly changing sounds of human speech.

Reticular Activating System

The reticular activating system (RAS) is another multifarious structure in the center of the brainstem that is involved in a range of central nervous system (CNS) activities (French, 1957). Filley (1995) stated that, because of indistinct boundaries of the ascending RAS, this system may be better thought of as a physiological concept rather than an anatomical entity. It is commonly described as a general alarm mechanism that, when activated by incoming sensory stimuli, arouses or alerts the brain to prepare to interpret the stimuli (Carpenter & Sutin, 1983) and further plays an important role in maintaining alertness (Filley, 1995). Magoun (1963) suggested that the RAS aids the cortex in determining which stimuli are important for transmission and which should be suppressed.

Evidence has indicated that the RAS and cortex must receive electrical impulses in a synchronous manner for efficient processing of information (Schnitker, 1972). Once again, timing of electrical information is a critical factor in efficient processing.

Auditory Cortex

Ascending fibers from the medial geniculate bodies project to a specific region in the temporal lobes. Whitfield (1967) and Brugge (1975) indicated that each hemisphere:

- Received projections from both ears, suggesting binaural representation of auditory signals
- Maintained the tonotopic organization of the cochlea and brainstem
- Had a primary area that received nerve fibers from the lower portions of the auditory pathway

Furthermore, hemispheric specialization suggests that whereas the mature left hemisphere has a relative affinity for the processing of linguistic, sequential, and analytic stimuli, the right hemisphere is relatively dominant for nonlinguistic functions (Kolb & Wishaw, 1990; Witelson, 1977).

Anatomical studies of the brains of individuals with dyslexia report an absence of ordinary hemispheric asymmetries in the planum temporale (Galaburda et al., 1985; Musiek & Reeves, 1990). Furthermore, Kaufman and Galaburda (1989) found a higher number of cellular abnormalities and clusters of ectopic neurons in brains of individuals with dyslexia.

The primary connection between the two hemispheres is a massive bundle of fibers known as the corpus callosum. Musiek et al. (1984) have shown that complete sectioning of the corpus callosum results in significantly poorer performance on auditory tasks that require interhemispheric transfer of information as in dichotic listening tasks. According to Gazzaniga and LeDoux (1978), these intracortical connections must also work in synchrony in the transfer of information between hemispheres.

CENTRAL AUDITORY PROCESSING TESTS

Early tests for CANS function were developed for adults to identify sites of CNS lesions. Specifically, they were meant to identify life-threatening lesions in central auditory pathways. Studies using these unique measures were instrumental to our understanding the complexity of the CANS (Bocca et al., 1954; Lynn & Gilroy, 1972, 1975, 1977; Matzker, 1959; Sinha, 1959). With the advent of electrophysiological tests and neuroimaging techniques, central auditory tests are not likely to be used as sole measures for site-of-lesion identification. Currently, they are used primarily for analysis of auditory function.

For reliable assessment of CAP, all tests must be administered according to strict guidelines, using consistency of presentation, environmental sound control, established pass-or-fail criteria, and control of other sensory input during testing. To control for test consistency, each measure is administered in either audio tape or CD formats. For more in-depth information on proper tape and recorder maintenance, see Willeford and Burleigh (1985). Many tests are currently available in CD format, which is more reliable and does not require the same maintenance as tape-recorded material.

Tests should always be administered in a soundproof room that has an acoustic environment suitable for threshold measurement and a calibrated audiometer (American National Standards Institute, 1989). Intensity of test stimuli should always be at levels specified in the test manual and relative to each individual's hearing. Furthermore, because of the maturation of the CANS, pass-or-fail criteria should be interpreted based on age norms specified in test manuals.

Audiologic measures of CANS function are

sometimes criticized for not directly assessing CAP difficulties that occur in real-life situations (Willeford & Burleigh, 1985). However, the use of noncontrolled measures of listening capabilities precludes definitive assessment of inefficiencies in the CANS. Therefore, it is important to control auditory input during evaluation. Furthermore, it is recommended that testing should minimize the need for motor responses and reduce visual input, both of which could compromise results.

Behavioral Assessment Measures

A variety of commercially available behavioral tests measure CANS function. Various tests assess different levels of function in the CANS and use different protocols. Tests for children and adults are fairly similar in design, but measures for young children have been adapted for language age and mode of response. For example, one test uses a picture-pointing response format for children with a receptive language of 3 years, and another, for children age 6 years of age and older, requires verbatim repetition of sentences.

There are basically three distinct classifications of behavioral tests for CAP, which involve:

- Presenting different speech stimuli to the two ears at the same time (dichotic tests)
- Presenting speech or frequency-specific signals to one ear at a time (monotic tests)
- Fusing, blending, or sequencing complementary speech stimuli presented to the two ears at different times or with a specified time-onset format (binaural interaction tests)

A detailed description of dichotic, monotic, and binaural interaction tests can be found in the Appendix to this chapter.

Screening Tools

Although screening tools have been used as sole indicators of CAPD, their use should be limited to identifying a need for more in-depth CANS assessment. A Screening Test for Auditory Processing Disorders (SCAN or SCAN-C, revised) (Keith, 1986; Keith, 1999; Keith et al., 1989) was developed for children. The 1986 version consists of three subtests: Filtered Words (FW), Auditory-Figure-Ground (AFG), and Competing Words (CW). A more recent, revised version uses a CD format and adds a Competing Sentence (CS) sub-

test. There is also an adult version of this screening tool.

Keith (1986) indicated that the SCAN does not need to be administered in a soundproof room through an audiometer. Rather, it can be presented with a stereo cassette or CD player with the volume controls set at the most comfortable loudness level for each ear.

Although this method allows for ease of presentation, it also contributes to a lack of control of auditory input. Emerson et al. (1997) reported differences in composite and AFG scores when the SCAN was administered in a school setting and in a soundproof room. No children received scores poorer than one standard deviation below the mean when it was administered in a soundproof room. In contrast, when the SCAN was administered in the school environment, two of six children showed performance poorer than one standard deviation below the mean for the composite score and AFG subtest. These authors suggested the need for normative data for subjects evaluated in an audiometric test suite. Perhaps another recommendation is that testing should always be performed in a controlled test environment (e.g., a soundproof room); however, the norming of this screening measure was done in an uncontrolled acoustic environment. Chermak and Musiek (1997) listed a number of other concerns regarding the use of the SCAN, including the small normative sample of 3- and 4-year-old children, lack of validation with individuals who have confirmed CANS lesions, and the exclusion of a test of temporal processing.

Another feature of the SCAN is that results from the two ears are averaged for both the FW and AFG subtests, giving the examiner a single performance score and making determination of ear differences impossible. The importance of determining ear differences is discussed in the management section of this chapter.

Test Battery Approach

Because a number of CAP tests have been shown to primarily assess specific areas of the CANS, use of a comprehensive test battery is the method of choice for CAPD assessment. A battery should embody tests shown to be sensitive to several areas of the CANS, including those that target both brainstem and cerebral cortex involvement. The intended focus for specific tests can be referenced in the Behavioral Measures Appendix at the end of this chapter.

Singer et al. (1998) showed that the Binaural Fusion and Filtered Speech tests of the Willeford Central Auditory Test Battery and Masking Level Differences represented the best battery for 147 children with learning disabilities. Although these tests may reflect the best battery for children with learning disabilities, other tests may be more discriminating with other groups. For example, Hurley and Musiek (1997) showed that the Auditory Duration Patterns Test (Musiek et al., 1990) and Dichotic Digits Test identified 85 and 75 percent, respectively, of individuals who had cerebral lesions confirmed by neurological or radiological assessment or surgery. They did not administer tests typically associated with brainstem level auditory function.

Electrophysiological Assessment

Although behavioral tests rely chiefly on methods in which recognition of speech stimuli can be made more challenging to the CANS, electrophysiological measures typically use methods by which evoked potential responses are obtained at the brainstem or cortical levels (or both). Work by Kraus et al. (1996) is intriguing in that it elicits changes in behavioral discrimination patterns for children with learning problems that originate in the auditory pathway that are not dependent on attention or a voluntary response paradigm. This gives rise to the possibility that electrophysiological assessment can be used to evaluate the CANS in difficult-to-test clients and for the assessment of hearing impaired individuals.

Current electrophysiological test procedures include auditory brainstem response (ABR), middle latency evoked response (MLR), N1 and P2 responses, the P300, and mismatched negativity (MMN) tests. Whereas the ABR test procedure is a measure of brainstem integrity, the MLR, N1, P2, P300, and MMN tests measure function of cortical and subcortical areas of the brain in response to acoustic signals. Also included in the objective test category are acoustic reflexes (AR).

Electrophysiological tests such as evoked potentials require more instrumentation, more expensive equipment, and more time for administration than do behavioral tests of CAP function. However, as outlined by Chermak and Musiek (1997), certain individuals, such as those with head injuries and neurological diseases that involve the brainstem, may be well suited for assessment using these procedures.

Various studies have investigated the hit rate or sensitivity of electrophysiological measures in individuals with confirmed CANS dysfunction (Hurley & Musiek, 1997; Musiek et al., 1990, 1992, 1994). Additional studies have addressed the use of electrophysiological measures as they relate to CAP function in children and adults who do not have a frank neurological deficit (Jirsa, 1992; Kraus et al. 1993; 1996; Protti, 1983). Findings of this research are equivocal and underscore the need for continued study regarding the usefulness of electrophysiological testing as an alternative to behavioral measures for identifying CAP inefficiency.

MANAGEMENT

A variety of approaches to managing the effects of CAPD have been described. Among the most commonly discussed approaches are strategies that can be placed into two categories: those that target therapeutic remediation and those involving compensatory intervention. A third approach to management incorporates the use of technology.

One use of technology has involved the enhancement of auditory signals in busy listening environments using frequency-modulated (FM) auditory systems. Recent advances in digital signal processing (DSP) offer another application of technology in CAP management. This novel approach involves technology that changes the way in which acoustic information is presented in order to facilitate more efficient processing. Some of these acoustic changes can be implemented in real time.

Therapeutic Approaches

Numerous manuals, books, and pamphlets outline therapeutic procedures and guidelines for children with auditory perception problems. These target a variety of areas for remediation, including language and reading (Katz & Harmon, 1981; Lindamood & Lindamood, 1969; Tallal et al., 1996), phoneme recognition (Sloan, 1986), and metacognition and metalinguistics (Chermak & Musiek, 1997).

Other programs are designed to target selected auditory deficits, presumed to be identified by a central auditory test battery (Bellis, 1996). Auditory integration methods developed by Berard (1993) and Tomatis (Gilmore et al., 1989) are based on a theory that listening to altered acoustic input can improve auditory processing. However, a well-controlled study by Yencer (1998) using the Berard program (1993) did not result in improved CAP test scores.

Although therapeutic programs enhance performance in specific skill areas such as language, phonemic recognition, reading, and spelling, there is a paucity of data demonstrating that they change underlying central auditory abilities. We believe that such programs are appropriate as long as they are used to target specific skill development, without an expectation that CANS function itself will be altered.

Based on the premise that if important acoustic cues in speech were emphasized and extended, phonological processing and language comprehension function should increase. Tallal et al. (1996) and Merzenich et al. (1996) used time-altered speech to aid speech discrimination and language comprehension abilities in children with language-learning impairments (LLI). Their approach, designed to increase temporal processing abilities, included between 8 and 16 hours of training exercises over a 20-day period using a computer game format. A two-step algorithm (or formula) expanded the speech signal by 50 percent while preserving its spectral and pitch quality and then increased the intensity of primary consonants by as much as 20 dB (Tallal et al., 1996). They applied the algorithm to speech and language exercises, children's stories, and educational CD-ROMs, resulting in sharply segmented auditory stimuli that had a staccato quality.

Seven children in a pilot program and then 22 children (mean chronological age, 7.4 years) demonstrated significant gains in speech and language improvement after completion of this therapy program. Their program is marketed under the Fast ForWord title and targets individuals with language and reading problems. The goal is to assist children in recognizing sounds and sound combinations for language and reading enhancement.

Compensatory Management and Strategies

The primary goal of compensatory management is to help individuals cope with a variety of demands in their listening environments (Ayres, 1972b).

We discuss several techniques, including teaching strategies, preferential seating and ear strength considerations, sound-attenuating devices, and classroom acoustics.

Teaching Strategies

Various researchers (Barr, 1972; Bellis, 1996; Lasky & Cox, 1983; Matkin, 1988; Willeford & Billger, 1978; Willeford & Burleigh, 1985) have recommended compensatory management programs to improve performance in academic, work, and social environments. Many of our recommendations that follow were developed in conjunction with teachers and special educators in a local school district.

The majority of adaptations made for students with CAPD assist all students. Providing clear verbal directions and a learning environment that fits the task and encouraging students to take responsibility for their needs generally result in improved performance. In addition, the following are particularly helpful to those working with children or adults with CAPD:

- Provide a quiet space with minimal background activity for work or study.
- Precede auditory information with a touch to the shoulder or speaking the person's name.
- Phrase verbal messages in more than one way.
- Ask individuals to cross-check or rephrase important concepts presented in class, at work, and at home.
- Use a multisensory (i.e., verbal and written) approach for directions and presentation of concepts. Place short written instructions on a chalkboard or overhead; create a handout for more lengthy directions. A course or unit syllabus can guide students' planning and facilitate assignment completion.
- Provide copies of another's notes or the services of a note taker. Note taking is often a very difficult task because subtle ambient noise hinders the reception of auditory information.
- Provide short breaks to give those with inefficient auditory systems a rest and time to regroup.
- Administer tests, including achievement (e.g., district-wide examinations) and aptitude tests in a separate quiet room. The latter requires an *a priori* request for adaptation.

- Allow students to preview new information to become familiar with vocabulary and concepts before presentation in class.
- Schedule course content that requires extensive listening early in the morning or afternoon.
- Provide structured, controlled classrooms for optimal learning environments.
- Encourage computer use. Computers provide immediate visual feedback and may facilitate writing.
- Conduct conversations in a quiet area.
- Provide additional support for foreign languages. Students may find learning a foreign language especially challenging. They may benefit from visual and written material and from taped texts generated in a quiet environment.
- Discourage the use of tape recorders. They are *not* recommended because they record background noise, making it difficult to transcribe information. Transcription is also very time consuming.

These general guidelines should be supplemented with recommendations specific to an individual's needs. For example, if a student has difficulty with spelling, he or she should take all spelling tests in a separate quiet environment.

Preferential Seating and Ear Strength Considerations

Preferential seating is often recommended for individuals with CAPD to improve performance and behavior. Preferred location should be based on an audiologist's determination of whether information is processed more accurately by one ear. If an ear strength is identified, students should sit in the front of the classroom, just to one side of the center, with the stronger ear toward the teacher or speaker and away from auditory distractions. The same is true when students are seated on the floor or when a teacher or special service provider is working individually with a student. For children who do not demonstrate a relative ear strength or measurable ear differences, seating directly in line with the speaker near the front of the classroom is preferred (Willeford & Billger, 1978; Willeford & Burleigh, 1985).

Seating near the teacher has several advantages: auditory input is more easily received; sup-

plementary visual cues are more accessible; and the teacher is better able to monitor listening problems such as auditory fatigue, distractions, or failure to understand instructions. Stimuli that are virtually unnoticed by other students (i.e., pencil sharpeners, heating fans, hall noise) may be extremely distracting to a student with CAPD.

Sound-Attenuating Devices

The use of sound-attenuating devices (e.g., earmuffs or earplugs) may be beneficial to children and adults with CAPD who have difficulty concentrating and processing auditory input in busy environments (Hasbrouck, 1980; Willeford, 1980; Willeford & Billger, 1978; Willeford & Burleigh, 1985). These devices may be implemented in two ways, depending on CAP test results and the classroom task demands.

The use of earmuffs or earplugs worn binaurally is one important modification that can reduce noise and improve concentration during silent reading and writing or during any quiet seatwork time. The earmuffs or earplugs, in this case, function to reduce extraneous auditory distractions and allow the student to focus on his or her work. We most commonly recommend earmuffs, either Howard Leight, model QM 24, or Peltor, model H6, at the Colorado State University Center for Central Auditory Research. Both are lightweight. Stigma associated with earmuffs may be reduced or eliminated by having a number of pairs available for any student. We also recommend custom-made filtered earplugs worn in a binaural arrangement for deskwork or silent reading for some children and adults.

Another way to implement the use of sound attenuating devices involves occluding only one ear (Hasbrouck, 1980; Willeford, 1980; Willeford & Billger, 1978; Willeford & Burleigh, 1985). Willeford and Burleigh (1985) hypothesized that bilateral integration of sound may be disrupted in an impaired CANS. They suggest that by reducing sound to the weaker ear, a reduction of neurological interference from the weak ear to the strong ear might occur, resulting in improved figure-ground when listening in a noisy environment. They suggested that in real life, listeners tend to depend on strategic body or head positioning to optimally process information from a speaker and ignore background noise when listening in noisy situations. Therefore, it appears logical that an individual with CANS dysfunction who has measured ear differences will compensate by maneuvering his or her stronger ear toward the source of sound and that selective use of an earplug worn in the weaker ear may address that issue.

Personnel at the Center for Central Auditory Research are investigating the use of custom filtered earplugs worn in only one ear by individuals who have atypical CANS function with obvious asymmetries. The filter minimally attenuates sounds in the speech frequency range while decreasing sounds in the higher frequencies to a greater extent and is particularly useful in noisy situations. This filter is fit so that hearing is still within normal limits, even in the targeted higher frequency range.

Filtered earplug data were collected at the Center for Central Auditory Research on a group of 22 individuals with confirmed atypical CANS function and a control group of 11 individuals who performed within normal limits on a CAP test battery. Three central findings were observed regarding the use of these filters worn by individuals with obvious asymmetries in CANS function:

1. Persons with normal CANS function perform significantly better in noise than individuals with CAPD.

2. Those without CANS dysfunction discriminate best with two ears in an unfiltered condition.

3. When a filter is fit appropriately in persons with defined CAP asymmetries, speech discrimination performance is significantly improved.

Data were collected for speech discrimination ability obtained in the sound field in noise in a soundproof room. As shown in Figure 6–4, whereas a mean score of 82 percent was obtained for those with normal CANS function, a mean score of 64 percent was recorded for those with CANS dysfunction without the use of filtered earplugs. Interestingly, when the normal CANS group used the filter system in either ear, their performance dropped significantly ($p < 0.01$). This decrease in speech discrimination performance suggests that those with normal CANS function best when using both ears in the presence of background noise.

The same is not true for persons with CAPD. As shown in Figure 6–5, significantly improved speech discrimination performance ($p < 0.001$) is observed when ear filters are fit in the preferred ear as designated by CAP tests. Mean improvement

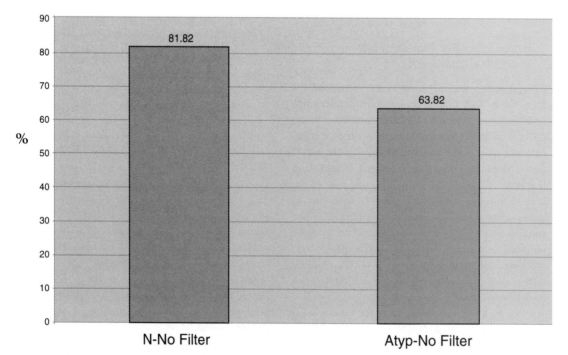

■ Figure 6–4 Auditory discrimination performance in persons with normal and atypical CANS function under noise condition with no ear filters (p<.0001).

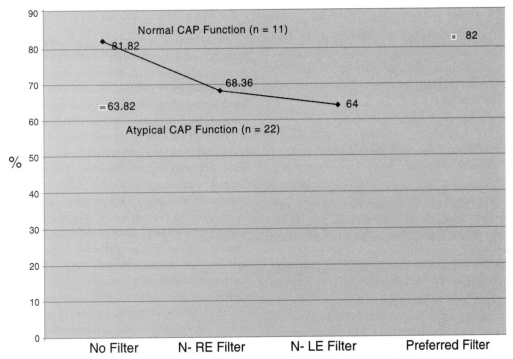

■ FIGURE 6-5 Auditory discrimination performance in persons with normal and atypical CAP function under noise condition with and without ear filters.

increased from 64 percent with no filters to more than 80 percent when using the preferred ear with the custom filter system. Interestingly, their performance with a filtered earplug in the preferred ear is similar to those with normal CANS function when using both ears in a noisy environment.

Mizushima and Burleigh (1997) presented a case study in which speech recognition ability increased 14 percent when using the filtered earplug over unoccluded performance in a noisy environment. The client reported less fatigue and improved ability to communicate when wearing the filter. However, care must be taken to determine which ear should be fitted with the customized filter to be worn when in difficult listening situations. Results have shown improvement in speech discrimination in an enclosed sound field when speech was presented at 40 dB greater than the individual's pure tone average (i.e., average of hearing thresholds at 500 Hz, 1000 Hz, 2000 Hz) and at a signal-to-noise ratio of +5.

Classroom Acoustics

Classroom acoustics have been of concern in the learning environment since the mid-1970s (Crum & Matkin, 1976; Finitzo-Hieber & Tillman, 1978),

but they have recently received a substantial increase in interest from educators. However, as research in the area of classroom acoustics suggests (Chermak & Musiek 1997; Crandell, 1992; Crandell & Smaldino, 1994), challenges remain in accomplishing an optimal environment for the reception of auditory information.

Several researchers (Crandell & Smaldino, 1994; Finitzo-Hieber, 1981; Sanders, 1965) have measured ambient noise in occupied and unoccupied classrooms and found that sound levels reflect adverse listening conditions in both. Furthermore, signal-to-noise ratios are often very low, which means that the intensity of the teacher's voice may be at or near the intensity level of noise in the classroom.

Sound absorption modifications of the classroom itself (e.g., drapes, carpeting, and sound-absorbing building materials) will likely benefit students with CAPD. However, according to Crandell and Smaldino (1994), consideration of noise levels before building a school is not typical. Acoustic modifications may not be given a high priority and are often considered after building completion. In addition, changes after construction may be costly and difficult to implement.

Technology

Advances in technology provide one of the most exciting emerging avenues for management. Novel ways of enhancing the efficiency of the auditory system will very likely be a target of future research and development.

Frequency-Modulated Assistive Listening Systems

In an effort to improve the signal-to-noise listening environment, classroom FM auditory systems have been recommended (Edwards, 1994; Flexer, 1994). FM auditory systems, both classroom amplification and personal units, are recommended for children with a variety of special needs, including CAPD (Blake et al., 1991; Crandell et al., 1994; Willeford & Billger, 1978).

Frequency-modulated systems consist of a wireless directional or omnidirectional microphone placed near the speaker's mouth in a lapel, lavaliere, or head-worn boom arrangement. The speaker's voice is amplified and transmitted, via FM radio waves, to a receiver worn by the listener (personal system) or placed close to the listener via loudspeaker (classroom system). The FM unit allows the speaker's voice to predominate while reducing background noise.

Rosenberg et al. (1995) used FM sound-field classroom amplification systems and reported improved listening and learning behaviors with 2054 kindergarten, first and second grade general education students. These investigators reported that the FM sound-field system aided listening and made it easier for the children to hear their teacher. Younger students showed more improvement in listening and learning performance than older children.

Audiologists traditionally recommend FM systems. Although their use has received considerable attention (Bellis, 1996; Chermak & Musiek, 1997; Stach et al., 1991; Willeford & Billger, 1978), we believe FM units should be used judiciously following guidelines for fitting and monitoring published by ASHA (1994). A trial with a personal system should precede its acquisition. Testing of performance with personal units should include speech recognition performance in quiet and noise. Tolerance for loud sounds should also be checked at specific volume control settings.

Digital Signal Processing

The advent of DSP technology has added greatly to the potential for exploring novel ways to enhance speech intelligibility in real-time. Wenndt (1991) and Wenndt et al. (1996) indicated that the use of linear time-rate expanded or slowed speech (i.e., all parts of speech expanded or slowed equally) shows promise for increasing intelligibility of speech in noisy situations for adults who have normal hearing acuity. Specifically, in the time-expansion paradigm, a 30 percent expansion or slowing of speech (compared with the average speaking rate) resulted in the greatest percentage of improvement. Burleigh (1996) showed that not only does time-rate linear expanded speech significantly enhance intelligibility for individuals with normal peripheral hearing and CANS function, but it also does so for individuals with atypical CANS function.

Craig (1997) described the development of a device (i.e., NHK Real-Time Speech Rate Conversion System) that allows for the manipulation of the rate of real-time speech without significantly changing the pitch, quality, or other suprasegmental characteristics of the speech signal. This device is targeted for potential use for aural (re)habilitative applications in an effort to increase the intelligibility of speech.

Burleigh et al. (1999) and Burleigh et al. (2000) presented a new approach for exploring CANS function while using DSP techniques for stimuli modification. Included in their studies was a method for accommodating a decrease in speech intelligibility in noise seen with CANS dysfunction. These authors' premise relied on the phenomenon of binaural asynchronies (BA) or differences in blending auditory information between ears for individuals with atypical CANS function. Their hypothesis was that these differences could be measured and accommodated in individuals with impaired CANS.

SUMMARY AND CONCLUSION

The wide variety of approaches to managing the various problems associated with CAPD can create confusion for practitioners seeking best management strategies for their clients. Practitioners must review a particular approach to critically evaluate its soundness and determine if it addresses the specific difficulties of individual clients. Practitioners must also review the purpose of the program and data that support claims of effectiveness.

The authors of this chapter believe that therapeutic approaches are important when specific skill areas such as phoneme recognition, reading, or spelling are targeted for remediation. However, when a CAPD (as defined in this chapter) is identified, consideration should be given to the likelihood that inefficiencies in the CANS affect the way in which acoustic information is being received by a learner, and therein underlie performance deficits across many areas of learning. In such cases, a management approach that focuses on novel ways of altering acoustic stimuli provides a means for more efficient processing of input, regardless of its content. Therefore, this approach may optimize learning of specific skills as well as facilitate learning in other skill areas. The use of compensatory strategies should also be considered a useful approach to any management program.

Central auditory processing in children and adults has received significant attention during the past two decades. Studies focusing on the manifestations of CAPD have led to increased insight into its broad ramifications. Children and adults with CAPD may have challenges in a number of sensory systems and behavioral areas. Because of the complex nature of CAPD, assessment cannot be done incidentally. Testing requires use of a comprehensive battery to reflect function at various levels of the CANS. Appropriate individualized management can be developed only after underlying function has been determined. Technology allows for the potential of changing acoustic input in novel ways so that efficient processing of acoustic events can be realized.

References

American National Standards Institute. (1989). *American national standards specifications for audiometers*. (ANSI S3.6-1989). New York.

American Psychiatric Association. (1994). *Diagnostic and statistical manual of mental disorders* (Ed. 4). Washington, DC.

American Speech Language Hearing Association. (1994, March). Guidelines for fitting and monitoring FM systems. *ASHA 36*(suppl. 12), 1–9.

American Speech Language Hearing Association. (1996). Central auditory processing: Current status of research and implications for clinical practice. *American Journal of Audiology, 5,* 41–54.

Ayres, A. J. (1972a). Improving academic scores through sensory integration. *Journal of Learning Disabilities, 5,* 338–343.

Ayres, A. (1972b). *Sensory integration and learning disorders*. Los Angeles: Western Psychological Services.

Barr, D. (1972). *Auditory perceptual disorders*. Springfield, IL: Charles C. Thomas.

Beasley, D., Forman, B., & Rintelmann, W. (1972a). Perceptions of time-compressed CNC monosyllables by normal listeners. *Journal of Auditory Research, 12,* 71–75.

Beasley, D., & Freeman, B. (1977). Time-altered speech as a measure of central auditory processing. In R. Keith (Ed.). *Central auditory dysfunction* (pp. 129–175). New York: Grune & Stratton.

Beasley, D., Schwimmer, S., & Rintelmann, W. (1972b). Intelligibility of time-compressed CNC monosyllables. *Journal of Speech and Hearing Research, 15,* 340–350.

Bellis, T. (1996). *Assessment and management of central auditory processing disorders in the educational setting: from science to practice*. San Diego: Singular Publishing Group.

Berard, G. (1993). *Hearing equals behavior*. New Canaan, CT: Keats.

Berlin, C., & McNeil, M. (1976). Dichotic listening. In N. Lass (Ed.). *Contemporary issues in experimental phonetics* (pp. 327–388). New York: Academic.

Blake, R., Field, B., Foster, C., Platt, F., & Wertz, P. (1991). Effect of FM auditory trainers on attending behaviors of learning-disabled children. *Language, Speech, and Hearing Services in Schools, 22,* 111–114.

Bocca, E., & Calearo, C. (1963). Central hearing processes. In J. Jerger (Ed.). *Modern developments in audiology* (pp. 337–370). New York: Academic.

Bocca, E., Calearo, C., & Cassinari, V. (1954). A new method for testing hearing in temporal lobe tumor. *Acta Otolaryngologica, 44,* 219–221.

Bornstein, S., & Musiek, F. (1992). Recognition of distorted speech in children with and without learning problems. *Journal of the American Academy of Audiology, 3,* 22–32.

Brugge, J. (1975). Progress in neuroanatomy and neurophysiology of auditory cortex. In E. Eagles (Ed.). *The nervous system, Vol. 3. Human communication and its disorders* (pp. 97–111). New York: Raven.

Burleigh, A. J., Skinner, B. K., & Norris, T. W. (1982, November). Central auditory processing disorders in children: A 5-year study. Paper presented at the convention of the American Speech Language Hearing Association, Toronto, Ontario.

Burleigh, J., Mangle, J., Sanders, J., Olson, L., & Buccafusca, O. (1995). Incidence of central auditory processing difficulties in children. Unpublished raw data.

Burleigh, J., Thompson, M., James, S., Peterson, M., Boardman, T., & McIntosh, K. (November 1999).

Interaural time differences and central auditory nervous system function. Paper presented at the meeting of the American Speech-Language-Hearing Association, Convention, San Francisco, CA.

Burleigh, J., Thompson, M., James, S., Peterson, M., McIntosh, K., & Boardman, T. (November 2000). Accommodation of interaural timing differences in central auditory processing disorders. Paper presented at the meeting of the American Speech-Language-Hearing Association Convention, Washington, DC.

Carpenter, M. (1972). *Core text of neuroanatomy*. Baltimore: Williams & Wilkins.

Carpenter, M., & Sutin, J. (1983). *Human neuroanatomy*. Baltimore: Williams & Wilkins.

Chermak, G. (1996). Central testing. In S. A. Gerber (Ed.). *Handbook of pediatric audiology* (pp. 206–253). Washington DC: Galludet University Press.

Chermak, G., & Musiek, F. (1997). *Central auditory processing disorders*. San Diego: Singular.

Craig, C. (1997). Spoken language processing. In G. D. Chermak & F. E. Musiek (Eds.). *Central auditory processing disorders: New perspectives* (pp. 71–90). San Diego: Singular.

Crandell, C. (1992). Classroom acoustics for hearing-impaired children. *Journal of the Acoustical Society of America, 92,* 2470.

Crandell, C., & Smaldino, J. (1994). An update on classroom acoustics for children with hearing impairment. *The Volta Review, 96,* 291–306.

Crandell, C., Smaldino, J., & Flexer, C. (1994). Speech perception in specific populations. In C. Crandell, J. Smaldino, & C. Flexer (Eds.). *Sound-field FM amplification: Theory and practical applications* (pp. 49–65). San Diego, CA: Singular.

Crum, M., & Matkin, N. (1976). Room acoustics: The forgotten variable. *Language, Speech & Hearing Services in the Schools, 7,* 106–110.

Dublin, W. (1985). The cochlear nuclei-pathology. *Otolaryngology of Head and Neck Surgery, 93,* 448–463.

Dunn, W. (1999). *Sensory profile user's manual*. San Antonio: Therapy Skill Builders.

Edwards, C. (1994). Listening strategies for teachers and students. In C. Crandell, J. Smaldino, & C. Flexer (Eds.). *Sound-field FM amplification: Theory and practical implications* (pp. 191–200). San Diego, CA: Singular.

Emerson, M., Crandall, K., Seikel, A., & Chermak, G. (1997). Observations on the use of SCAN to identify children at risk for central auditory processing disorder. *Language Speech & Hearing Services in Schools, 28*(1), 43–49.

Filley, C. M. (1995). *Neurobehavioral anatomy*. Niwot, CO: University Press of Colorado.

Finitzo-Hieber, T. (1981). Classroom acoustics. In R. Roeser & M. Downs (Eds.). *Auditory disorders in school children: The law, identification, remediation* (pp. 250–262). New York: Thieme-Stratton.

Finitzo-Hieber, T., & Tillman, T. (1978). Room acoustics effects on monosyllabic word discrimination ability for normal and hearing impaired children. *Journal of Speech and Hearing Research, 21,* 440–458.

Fisher, A. G., Murray, E. A., & Bundy, A. C. (1991). *Sensory integration: Theory and practice*. Philadelphia: F. A. Davis.

Flexer, C. (1994). Rational for the use of sound-field FM amplification systems in classrooms. In C. Crandell, J. Smaldino, & C. Flexer (Eds.). *Sound-field FM amplification: Theory and practical applications* (pp. 3–16). San Diego, CA: Singular.

French, J. (1957). The reticular formation. *Scientific American, 196,* 54–60.

Gade, P., & Mills, C. (1989). Listening rate and comprehension as a function of preference for and exposure to time-altered speech. *Perceptual and Motor Skills, 68,* 531–538.

Galaburda, A. (1994a). Developmental dyslexia and animal studies: At the interface between cognition and neurology. *Cognition, 50,* 133–149.

Galaburda, A. (1994b, August 16). *The New York Times*, section C, p. 1.

Galaburda, A., Menard, M., & Rosen, G. (1994). Evidence for aberrant auditory anatomy in developmental dyslexia. *Proceedings of the National Academy of Sciences, 91,* 8010–8013.

Galaburda, A., Sherman, G., Rosen, G., Aboitiz, F., & Geschwind, N. (1985). Developmental dyslexia: Four consecutive patients with cortical anomalies. *Annuals of Neurology, 18,* 222–233.

Gazzaniga, M., & LeDoux, J. (1978). *The integrated mind*. New York: Plenum.

Gilmore, T., Madaule, P., & Thompson, B. (1989). *About the Tomatis method*. Toronto: Listening Centre.

Goldstein, R. (January 1967). Hearing disorders in children. Paper presented at the University of Oklahoma Symposium.

Hasbrouk, J. (1980). Performance of students with auditory figure-ground disorders under conditions of unilateral and bilateral ear occlusion. *Journal of Learning Disabilities, 13,* 548–551.

Hurley, R. M., & Musiek, F. E. (1997). Effectiveness of three central auditory processing (CAP) tests in identifying cerebral lesions. *Journal of American Academy of Audiology, 8,* 257–262.

Ivey, R. (1969). Tests of CNS function. Unpublished master's thesis, Colorado State University, Fort Collins.

Jerger, J. (1960). Audiological manifestations of lesions in the auditory nervous system. *Laryngoscope, 70,* 417–425.

Jerger, J., & Jerger, S. (1974). Auditory findings in brainstem disorders. *Archives of Otolaryngology, 99,* 342–350.

Jerger, J., & Jerger, S. (1975). Clinical validity of central auditory tests. *Scandinavian Audiology, 4,* 147–163.

Jerger, S., Jerger, J., & Abrams, S. (1983). Speech audiometry in the young child. *Ear and Hearing, 4*(1), 56–66.

Jirsa, R. (1992). The clinical utility of the P3 AERP in children with auditory processing disorders. *Journal Speech & Hearing Research, 35,* 903–912.

Katz, J. (1962). The use of staggered spondaic words for assessing the integrity of the central auditory system. *Journal of Auditory Research, 2,* 327–337.

Katz, J. (1968). The SSW test—an interim report. *Journal Speech Hearing Disorders, 33,* 132–146.

Katz, J. (1992). Classification of auditory processing disorders. In J. Katz, N. Stecker, & D. Henderson (Eds.). *Central auditory processing: A transdisciplinary view* (pp. 81–91). St. Louis: Mosby Year Book.

Katz, J., & Harman, C. (1981). Phonemic synthesis: testing and training. In R. Keith (Ed.). Central auditory and language disorders in children (pp. 145–159). Houston: College-Hill.

Katz, J., Stecker, N., & Henderson, D. (1992). *Central auditory processing: A trans-disciplinary view.* St. Louis: Mosby Year Book.

Kaufmann, W., & Galaburda, A. (1989). Cerebrocortical microdysgenesis in neurologically normal subjects: A histopathologic study. *Neurology, 39,* 238–244.

Keith, R. (1986). *SCAN: A screening test for auditory processing disorders.* San Antonio: Psychological Corporation.

Keith, R. (1999). SCAN-C: Test for Auditory Processing Disorders in Children-Revised. San Antonio: Psychological Corp.

Keith, R., Rudy, J., Donahue, P., & Katbamna, B. (1989). Comparison of SCAN results with other auditory and language measures in a clinical population. *Ear & Hearing, 10,* 382–386.

Keller, W. (1992). Auditory processing disorder and attention deficit disorder? In J. Katz, N. A. Stecker & D. Henderson (Eds.). *Central auditory processing: a transdisciplinary view* (pp. 107–114). St Louis: Mosby Year Book.

Kiang, N. (1975). Stimulus representation in the discharge patterns of auditory neurons. In E. Eagles (Ed.). *The nervous system* (Vol. 3, pp. 81–96). *Human communication and its disorders.* New York: Raven.

Kolb, B., & Wishaw, I. Q. (1990). *Fundamentals of human neuropsychology* (3rd ed.). New York: W.H. Freeman and Company.

Konkel, D., Beasley, D., & Bess, F. (1977). Intelligibility of time-altered speech in relation to chronological aging. *Journal of Speech and Hearing Research, 20,* 108–115.

Kraus, N., McGee, T., Carrell, T. , Zecker, S., Nicol, T., & Koch, D. (1996). Auditory neurophysiologic responses and discrimination deficits in children with learning problems. *Science, 273,* 971–973.

Kraus, N., McGee, T., Ferre, J., Hoeppner, J., Carrell, T., Sharma, A., & Nicol, T. (1993). Mismatch negativity in the neurophysiologic/behavioral evaluation of auditory processing deficits: A case study. *Ear & Hearing, 14,* 223–234.

Lasky, E., & Cox, L. (1983). Auditory processing and language interaction: Evaluation and intervention strategies. In E. Z. Lasky & J. Katz (Eds.). *Central auditory processing disorders: Problems of speech, language, and learning* (pp. 243–268). Baltimore: University Park.

Lindamood, C., & Lindamood, P. (1969). *Auditory discrimination in depth.* Boston: Teaching Resource.

Lynn, G., & Gilroy, J. (1972). Neuro-audiological abnormalities in patients with temporal lobe tumors. *Journal of Neurological Science, 17,* 167–184.

Lynn, G., & Gilroy, J. (1975). Effects of brain lesions on the perception of monotic and dichotic speech stimuli. In M. Sullivan (Ed.). *Proceedings of Symposium on Central Auditory Processing Disorders* (pp. 47–83). Omaha: University of Nebraska Medical Center.

Lynn, G., & Gilroy, J. (1976). Central aspects of audition. In J. Northern (Ed.). *Hearing disorders* (pp. 102–116). Boston: Little, Brown and Company.

Lynn, G., & Gilroy, J. (1977). Evaluation of central auditory dysfunction in patients with neurological disorders. In R. Keith (Ed.). *Central auditory dysfunction* (pp. 177–221). New York: Grune & Stratton.

Lynn, G., Gilroy, J., Taylor, P., & Leiser, R. (1981). Binaural masking level differences in neurological disorders. *Archives of Otolaryngology, 107,* 357–362.

Magoun, H. (1963). The waking brain (2nd ed.). Springfield, IL: Charles C. Thomas.

Matkin, N. (Sept 1988). Guidelines for classroom management of children with auditory processing deficits. Paper presented at Central Auditory Processing Workshop, Frisco, CO.

Matzker, J. (1959). Two new methods for the assessment of central auditory functions in cases of brain disease. *Annals of Otology, Rhinology, & Laryngology, 68,* 1185–1197.

Merzenich, M., Jenkins, W., Johnston, P., Schreiner, C., Miller, S., & Tallal, P. (1996). Temporal processing deficits of language-learning impaired children ameliorated by training. *Science, 271,* 77–81.

Mizushima, M., & Burleigh, J. (November 1997). Evaluation and management post eosinophilia–myalgia syndrome: A case study. Poster session presented at the annual meeting of the American Speech Language Hearing Association, Boston, MA.

Morales-Garcia, C., & Poole, J. (1972). Masked speech audiometry in central deafness. *Acta Otolaryngologica, 74,* 307–316.

Musiek, F. (1983). Results of three dichotic speech tests on subjects with intracranial lesions. *Ear and Hearing, 4,* 318–323.

Musiek, F., & Baran, J. (1986). Neuroanatomy, neurophysiology, and central auditory assessment. Part 1. *Brain Stem, Ear and Hearing, 7,* 207–219.

Musiek, F., Baran, J., & Pinheiro, M. (1990). Duration pattern recognition in normal subjects and patients with cerebral and cochlear lesions. *Audiology, 29,* 304–313.

Musiek, F., Baran, J., & Pinheiro, M. (1992). P300 results in patients with lesions of the auditory areas of the cerebrum. *Journal of American Academy of Audiology, 3,* 5–15.

Musiek, F., Baran, J., & Pinheiro, M. (1994). *Neuroaudiological case studies.* San Diego: Singular.

Musiek, F., & Geurkink, N. (1980). Auditory perceptual problems in children: considerations for the otolaryngologist and audiologist. *Laryngoscope, 90,* 962–971.

Musiek, F., Geurkink, N., & Keitel, S. (1982). Test battery assessment of auditory perceptual dysfunction in children. *Laryngoscope, 92,* 251–257.

Musiek, F., Kibbe, K., & Baran, J. (1984). Neuroaudiological results from split-brain patients. *Seminars in Hearing, 5,* 219–241.

Musiek, F., & Lamb, L. (1992). Neuroanatomy and neurophysiology of central auditory processing. In J. Katz, N. Stecker, & D. Henderson (Eds.). *Central auditory processing: A transdisciplinary view* (pp. 11–37). St. Louis: Mosby Year Book.

Musiek, F., & Pinheiro, M. (1985). Dichotic speech tests in the detection of central auditory dysfunction. In M. Pinheiro & F. Musiek (Eds.). *Assessment of central auditory dysfunction: Foundations and clinical correlates* (pp. 201–217). Baltimore: Williams & Wilkins.

Musiek, F., & Pinheiro, M. (1987). Frequency patterns in cochlear, brainstem and cerebral lesions. *Audiology, 26,* 79–88.

Musiek, F., & Reeves, A. (1990). Asymmetries of the auditory areas of the cerebrum. *Journal of American Academy of Audiology, 1,* 240–245.

Musiek, F., & Wilson, D. (1979). SSW and dichotic digit results pre- and post-commissurotomy: A case report. *Journal of Speech and Hearing Disorders, 44,* 528–533.

Musiek, F., Wilson, D., & Pinheiro, M. (1979). Audiological manifestations in split-brain patients. *Journal of the American Auditory Society, 5,* 25–29.

Noback, C. (1985). Neuroanatomical correlates of central auditory function. In M. Pinheiro & F. Musiek (Eds.). *Assessment of central auditory dysfunction: Foundations and clinical correlates* (pp. 7–21). Baltimore: Williams & Wilkins.

Noffsinger, D., Olsen, W., Carhart, R., Hart, C., & Sahgal, V. (1972). Auditory and vestibular aberrations in multiple sclerosis. *Acta Otolaryngologica, 303* (Suppl.), 1–63.

Oertel, D. (1997). Activation of the ascending pathways of the cochlear nuclei. Proceedings of the Second Biennial Hearing Aid Research and Development Conference, Bethesda, MD.

Oliver, D., & Morest, D. (1984). The central nucleus of the inferior colliculus in the cat. *Journal of Comparative Neurology, 222,* 237–264.

Olsen, W., Noffsinger, D., & Carhart, R. (1976). Masking level differences encountered in clinical populations. *Audiology, 15,* 287–301.

Olsen, W., Noffsinger, D., & Kurdziel, S. (1975). Speech discrimination in quiet and in white noise by patients with peripheral and central lesions. *Acta Otolaryngologica, 80,* 375–382.

Pinheiro, M. (1977). Tests of central auditory function in children with learning disabilities. In R. W. Keith (Ed.). *Central auditory dysfunction* (pp. 223–256). New York: Grune & Stratton.

Pinheiro, M., Jacobson, G., & Boller, F. (1982). Auditory dysfunction following a gunshot wound of the pons. *Journal of Speech and Hearing Disorders, 47,* 296–300.

Protti, E. (1983). Brainstem auditory pathways and auditory processing disorders. In E. Lasky & J. Katz (Eds.). *Central auditory processing disorders: Problems of speech, language, and learning* (pp. 117–139). Baltimore: University Park.

Riccio, C., Hynd, G., Cohen, M., Hall, J., & Molt, L. (1994). Comorbidity of central auditory processing disorders and attention deficit hyperactivity disorder. *Journal of American Academy of Child Adolescent Psychiatry, 33,* 849–857.

Rose, J., Gross, N., Geisler, C., & Hind, J. (1966). Some neural mechanisms in the inferior colliculus of the cat which may be relevant to the localization of a sound source. *Journal of Neurophysiology, 29,* 288–314.

Rosenberg, G., Blake-Rahter, P., & Heavner, J. (December 1995). Enhancing listening and learning environments with FM soundfield classroom amplification. Paper presented at the annual meeting of the American Speech-Language-Hearing Association, Orlando, Florida.

Sanders, D. (1965). Noise conditions in normal school classrooms. *Exceptional Children, 31,* 344–353.

Schmitt, J., & McCroskey, R. (1981). Sentence comprehension in elderly listeners: The factor of rate. *Journal of Gerontology, 36,* 441–445.

Schnitker, M. (1972). *The teacher's guide to the brain and learning.* San Rafael, CA: Academic Therapy.

Singer, J., Hurley, R., & Preece, J. (1998). Effectiveness of central auditory processing tests with children. *American Journal of Audiology, 7*(2), 73–84.

Sinha, S. (1959). *The role of the temporal lobe in hearing.* Unpublished master's thesis, McGill University, Montreal, Canada.

Sloan, C. (1986). *Treating auditory processing difficulties in children.* San Diego: College-Hill.

Speaks, C., & Jerger. J. (1965). Method for measurement of speech identification. *Journal of Speech and Hearing Research, 8,* 185–194.

Stach, B., Loiselle, L., & Jerger, J. (1991). Special hearing aid considerations in elderly patients with auditory processing disorders. *Ear & Hearing, 12*(suppl), 131–138.

Tallal, P., Miller, S., Bedi, G., Byma, G., Wang, X., Nagarajan, S., Schreiner, C., Jenkins, W., & Merzenich, M. (1996). Language comprehension in language-learning impaired children improved with acoustically modified speech. *Science, 271,* 81–84.

Tobin, H. (1985). Binaural interaction tasks. In M. Pinheiro & F. Musiek (Eds.). *Assessment of central*

auditory dysfunction: Foundations and clinical correlates (pp. 155–171). Baltimore: Williams & Wilkins.

Webster, D. (1971). Projection of the cochlea to cochlear nuclei in Merriam's kangaroo rat. *Journal of Comparative Neurology, 143,* 323–340.

Wenndt, S. (1991). *Novel signal processing for the enhancement of speech intelligibility.* Unpublished master's thesis, Colorado State University, Fort Collins.

Wenndt, S., Burleigh, J., & Thompson, M. (1996). Pitch adaptive time-rate expansion for enhancing speech intelligibility. *Journal of the Acoustical Society of America, 99,* 3853–3856.

Whitfield, I. (1967). *The auditory pathway.* Baltimore: Williams & Wilkins.

Willeford, J. (1977). Assessing central auditory behavior in children: A test battery approach. In R. Keith (Ed.). *Central auditory dysfunction* (pp. 43–72). New York: Grune & Stratton.

Willeford, J. (1980). Central auditory behaviors in learning-disabled children. *Seminars in Speech, Language and Hearing, 1,* 127–140.

Willeford, J. (1985a). Assessment of central auditory disorders in children. In M. Pinheiro & F. Musiek (Eds.). *Assessment of central auditory dysfunction:*

Foundations and clinical correlates (pp. 239–255). Baltimore: Williams & Wilkins.

Willeford, J. (1985b). Sentence procedures in central testing. In J. Katz (Ed.). *Handbook of clinical audiology* (ed. 3, pp. 404–420). Baltimore: Williams & Wilkins.

Willeford, J., & Billger, J. (1978). Auditory perception in children with learning disabilities. In J. Katz (Ed.). *Handbook of clinical audiology* (2nd ed., pp. 410–425). Baltimore: Williams & Wilkins.

Willeford, J., & Burleigh, J. (1985). *Handbook of central auditory processing disorders in children.* New York: Grune & Stratton.

Willeford, J., & Burleigh, J. (1994). Sentence procedures in central testing. In J. Katz (Ed.). *Handbook of clinical audiology* (4th ed., pp. 256–268). Baltimore: Williams & Wilkins.

Witelson, S. (1977). Early hemispheric specialization and interhemisphere plasticity: An empirical and theoretical review. In S. Segalowitz & F. Gruber (Eds.). *Language development and neurological theory* (pp. 213–287). New York: Academic.

Yencer, K. (1998). The effects of auditory integration training for children with central auditory processing disorders. *American Journal of Audiology, 7*(2), 32–44.

■■ Appendix 6–1
Behavioral Measures

Dichotic Tests

Tests that use a dichotic format, shown in Appendix Table 6–1, typically use a variety of speech stimuli presented in different formats. These tests are thought to be most sensitive to cortical or hemispheric functions. Cortical or hemispheric lesions classically result in deficits for dichotic speech in the ear contralateral to the lesion or involved hemisphere (Lynn & Gilroy, 1975, 1976, 1977; Musiek, 1983; Musiek & Pinheiro, 1985). However, when damage occurs to the transverse interhemispheric auditory pathways in the region of the corpus callosum, the deficits may be ipsilateral (Lynn & Gilroy, 1972).

Dichotic tests typically rely on one of two general formats: binaural integration and binaural separation. In tests using a binaural integration format, listeners respond to stimuli presented to both ears. For example, a listener may be presented with different digits to each ear and asked to repeat both numbers. Other stimuli include dichotic words, consonant-vowel syllables or words, natural and synthetic sentences, and staggered spondaic words (i.e., two-syllable words with equal emphasis on each syllable). Detailing all the tests that fall within various central auditory test parameters is beyond the scope of this chapter. However, a brief description of each type is provided.

Tests that involve dichotic digits or words have been used both clinically and experimentally for a number of years. One of the more recent, the Dichotic Digits Test (Musiek, 1983; Musiek & Wilson, 1979; Musiek et al., 1979), is composed of four spoken numbers (from 1 through 10), two presented to each ear simultaneously. For example, digits 2 and 5 may be presented to the subject's right ear, and 6 and 10 may be presented to the left. Clients are asked to repeat all the digits they heard in any order. According to Musiek et al. (1994), the dichotic digits test is fairly sensitive to intracortical involvement. Although less sensitive to brainstem involvement, abnormal findings have been reported (Musiek, 1983).

Consonant-vowel tests have been used mainly for experimental, rather than clinical, purposes. The most common format for this measure uses six consonant-vowel combinations (pa-ba-ga-ka-ta-da), presented in all combinations and in 30 paired items per test (Berlin & McNeil, 1976). Clients are asked to repeat what they hear in both ears.

The Staggered Spondaic Word Test (Katz, 1962; 1968) is designed so that two spondaic words partially overlap. The second syllable of the first word overlaps with the first syllable of the second word presented in the opposite ear to form a completely new word. Clients are asked to repeat the two-syllable words presented to both ears.

A second type of dichotic protocol includes binaural separation tasks. Clients respond to words or sentences presented to one ear while ignoring input presented to the other ear (a competing sentence paradigm). One such test, designed by Willeford and his graduate students in 1968, is part of the Willeford Central Auditory Test Battery (Willeford, 1977). This test involves dichotically presented natural sentence materials that have similar length and linguistic content (Willeford, 1977, 1980). The primary sentence (i.e., the sentence to be repeated) is presented to the target ear at a softer intensity level than that of a competing sentence. Clients are asked to repeat the sentence heard in the target ear.

The Synthetic Sentence Identification with Contralateral Competing Message (Jerger & Jerger, 1974, 1975; Speaks & Jerger, 1965) is composed of third-order approximations of real language arranged in 10 target nonsense sentences that are seven words long. Each nonsense sentence is paired with a historical monologue about the life of Davy Crockett, presented in the contralateral ear. Clients indicate what nonsense sentence they heard in the target ear from a list of 10 nonsense sentences. All subjects are given a sheet with these

■ Appendix Table 6–1 **Dichotic Tests***

Digits: Different digits, presented in competition
Words (Consonant-Vowel-Consonant (CVCs): spondees): Monosyllabic or bisyllabic words presented in competition
Nonsense Sentences vs. Discourse: Nonsense sentences competing against continuous discourse
Real Sentences vs. Real Sentences
Consonant-Vowels (CVs): Different CV pairs in competition

*Dichotic tests present different messages to the two ears simultaneously. In some test designs, the listener is required to repeat both messages. In others, response is to one ear only while attempting to ignore the competing message in the other ear. Test protocols vary widely in terms of message-to-competition ratios.
Source: Willeford, J., & Burleigh, J. *Handbook of central auditory processing disorders in children.* Grune & Stratton, 1985, with permission.

sentences and are instructed to respond either by giving the number shown by each sentence or by repeating the nonsense sentences. Because the test requires reading, it cannot be given to children who have not yet learned to read.

The Pediatric Speech Intelligibility Test (Jerger et al., 1983) was specifically designed for children with language ages of 3 to 6 years. This dichotic test uses a picture-pointing format that pairs a target picture with a competing sentence directed to the opposite ear.

Monotic Tests

Tests that are presented in only one ear at a time are considered to be monotic tests. They take a variety of forms and are shown in Appendix Table 6–2.

Frequency limiting of speech stimuli or degraded speech (i.e., omitting certain frequencies in words) has been shown to limit intelligibility, especially for persons with impaired temporal lobe function (Lynn & Gilroy, 1972, 1975, 1976, 1977). Reduced word recognition is generally associated with monaurally presented low-pass filtered speech (only certain low frequencies are heard) in the ear contralateral to a temporal lobe lesion (Lynn & Gilroy, 1972, 1975, 1977). Various investigators have used a variety of filtering characteristics with differing results.

The ipsilateral version of the Synthetic Sentence Identification Test is sensitive to either brainstem or temporal lobe lesions; however, abnormal performance is most commonly observed in individuals with brainstem involvement (Jerger & Jerger, 1974, 1975). In this test, each nonsense sentence is paired with the narrative about Davy Crockett and is presented in the ipsilateral ear at progressively more difficult signal-to-competition ratios. The Pediatric Speech Intelligibility Test and the Ipsilateral Contralateral Competing Sentence Test also use an ipsilateral format (Willeford, 1985a, 1985b; Willeford & Burleigh, 1994).

Another monaural format involves sequencing and temporal ordering of acoustic stimuli. The Pitch Pattern Sequence Test, developed by Pinheiro (1977), requires clients to sequence high (H) and low (L) auditory tones presented in six different formats: HLH, LHL, HLL, LLH, HHL, LHH. These "high-low" tones are presented in one ear at a time in 500-ms tone combinations separated by 300-ms silent intervals. Clients give either a verbal or hummed response to a series of tones. This test has been most often associated with cerebral cortex functioning (Musiek & Geurkink, 1980; Musiek et al., 1982; Musiek & Pinheiro, 1987; Pinheiro, 1977).

Compressed or accelerated speech, in which the frequency or pitch spectrum is held constant, has also been used to assess CANS function. The most common compression rate is 60 percent. Disruption of the temporal pattern of speech is a charac-

■ Appendix Table 6–2 **Monotic Tests***

Frequency Limiting: Filtering out certain frequency content
Time Altered: Accelerating the rate of speech stimuli
Pattern Recognition: Identification of changes in pitch
Ipsilateral Competing Signals: Intelligibility of speech in competition with speech or noise signals

*Monotic tests present messages to only one ear.
Source: Adapted from Willeford, J., & Burleigh, J. *Handbook of central auditory processing disorders in children.* Grune & Stratton, 1985, with permission.

■ ☐ APPENDIX TABLE 6–3 BINAURAL INTERACTION TESTS

Binaural Fusion: Combining high-frequency bands in one ear with low-frequency bands of the same signal in the other ear
Rapidly Alternating Speech: Bursts of continuous sequential signals alternating between the two ears.
Masking Level Differences: Comparison of two binaural signals when in and out of phase

(Source: From Willeford, J. and Burleigh, J. *Handbook of central auditory processing disorders in children.* Grune & Stratton, 1985, with permission.)

teristic observed in some individuals with cortical involvement. The effect of compression on intelligibility has been explored extensively (Beasley et al., 1972a, 197b; Beasley & Freeman, 1977; Bornstein & Musiek, 1992; Gade & Mills, 1989; Konkle et al., 1977; Schmitt & McCroskey, 1981).

Another test paradigm pairs single-syllable words with competing noise. The task is to repeat the target words. Researchers (Morales-Garcia & Poole, 1972; Noffsinger et al. 1972; Olsen et al., 1975; Sinha, 1959) have indicated that noise presented monaurally decreases speech recognition of individuals with both temporal lobe and brainstem involvement.

Binaural Interaction Tests

The designs of binaural interaction tests vary. These measures are described below and listed in Appendix Table 6–3.

Tests of binaural fusion involve presentation of bisyllabic words that are filtered and then presented to both ears simultaneously (Ivey, 1969; Willeford, 1977, 1980). This technique was developed and described by Matzker (1959). One ear receives the low-frequency (i.e., only 500 to 700 Hz) segment of a word while the opposite ear receives its high-frequency (i.e., only 1900 to 2100 Hz) complement. Listeners combine the two relatively unintelligible segments of a two-syllable word to perceive a meaningful word. This test has been shown to be sensitive to brainstem involvement (Lynn & Gilroy, 1975; Pinheiro et al., 1982).

Another test that uses a binaural interaction test paradigm is rapidly alternating speech. A sequence of speech bursts in a sentence format is presented alternately to the two ears. The individual repeats each sentence. Lynn and Gilroy (1977) reported that this test paradigm is sensitive to lesions in the low pons and cerebello-pontine angle regions in adults.

One of the procedures most commonly used for assessing brainstem level auditory function is masking level differences (MLD). The examiner presents pure tone (500 Hz) and speech stimuli (e.g., two-syllable words) in or out of phase with either narrow band noise (i.e., filtered white noise with only selected frequencies present) or white noise (i.e., containing all the frequencies in the audible spectrum). Abnormal results are thought to reflect low brainstem involvement when hearing is within normal limits (Lynn et al., 1981; Olsen et al., 1976).

PART II

Assessment and Intervention

Assessing Sensory Integrative Dysfunction

Anita C. Bundy, ScD, OTR, FAOTA

Purpose should always drive the . . . assessment process, not the latest or most popular instrument. The primacy of purpose should draw one back to look at previous approaches . . . , to consider approaches that may seem too simple to be acceptable to others . . . , and to carefully examine current practice (Burton & Miller, 1998, p. 332)

In the process of gathering data, theory should provide a systematic way of looking for information (Kielhofner & Mallinson, 1995, p. 191)

This chapter is divided into four sections. The first section discusses the relationship of the assessment of sensory integration to functional evaluation. The second section describes the development and psychometric properties of the Sensory Integration and Praxis Tests (SIPT) (Ayres, 1989). The third section reviews information that is complementary to the SIPT and necessary for a complete assessment of sensory integration, including obtaining a relevant client history, making clinical observations of neuromotor behavior, and assessing sensory modulation. Finally, although the SIPT remain the most comprehensive and statistically sound measures of sensory integration, their use is not always possible or practical. Thus, in the fourth section

of this chapter, we suggest alternative methods for examining sensory integration.

SENSORY INTEGRATION AND FUNCTIONAL ASSESSMENT

Sensory integrative dysfunction is widely believed to affect individuals' performance in daily life roles and tasks. However, the presence of sensory integrative dysfunction does not ensure that function will be impaired any more than its absence ensures that function will be intact. Because occupational therapy practitioners are concerned primarily with occupational and role performance, we should situate the assessment of sensory integration (or any performance component) in the context of an overall evaluation of daily life roles and tasks. This approach to assessment commonly is referred to as the "top-down" approach (Burton & Miller, 1998; Coster, 1998; Fisher & Short DeGraff, 1993; Mathiowetz, 1993, Mathiowetz & Haugen, 1995; Trombly, 1993). Typically, authors depict role and occupational performance and performance components as a three-level hierarchy that occupies spaces within an isosceles triangle (e.g., Mathiowetz, 1993) (see Fig. 1–9)

In a top-down approach, practitioners *begin* by assessing individuals' abilities to carry out daily life tasks (occupational performance) (Coster, 1998). When clients are adults, we begin by examining the roles they assume (Trombly, 1993). Only after we have established specific areas in which individuals have difficulty do we seek to understand ways in which performance components (e.g., sensory integration) interfere with occupational and role performance. Burton and Miller (1998) argued convincingly that:

> . . . there are numerous advantages to a top-down strategy for assessment and . . . intervention. First, evaluating an individual's . . . skills in the highest-level functional context possible at the outset provides a preassessment relative to the ultimate goal of the . . . intervention. Second, the content validity of the preassessment is clearly established because it matches exactly to the ultimate goal of the . . . intervention. Third, such a preassessment should minimize the amount of time spent on skills the individual is already able to perform competently. The preassessment should also help [clients] to see their own needs in light of their own functional performances. And fourth, these advantages should make . . . intervention not only more efficient in terms of time, than a broad-based bottom-up approach, but also more motivating to the individual (p. 307).

Top-down assessment makes sense for all the reasons Burton and Miller (1998) have enumerated; it also makes sense in an era of tightening budgets in which minimal funds are available to pay for therapeutic assessment and intervention.

Assessment of individuals with suspected sensory integrative dysfunction has tended to focus on the performance component. This represents a bottom-up approach in which the assumption is made that performance components must be in-

tact for individuals to successfully perform meaningful activities. The bottom-up approach has several distinct disadvantages (Burton & Miller, 1998). Among them is a lack of clear relevance of the assessment or intervention to clients' lives (Burton & Miller, 1998; Trombly, 1993). For example, the relevance of assessing prone extension or intervening to improve the ability to do it are not obvious to caregivers or professionals who are not trained in sensory integration theory.

Practitioners' use of a bottom-up approach has been partially fueled by a preponderance of assessments that target performance components and a dearth of assessments that focus on occupational and role performance. Although there is a clear need for more assessments that support a top-down approach, such assessments are increasingly available. A list of all such formal assessments is beyond the scope of this chapter; readers are referred to Law et al. (2000) for a more complete discussion.

Although Burton and Miller (1998) argued *for* the top-down approach, they argued *against* hierarchical depictions (i.e., the isosceles triangle). However unintentionally, such depictions contribute to the idea that role and occupational performance are dependent on proficiency in performance components. Writing specifically about motor skills, Burton and Miller suggested a nonhierarchical model for depicting relationships among skills. Their model is shown in Figure 7–1. Although Burton and Miller's model is not directly translatable into the breadth of skills required for all occupational and role performance, it is worth considering the place of assessment of sensory integration, as it is typically conducted, even in such a limited model; this is also depicted in Figure 7–1.

At this stage of our profession's development, it may not always be possible to conduct formal top-down assessment. However, we *can* always keep in mind *where* our assessments lie with respect to the big picture of function in clients' lives.

SENSORY INTEGRATION AND PRAXIS TESTS

When practitioners deem it appropriate to examine clients' sensory integrative functioning, the SIPT (Ayres, 1989) is the most comprehensive and statistically sound means for assessing some important aspects of sensory integration, most notably praxis and tactile discrimination. In addition to the SIPT, giving clinical observations of

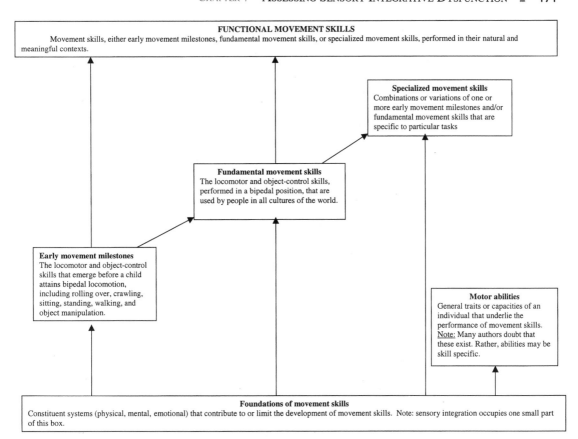

FUNCTIONAL MOVEMENT SKILLS
Movement skills, either early movement milestones, fundamental movement skills, or specialized movement skills, performed in their natural and meaningful contexts.

Specialized movement skills
Combinations or variations of one or more early movement milestones and/or fundamental movement skills that are specific to particular tasks

Fundamental movement skills
The locomotor and object-control skills, performed in a bipedal position, that are used by people in all cultures of the world.

Early movement milestones
The locomotor and object-control skills that emerge before a child attains bipedal locomotion, including rolling over, crawling, sitting, standing, walking, and object manipulation.

Motor abilities
General traits or capacities of an individual that underlie the performance of movement skills. Note: Many authors doubt that these exist. Rather, abilities may be skill specific.

Foundations of movement skills
Constituent systems (physical, mental, emotional) that contribute to or limit the development of movement skills. Note: sensory integration occupies one small part of this box.

■ FIGURE 7–1 Taxonomy of movement skills. (Adapted from Burton & Miller, 1998.)

neuromotor performance and an assessment of sensory modulation (e.g., Dunn, 1999) provides a more complete evaluation of sensory integration. Clinical observations provide additional information, particularly about vestibular and proprioceptive processing. Assessing sensory modulation provides information about sensory defensiveness, gravitational insecurity, aversive responses to sensory information, and sensory registration (see Chapter 4).

In this section, we describe the development, standardization, and psychometric properties of the SIPT (Ayres, 1989). A more complete discussion of the SIPT can be found in Appendix B of this text and in the SIPT manual. In subsequent sections, clinical observations of neuromotor performance and assessments of sensory modulation are described.

The SIPT were designed for children ages 4 to 8 years with mild to moderate learning or motor difficulties. Each of the 17 tests in the SIPT is individually administered; the entire battery generally can be completed in 1.5 to 2 hours. The test's primary use is to contribute to understanding a child's difficulties and planning intervention. The SIPT can be categorized into four overlapping groups:

1. Form and space, visual-motor coordination, and constructional ability
2. Tactile discrimination
3. Praxis
4. Vestibular and proprioceptive processing

A description of each of the SIPT, by group, is shown in Table 7–1.

To attain standard scores, a child's raw scores are entered into a computer. The computer plots the child's scores (Fig. 7–2) and likens them to one or more of the typical patterns observed in six different cluster groups in the normative sample; this facilitates interpretation. However, because the computer does not have access to information regarding posture or sensory modulation, two important components of sensory integration, practitioners must reinterpret the data, considering all available information.

■ Table 7–1 Functions Measured by the SIPT

Primary Domain	Test	Description
Form and space, visual-motor coordination, construction	Space Visualization (SV)	Motor-free visual form and space perception, mental manipulation of objects
	Figure-Ground Perception (FG)	Motor-free visual perception of figures on a rival background
	Design Copying (DC)	Ability to copy simple and complex 2-dimensional designs and manner of approach for copying
	Constructional Praxis (CPr)	Ability to relate objects to each other in 3-dimensional space
	Motor Accuracy (MAC)	Eye–hand coordination and control of movement
Tactile discrimination	Finger Identification (FI)	Discrimination of individual fingers
	Localization of Tactile Stimuli (LTS)	Perception of specific stimuli applied to arms or hands
	Manual Form Perception (MFP)	Matching of block held in hand with visual counterpart or block held in other hand
	Graphesthesia (GRA)	Perception and replication of designs drawn on a hand
Praxis	Bilateral Motor Coordination (BMC)	Ability to move both hands and both feet in smooth and integrated patterns
	Sequencing Praxis (SPr)	Ability to repeat a series of hand and finger movements
	Postural Praxis (PPr)	Ability to plan and execute body positions demonstrated by the examiner
	Oral Praxis (Opr)	Ability to plan and execute lip, tongue, and jaw movements
	Praxis on Verbal Command (PrVC)	Ability to plan and execute postures on the basis of verbal commands
Vestibular and proprioceptive processing	Kinesthesia (KIN)	Perception of passive hand and arms movements
	Standing and Walking Balance (SWB)	Static and dynamic balance on one or both feet with eyes open or closed
	Postrotary Nystagmus (PRN)	Duration of vestibulo-ocular reflex

Adapted from Ayres (1989)

The SIPT were based on 12 tests from the Southern California Sensory Integration Tests (SCSIT; Ayres, 1980) and the Southern California Postrotary Nystagmus Test (SCPNT; Ayres, 1975). In addition, Ayres (1989) developed four new praxis tests.

The SIPT were standardized on a sample of approximately 2000 North American children. Children in the normative sample were representative of the population distribution characteristics from the 1980 US Census. A number of Canadian children were also included.

Preliminary analyses of the normative data indicated significant gender and age differences on all SIPT tests except Manual Form Perception and Postrotary Nystagmus. Therefore, Ayres (1989) computed separate means and standard deviations for boys and girls in each of 12 age groups. Children's standard scores provide an index of the degree to which their performance differs from the average performance of children of the same age and gender.

Validity and Reliability of the SIPT

Evidence of a test's validity and reliability determines whether it is a "good" test. *Validity* is the ability to draw meaningful inferences from test scores, and *reliability* is the consistency of scores. We provide evidence for construct-related validity and two types of reliability (i.e., interrater and test-retest).

Evidence of Construct Validity

Construct validity is the conceptual or theoretical basis for using an assessment to make a particular interpretation (Burton & Miller, 1998). One of the most common ways to examine construct validity is with factor and cluster analyses, used to determine how many factors (i.e., test groupings; factor analysis) or clusters (i.e., groupings of people, cluster analysis) are included within a construct.

Another way of examining construct validity on tests such as the SIPT is to determine whether children with known impairments score signifi-

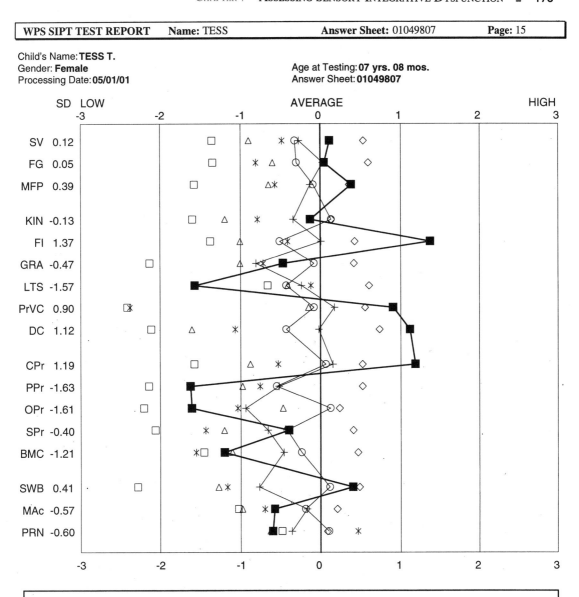

FIGURE 7-2 Sensory Integration and Praxis Tests (SIPT).

cantly lower than children without known impairments (Burton & Miller, 1998). We review both factor and cluster analyses conducted with SIPT data and research comparing SIPT scores of children with and without disabilities.

Ayres (1965, 1966a, 1966b, 1969, 1972b, 1977, 1989) conducted a number of factor analytic studies with data from the SCSIT and related measures and factor and cluster analyses with SIPT data from children with and without dysfunction. She labeled six patterns that described various types of sensory integrative dysfunction:

1. Somatosensory processing deficits
2. Poor BIS
3. Somatodyspraxia
4. Poor praxis on verbal command (not a disorder of sensory integration)
5. Form and space, visual-motor coordination, and visual construction
6. Generalized sensory integrative dysfunction, which seemed to represent extreme cases of the listed patterns

The results of these factor and cluster analyses are summarized in more detail in Chapter 1 and Appendix B at the back of the book. However, Ayres derived her factor labels from analyses that included different tests. Thus, no study was a true replication of any other. For this and other valid reasons, her studies have been criticized.

More recently, Mulligan (1998) used confirmatory factor analysis with SIPT data from more than 10,000 children in an attempt to confirm a five-factor structure of sensory integrative dysfunction. These factors consisted of BIS; postural ocular movements; somatosensory processing; somatopraxis; and form and space, visual-motor, and constructional ability. Mulligan did not consider sensory modulation because the SIPT did not provide evidence of this or praxis on verbal command because it was thought to reflect left hemisphere functioning.

Although Mulligan found a reasonable fit to the data using the five-factor model, she also found numerous weaknesses. Thus, she conducted exploratory factor analysis and found the best fit to the data with a second-order, four-factor model. She labeled the higher-order factor "generalized dysfunction" and the four first-order factors visuoperceptual, BIS, somatosensory, and praxis. Mulligan's model is shown in Figure 1–7.

Mulligan (1998) conducted confirmatory factor analyses using both the original data set and a subset of approximately 1000 children with learning disabilities. The results were similar to her original findings. Thus, she concluded that her model represented the best available model of sensory integration. Mulligan's (1998) results raised a number of interesting points.

- No pattern related to posture emerged. This is likely because of the absence of measures on the SIPT to discriminate such a function. These results confirmed the need to include clinical observations of posture in the assessment of sensory integration (Fisher & Bundy, 1991).
- Mulligan found no evidence of a somatodyspraxia factor. This result was surprising because Ayres emphasized the associations between praxis and somatosensory measures. Mulligan concluded that children with poor scores on both tactile and praxis measures would be described most accurately as "having generalized . . . dysfunction with weaknesses in the areas of praxis and somatosensory processing" (p. 825). [Editor's note: We believe it is *always* best to describe both the practic problem and its apparent underlying basis in any report of sensory integrative functioning.]
- Finally, Mulligan discussed the possibility of a shorter test to measure sensory integration. She found that Postrotary Nystagmus (PRN), Kinesthesia (KIN), Standing and Walking Balance (SWB), and Motor Accuracy (MAC) failed to support any patterns. In addition, she believed that eliminating some of the visual perceptual tests would make testing more efficient. Because of its poor test-retest reliability, Figure-Ground Perception (FG) seemed a likely candidate for elimination.

Mulligan's (1998) study represented the largest study to date of SIPT patterns. Thus, her results must be considered carefully. However, because she used the same sample for both exploratory and confirmatory factor analyses, her work must also be viewed with caution until it is replicated. Clearly, further research is indicated.

Comparing SIPT Scores of Children with and Without Disabilities

Children representing eight different diagnostic groups (i.e., children with learning disabilities, sensory integrative dysfunction, reading disorder, language disorder, cognitive impairments, spina bifida, traumatic brain injury, and cerebral palsy) participated in studies comparing their performance on the SIPT with that of the normative sample. The mean scores of all eight groups combined were below average on all of the SIPT. Although the test scores for some of the groups reflected logical patterns given the difficulties associated with their diagnoses, some of these groups had frank central nervous system damage (e.g., children with cerebral palsy). Thus, their low SIPT scores did not necessarily reflect sensory integrative dysfunction. Rather, they likely suggested that the SIPT were sensitive to functions compromised by CNS dysfunction or damage.

Evidence of Reliability

Interrater reliability indicates the extent to which individuals' test scores are the same when different examiners evaluate their performance. *Test-retest reliability* indicates the extent to which test scores for individuals are consistent over time.

Ayres found that, although most of the SIPT had acceptable test-retest reliability, the praxis tests had the highest test-retest coefficients. Only Postrotatory Nystagmus, Kinesthesia, Localization of Tactile Stimuli, and Figure-Ground Perception had low reliability. Furthermore, all interrater reliability coefficients were very high, ranging from 0.94 to 0.99. The reliability statistics for the SIPT are shown in Appendix B.

A COMPLETE ASSESSMENT: COMPLEMENTING THE SIPT

The SIPT are useful for detecting problems with praxis, tactile processing, form and space perception, visuomotor coordination, and constructional abilities. However, even setting aside occupational performance for the moment, SIPT results should never be used as the sole source of information when making diagnostic judgments. To do an adequate job of uncovering the nature of clients' sensory integrative dysfunction, practitioners should have:

- General knowledge of their development, intellectual capacity, and primary diagnoses
- Clinical observations, especially those of postural responses (i.e., reflective of vestibular and proprioceptive processing)
- Assessment of sensory modulation (e.g., defensiveness, gravitational security)

SIPT scores should be interpreted in light of all of these additional sources of information.

Supplementary Information: Knowledge of Development, Cognition, and Primary Diagnoses

Sensory integrative dysfunction is a diagnosis of exclusion. Clients who have difficulties with motor planning or sensory modulation *in the absence of any other known cause* may be diagnosed with sensory integrative dysfunction. Thus, knowledge of the presence of primary medical or psychological diagnoses may be particularly germane to whether clients' difficulties are considered to be the result of sensory integrative dysfunction.

Careful interview of adult clients and caregivers (e.g., parents, teachers) can be very helpful in determining the direction of assessment. For example, children who achieved motor milestones (e.g., sitting, walking) at an appropriate age but who experienced difficulty with complex tasks (e.g., riding a bike, buttoning a shirt) would be likely candidates for assessment of motor planning, possibly including the SIPT. Clients who have increased activity level and decreased attention but who have no difficulty with motor tasks might also have sensory integrative dysfunction. However, less will be learned by giving that child a SIPT because the SIPT contains no measures of sensory modulation. More appropriate measures of sensory modulation are discussed later in this chapter.

Clinical Observations of Postural Movements

Frequently, the SIPT are supplemented by clinical observations of neuromotor performance. Generally, these are fairly standard observations that, for various reasons, lack normative data. Thus, examiners' skills and knowledge of typical development determine the inferences made from these observations. (See Appendix 7–1 for scoring of common clinical observations.)

The area in which clinical observation is most critical is posture, which is thought to be the behavioral manifestation of vestibular and proprioceptive processing underlying praxis. (Poor vestibular and proprioceptive processing may underlie difficulties with praxis *or* sensory modulation. However, we discuss gravitational insecurity and aversive responses to movement when we discuss assessing sensory modulation disorders.)

Although Ayres and others have placed significant emphasis on the role of the vestibular and proprioceptive systems, the SIPT contain only three measures of vestibular or proprioceptive functioning: the PRN, SWB, and KIN tests.

However, Mulligan (1998) did not find that PRN, SWB, or KIN loaded together *or* contributed significantly to any factor reflecting practic dysfunction. The reason for this is unclear. However, Ayres indicated, "I suspect one of the reasons Kinesthesia of the SIPT does not show a stronger loading is that it is not really a good test" (A. J. Ayres, personal communication, March 11, 1988). Because examiners move children's arms, no efference copy is generated; thus, one might question whether KIN actually is a measure of kinesthesia. PRN is fraught with its own difficulties. These are discussed below.

Thus, we supplement the SIPT with clinical observations reflective of vestibular and proprioceptive processing. In the assessment of posture, as in all assessment related to sensory integration, practitioners are looking at clients' performance on *meaningful clusters* of observations. The observations commonly associated with posture include:

- The inability to assume or maintain prone extension
- Difficulty flexing the neck when assuming supine flexion
- Low extensor muscle tone
- Poor proximal joint stability
- Deficient postural adjustments or background movements
- Poor equilibrium

In addition, observation and careful interview often reveal evidence of concomitant deficits in body schema and awareness of body position or movement in space.

Prone Extension

The ability to assume and maintain prone extension is an indication of the strength of tonic postural extension; Ayres stated that it is a strong indicator of vestibular and proprioceptive functioning (A. J. Ayres, personal communication, March 11, 1988). When vestibular and proprioceptive inputs to extensor muscles, especially of the neck and upper trunk, are diminished, the ability to assume prone extension may be affected. Prone extension is evaluated first by demonstrating the desired posture and then by asking the client to assume the position independently (Fig. 7–3). Verbal and physi-

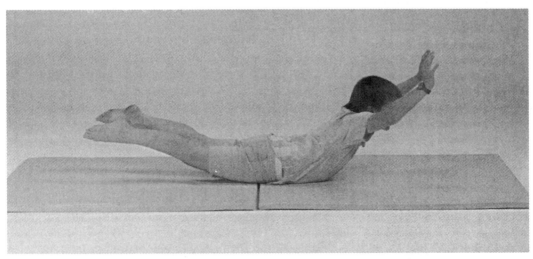

■ FIGURE 7–3 Normal prone extension position.

cal assistance may be given to ensure that the client understands what is expected. The quality of the response is graded based on the ability to

- Assume the whole position quickly (i.e., nonsegmentally).
- Hold the head steady and within 45 degrees of a vertical position.
- Lift the shoulders, chest, and arms off the floor.
- Raise the distal one third of both thighs off the floor.
- Maintain the knees in less than 45 degrees of flexion.
- Talk out loud (i.e., not hold breath).

Individuals age 6 years and older should be able to assume prone extension and hold it for 30 seconds (Harris, 1981; Wilson et al., 2000). However, individuals with tight hip flexors may have difficulty lifting their thighs or assuming the position without flexing their knees more than 30 degrees (Fisher & Bundy, 1989).

Neck Flexion During Supine Flexion

When assuming supine flexion, vestibular inputs (especially those originating from the utricle) facilitate righting of the head and upper trunk. Although individuals with poor vestibular processing usually find supine flexion easier than prone extension, a tendency to lead with the chin (i.e., head lag) may reflect diminished vestibular input to neck flexors.

Low Extensor Muscle Tone

Vestibular processing influences extensor muscle tone. Low muscle tone cannot be measured directly. Therefore, identification of low extensor muscle tone is based on a meaningful cluster of:

- Hyperextensibility of distal joints
- A standing posture characterized by lordosis and hyperextended or locked knees
- "Mushiness" of muscles when palpated

Before concluding that an individual has low extensor muscle tone, it is necessary to rule out the presence of joint laxity, lordosis compensatory to tight hip flexors, and lordotic posture normally seen in toddlers (Fisher & Bundy, 1989).

Proximal Joint Stability

Joint stability refers to the ability of tonic postural extensor muscles to contract so as to stabilize proximal joints during weight bearing. One of the best ways to evaluate for proximal stability is in quadruped, where we can observe for lordosis, hyperextension or locking of the elbows, raising of the medial border of the scapulae, and excessive scapular abduction (Fisher & Bundy, 1989). As with the evaluation of prone extension, verbal and physical cues may ensure that the client understands what is expected.

Postural Adjustments or Background Movements

Postural background movements are appropriate postural adjustments made during the performance of adaptive behaviors. Poor postural background movements are exaggerated, awkward, inappropriate, or diminished postural adjustments; they can be associated with low postural tone, deficient equilibrium reactions, or poor tonic proximal stability. There are no standard methods of evaluating postural background movements. However, they are readily observed as clients attempt to get into position to use their limbs effectively (Fisher & Bundy, 1989).

Equilibrium Reactions

One of the best methods of assessing vestibular and proprioceptive contributions to posture is through the evaluation of equilibrium. However, because of the low correlations among different assessments, thorough evaluation requires that a variety of equilibrium tests be administered (Fisher et al., 1988).

In addition to clinical observation, several standardized tools are available. The SWB Test of the SIPT tests the ability to perform a series of balance tasks (Ayres, 1989). Others appropriate for older children and adults include the Bruininks-Oseretsky balance subtest (Bruininks, 1978), portions of the Movement Assessment Battery for Children (MABC) (Henderson & Sugden, 1992), and the floor ataxia test battery (Fregly & Graybiel, 1968). Although these assessments are standardized, most provide limited information about the qualitative aspects of equilibrium.

Fisher (1989), Fisher & Bundy (1989), and

Fisher et al. (1988) developed three objective tests of the quality of equilibrium that have been useful for identifying individuals with vestibular deficits. The three tests are the Tilt Board Tip, Flat Board Reach, and Tilt Board Reach.

During the Tilt Board Tip Test, individuals age 5 years and older should maintain the head and upper trunk in the vertical position, demonstrate an increased support reaction in the downhill leg, and flex the hip and knee of the uphill leg (Figs. 7–4 to 7–6). The Flat Board Reach and Tilt Board Reach tests are measures of the ability to maintain balance during lateral reach while standing on a stable and an unstable surface, respectively. Children younger than age 7 years may not lift the uphill foot from the support surface (Fig. 7–7). By age 7 years, normal individuals extend and abduct the uphill arm and lift the uphill foot from the support surface; most individuals extend and abduct the uphill leg at least 30 degrees from the original starting position (Fig. 7–8). Persistence in not lifting the uphill foot from the support surface or the presence of uphill arm or leg flexion is suggestive of dysfunction, as shown in Figure 7–9 (Fisher, 1989). Interrater reliability of all three tests is high ($r > 0.90$); test–retest reliability of the reaching tasks is also high ($r > 0.90$).

Crowe et al. (1990), Deitz et al. (1991), and Richardson et al. (1992) adapted the Pediatric Clinical Test of Sensory Interaction for Balance

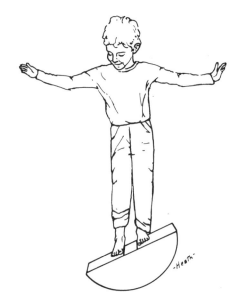

■ FIGURE 7–5 Abnormal or immature response on the Tilt Board Tip Test: arms raised in a "high guard" position, uphill hip and knee not flexed, and gaze directed toward the floor.

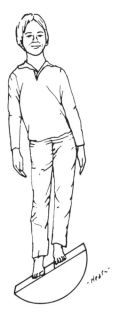

■ FIGURE 7–6 Abnormal or immature response on the Tilt Board Tip Test with lack of hip and knee flexion of the uphill leg.

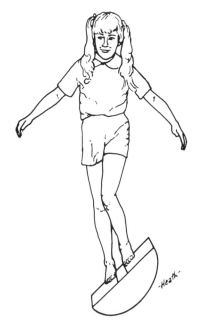

■ FIGURE 7–4 Normal response on the Tilt Board Tip Test.

(P-CTSIB) from Shumway-Cook and Horak (1986). The P-CTSIB is an assessment of the ability to maintain balance under conditions of sensory conflict. Examiners measure the amount of postural sway and duration of time maintaining a position (i.e., standing with feet together, standing heel

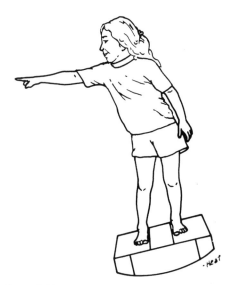

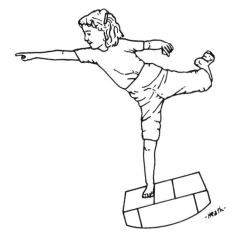

■ FIGURE 7-9 Abnormal response on the Tilt (or Flat) Board Reach Test; the uphill arm and leg flex more than 30 degrees.

■ FIGURE 7-7 Uphill foot remains in contact with the support surface of the Tilt (or Flat) Board Reach Test.

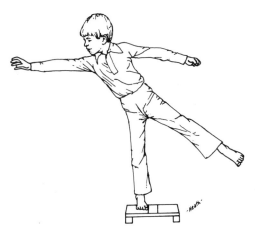

■ FIGURE 7-8 Mature response on the Flat (or Tilt) Board Reach Test; uphill arm and leg extend and abduct.

to toe) under conditions of normal, absent, and altered (i.e., present but distorted) visual or support surface information.

Postrotary Nystagmus: Some Comments

Postrotary Nystagmus (PRN) is a standardized test of vestibular processing rather than a clinical observation. However, because of the inordinate amount of attention given to the evaluation of postrotary nystagmus, we will discuss the PRN in some detail.

Depressed duration of postrotary nystagmus is defined as a score on the PRN test of more than 1.0

standard deviation below the mean (< -1.0) (Ayres, 1989). Polatajko (1983) and Cohen (1989) questioned the validity of PRN, in part because it is administered in the light; thus, both the vestibulo-ocular reflex and optokinetic nystagmus are elicited. When tested in the light, duration of postrotary nystagmus is shorter than when it is tested in the dark. Furthermore, postrotary nystagmus can be suppressed by visual fixation. Other factors that might contribute to a shortened time course of postrotary nystagmus (whether tested in the light or in the dark) include habituation as a result of repeated vestibular stimulation, alertness, or tilt suppression (i.e., neck flexion upon termination of the per-rotary stage of testing).

Polatajko (1983) and Cohen (1989) presented several valid reasons why typically developing children could have depressed scores on PRN. Thus, when a depressed score occurs in the absence of postural indicators, it probably is not evidence of dysfunction. A conservative interpretation of PRN is also warranted by its relatively low test–retest reliability (Ayres, 1989; Morrison & Sublett, 1983).

Clinical Observations Associated Directly with Praxis

Although the SIPT provide a relatively complete picture of the motor difficulties associated with somatodyspraxia and BIS deficits, many practitioners supplement them with relevant clinical observations. We have described a few such observations by category and discussed the rationale for their use.

Bilateral Integration

Deficits in bilateral integration are supported by clinical observation of poor coordination of two body sides; avoidance of crossing the midline; failure to develop a preferred hand; and possibly, right–left confusion.

Bilateral coordination can be observed in a variety of tasks, but observation of age-appropriate hopping, skipping, and jumping with both feet together are among the better measures. Jumping jacks and symmetrical and reciprocal stride jumping are also helpful tools used to evaluate bilateral motor coordination. Magalhaes et al. (1989) reported preliminary norms and a rating scale for 5- to 9-year-old children. The ability to perform jumping jacks, the most reliable of the assessments, appeared to mature by age 7. Reciprocal stride jumps were found to be the more difficult; few of the 9-year-old children obtained near-perfect scores. Symmetrical and reciprocal stride jumps are also included as items on the Bruininks-Oseretsky Test of Motor Proficiency (BOTMP; Bruininks, 1978).

Avoidance of crossing the midline is best observed during performance of unstructured tasks. Contrived situations (e.g., placing cones on the floor on either side of a child and asking the child to place rings over the cones) do not provide good opportunities for observation. Children have a *tendency,* not an inability, to cross.

The development of hand preference has also been associated with bilateral integration. Tan (1985) found that children as young as age 4 years who had not yet established hand preference had lower scores on gross and fine motor tests than children with well-established preferences, supporting the observation that inconsistent hand preference may be associated with poor coordination.

Finally, right–left confusion is often considered to reflect poor bilateral integration. The rationale is that a part of bilateral integration is intuitive awareness of right and left body sides that meet in the middle. However, the most common evaluations of right–left knowledge involve labeling body parts, which is heavily dependent on the ability to assign verbal labels to body sides.

Projected Action Sequences

Two of the better methods of evaluating the ability to plan and produce projected action sequences are catching a bouncing ball and jumping in a series of defined spaces. In the latter case, bilateral motor coordination is indicated by the ability to jump with both feet together. Difficulty initiating, sequencing, and terminating the sequence suggests poor ability to perform projected actions; anticipation is an important factor. Difficulty learning to perform jumping jacks and symmetrical and reciprocal stride jumping, even with demonstration, may also reflect deficits in planning and producing projected action sequences (Magalhães et al., 1989). Other methods that can be used to evaluate the ability to plan and produce projected action sequences include kicking a rolling ball or stepping over a rolling stick without breaking stride. Although relatively easy, these two tasks are more difficult when the examiner rolls the object after the client has begun moving.

Somatodyspraxia

Several clinical observations are commonly associated with somatodyspraxia:

- Inadequate supine flexion
- Difficulty with sequential finger touching
- Impaired ability to perform slow, controlled (ramp) movements
- Difficulty with rapidly alternating movements
- Impaired haptic exploration and in-hand manipulation

Although the ability to flex the neck against gravity when assuming supine flexion is associated with postural deficits and vestibular processing, the ability to assume the *whole* posture, quickly and nonsegmentally, and maintain it for 20 to 30 seconds is associated with somatodyspraxia. Most children age 6 years and older can assume and maintain supine flexion without excessive effort. Wilson et al. (2000) offered specific guidelines for scoring the neck, upper trunk, hips, and knees.

Sequential finger touching involves touching each successive finger (index to little and back) with the thumb, quickly and rhythmically. There are many variations on this basic task. These include eyes open versus eyes closed, unilateral versus bilateral, and whether individuals are instructed to touch the index and little fingers one or two times. Sequential finger touching is an item on the BOTMP (Bruininks, 1978).

The ability to perform slow, controlled (ramp) movements is generally examined by having the client mirror the slow, smooth, controlled arm movements of the examiner. The client should begin with his or her shoulders in abduction, elbows fully extended, wrists in neutral, and fingers comfortably extended. Then he or she should move the hands slowly toward the shoulders (Wilson et al., 2000). These authors indicated that the movement optimally takes 5 or more seconds for children age 5 years and older.

The ability to perform rapidly alternating movements (i.e., diadokokinesis) is generally assessed with forearm pronation and supination. The client gently touches the palm and dorsum of the hand alternately and rhythmically on the thigh. The task is done both unilaterally and bilaterally. Wilson et al. (2000) indicated that children age 5 years and older should be able to perform nine or more rotations in 10 seconds.

Haptic manipulation, generally assessed through stereognosis tasks (including Manual Form Perception), reflects practic abilities, perhaps because it has both tactile and motor components. We observe how clients initiate active, exploratory manipulation. Several researchers (Abravanel, 1972a, 1972b; Hoop, 1971a, 1971b; Jennings, 1974; Kleinman, 1979; Wolff, 1972; Zaporozhets, 1965, 1969) have demonstrated a developmental progression in the acquisition of haptic manipulation strategies; the accuracy of object identification is related to the level of the client's haptic manipulation strategies. Contour following (i.e., moving the fingers around the edge of an object), which develops between age 6 and 7 years, is the optimum strategy for identifying shapes (Lederman & Klatzky, 1987). Before age 4 years, children may grasp or touch the object, but the palm remains still. By about age 5 years, children begin exploring with both the palm and fingers (Piaget & Inhelder, 1948; Zaporozhets, 1965, 1969).

Closely related to haptic perception is in-hand manipulation, the ability to use intrinsic hand movements to position an already-grasped object for use. In-hand manipulation is commonly included as a clinical observation associated with somatodyspraxia. Exner (1992, 2001) has developed a standard assessment of in-hand manipulation. The following guidelines are drawn from her test.

There are three major categories of in-hand manipulation skills. These are translation, shift, and rotation. *Translations* are linear movements from finger surfaces to the palm or the palm to finger surfaces. *Rotations* represent movement of the object around one or more of its axes. The movement is a *simple rotation* if it is less than 180 degrees (usually less than 90 degrees) and a *complex rotation* if it is more than 180 degrees. Finally, *shifts* are small linear movements at the thumb and fingertips. Each of these types of in-hand manipulations can be done *with or without stabilization*. If the individual is simultaneously stabilizing one or more other objects with the ulnar fingers, the in-hand manipulation is done *with stabilization*. If no other objects are in the hand, the in-hand manipulation is done *without stabilization*. Manipulations done with stabilization always are more difficult than their counterparts without stabilization (Exner, 1992, 2001).

In-hand manipulation skills begin to develop around age 18 months. All types are present, but not fully developed, at age 7 years. Children younger than age 2 years cannot do manipulations with stabilization. Three-year-old children can do all of the manipulations without stabilization. In general, translations and simple rotations are the easiest in-hand manipulations and shifts and complex rotations are the hardest (Exner, 1992, 2001).

Assessing Sensory Modulation

Poor ability to modulate sensation may be manifested in a number of different ways. We have discussed

- Sensory defensiveness
- Gravitational insecurity
- Aversive response to movement
- Poor registration (i.e., hyporesponsiveness) to sensation

Knowledge of sensory modulation disorders is relatively limited and not very sophisticated. As assessment becomes more refined, no doubt knowledge will also become more complete. Miller and her colleagues (Miller et al., 1999; McIntosh et al., 1999) are doing exciting new work in the area of modulation.

Assessment of sensory modulation is often done through observation and history taking (i.e., interview or questionnaire). Although both observation and history taking can be revealing, both methods can also be problematic. New assessments, such as the Sensory Profile (Dunn, 1999) and the Evaluation of Sensory Processing (Parham & Ecker; see Appendix 7–1 for a copy) provide valid and reliable information regarding sensory modulation.

Observation

When observation is used, practitioners set up situations likely to elicit problems with modulation and observe clients' responses.

Tactile defensiveness is a fight-or-flight reaction to unexpected light touch. It tends to be cumulative and gets worse after repeated exposure. Thus, the tactile tests from the SIPT provide a good opportunity to observe for indicators of tactile defensiveness.

Similarly, *gravitational insecurity* (i.e., excessive fear in response to movement, being out of the upright, or having one's feet off the ground) may be observed as clients attempt to assume a position on unstable or suspended equipment. May (1988) reported on an observational assessment that involved the performance of 15 potentially fear-inducing activities scored on a three-point scale for avoidance, emotional responses, and postural responses. May used her scale to differentiate between children who were gravitationally insecure and those who were not.

Intolerance or aversive responses to movement, defined as autonomic nervous system reactions to movement, *may* be observed during the PRN test or while clients are on suspended equipment. However, because nausea is a common indicator of aversive responses, assessment is accomplished best through history taking.

One disadvantage of observation as a part of formal assessment is that practitioners generally record only the presence or absence of behaviors; nothing is known about how these affect clients' real lives.

History Taking

Although some circumstances likely to result in poor modulation occur during the SIPT or may be set up as a part of clinical observations, observation of problematic circumstances in clients' lives, which would be most informative, is not generally practical. Thus, in an attempt to learn about clients' reactions to sensation in everyday life, practitioners have resorted to questionnaires.

Unfortunately, until very recently, practitioners devised most of those tools informally, and nothing was known about their validity or reliability.

The single exception was Royeen and Fortune's (1990) Touch Inventory for Elementary School-Aged Children (TIE). The TIE focuses on the responses of children to 26 questions that reflect tactile defensiveness. Normative data, expressed in percentiles of children who answered with responses *less* associated with tactile defensiveness (see Appendix 7–1).

Although the TIE provides a valuable perspective on tactile defensiveness—that of the child—it is appropriate only for children within a limited age range. Furthermore, it pertains only to tactile defensiveness; no other sensory modulation disorders are addressed. Professionals who work with children generally believe that parents are better reporters than are children. Parents experience their child's behavior in a number of situations but from an outside perspective. In addition, parents usually have a larger vocabulary and a longer attention span, so they can respond to greater numbers of more complicated questions. Nonetheless, parents are second-hand reporters of their children's experiences.

More recently, Dunn (1999) published a parent questionnaire of sensory processing, the Sensory Profile. It consists of approximately 100 statements of a child's responses to sensory experiences or situations. Using a five-point Likert scale, parents respond about how frequently the statements are true of their children. The statements are categorized by sensory system and include sensory modulation as well as emotional and fine motor behavior. Parham and Ecker (see Appendix 7–1) have developed another questionnaire, the Evaluation of Sensory Processing (ESP), which focuses more specifically on sensory modulation.

Based partly on factor analysis with Sensory Profile data from more than 1000 children who were typically developing, Dunn (1997) offered a working model in which she set children's responses to sensory events in daily life in the context of a continuum representing neurological thresholds. Dunn's model provides practitioners with a means for thinking about the responses of their clients to situations and sensory information and for conceptualizing intervention strategies.

Dunn identified two relevant continua, a neurological threshold continuum ranging from high (habituation) to low (sensitization) and a behavioral response continuum ranging from responds in *accordance with* threshold to responds to *counteract* threshold. By situating the two continua perpendicular to one another, Dunn created quadrants. She labeled the extreme corners of each quadrant *poor registration, sensation seeking, sensitivity to stimuli, and sensation avoiding.* Dunn's model is shown in Table 7–2.

Dunn and Brown's (1997) factor analysis revealed nine factors that Dunn (1997) indicated were "like behavioral patterns seen in children with disabilities" (p. 27). She speculated that eight of the nine factors could be used to situate a child in a quadrant of her working model. The factors associated with each quadrant are shown in Table 7–3.

ASSESSING SENSORY INTEGRATIVE DYSFUNCTION WITHOUT THE SIPT

Although the SIPT remain the most comprehensive and psychometrically sound means to assess praxis in children, their use is not always possible or practical. One important reason for not using the SIPT is that the level of detail it provides often far exceeds that necessary for the type of intervention that will be provided. For example, if a practitioner wished to consult with a teacher to minimize difficulties the teacher experienced while instructing a particular child, it is not necessary to know the child's scores on the SIPT. Nonetheless, practitioners might wish to know if sensory integrative dysfunction was a factor in the child's difficulties. They might also want to know something about the extent of the child's dysfunction.

Another place in which the SIPT might be impractical is outside North America; the tests require extensive training and are expensive to administer and score. Because no norms have been developed for children outside North America, the results must be interpreted cautiously. Although no norms are available for children outside North America on many tests, few are as expensive to administer as the SIPT. Uncertain interpretation of the SIPT makes the expense of the test even less appealing outside North America.

Although few formal assessments are available to aid in diagnosis, practitioners outside North America commonly use sensory integration theory in intervention. For intervention to be optimally effective and efficient, these practitioners must hone their observation, interview, and assessment skills to a very high degree.

All practitioners have a responsibility to contribute to the development of valid and reliable assessments. However, test development is a long-term project, often one's life's work. The dearth of meaningful assessments (particularly those examining occupational and role performance) is a worldwide problem, not one experienced only outside North America.

In this section, we return to the model of sensory integration presented in Chapter 1 to suggest ways for practitioners to determine the presence of sensory integrative dysfunction and something about its characteristics in the absence of the SIPT. Although we do not explore assessments of occupational or role performance, we believe that

■ TABLE 7–2	DUNN'S MODEL DESCRIBING RELATIONSHIPS BETWEEN BEHAVIORAL RESPONSES AND NEUROLOGICAL THRESHOLDS	
	Behavioral Response Continuum	
Neurologic Threshold Continuum	**Acting in ACCORDANCE with the threshold**	**Acting to COUNTERACT the threshold**
High (habituation)	Poor registration	Sensation seeking
Low (sensitization)	Sensitivity to stimuli	Sensation avoiding

Adapted from Dunn (1999); reproduced with permission.

■ Table 7–3 Summary of Interpretation Using Dunn's Theoretical Model of Sensory Processing.

Model Category	Associated Factors	Related Section Headings	Behavior Indicators
Poor registration	Low endurance or tone Poor registration Sedentary*	Sensory processing related to endurance or tone Modulation of movement affecting activity*	Uninterested Dull affect Withdrawn "Overly tired" Apathetic Self-absorbed
Sensitivity to stimuli	Oral sensory sensitivity Inattention or distractibility Sensory sensitivity	Auditory processing Oral sensory processing	Distractible Hyperactive
Sensation seeking	Sensory seeking	Modulation related to body position and movement	Active Continuously engaging Fidgety excitable
Sensation avoiding	Emotionally reactive Sedentary*	Behavioral outcomes of sensory processing	Resistant to change Reliant on rigid rituals

*Indicates section and factors that need further interpretation to determine to which model category they contribute.
Adapted from Dunn (1999).

such assessment, formal or informal, should always *precede* examination of any performance component, including sensory integration. Once again, readers are referred to Law et al. (2000) for a review of assessments.

Sensory Integration Theory Revisited

Chapter 1 proposed a model of sensory integration in which two major types of dysfunction are represented, poor praxis and poor modulation of sensation. Multiple types of sequelae comprise both praxis and modulation disorders. Sensory integrative–based practic dysfunction can be manifested as poor BIS or somatodyspraxia. Modulation problems can be manifested as sensory defensiveness, gravitational insecurity, or aversive responses to movement.

We have associated each sequela with difficulty processing one or more types of sensation (see Fig. 1–3). The important point is that what separates sensory integration theory from other theories that describe causes of motor incoordination or poor attention is Ayres' (1972a) hypothesis that poor ability to process and interpret sensation (specifically, vestibular, proprioceptive, or tactile) is at the root of sensory integrative dysfunction.

If the theory of sensory integration is sound, the results of any valid, reliable measures of the constructs described (e.g., posture, tactile discrimination, bilateral integration) should provide information about one or more aspects of sensory

integrative functioning. Of course, assessments are valid and reliable only within their own intrinsic limitations. Practitioners who use assessments must be aware of the qualifying factors associated with the tools. This information is available in test manuals and in reports of research examining the test properties.

To say that individuals have sensory integrative dysfunction, we must find meaningful clusters that relate a particular coordination or attention problem to poor sensory processing. Thus, for example, it is not enough to identify a problem with bilateral coordination. If the problem is truly sensory integrative in nature, there should also be evidence of poor processing of vestibular or proprioceptive information (e.g., low muscle tone, poor prone extension). If the problem is distractibility, then there should be evidence of poor processing of tactile, vestibular, or proprioceptive sensation. In Figure 7–10, we have embellished the model of sensory integration presented in Chapter 1 by proposing some common assessments that might be used to examine the constructs. Table 7–4 contains a key to the assessments appearing in Figure 7–10.

Assessing Praxis

In the evaluation of praxis, we have relied heavily on two assessments: the BOTMP (Bruininks, 1978) and the MABC (Henderson & Sugden, 1992), which includes both a performance test and an accompanying checklist.

There is some support for using the BOTMP as a

■   TABLE 7–4   TESTS CITED IN FIGURE 7–10

Acronym	Test Name	Comments
BOTMP	Bruininks Oseretsky Test of Motor Proficiency	Several subtests are included: Balance, Bilateral Coordination, Upper Limb (UL) Speed and Dexterity, Visual-motor Control, Running Speed & Agility
MABC	Motor Assessment Battery for Children	Contains both a performance assessment and a checklist; specific items associated with each construct are listed in Table 7–5
CTSIB	Clinical Test of Sensory Interaction with Balance	Assessment of the ability to maintain balance under conditions of sensory conflict
Cos	Clinical Observations of Neuromotor Performance	Informal assessment often included in the evaluation of sensory integrative function; many versions of these are available; specific observations cited are prone extension, extensor muscle tone, postural stability, supine flexion, head flexion in supine
SCSIT	Southern California Sensory Integration Tests	Some of the somatosensory tests are listed: Localization of Tactile Stimuli (LTS), Finger Identification (FI), Graphesthesia (GRA), Manual Form Perception (MFP), Kinesthesia (KIN) (because reliability of KIN is not high, it is shown in parentheses)
SP	Sensory Profile	Parent report of children's reactions to sensory events; this is the only one of the assessments of sensory modulation that addresses the full range of modulation disorders. However, the SP pertains to processing, a construct larger than modulation.
ESP	Evaluation of Sensory Processing	Parent report of children's reactions to sensory events; pertains to sensory modulation
TIE	Touch Inventory for Elementary School-Aged Children	Child report of reactions to various tactile events

part of an evaluation of praxis. Relating composite BOTMP scores with individual tests from the SCSIT (Ayres, 1972) (Ziviani et al., 1982) found 14, 6, and 9 statistically significant correlations ($p < 0.01$) between the SCSIT scores and the BOTMP fine motor composite, the gross motor composite, and the battery composite, respectively.

The MABC performance assessment includes items designed to assess manual dexterity, ball skills, and balance. Table 7–5 shows how these items reflect the sensory integrative constructs of BIS and somatodyspraxia, as well as postural deficits.

The checklist included in the MABC has parents rate their children on a variety of daily life activities. In developing this checklist, Henderson and Sugden (1992) applied the hierarchy of difficulty of movement tasks described by Gentile et al. (1975) and Keogh and Sugden (1985). This hierarchy is based on both the amount of movement of a target object and the amount of movement required of the individual to act on the object and reflects the construct of praxis as a continuum. (See Chapter 3 for more detailed discussion of the hierarchy and its relation to praxis.)

Assessment of Sensory Discrimination

For the evaluation of sensory discrimination, on which a diagnosis of sensory integrative–based practic dysfunction is based, we have listed:

- Several somatosensory tests from the SCSIT (Ayres, 1980)
- The balance subtest from the BOTMP and items from the MABC
- The CTSIB
- Standard clinical observations of neuromotor performance

Few standardized tests of tactile discrimination exist. We have cited tests from the SCSIT (Ayres, 1980) because these have published norms for children between age 4 and 9 years. However, these tactile tests are known to ceiling early, and several are associated with large errors and relatively poor test–retest reliability. Furthermore, the SCSIT was standardized more than 30 years ago and is no longer available commercially. Because of the questionable psychometric properties of the SCSIT tactile tests, readers are urged

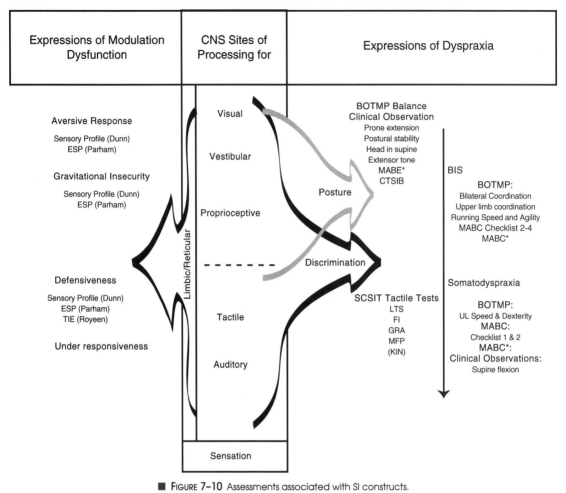

■ FIGURE 7–10 Assessments associated with SI constructs.

■□ TABLE 7–5 HYPOTHESIZED RELATIONSHIP OF MOTOR ASSESSMENT BATTERY FOR CHILDREN ITEMS TO SENSORY INTEGRATIVE CONSTRUCTS

Age, years	MABC Subtest	SI	MABC Subtest	SI	MABC subtest	SI
	Manual Dexterity	SD	Ball Skills	BIS	Balance	Posture
4–6	Posting coins	SD	Catching bean bag	BIS	One-leg balance	Posture
	Threading beads	SD	Rolling ball into goal	SD/BIS	Jumping over cord	BIS
	Bicycle trail	SD or BIS			Walking heels raised	Posture
7–8	Placing pegs	SD	One-hand bounce and	BIS	Stork balance	Posture
	Threading lace	SD	catch	SD or BIS	Jumping in squares	BIS
	Flower trail	SD or BIS	Throwing bean bag into		Heel-to-toe walking	Posture
			box			
9–10	Shifting pegs by	SD	Two-hand catch (off	BIS	One-board balance	Posture
	rows	SD	wall)	SD or BIS	Hopping in squares (1	BIS
	Threading nuts on	SD or BIS			foot)	Posture
	bolt				Ball balance	
	Flower trail					
11–12	Turning pegs	SD	One-hand catch (off wall)	BIS	Two-board balance	Posture
	Cutting out ele-	SD or BIS	Throwing at wall target	SD/BIS	Jumping & clapping	BIS
	phant picture	SD or BIS			Walking backwards	Posture
	Flower trail					

not to report standard scores in documentation. Rather, consider scores above 1 standard deviation below the mean (> -1.0) to reflect typical functioning and scores below that to be indicative of performance markedly below that of most children of a given age. Clearly, these results should be used with caution.

As mentioned earlier in this chapter, the measures of vestibular and proprioceptive processing in the SIPT are weak, and we supplement these measures with clinical observations of neuromotor behavior. These observations can also be used when assessing sensory integration without the SIPT. Additionally, the BOTMP balance subtest provides a measure of vestibular and proprioceptive processing, as do several balance subtest items of the MABC (see Table 7–5 for the specific items). Earlier we described the CTSIB, a relatively new assessment of equilibrium. All three of these assessments are standardized and can be used as behavioral measures of processing of vestibular and proprioceptive sensation.

Assessment of Sensory Modulation Disorders

For an evaluation of modulation disorders, we cite three assessments: the Sensory Profile (Dunn, 1999), The TIE mentioned previously, and the Evaluation of Sensory Processing. There is considerable support for the use of these modulation tests. These tests are among the few means for testing modulation formally; one or more of them should be a part of any comprehensive assessment of sensory integration. The SIPT provide only an opportunity for clinical observation of sensory defensiveness; no standard scores are available to validate such a diagnosis. The Sensory Profile (Dunn, 1999), in particular, has undergone rigorous psychometric testing and has been found to differentiate successfully between typically developing and children with attention deficit hyperactivity disorder (ADHD) and autism (Ermer & Dunn, 1998; Kientz & Dunn, 1997). Similarly, although the ESP is in early stages of development, preliminary examination of its reliability and validity have been promising (Lacroix, 1993; Lacroix & Mailloux, 1995), including its ability to discriminate between children with and without autism and children with and without SI dysfunction (Diane Parham, personal communication, January 26, 2001).

Limitations of Using Alternative Tests

Although the suggested measures may provide the basis for assessment in situations where the SIPT are impractical or impossible, there are several limitations inherent to their use, particularly with regard to praxis. First, they frequently use items or subtests excerpted from a total test battery. This most certainly affects the reliability and, thus, the validity, of the items. However, Wilson et al. (1995) have recommended the use of subtests of the BOTMP for diagnostic purposes, citing four (Running Speed and Agility, Balance, Visual-Motor Coordination, and Upper Limb Speed and Dexterity) as particularly good predictors of mild motor problems. Because the interrater reliability of the BOTMP has been addressed for only one subtest, Wilson et al. (1995) have also recommended that the same examiner administer all tests, especially when scores are used for examination of the effectiveness of intervention.

Second, terminology may be a problem. The proposed alternative testing was developed from a blend of knowledge about sensory integrative dysfunction with an analysis of demands of test items. Although the names of subtests, especially those associated with the MABC, may appear to reflect one construct of sensory integration, analysis sometimes suggested that an item was a better measure of a different construct. In some cases, items within subtests appear to reflect different constructs.

Third, both the BOTMP and the MABC performance test are thought to be tests of motor abilities (Burton & Miller, 1998). Burton and Miller have argued that motor abilities may not exist— that is, abilities that are inferred from tests such as the BOTMP may be skill specific rather than reflecting general underlying capacities. Burton and Miller believed that a far preferable method for evaluating performance was to assess functional movement skills (i.e., those done within the context of everyday activity). Of the tests described in this chapter, the MABC Checklist is the only assessment that falls in that category.

Finally, an accurate assessment of sensory integrative dysfunction is dependent on valid testing of sensory processing. However, the tests that reflect sensory discrimination are weak because few standardized and psychometrically sound tools exist for assessment of these functions. Thus, results of the tests proposed must be used cautiously.

SUMMARY AND CONCLUSION

This chapter discussed assessment of sensory integration within the context of a top-down approach to evaluation. It also reviewed the development of the SIPT and existing evidence of their construct validity and inter- and intrarater reliability. The third section presented formal and informal assessments complementary to the SIPT and necessary for a complete evaluation of sensory integration. Finally, the text proposed a means of assessing sensory integration in the absence of the SIPT.

References

Abravanel, E. (1972a). How children combine vision and touch when perceiving the shape of objects. *Perception and Psychophysics, 12,* 171–175.

Abravanel, E. (1972b). Short-term memory for shape information processed intra- and intermodally at three ages. *Perceptual and Motor Skills, 35,* 419–425.

Ayres, A. J. (1965). Patterns of perceptual-motor dysfunction in children: A factor analytic study. *Perceptual and Motor Skills, 20,* 335–368.

Ayres, A. J. (1966a). Interrelation among perceptual-motor functions in children. *American Journal of Occupational Therapy, 20,* 68–71.

Ayres, A. J. (1966b). Interrelationships among perceptual-motor functions in children. *American Journal of Occupational Therapy, 20,* 288–292.

Ayres, A. J. (1969). Relation between Gesell developmental Quotients and later perceptual-motor performance. *American Journal of Occupational Therapy, 23,* 11–17.

Ayres, A. J. (1972a). *Sensory integration and learning disorders.* Los Angeles: Western Psychological Services.

Ayres, A. J. (1972b). Types of sensory integrative dysfunction among disabled learners. *American Journal of Occupational Therapy, 26,* 13–18.

Ayres, A. J. (1975). *Southern California Postrotary Nystagmus Test manual.* Los Angeles: Western Psychological Services.

Ayres, A. J. (1977). Cluster analyses of measures of SI. *American Journal of Occupational Therapy, 31,* 362–366.

Ayres, A. J. (1980). *Southern California Sensory Integration Tests manual: Revised 1980.* Los Angeles: Western Psychological Services.

Ayres, A. J. (1989). *Sensory Integration and Praxis Tests manual.* Los Angeles: Western Psychological Services.

Bruininks, R. H. (1978). *Bruininks-Oseretsky Test of Motor Proficiency manual.* Circle Pines, MN: American Guidance Services.

Burton, A. W., & Miller, D. E. (1998). *Movement skill assessment.* Champaign, IL: Human Kinetics.

Cohen, H. (1989). Testing vestibular function: Problems with the Southern California Postrotary Nystagmus Test. *American Journal of Occupational Therapy, 43,* 475–477.

Coster, W. (1998). Occupation-centered assessment of children. *American Journal of Occupational Therapy, 52,* 337–344.

Crowe, T. K., Deitz, J., Richardson, P., & Atwater, S. (1990). Interrater reliability of the Pediatric Clinical Test of Sensory Interaction for Balance. *Physical and Occupational Therapy in Pediatrics, 10*(4), 1–27.

Deitz, J., Richardson, P., Atwater, S., Crowe, T., & Odiorne, M. (1991). Performance of normal children on the Pediatric Clinical Test of Sensory Interaction for Balance. *Occupational Therapy Journal of Research, 11,* 336–356.

Dunn, W. (1997). The impact of sensory processing abilities on the daily lives of young children and their families: A conceptual model. *Infants and Young Children, 9,* 23–35.

Dunn, W. (1999). *Sensory Profile User's Manual.* San Antonio: Psychological Corporation.

Dunn, W., & Brown, C. (1997). Factor analysis on the Sensory Profile from a national sample of children without disabilities. *American Journal of Occupational Therapy, 51,* 490–495.

Ermer, J., & Dunn, W. (1998). The Sensory Profile: A discriminant analysis of children with and without disabilities. *American Journal of Occupational Therapy, 52,* 283–290.

Exner, C. E. (1992). In-hand manipulation skills. In J. Case-Smith & C. Pehoski (Eds.). *Development of hand skills in the child* (pp. 35–46). Bethesda, MD: American Occupational Therapy Association.

Exner, C. E. (2001). In hand-manipulation skills. In J. Case-Smith (Ed.). *Occupational therapy for children* (pp. 289–328). Philadelphia: Lippincott Williams & Wilkins.

Fisher, A. G. (1989). Objective measurement of the quality of response during two equilibrium tests. *Physical and Occupational Therapy in Pediatrics, 9,* 57–78.

Fisher, A. G., & Bundy, A. C. (1989). Vestibular stimulation in the treatment of postural and related disorders. In O. D. Payton, R. P. Difabio, S. V. Paris, E. J. Protas, & A. F. Van Sant (Eds.). *Manual of physical therapy techniques* (pp. 239–258). New York: Churchill Livingstone.

Fisher, A. G., & Bundy, A. C. (1991). SI. In H. Forssberg & H. Hirschfeld (Eds.). *Movement disorders in children* (pp. 16–20). New York: Karger.

Fisher, A. G., & Short De Graff, M. (1993). Improving functional assessment in occupational therapy: Recommendations and philosophy for change. *American Journal of Occupational Therapy, 47,* 199–201.

Fisher, A. G., Wietlisbach, S. E., Wilbarger, J. L. (1988). Adult performance on three tests of equilibrium. *American Journal of Occupational Therapy, 42,* 30–35.

Fregly, A. R., & Graybiel, A. (1968). An ataxia

battery not requiring rails. *Aerospace Medicine, 39,* 277–282.

Gentile, A. M., Higgins, J. R., Miller, E. A., & Rosen, B. M. (1975). The structure of motor tasks. *Movement, 7,* 11–28.

Harris, N. P. (1981). Duration and quality of prone extension in 4, 6, and 8-year-old normal children. *American Journal of Occupational Therapy, 35,* 26–30.

Henderson, S. E., & Sugden, D. A. (1992) *Movement Assessment Battery for Children manual.* New York: Psychological Corporation.

Hoop, N. H. (1971a). Haptic perception in preschool children, part I: Object recognition. *American Journal of Occupational Therapy, 25,* 340–344.

Hoop, N. H. (1971b). Haptic perception in preschool children, part II: Object manipulation. *American Journal of Occupational Therapy, 25,* 415–419.

Jennings, P. A. (1974). Haptic perception and form reproduction in kindergarten children. *American Journal of Occupational Therapy, 28,* 274–280.

Keogh, J. F., & Sugden, D. A. (1985). *Movement skill development.* New York: MacMillan.

Kientz M. A. & Dunn W. (1997). A comparison of the performance of children with and without autism on the Sensory Profile. *American Journal of Occupational Therapy, 51,* 530–537.

Kielhofner, G., & Mallinson, T. (1995). Application of the model in practice: Case illustrations. In G. Kielhofner (Ed.). *A model of human occupation: Theory and application* (2nd ed., pp. 271–342). Baltimore: Williams & Wilkins.

Kleinman, J. J. (1979). Developmental changes in haptic exploration and matching accuracy. *Developmental Psychology, 15,* 480–481.

Johnson, C. L. (1996). A study of a pilot Sensory History Questionnaire using contrasting groups. Unpublished master's thesis, University of Southern California, Los Angeles.

Lacroix, J. E. (1993). A study of content validity using the Sensory History Questionnaire. Masters thesis, University of Southern California, Los Angeles.

Lacroix, J. E., & Mailloux, Z. (1995, April). Evaluation of sensory processing. Paper presented at the annual conference of the American Occupational Therapy Association, Denver.

Law, M., Baum, C., & Dunn, W. (2000). *Measurement of occupational therapy performance: Supporting best practice in occupational therapy.* Thorofare, NJ: Slack.

Lederman, S. J., & Klatzky, R. L. (1987). Hand movements: A window into haptic object recognition. *Cognitive Psychology, 19,* 342–368.

Magalhães, L. C., Koomar, J., & Cermak, S. A. (1989). Bilateral motor coordination in 5- to 9-year-old children: A pilot study. *American Journal of Occupational Therapy, 43,* 437–443.

Mathiowetz, V. (1993). Role of physical performance component evaluation in occupational therapy functional assessment. *American Journal of Occupational Therapy, 47,* 225–230.

Mathiowetz, V., & Haugen, J. B. (1995). Evaluation of motor behavior: Traditional and contemporary views. In C. A. Trombly (Ed.). *Occupational therapy for physical dysfunction* (pp. 157–185). Baltimore: Williams & Wilkins.

May, T. (1988). Identifying gravitational insecurity in children with sensory integrative dysfunction. Unpublished master's thesis, Boston University.

McIntosh, D. N., Miller, L. J., Shyu, V., & Dunn, W. (1999). Overview of the Short Sensory Profile (SSP). In W. Dunn (Ed.). *Sensory profile: User's manual* (pp. 59–73). San Antonio, TX: Psychological Corporation.

Miller, L. J., McIntosh, D. N., McGrath, J., Shyu, V., Lampe, M., Taylor, A. K., Tassone, F., Neitzel, K., Stackhouse, T., & Hagerman, R. J. (1999). Electrodermal responses to sensory stimuli in individuals with Fragile X Syndrome. *American Journal of Medical Genetics, 83,* 268–279.

Morrison, D., & Sublett, J. (1983). Reliability of the Southern California Postrotary Nystagmus Test with learning disabled children. *American Journal of Occupational Therapy, 37,* 694–698.

Mulligan, S. (1998). Patterns of SI dysfunction: A confirmatory factor analysis. *American Journal of Occupational Therapy, 52,* 819–828.

Parham, L. D. (April 1997). Sensory questionnaire validity for children with autism. Paper presented at the annual conference of the American Occupational Therapy Association. Orlando, FL.

Piaget, J., & Inhelder, B. (1948). *The child's conception of space.* New York: Norton.

Polatajko, H. (1983). The Southern California Postrotary Nystagmus Test: A validity study. *Canadian Journal of Occupational Therapy, 50,* 119–123.

Richardson, P. K., Atwater, S. W., Crowe, T. K., & Deitz, J. C. (1992). Performance of preschoolers on the Pediatric Clinical Test of Sensory Interaction for Balance. *American Journal of Occupational Therapy, 46,* 793–800.

Royeen, C. B., & Fortune, J. C. (1990). TIE: Touch inventory for school aged children. *American Journal of Occupational Therapy, 44,* 165–170.

Shumway-Cook, A., & Horak, F. (1986). Assessing the influence of sensory interaction on balance. *Physical Therapy, 66,* 1548–1550.

Tan, L. E. (1985). Laterality and motor skills in four-year-olds. *Child Development, 56,* 119–124.

Trombly, C. (1993). Anticipating the future: Assessment of occupational function. *American Journal of Occupational Therapy, 47,* 253–257.

Wilson, B. N., Polatajko, H. J., Kaplan, B. J., & Faris, P. (1995). Use of the Bruininks-Oseretsky Test of Motor proficiency in occupational therapy. *American Journal of Occupational Therapy, 49,* 8–17.

Wilson, B., Pollock, N., Kaplan, B. J., Law, M., & Faris, P. (2000). *Clinical observations of motor and postural skills.* Framingham, MA: Therapro.

Wolff, P. (1972). The role of stimulus-correlated activity in children's recognition of nonsense forms. *Journal of Experimental Child Psychology, 24,* 427–441.

Zaporozhets, A. V. (1965). The development of perception in the preschool child. *Monographs of the Society for Research in Child Development, 30,* 82–101.

Zaporozhets, A. V. (1969). Some of the psychological problems of sensory training in early childhood and the preschool period. In A. R. Leont'ev & A. R. Luria (Eds.). *A handbook of contemporary Soviet psychology* (pp. 86–120). New York: Basic.

Ziviani, J., Poulsen, A., & O'Brien, A. (1982). Correlation of the Bruininks-Oseretsky Test of Motor Proficiency with the Southern California SI Tests. *American Journal of Occupational Therapy, 36,* 519–523.

■■ Appendix 7–1

Clinical Observations of Neuromotor Performance, Evaluation of Sensory Processing, and Touch Inventory for Elementary School Children

Clinical Observations of Neuromotor Performance

NAME_____   TEST DATE: _____

BIRTH DATE: _____

AGE: _____

Poor Sensory Modulation

1. GRAVITATIONAL INSECURITY
   − Normal reaction to change in body position
   +Fear reaction out of proportion to actual danger
2. AVERSIVE RESPONSE TO MOVEMENT
   − No evidence of aversive responses
   +Feelings of discomfort (nausea, vomiting, vertigo, dizziness) to movement
3. TACTILE DEFENSIVENESS
   − Tolerates variety of tactile stimuli
   +Overreacts or aversion to tactile stimuli
4. AVOIDANCE OF SENSORY EXPERIENCES
   − Seeks new and challenging experiences
   +Avoids unfamiliar activities or sensory stimuli
5. HYPERRESPONSIVE TO SMELL
   − No evidence of aversive responses
   +Overreacts or aversive response to smell
6. HYPERRESPONSIVE TO SOUND
   − No evidence of aversive responses
   +Overreacts or aversion to noise
7. DISTRACTIBILITY
   − No evidence of unusual tendency to attend to irrelevant stimuli
   +Attends to irrelevant stimuli; difficulty attending to task
8. LEVEL OF ACTIVITY
   − Level of motor and verbal activity appropriate to situation
   +Unusually high levels of activity or difficulty transitioning from active to quiet activities

DIFFICULTY WITH POSTURE

1. PRONE EXTENSION
   − Extends body against gravity easily for 20–30 s
   +Difficulty extending body against gravity

2. PROXIMAL STABILITY IN QUADRUPED
   − Stabilize scapulae, back, elbows during weight bearing
   +Lordosis, hyperextends or locks elbows or scapulae wing.
3. EXTENSOR MUSCLE TONE
   − No evidence of low tone
   +Lordosis and hyperextended knees in standing, "mushy" muscles when palpated
4. EQUILIBRIUM
   − Makes postural adjustments of uphill limbs and maintains head or upper trunk upright
   +Does not maintain head or upper trunk upright or make postural adjustments of uphill limbs to maintain balance
5. NECK FLEXION IN SUPINE
   − Flexes neck and no head lag when assuming supine flexion
   +Head lag (leads with chin) when assuming supine position
6. POSTURAL ADJUSTMENT
   − Appropriate postural adjustments to support limb movements
   +Exaggerated, awkward, inappropriate, or diminished postural adjustments

POOR BILATERAL INTEGRATION AND SEQUENCING (BIS)

1. MIXED HAND PREFERENCE
   − Consistently uses the same hand for given task
   +Sometimes uses right and sometimes uses left hand to perform the same task (or history of doing so)
2. CROSSING BODY MIDLINE
   − Spontaneously crosses midline of body
   +Avoids crossing midline
3. RIGHT-LEFT CONFUSION
   − Correctly identifies right and left or knows but cannot label correctly
   +Confuses right and left
4. PROJECTED ACTION SEQUENCES AND BILATERAL MOTOR SKILLS
   a. CATCHING A BOUNCED BALL
      − Able to catch bounced ball when force or direction varies
      +Difficulty catching bounced ball when force or direction varies
   b. HOPPING/JUMPING IN SERIES OF CIRCLES
      − Able to jump in a series with both feet together, without stopping
      +Cannot jump with feet together, breaks task apart into separate jumps, difficulty terminating series
   c. SKIPPING
      − Skips in a fluid, reciprocal manner
      +Unable to skip; breaks into step-hop pattern
   d. JUMPING JACKS
      − Able to simultaneously open and close arms and legs and jump in smooth series
      +Moves arms or legs segmentally while jumping or difficulty performing a series of jumps
   e. SYMMETRICAL STRIDE JUMPING
      − Simultaneously swings ipsilateral arm and leg forward and backward while performing a series of jumps
      +Unable to move ipsilateral arm and leg simultaneously, segments jumps, unable to perform a series of jumps
   f. RECIPROCAL STRIDE JUMPING
      − Simultaneously swings contralateral arm and leg forward and backward while performing a series of jumps
      +Unable to move contralateral arm and leg simultaneously, segments jumps, unable to perform a series of jumps

g. STEPPING OVER A MOVING OBJECT
   − Able to plan and execute movement over moving object without object hitting client
   + Object hits client with attempt to step over moving object

Comments:

SOMATODYSPRAXIA

1. SUPINE FLEXION
   − Able to assume and maintain body in total flexion easily 20–30 sec
   +Unable to assume or maintain position
2. SEQUENTIAL FINGER TOUCHING
   − Able to oppose thumb to each finger bilaterally in smooth sequence
   +Unable to touch thumb to fingers in smooth sequence, visual monitoring required
3. IN-HAND MANIPULATION
   − Able to manipulate objects within hand
   +Must use two hands or place object on table to manipulate objects
4. DIADOKOKINESIA
   − Pronation or supination in continuous bilateral sequence
   +Segmented movements, poor bilateral coordination

OTHER CLINICAL OBSERVATIONS THAT MAY SUGGEST CNS IMMATURITY OR BE COMMON IN INDIVIDUALS WITH SENSORY INTEGRATIVE DYSFUNCTION

1. ASSOCIATED MOVEMENTS
   − No evidence of extraneous movements or overflow when performing developmentally appropriate tasks; some overflow when performing difficult tasks
   +Excessive extraneous movements or overflow when performing developmentally appropriate tasks
2. FINGER TO NOSE
   − Alternately and accurately touches nose with finger
   +Diminished accuracy touching nose; over- or undershoots
3. SLOW (RAMP) MOVEMENTS
   − Able to flex and extend elbows in smooth, bilateral, symmetrical pattern
   +Moves arms segmentally or unable to move both arms simultaneously
4. PROTECTIVE EXTENSION OR SUPPORT REACTIONS
   − Extends downhill limb when balance is lost; supports weight on "weight-bearing" limb
   +Delayed extension of downhill limbs when balance is lost; difficulty shifting weight onto "weight-bearing" limbs

VISUALLY CONTROLLED EYE MOVEMENTS

1. TRACKING
   − Able to easily follow small object with eyes
   +Loses object; eyes not well coordinated; tires easily
2. CONVERGENCE OR DIVERGENCE
   − Able to easily follow small object with eyes
   +Eyes not well coordinated; tires easily
3. QUICK LOCALIZATION
   −Able to easily follow small object with eyes
   +Eyes not well coordinated; tires easily

+ *indicates evidence of difficulty or dysfunction*
− *indicates NO evidence of difficulty or dysfunction*

These observations are helpful in the evaluation of clients with suspected sensory integrative dysfunction. Judgment of performance should be based on *knowledge of normal development.*

EVALUATION OF SENSORY PROCESSING*

ESP Research Version 4
Child's Name: _____
Child's Age: _____ years _____ months
Name of adult completing this form: _____
Relationship to child: _____
Date: _____

A = Always
O = Occasionally
S = Sometimes
R = Rarely
N = Never

	A	O	S	R	N
Auditory System					
1. Does your child have trouble understanding what other people mean when they say something?					
2. Is your child bothered by any household or ordinary sounds, such as the vacuum, hair dryer, or toilet flushing?					
3. Does your child respond negatively to loud noises as in running away, crying, or holding hands over ears?					
4. Does your child appear to not hear certain sounds?					
5. Is your child distracted by sounds not usually noticed by other people?					
6. Is your child frightened of sounds that do not usually convey alarm to other children the same age?					
7. Does your child seem to underreact to loud noises?					
8. Does your child have trouble interpreting the meaning of simple or common words?					
9. Is your child easily distracted by irrelevant noises such as a lawn mower outside, children talking in the back of the room, crinkling paper, an air conditioner, a refrigerator, or fluorescent lights?					
10. Does your child seem too sensitive to sounds?					
Gustatory or Olfactory System					
1. Does your child gag, vomit, or complain of nausea when smelling odors such as soap, perfume, or cleaning products?					
2. Does your child complain that foods are too bland or refuse to eat bland foods?					
3. Does your child prefer very salty foods?					
4. Does your child like to taste nonfood items such as glue or paint?					
5. Does your child gag when anticipating an unappealing food such as cooked spinach?					
Proprioception System					
1. Does your child grasp objects so tightly that it is difficult to use the object?					
2. Does your child grind his or her teeth?					
3. Does your child seem driven to seek activities such as pushing, pulling, dragging, lifting, and jumping?					
4. Does your child seem unsure of how far to raise or lower his or her body during movement such as sitting down or stepping over an object?					
5. Does your child grasp objects so loosely that it is difficult to use the object?					
6. Does your child seem to exert too much pressure for a task, such as walking heavily, slamming doors, or pressing too hard when using pencils or crayons?					
7. Does your child jump a lot?					
8. Does your child have difficulty playing with animals appropriately, such as petting them with too much force?					
9. Does your child have difficulty positioning him- or herself in a chair?					

	A	O	S	R	N
10. Does your child bump or push other children?					
11. Does your child seem generally weak?					
12. Does your child chew on toys, clothes, or other objects more than other children do?					

Tactile System

	A	O	S	R	N
1. Does your child pull away from being touched lightly?					
2. Does your child seem to lack the normal awareness of being touched?					
3. Does your child react negatively to the feel of new clothes?					
4. Does your child show an unusual dislike for having his or her hair combed, brushed, or styled?					
5. Does your child prefer to touch rather than be touched?					
6. Does your child seem driven to touch different textures?					
7. Does your child refuse to wear hats, sunglasses, or other accessories?					
8. Does it bother your child to have his or her finger or toe nails cut?					
9. Does your child struggle against being held?					
10. Does your child have a tendency to touch things constantly?					
11. Does your child avoid or dislike playing with gritty things?					
12. Does your child prefer certain textures of clothing or particular fabrics?					
13. Does it bother your child to have his or her face touched?					
14. Does it bother your child to have his or her face washed?					
15. Does your child resist or dislike wearing short-sleeved shirts or short pants?					
16. Does your child dislike eating messy foods with his or her hands?					
17. Does your child avoid foods of certain textures?					
18. Does your child mind getting his or her hands in finger paint, paste, sand, clay, mud, glue, or other messy things?					
19. Does it bother your child to have his or her hair cut?					
20. Does your child overreact to minor injuries?					
21. Does your child have an unusually high tolerance for pain?					

Vestibular System

	A	O	S	R	N
1. Does your child seem excessively fearful of movement, as in going up and down stairs or riding swings, teeter totters, slides, or other playground equipment?					
2. Does your child demonstrate distress when he or she is moved or riding on moving equipment?					
3. Does your child have good balance?					
4. Does your child avoid balance activities such as walking on curbs or on uneven ground?					
5. Does your child like fast, spinning carnival rides, such as merry-go-rounds?					
6. When your child shifts his or her body, does he or she fall out of the chair?					
7. Is your child unable to catch him- or herself when falling?					
8. Does your child seem to not get dizzy when others usually do?					
9. Does your child seem generally weak?					
10. Does your child spin and whirl his or her body more than other children?					
11. Does your child rock him- or herself when stressed?					
12. Does your child like to be inverted or tipped upside down or enjoy doing activities that involve inversion, such as hanging upside down or doing somersaults?					
13. Was your child fearful of swinging or bouncing as an infant?					
14 Compared with other children the same age, does your child seem to ride longer or harder on certain playground equipment, such as a swing or merry-go-round?					

	A	O	S	R	N
15 Does your child demonstrate distress when his or her head is in any other position than upright or vertical such as having the head tilted backward or upside down?					

Visual System

	A	O	S	R	N
1. Does your child have trouble telling the difference between printed figures that appear similar, for example, differentiating between *b* and *p* or + and *x*?					
2. Is your child sensitive to or bothered by light, especially bright light (blinks, squints, cries, or closes eyes)?					
3. When looking at pictures, does your child focus on patterns or details instead of the main pictures?					
4. Does your child have difficulty keeping his or her eyes on the task or activity at hand?					
5. Does your child become easily distracted by visual stimuli?					
6. Does your child have trouble finding an object when it is amid a group of other things?					
7. Does your child close one eye or tip his or her head back when looking at something or someone?					
8. Does your child have difficulty with unusual visual environments such as a bright, colorful room or a dimly lit room?					
9. Does your child have difficulty controlling eye movement when following objects like a ball with his or her eyes?					
10. Does your child have difficulty naming, discriminating, or matching colors, shapes or sizes? If your child is 6 years of age or older, please answer the following 3 questions.					
11 Did your child make reversals in words or letters when writing or copying or read words backwards (such as reading saw for was) after the first grade?					
12. Does your child lose his or her place on a page while reading, copying, solving problems, or performing manipulations?					
13. In school, does your child have difficulty shifting gaze from the board to the paper when copying from the board?					

*Courtesy of L. D. Parham and C. Ecker

TOUCH INVENTORY FOR ELEMENTARY SCHOOL CHILDREN*

Equipment

Two chairs and a table are required, as well as a copy of the instrument and three blocks made of poster board. Each block has one of the response choices inscribed on it with large black letters: "No" on a 2-inch by 2-inch reponse card, "A little" on a 2-inch by 3-inch response card, and "A lot" on a 2-inch by 4-inch reponse card.

Procedure

The scale takes less than 10 minutes to administer. The subject (S) and the examiner (Ex) sit across from each other. Ex uses a shield to cover the instrument in order to reduce distraction for S.

Ex orients S to the task. Ex explains that they will be playing a gaine in which there are no "right" answers and no "wrong" answers. The game is being played so that the Ex can learn more about S.

Ex explains the response format to S. Ex says:

"I will ask you questions and you are to answer them saying either 'No,' 'A little,' or 'A lot'."

Ex is to point to each of the three blocks inscribed with the phrases while saying them aloud. Ex continues, saying:

"Let's practice the game for you to learn how to play it. I will ask you a question—'Do you like ice cream?' You answer by saying either 'No,' 'A little,' or 'A lot'."

Ex points to the blocks again when stating choices for response. Ex continues:

"Remember to point to the block that is your choice. You don't have to say which one it is, just point to it."

In the beginning, S is required to point to the block which is his or her choice. S may also state

TOUCH INVENTORY FOR ELEMENTARY SCHOOL-AGED CHILDREN (TIE)
By Charlotte Brasic Royeen

Date: _____

Subject: _____

Examiner: _____

Procedure: Administer the scale according to standard instructions. Reponse of "No" is scored "1"; a response of "A Little" is scored "2"; and a response of "A Lott" is scored "3".

Response (Check)			No.	Question
1	2	3		
[ ]	[ ]	[ ]	1.	Does it bother you to go barefooted?
[ ]	[ ]	[ ]	2.	Do fuzzy shirts bother you?
[ ]	[ ]	[ ]	3.	Do fuzzy socks bother you?
[ ]	[ ]	[ ]	4.	Do turtleneck shirts bother you?
[ ]	[ ]	[ ]	5.	Does it bother you to have your face washed?
[ ]	[ ]	[ ]	6.	Does it bother you to have your nails cut?
[ ]	[ ]	[ ]	7.	Does it bother you to have your hair combed by someone else?
[ ]	[ ]	[ ]	8.	Does it bother you to play on a carpet?
[ ]	[ ]	[ ]	9.	After someone touches you, do you feel like scratching that spot?
[ ]	[ ]	[ ]	10.	After someone touches you, do you feel like rubbing that spot?
[ ]	[ ]	[ ]	11.	Does it bother you to walk barefooted in the grass and sand?
[ ]	[ ]	[ ]	12.	Does getting dirty bother you?
[ ]	[ ]	[ ]	13.	Do you find it hard to pay attention?
[ ]	[ ]	[ ]	14.	Does it bother you if you cannot see who is touching you?
[ ]	[ ]	[ ]	15.	Does fingerpainting bother you?
[ ]	[ ]	[ ]	16.	Do rough bedsheets bother you?
[ ]	[ ]	[ ]	17.	Do you like to touch people, but it bothers you when they touch you back?
[ ]	[ ]	[ ]	18.	Does it bother you when people come from behind?
[ ]	[ ]	[ ]	19.	Does it bother you to be kissed by someone other than your parents?
[ ]	[ ]	[ ]	20.	Does it bother you to be hugged or held?
[ ]	[ ]	[ ]	21.	Does it bother you to play games with your feet?
[ ]	[ ]	[ ]	22.	Does it bother you to have your face touched?
[ ]	[ ]	[ ]	23.	Does it bother you to be touched if you don't expect it?
[ ]	[ ]	[ ]	24.	Do you have difficulty making friends?
[ ]	[ ]	[ ]	25.	Does it bother you to stand in line?
[ ]	[ ]	[ ]	26.	Does it bother you when someone is close by?

[ ]   (no. of reponses scored "1") $\times$ 1 = [   ]

+ [ ]   (no. of reponses scored "2") $\times$ 2 = [   ]

+ [ ]   (no. of reponses scored "3") $\times$ 3 = [   ]

Total Score = [   ]

Percentile Score = [   ]

his or her answer aloud but that is not required. The purpose of the blocks is to aid S in remembering the three response items. Thus, it is all right if after doing the test for a few items the subject stops pointing to the blocks. The purpose of the practice session is to teach the child the response format. Therefore, the procedures should be repeated until Ex is certain that S understands how to answer the questions. Suggested questions to use if further practuce is required follow:

"Do you like snakes?", "Do you like turtles?", "Do you like vegetables?", "Do you like school?"

Once S understands the task and the required response style, Ex says:

"Now we will play the game."

Ex may restate or explain the item until S understands it. If S asks Ex to repeat an item or states that he or she does not understand the question. Ex should read the question and wait for S to respond. If S does not respond or needs prompting, Ex may say:

"Which answer do you want?" and then point to the three answers on the response cards, "No," "A Little," or "A Lot."

Ex records S's answers and notes any pertinent

observations. Upon completion of the session, Ex praises S for his participation.

Scoring and interpreting the tie

The TIE is easily scored by summing the child's response scores (i.e., adding the scores from items 1 through 26). The child's score is then compared to the normative data supplied in Table 7–A.

Proper interpretation of Table 7–A is contingent upon understanding that a high raw score does not mean a better performance on part of the child. Recall that the response format for the TIE is 1 = no, 2 = a little, and 3 = a lot. Therefore, a child who responds with "a lot" for many of the test items will receive a higher raw score than the child who answers with "a little" for many of the test items. Thus, *the higher the score, the more the child's self-reported behaviors are associated with behaviors indicative of tactile defensiveness.* Conversely, *the lower the score, the less the subject's self-reported behaviors are associated with behaviors indicative of tactile defensiveness.*

Conversion of raw scores into corresponding percentile scores using Table 7–A provides a stan-

■□ TABLE 7–A	DATA FOR SCORING THE TOUCH INVENTORY FOR ELEMENTARY SCHOOL CHILDREN

Percentile Score	Raw Score
100	60
90	51
75	45
50	40
25	35
10	31
0	25

Percentile Score   0 10 25 50 75 90 100
Raw Score   25 30 35 40 45 50 60
Mean score = 41; standard deviation = 7.8; standard error of the mean = 0.38.

dard reference for how a given child responds to test items compared to the normative sample. Again, it is important to note that a higher percentile score does not mean a better test performance. Rather, a higher percentile score, for example, the range of the 75th percentile and above, means that at least 75 percent of the normative sample answered the responses *less* associated with tactile defensiveness: Only 25 percent of the normative sample answered with responses *more* associated with tactile defensiveness.

Source: Royeen, C.B., & Fortune, J.C. (1990). TIE: Touch inventory for school aged children. *American Journal of Occupational Therapy, 44,* 165–170, with permission.

8

Interpreting Test Scores and Observations: A Case Example

Anita C. Bundy, ScD, OTR, FAOTA

Anne G. Fisher, ScD, OTR, FAOTA

> *Interpret 1: to explain or tell the meaning of: present in understandable terms*
> *2: to conceive in the light of individual belief, judgement, or circumstance.*
> —*C. & G. Merriam, 1981*
>
> *The utilization of interpretive models for the treatment of individual [clients] is a basic characteristic of all clinical practice, whether the clinician is an [occupational therapist], internist, psychiatrist, spiritualist healer, Chinese shaman or Iranian prayer writer.*
> —*Good & Good, 1981, p. 177*

PURPOSE AND SCOPE

Chapter 7 presented a description of the evaluation of sensory integration, including the Sensory Integration and Praxis Tests (SIPT) (Ayres, 1989), related clinical observations, and measures of sensory modulation dysfunction. This chapter demonstrates how evaluation data are interpreted. A case report of Kyle, a 6½-year-old boy, is presented. The chapter recounts the process of determining:

- That Kyle had sensory integrative dysfunction

- The specific nature of his dysfunction
- The ways in which sensory integrative dysfunction interfered with his daily life

Finally, the text demonstrates how the results of an evaluation can be presented to parents and teachers.

Evaluation involves gathering relevant information, and this process yields both quantitative and qualitative data. Interpretation entails making meaning. When appropriate, we seek to use sensory integration theory to explain clients' presenting problems. We use the results of the SIPT, clinical observations, and measures of sensory modulation together with relevant information obtained from clients and caregivers. We also consider additional data provided by other professionals.

Interpretation is an art that is based on a thorough understanding of the strengths and limitations of sensory integration theory and the evaluation process. This chapter examines test scores and observations for groupings suggestive of sensory integrative dysfunction; the term *meaningful clusters* is used to explain presenting problems and as a foundation for intervention planning. If meaningful clusters cannot be identified, or when there are important presenting problems that we cannot explain, we acknowledge that sensory integration is not the best theoretical framework for understanding the client.

THE REFERRAL AND DEVELOPMENTAL HISTORY

Kyle was 6½ years old when his mother, Mrs. P., initiated a referral to occupational therapy for evaluation of suspected sensory integrative dysfunction. Mrs. P.'s sister was an occupational therapist living in a different state. When Mrs. P.'s sister learned about Kyle's difficulties, she urged Mrs. P. to have him evaluated.

Kyle's mother began by saying, "l don't know what any of this means, but l want to tell you how Kyle is different from my other three children." Mrs. P. then related the story of Kyle's development from the time of his birth. We asked questions to help focus her story on relevant aspects of Kyle's childhood and the effect of his problems on his daily life. We listened carefully for evidence that an evaluation of sensory integrative functioning was warranted.

Kyle was a full-term infant, and his birth was uncomplicated. From the time of his first feeding, however, Mrs. P. felt that he was different. He was cranky and irritable, and he seemed to dislike cuddling and handling. He had difficulty nursing because of a weak suck. His sleep cycles were erratic; he did not sleep more than 4 hours until he was almost 2 years old. Even at age 6 years, he seldom slept more than 6 hours a night.

Kyle's crankiness and difficulty sleeping were complicated by chronic ear infections. Kyle's mother had attributed all of his problems to this problem. However, even when tubes reduced the frequency of the ear infections, Kyle persisted in being somehow different from his siblings.

Although Kyle's behavior was problematic, he attained most motor milestones at the later end of "normal." He sat independently at age 8 months and walked at age 15 months, although he never had crawled on his hands and knees.

Before he learned to walk, Kyle seemed frustrated by his inability to get around and cried a lot. Mrs. P. remembered feeling relieved when Kyle learned to walk because his disposition improved. However, her relief was short lived. The ambulatory Kyle was in constant motion. He was into everything; he fell frequently, bumped into things, and knocked things over.

Despite Kyle's difficult behaviors, Mrs. P. described him as a loving and lovable child. He seemed bright, his language skills developed early, and he had a highly developed sense of humor.

As he grew older, Kyle's differences became more apparent. He was the second of four children. Although all the children were active, Kyle's activity often seemed without purpose. He ran from place to place and thing to thing without stopping to engage for more than a few seconds. Kyle's behavior became markedly worse when there were a lot of people or noise present. The family stopped taking him to shopping malls and avoided most restaurants. They noticed that when he ate certain foods, he became even more active, so they controlled his diet.

When Kyle was 5 years old, ready to enter kindergarten, Mrs. P. noticed that he tended to use whichever hand was closest to an object. He looked awkward when he walked and ran. He bumped into things and fell a lot. He was unable to catch or throw a ball even as well as his 3-year-old brother. He could not pump himself on a swing (although he loved to be pushed and would swing for hours). He had difficulty pedaling a small bicycle with training wheels.

Although Kyle expressed interest in coloring, artwork, and puzzles, he was not as good at them as his 4-year-old sister. Kyle often laid his upper body on the table; sometimes he fell off the chair. Whenever he got his hands even slightly dirty, he washed them immediately. Further questioning clarified that Kyle often responded adversely to light touch. Mrs. P. felt that his dislike of glue and finger paint was related to sensitivity to touch.

Mrs. P. expressed her concerns to the pediatrician when Kyle went for his kindergarten physical examination. The physician recommended trying a small dose of Ritalin. The medication seemed to help Kyle attend to tasks, and Mrs. P. believed it was beneficial. However, although he was able to focus, his activity level remained very high, he continued to be overly sensitive to touch and noise, and his coordination was not improved.

Kyle entered kindergarten at age 5½ years. His teacher really enjoyed his sense of humor and genuinely liked him. Because she seemed to understand his needs and easily accommodated for them, Kyle's kindergarten year was a success. Mrs. P. was delighted, but she worried that he was getting further behind his peers in motor and preacademic skills and his activity level had not diminished. Although he played with his brother and sisters, he did not have any other friends.

Mrs. P. was concerned that Kyle would not succeed in first grade when he had to go to school for a whole day and the demands increased. She feared that a new teacher might not understand his needs and make the necessary adaptations. The school personnel were more optimistic and assured Mrs. P. that Kyle was bright and would do fine in first grade.

Mrs. P.'s concerns were warranted, however. Kyle's early days in first grade were a "disaster." He hated school; he developed stomachaches and found many excuses to remain at home. His work was poor, and his behavior was worse. His teacher wrote notes indicating that he was not finishing his work, his printing was illegible, and he erased until there were holes in the paper. Sometimes he would get frustrated and tear up his papers. Kyle's teacher wondered about having him tested for special education services. At that point, Mrs. P. discussed Kyle with her sister, who recommended that an occupational therapist evaluate him.

When asked what hindered Kyle the most, Mrs. P. replied, "His poor self-esteem." She felt distractibility, clumsiness, lack of friends, and feelings that he could not do anything right contributed to his negative self-image.

THE EVALUATION

We scheduled an evaluation because Mrs. P.'s description suggested that sensory integrative dysfunction might be the basis for Kyle's motor difficulties, distractibility, and increased activity.

CLASSROOM OBSERVATION

We made arrangements to observe at school and spend time with Kyle's teacher to enhance our ability to interpret test results and plan intervention. We observed during reading, arithmetic, lunch, and recess, paying careful attention to the effects of various environments on Kyle's performance.

The first grade classroom was a busy place. Kyle was one of 33 students. Because he had difficulty attending, his seat was beside the teacher's desk, and a steady stream of children passed his desk to get help or instruction. On several occasions, Kyle followed directions given to other children. Because his seat was on a major traffic route, children occasionally brushed into him. Once when this happened, Kyle hit the child and was disciplined.

Kyle's arithmetic assignment involved cutting out squares with numbers on them and pasting them on a piece of paper. Kyle's skills with the scissors, although slow and labored, were adequate. However, after he pasted the first square, he became so preoccupied with the paste on his fingers that he did not complete the assignment. Instead, he picked paste off his fingers and watched the other students.

His performance in reading group was markedly better. Kyle, his teacher, and four classmates gathered in a corner, their backs to the class. Kyle contributed to the group appropriately. However, he fell out of his chair twice and was reprimanded for his sitting posture.

At lunch, Kyle seemed completely overwhelmed by the noise and the number of children in the cafeteria. He had difficulty opening his milk container and finally used so much force that he spilled the milk. Although he sat with his classmates, he did not interact with them. Instead, he spent most of his time looking around. When lunch was over, he had eaten only half his sandwich and one bite of fruit.

When Kyle and his classmates went outside for recess, Kyle raced around the playground, seemingly without purpose. He did not interact with any classmates or join in organized games, and none of his classmates asked him to play.

When we talked with the teacher, she indicated

that the morning's activities were typical. She expressed frustration because she believed Kyle could do better if he tried harder. Her greatest concerns pertained to his behavior, especially his distractibility and activity level and not finishing his work.

Sensory Integration and Praxis Tests

The following week, we evaluated Kyle using the SIPT and the related clinical observations. Kyle's scores are shown in Table 8–1.

Additional Testing and Observation

Kyle found it difficult to sit for prolonged periods. He particularly disliked the tactile tests and rubbed his arms and hands in response to the stimuli. He made a number of excuses to stop.

Kyle's mother completed the Sensory Profile (SP) (Dunn, 1999). His total score of "definite difference" suggested that sensory processing difficulties, particularly poor modulation in the tactile and auditory systems, interfered with daily life functioning. Modulation difficulties appeared to be affecting his activity level. He scored in the "probable difference" category for emotional and social responses, suggesting that poor modulation was influencing his self-esteem, frustration

■ TABLE 8–1 **KYLE'S SIPT RESULTS**

Test	SD Score
Space Visualization (SV)	−1.47
SV Contralateral Use	−1.05
SV Preferred Hand Use	0.62
Figure-Ground Perception	0.67
Manual Form Perception	−1.25
Kinesthesia	−0.24
Finger Identification	−0.81
Graphesthesia	−2.13
Localization of Tactile Stimuli	1.34
Praxis on Verbal Command	0.92
Design Copying	−1.69
Constructional Praxis	−2.32
Postural Praxis	−1.52
Oral Praxis	−2.72
Sequencing Praxis	−3.00*
Bilateral Motor Coordination	−2.21
Standing and Walking Balance	−2.04
Motor Accuracy	−1.42
Postrotary Nystagmus	−1.43

*Scores lower than −3.0 are reported by Western Psychological Services as −3.0.

level, social interactions, and sensitivity to criticism.

Kyle had difficulty with many clinical observations associated with vestibular and proprioceptive processing. When he tried to assume prone extension, his head was not vertical and his neck hurt; he flexed his legs sharply at the knees after only a few seconds. He maintained this approximation of prone extension for about 8 seconds.

Kyle was slightly better at performing supine flexion. He assumed the posture without assistance; however, his head lagged as he did so. He maintained supine flexion for 12 seconds. Most 6-year-old children can maintain prone extension and supine flexion for 30 seconds without excessive effort (Wilson et al., 2000).

Not surprisingly, Kyle also demonstrated low tone in his extensor muscles. He stood with a marked lordosis and locked knees. His proximal stability, observed in quadruped, was also poor; his scapulae winged bilaterally, and he locked his elbows and externally rotated at the shoulders to improve stability. His trunk sagged slightly. Additionally, he had difficulty modulating force in a number of tasks. He tended to use a great deal more force than necessary.

When seated on a large ball, he moved his trunk and limbs to prevent falling. He particularly liked this activity and asked to repeat it several times. When asked to stand on either a flat board or a tilt board and reach for an object at shoulder height, but slightly out of reach, he was able to lift one foot off the board but flexed it at the knee (see Fig. 7–9). When tilted on a small tilt board, he did not flex his uphill leg (see Fig. 7–6). Both flexing the knee while reaching and failing to bend the uphill leg when tilted are immature patterns suggesting difficulty with equilibrium (Fisher, 1989). However, overall, Kyle's equilibrium was slightly better than his ability to maintain tonic postures.

Kyle demonstrated no signs of gravitational insecurity. He enjoyed riding on moving equipment and being tipped upside down or placed in precarious positions. He also demonstrated no evidence of an aversive response to vestibular stimulation.

We observed for difficulty with bilateral coordination and projected action sequences as Kyle tried to catch a tennis ball and hop through a series of hoops. Kyle never caught the ball unless it was thrown directly into his outstretched hands. He was unable to make both feet land at precisely the same time or execute a series of smooth jumps; he stopped after each one. His performance on jumping jacks and symmetrical and reciprocal stride jumps was poor. Also, he hesitated when crossing the midline, more with the left than the right.

We observed Kyle's performance on several tasks associated with somatodyspraxia, including in-hand manipulation and diadokokinesia. Both skills were within normal limits (Exner, 1992, 2001; Wilson et al., 2000).

We asked Kyle about his most and least favorite things at school and home. He could not easily articulate his likes and dislikes. He said he really did not like school but if he had a favorite subject, it was reading. He could not specify any play activity he really enjoyed except for using the swings. He said he was the last person chosen for teams. He did not like going to the mall. When asked the name of his best friend, he mentioned his younger sister.

Other Information

The findings of other professionals can be very helpful when interpreting the results of an assessment of sensory integration. Kyle had been given the Weschler Intelligence Scale for Children-Revised (WISC-R) by the school psychologist. His score was 130 on the verbal portion and 114 on the performance portion. These scores suggested that Kyle's difficulties on SIPT tests could not be explained by cognitive limitations.

INTERPRETING THE RESULTS

Our goal was to determine if sensory integrative dysfunction explained some of Kyle's difficulties. We had quite a lot of information to organize and interpret. In Table 8–2, we separated Kyle's presenting problems and sensorimotor history, relevant background information, and information obtained from testing.

Next, we examined the test results (see Tables 8–1 and 8–2) to look for meaningful clusters suggestive of specific types of sensory integrative dysfunction. We were aware that some of Kyle's test results would not fit into clusters reflective of sensory integrative dysfunction, and we remained cognizant that such isolated observations would not help us clarify Kyle's problems from the perspective of sensory integration theory.

To facilitate the process of looking for mean-

■ TABLE 8–2   **SUMMARY OF RELEVANT INFORMATION OBTAINED BY REPORT AND THROUGH OBSERVATION**

Kyle's Presenting Problems

Parental and Teacher Concerns
Believes he can't do anything right and is developing a poor self-image
Distractible
Behavior becomes worse in crowded or noisy situations
Follows directions given to other children standing close to his desk
Easily disrupted or distracted by other children
Increased activity
Ambulatory Kyle in constant motion
Runs from place to place without stopping to engage in activity
Behavior becomes worse in crowded or noisy situations
Races around playground seemingly without purpose
Difficulty sitting still for prolonged periods
Clumsiness (see Sensorimotor development)
Lack of friends
Not finishing his schoolwork

Related Behavior
Hates school; developed stomachaches and excuses to remain at home
Gets frustrated and tears up papers
Does not play or interact with friends or classmates

Sensorimotor Development
Difficulty nursing; weak suck; tired quickly
Sat independently at age 8 months, walked at age 15 months; never crawled
Fell frequently, bumped into things, knocked over things
Seemed to prefer right hand but tended to use hand closest to objects
Awkward when he walked and ran
Unable to catch; throwing awkward, inaccurate
Did not know how to pump swing
Loved to be pushed on swing, would swing for hours
Difficulty propelling bicycle (with training wheels)
Problems with coloring, artwork, and puzzles
Laid his upper body on the table when coloring, etc.
Fell off chair
Illegible handwriting
Erased his papers until there were holes in them

Related Background Information

Developmental History
Full-term, uncomplicated birth
Cranky, irritable baby who disliked cuddling and handling
Erratic sleep cycles, did not sleep for more than 4 hours at a time until age 2 years
Seldom sleeps more than 6 hours
History of chronic ear infections

Strengths
Loving and lovable child
Mother believes he is bright
Language skills developed ahead of schedule
Sense of humor

Related Test Results
Verbal IQ, 130; performance IQ, 114 (WISC-R)

continued on following page

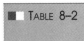

TABLE 8–2 Summary of Relevant Information Obtained by Report and Through Observation (Continued)

Evaluation of SI Functioning

Behaviors Observed at School
Scissors skills slow and labored but adequate for task
Fell out of chair
Difficulty opening milk container

Clinical Observations of Posture
Poor prone extension posture
Head lag when assuming supine flexion
Hypotonia of extensor muscles
Lordotic standing posture, tendency to lock his knees
Poor proximal stability in quadruped
Equilibrium better than static, controlled postures
Deficient tilt board response
Used too much force to open milk container

Clinical Observations of BIS
Difficulty with bilateral and projected action sequences
  (e.g., catching a ball, jumping with two feet together,
  doing jumping jacks)
Difficulty crossing the midline

Clinical Observations of Somatopraxis
Unable to maintain supine flexion

Indicators of Poor Sensory Modulation
Responded aversely to light touch stimuli
Dislike of glue or finger paint on his fingers
Sensitive to noise
Rubbed arms and hands after application of tactile stimuli
Made excuses to quit testing during tactile tests
SP total "definite difference"
No gravitational insecurity
No evidence of an aversive response to vestibular
  stimulation

ingful clusters, we used the SIPT Interpretation Worksheet, marking a plus (+) where there was evidence of a problem and a minus (−) where there was none (Table 8–3). We left the space blank if we had not assessed a specific behavior. Evidence of possible dysfunction was defined as a SIPT score below −1.0 SD or a clinical observation considered problematic for a 6½-year-old child (see also Chapter 7).

After Kyle's test results were recorded on the Interpretation Worksheet, we examined the pattern of pluses and minuses in each box (see Table 8–3). Pluses predominated in every instance. However, a predominance of pluses, when interpreted appropriately, did not mean that Kyle had dysfunction in every domain.

Meaningful Clusters

Only one rule exists with regard to meaningful clusters. With one exception, tests and observations listed in the sensory modulation category, no single "plus" constitutes a cluster. All pluses in sensory modulation reflect multiple observations and, therefore, qualify as clusters. Otherwise, the number of test scores that must be low or observations that must be present to conclude there is evidence of a meaningful cluster is a matter of clinical judgment. To say that a meaningful cluster exists, we attempt to capture the most important aspects of a construct. We provide an example of the reasoning associated with the determination of meaningful clusters below.

Using the Interpretation Worksheet

To conclude that sensory integrative dysfunction was the source of Kyle's difficulties, we needed to find evidence of a sensory processing deficit. Kyle had several scores that suggested central vestibular and proprioceptive processing deficits. They can be seen in the category labeled "postural deficits." As is always the case when identifying vestibular-proprioceptive processing deficits, our interpretation relied heavily on clinical observations. Although his score on the Kinesthesia test was within normal limits, this test is a measure of passive joint movement, which is not the best measure of proprioception (see Chapter 7).

When we examined Kyle's tactile testing, the results were less clear. Two scores, Graphesthesia (GRA) and Manual Form Perception (MFP), were below −1.0 SD. However, Ayres found associations between GRA and bilateral integration and sequencing (BIS) deficits, and MFP is also a test of form and space perception. (Although GRA also has a form and space component, Ayres never found it to load strongly on that factor.) Because both of Kyle's more "pure" tactile discrimination test scores, Localization of Tactile Stimuli and Finger Identification, were within normal limits, we examined the categories of BIS and form and space perception before deciding whether or not Kyle's low MFP and GRA scores reflected poor tactile discrimination.

Given the number of indicators of deficits in BIS, we believed Kyle's GRA score was likely reflective of dysfunction in that area. Similarly, because he had several other indicators of form

▪ TABLE 8–3   SIPT INTERPRETATION WORKSHEET

Postural Dysfunction	+/−	Poor Tactile Discrimination	+/−	Sensory Modulation Dysfunction*	+/−
Standing and Walking Balance	+	Localization of Tactile Stimuli	−	Sensory Profile	+
Other standardized balance tests		Finger Identification	−	Evaluation of Sensory Processing (ESP)	
CO: Prone Extension	+	Manual Form Perception	+	Touch Inventory (TIE)	+
CO: Proximal joint stability	+	Graphesthesia	+	Hx/CO: Gravitational insecurity	−
CO: Extensor muscle tone	+			Hx/CO: Aversive response to mvt	−
CO: Equilibrium	+			Hx/CO: Sensory defensiveness (i.e., tactile, auditory, visual, olfactory)	+
CO: Neck flexion in supine	+			Avoidance of sensory experiences	+
CO: Postural Adjustments	+			Distractibility, increased activity	+
CO: Poor modulation of force	+			Withdrawn	−
CO: Awareness of position or movement	+			Sensory seeking	+
Postrotary Nystagmus	+				
[Kinesthesia]	−				

Bilateral Integration and Sequencing (BIS) Dyspraxia**	+/−	Somatodyspraxia**	+/−	Dyspraxia on Verbal Command	+/−
Meaningful Postural Cluster	+	Meaningful tactile discrimination cluster	−	Praxis on Verbal Command	−
Bilateral Motor Coordination	+	[Meaningful posture cluster]	+	Postrotary Nystagmus (prolonged)	−
Sequencing Praxis	+	Meaningful BIS cluster	+	[Bilateral Motor Coordination]	+
[Oral Praxis]	+	Postural Praxis	+	[Sequencing Praxis]	+
[Graphesthesia]	+	[Oral Praxis]	+	[Standing and Walking Balance]	+
SV Contralateral Use	+	[Graphesthesia]	+	[Oral Praxis]	+
SV Preferred Hand Use	−	[Design Copying]	+		
Hx/CO: Mixed/delayed hand pref	+	CO: Supine flexion	+		
CO: Crossing midline	+	CO: Sequential finger touching			
CO: Right-left confusion	−	CO: In-hand manipulation	−		
CO: Projected action sequences	+	CO: Diadochokinesia			
CO: Bilateral motor skills	+				

Form and Space Perception	+/−	Construction	+/−	Visual Motor Coordination	+/−
Space Visualization	+	Design Copying	+	Motor Accuracy	+
Figure-Ground Perception	−	Constructional Praxis	+	Design Copying	+
Constructional Praxis	+	Other construction tests		Other visual motor tests	
Design Copying	+				
Manual Form Perception	+				
Other visual perceptual tests					

+ = score that suggests that dysfunction is present (positive sign); − = score that refutes the presence of dysfunction (negative sign); [ ] = Not a major indicator of construct; often reflects more than one construct; CO = clinical observation; Hx = history; * = Any + above dotted line interpreted as a meaningful cluster; ** = In the absence of evidence of poor sensory processing, a cluster here would be labeled "dyspraxia with no sensory integrative basis."

and space deficits, we interpreted his low MFP score as reflective of that category. As a result, we concluded that Kyle did not have a meaningful cluster suggestive of deficits in tactile discrimination.

Kyle did not have a problem with modulation of

vestibular or proprioceptive sensation; he demonstrated no evidence of gravitational insecurity or aversive responses to movement. However, our observations and Kyle's SP score confirmed that he had a sensory modulation dysfunction, with overresponsiveness in the tactile and auditory systems. Through the SP, these modulation difficulties were linked to lowered self-esteem as well as low frustration tolerance when tasks became difficult. Kyle's modulation difficulties also appeared to influence his activity level.

Having found evidence of deficits in sensory processing, we looked for difficulties in other domains assessed by the SIPT that might result from poor sensory processing (see Table 8–3). Assessment of BIS revealed evidence of dysfunction by low scores on Bilateral Motor Coordination and Sequencing Praxis and clinical observations.

We then examined evidence for somatodyspraxia, for which there are two major distinguishing characteristics. These included deficits in both bilateral projected action sequences *and* more feedback-dependent motor actions and tactile or proprioceptive (somatosensory) processing (see Chapter 3).

Postural Praxis (PPr) is the best indicator of somatodyspraxia. Kyle's PPr score was −1.52. However, both Ayres and Mulligan found weak loadings of PPr on the BIS factor (see Chapters 1 and 7 and Appendix B). Furthermore, because Kyle did not have a deficit in tactile discrimination, we had to reject the possibility that he had somatodyspraxia.

The conclusion that Kyle did not have a deficit in praxis on verbal command was much easier. This dysfunction is characterized by prolonged Postrotary Nystagmus (i.e., score > +1.0) and a low Praxis on Verbal Command (PrVC) score. Kyle had *depressed* nystagmus and a normal PrVC score. In fact, Kyle had a relative strength in translating verbal commands into motor actions.

So far, we had concluded that Kyle had deficits in interpreting sensation derived from active movement (i.e., vestibular and proprioceptive sensation); these deficits, in turn, resulted in difficulty planning and producing bilateral and projected action sequences (see Table 8–3). Kyle did not have difficulty with praxis tasks that relied on feedback, as would have been seen with somatodyspraxia. We had identified overresponsiveness to the sensations of touch and sound but had also found that Kyle had adequate modulation of other sensations. Mod-

ulation difficulties were linked to increased activity level and sensory seeking and had a negative influence on his self-esteem and ability to make friends. Furthermore, we had identified strength in translating verbal commands into motor actions. We then examined evidence of difficulty in any of the common end products of sensory integrative dysfunction: form and space perception, visual motor coordination, or construction.

Although Kyle's Figure-Ground (FG) score suggested a relative strength, the other test scores in these areas revealed difficulties in all three end product areas. Unlike the other tests in this category, FG is entirely a test of form perception; thus, it is not surprising that if one test result were different from the others, it would be FG (see Chapter 5).

The Final Stage of Interpretation

We used the model in Figure 8–1 for the final stage of interpretation. We placed a plus or a minus above each construct to reflect whether there was meaningful cluster providing evidence of dysfunction. We placed pluses above each of the constructs for Kyle:

- Vestibular processing
- Proprioceptive processing
- Tactile processing
- Auditory processing
- Posture
- BIS
- Defensiveness
- Clumsiness
- Avoidance of motor behavior
- Exaggerated force
- Distractability activity
- Sensory seeking

In determining whether meaningful clusters existed, we addressed two bigger questions: Is there evidence of sensory integrative dysfunction? And, if so, what is the nature of the dysfunction? The latter question ultimately leads to a third question: What will intervention look like? More specifically, what type (or types) of enhanced sensation will we include? What will be the desired characteristics of adaptive interactions?

REPORTING THE RESULTS

Reporting the results of Kyle's evaluation involved communicating in a manner that was meaningful

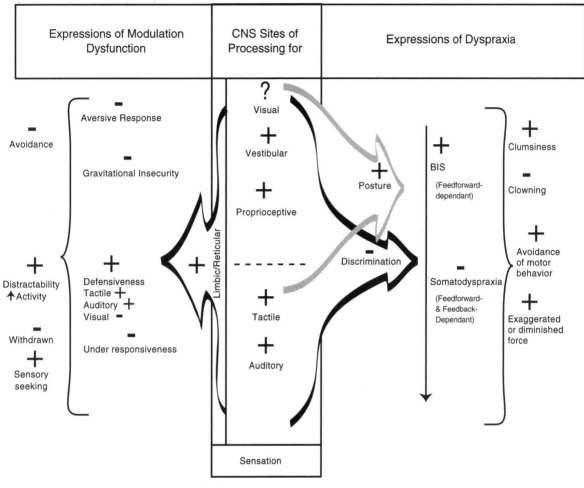

Figure 8-1 Kyle's sensory integration profile.

to his parents and teacher and that would help them reframe many of his real life difficulties in terms of sensory integrative dysfunction. We prepared a written report and met with Mrs. P. to discuss it.

Both Kyle's parents' and teacher's greatest concerns were his distractibility and activity level. Therefore, we began with a discussion of sensory modulation deficits. Individuals who have sensory integrative dysfunction have difficulty with the meaningful interpretation of sensation. Often they seem unable to "screen out" irrelevant details. Thus, they behave as though they are paying attention to everything around them. For example, all of us wear clothing that provides a source of continual sensory stimulation. However, we screen out that stimulation unless, for some reason, we begin to think about clothing. Similarly, although there may be noise in the hallway, we are able to concentrate

on our conversation and screen out the irrelevant noise.

The results of Kyle's testing suggested that he had difficulty screening out irrelevant sensations and attending only to important information (e.g., instructions, schoolwork, a particular game). Thus, he appeared to be highly distractible. Because his distractibility was caused, at least in part, by an inability to screen out irrelevant stimuli, it became markedly worse when stimulation increased. Thus, it was understandable that his behavior deteriorated in busy places such as shopping malls or crowded restaurants. Similar difficulties occurred when Kyle's classmates congregated around the teacher's desk, all waiting for different instructions.

Kyle's negative reactions to touch likely came from a similar source. When Kyle became stressed, he translated light touch negatively. The more people touched him, either accidentally or to control his behavior, the less able he was to cope with it. Thus, his distractibility and increased activity, caused by his inability to screen out irrelevant stimulation, became a part of a vicious cycle. Kyle's "lashing out" at other children also seemed to be related to his inability to meaningfully interpret the affective aspects of touch.

Mrs. P. worried that Kyle was growing up feeling he could not do anything right. She believed that his negative self-concept was caused, in part, by all the reprimands he received during a typical day. Although his parents tried hard to emphasize Kyle's accomplishments, they also had to control his behavior. Thus, they found themselves saying, "don't do that" far more often than they liked. This situation was even worse at school.

Mrs. P. believed that Kyle also felt bad about himself because he knew that he was poorly coordinated. The evaluation suggested that this might be related to his sensory processing difficulties as well. Kyle was aware that he had no friends and was never included in games because no one wanted him on their team. Mrs. P. was at a loss to deal with this problem; Kyle's appraisal of his motor skills was fairly accurate. She hoped she could come to understand his motor incoordination and find ways to help him improve it.

Without launching into a major description of vestibular-proprioception or factor analysis, we explained that many children who had poor motor planning abilities seemed to demonstrate coordination problems similar to Kyle's. Kyle's difficulties with catching and throwing a ball, jumping, knowing how much force to use, and deciding which hand to use were all related to his difficulties interpreting sensation about the position and movement of his body in space.

Because Mrs. P. seemed particularly interested in intervention to minimize Kyle's difficulties, we discussed different ways that an occupational therapist could provide services and the benefits generally associated with each type of intervention. If we were to provide direct intervention using the principles of sensory integration theory, we would involve Kyle in activities that involved enhanced sensation and required Kyle to attempt new skills and master those that were emerging. We would carefully construct activities so they addressed Kyle's needs.

Although we believed Kyle's skills would improve markedly, all of us (i.e., Kyle, the occupational therapist, family, and teacher) would have to work very hard to improve Kyle's self-image. An improvement in Kyle's skills would not automatically result in a better self-concept. Mrs. P. expressed her willingness to think of creative ways to facilitate Kyle's participation with children in the neighborhood. We believed that the services of a consultant would be invaluable to Kyle's success at school, and we recommended that the occupational therapist there assume that role. In much the same way that we had interpreted Kyle's difficulties for Mrs. P., the consultant would explain Kyle's sensory integrative dysfunction to his teacher and help her develop new strategies for teaching him.

The consultant might help the teacher rearrange the classroom or adapt assignments. Perhaps Kyle's desk could be moved from a high traffic area and his arithmetic answers could be written rather than glued into place. We planned to share the results of the evaluation with the school occupational therapist.

Mrs. P. seemed relieved that our explanation "fit" so well. She planned to discuss the report and recommendations with her husband. Together, they would decide how to proceed. Although we made numerous recommendations, the decisions rested with Kyle's family. We encouraged her to call with any questions.

SUMMARY AND CONCLUSION

We have presented the process of interpreting the results of an occupational therapy evaluation of sensory integration. An important component of the process was to reframe presenting problems in terms easily understood by families and in keeping with the unique perspectives of occupational therapy and sensory integration theory. We interpreted by examining test scores for meaningful clusters. When clusters were identified, they formed the basis for reframing and planning intervention. In subsequent chapters, we discuss setting goals (Chapter 9) and providing intervention using direct service (Chapters 9, 11, and 12) and consultation (Chapter 13).

When we talked with Mrs. P. the next week, she told us that she had requested occupational therapy services for Kyle at school. She was eager to make an appointment to develop goals. That process is the focus of Chapter 9.

References

Ayres, A. J. (1989). *Sensory Integration and Praxis Tests manual.* Los Angeles: Western Psychological Services.

C. & G. Merriam. (1981). *Webster's new collegiate dictionary.* Springfield, MA: Merriam.

Dunn, W. (1999). *Sensory Profile.* San Antonio: Psychological Corporation.

Exner, C. E. (1992). In-hand manipulation skills. In J. Case-Smith & C. Pehoski (Eds.). *Development of hand skills in the child* (pp. 35–46). Bethesda, MD: American Occupational Therapy Association.

Exner, C. E. (2001). Development of hand skills. In J. Case-Smith (Ed.). *Occupational therapy for children* (ed. 4, pp. 289–328). Philadelphia: Lippincott, Williams & Wilkins.

Fisher, A. G. (1989). Objective measurement of the quality of response during two equilibrium tests. *Physical and Occupational Therapy in Pediatrics, 9,* 57–78.

Good, B., & Good, M. D. (1981). The meaning of symptoms: A cultural hermeneutic model for clinical practice. In I. Eisenberg & A. Kleinman (Eds.). *The relevance of social science for medicine* (pp. 165–196). Boston: Reidel.

Wilson, B., Pollock, N., Kaplan, B. J., & Law, M. (2000). *Clinical observations of motor and postural skills.* Framingham, MA: Therapro.

The Process of Planning and Implementing Intervention

Anita C. Bundy, ScD, OTR, FAOTA

"Would you tell me, please," [asked Alice,] "which way I ought to walk from here?"
"That depends a good deal on where you want to get to," said the Cat.
"I don't much care where," said Alice.
"Then it doesn't matter which way you walk," said the Cat.
"—so long as I get somewhere," Alice added as an explanation.
"Oh, you're sure to do that," said the Cat, "if you only walk long enough."

—Carroll, 1923, p. 69

Intervention consists of two phases, planning and implementation. Each one depends on the other for effectiveness. That is, unless implementation is preceded by well-constructed plans, intervention becomes haphazard at best and chaotic or harmful at worst. Similarly, unless planning is followed by skillful implementation, the plan dies.

Developing a plan to address the specific needs of clients with sensory integrative dysfunction is the most essential component of the intervention process. The plan has three parts:

1. Setting goals and objectives
2. Determining the type (or types) of service delivery (e.g., direct service, consultation)
3. Developing preliminary ideas about intervention

Having a plan ensures that intervention is carried out in a way that is mutually agreeable to clients, caregivers or significant others, and the therapist. It also ensures that the intervention is conducted in an orderly, efficient, and effective fashion.

While developing the plan, therapists think in a logical, deductive manner (Rogers & Masagatani, 1982). Based on a synthesis of information gathered during the evaluation and knowledge of occupational therapy practice models, we collaborate with the clients and caregivers to set goals to minimize or eliminate the presenting problems.

Having established general goals, we engage clients and caregivers in a discussion to determine objectives representative of those goals. That is, we seek to learn, specifically, how the clients would *behave* differently or what they would like to be able to *do* after intervention that they cannot currently do. Based on the goals and objectives and on the constraints of the systems in which we work, we recommend an intervention plan to meet the goals.

We reason that, although certain goals can best be met by consultation, others can be met better through direct service (Bundy, 1995). Furthermore, we develop a general idea about activities to meet the goals and the characteristics of the intervention environment. If, for example, a client has low postural muscle tone and decreased postural stability from vestibular and proprioceptive processing deficits, we may create activities that provide enhanced vestibular sensation in direct intervention. If the same child is also distractible at school, we may work with the teacher to modify the classroom. Clients and their caregivers, having helped to shape each decision, respond to our recommendations by stating their own constraints (e.g., finances, time). We modify the recommendations until a working plan is established.

Intervention proceeds in the manner suggested by the plan. Although this idea may seem rather simplistic, the process of translating the plan into action requires a kind of reasoning quite different from that used during the development of the plan.

Although the logic demanded by the planning process is fairly linear, the logic used for conducting intervention is more dialogic, a kind of ongoing "conversation" between a therapist and a client (Mattingly & Fleming, 1994). To a great extent, this conversation is a nonverbal exchange.

We set up the environment in such a way as to encourage collaborative, therapeutic interactions. In direct intervention, we follow a client's lead to create activities that promote development and self-actualization. In consultation, we foster the development of strategies. We reflect on the actions of all the players and modify accordingly (Schön, 1983, 1987). Guided by the client or consultee, we shape activities and interactions and examine the results, asking ourselves whether the changes produced the desired results.

PURPOSE AND SCOPE

In this chapter, we illustrate the development of an intervention plan and its implementation with Kyle, the child whose evaluation data we presented in Chapter 8. We discuss not only aspects of the intervention that went "according to plan," but also some of the difficulties we encountered. We demonstrate how therapists reflect both in-action and on-action (Schön, 1983, 1987).

KYLE REVISITED

Kyle was a 6½-year-old boy who lived with his parents, brother, and two sisters; he was the second child. Kyle's parents, Mr. and Mrs. P., were very sensitive to the subtle differences between Kyle's behavior and that of his brother and sisters. His mother provided a clear description of Kyle and described her concerns. She believed that Kyle had two primary areas of difficulty, his distractible and overly active behavior and his poor motor coordination. She thought that these two problem areas resulted in Kyle's feeling bad about himself and having few friends. Kyle's negative self-concept was Mrs. P.'s greatest concern.

We have evaluated Kyle using the Sensory Integration and Praxis Tests (SIPT) (Ayres, 1989), the Sensory Profile (SP) (Dunn, 1999), and related clinical observations. We also observed Kyle at school. We concluded that Kyle's difficulties were based, at least in part, on sensory integrative dysfunction. More specifically, Kyle appeared to have a vestibular and proprioceptive processing disorder that was manifested in postural difficulties. His poor vestibular and proprioceptive processing appeared to have resulted in bilateral integration and sequencing (BIS) deficits and likely contributed to poor visuomotor skills, constructional abilities, and form and space perception. Furthermore, Kyle showed sensory modulation dysfunction in the form of tactile defensiveness and, to some extent, with the modulation of auditory input. The SP also identified the presence of behavioral and emotional issues (i.e., lowered self-esteem and poor frustration tolerance). Both the SP and clinical observations indicated that Kyle was highly distractible and overly active. We explained our findings to Mrs. P. and interpreted her concerns in light of these findings (see Chapter 8 for additional information).

When we completed our evaluation, we specified options for intervention and made certain preliminary recommendations. We recommended that Kyle obtain direct intervention in a clinic setting, and we encouraged Mrs. P. to seek consultation services from the occupational therapist at Kyle's school. Mr. and Mrs. P. spent a couple of days thinking about our report and discussing our recommendations. We then made an appointment to formulate goals and develop a specific plan.

SETTING GOALS AND DEVELOPING OBJECTIVES

We began our meeting by asking Mr. and Mrs. P. about the specific things they wanted Kyle to be able to do after intervention. We set a 6-month time frame as a guide for these predictions. We reiterated the things they had expressed as major concerns. We offered explanations for and links between their concerns and asked for confirmation, clarification, and correction of our perceptions.

We believed that the major concern was that Kyle did not feel very good about himself or his skills. His parents worried about the effect that a negative sense of self would have as Kyle grew older. We speculated that two things contributed to Kyle's negative beliefs about himself. These were:

1. Poor motor coordination, which interfered with his ability to perform the same kinds of skilled activities that his peers easily performed
2. Distractibility and increased activity, which resulted in Kyle's being reprimanded more frequently than his peers or his brother and sisters

Mr. and Mrs. P. agreed with this assessment. We determined that our goals should reflect each of these major areas of concern

Modifying Kyle's Expectations about Himself

Kyle's expectations that he would fail seemed to be both a cause of some his difficulties and a result of others. Because he knew he lacked skills, he avoided certain activities. In avoiding them, he deprived himself of the opportunity to practice. He fell further and further behind his peers and came to believe, even more firmly, that he was "no good." When he was forced to do activities

that he knew he could not do well (e.g., handwriting), he became anxious about performing, and his performance deteriorated. When he became anxious, he also became overly active and overwhelmed. His behavior further deteriorated and he was reprimanded for bad behavior. As a result, he had more reason to believe he was "bad" and that others also viewed him that way.

Mr. and Mrs. P. concurred with this line of reasoning. They punctuated our conversation with examples that illustrated our developing "theory" of Kyle's beliefs and behavior.

Based on our jointly held perceptions, we proposed that one general goal for our intervention would be to help Kyle to develop a belief that he would succeed at activities that he valued and that were appropriate for his age. Kyle's parents thought this was an important goal. However, we wanted to be sure that we could evaluate Kyle's progress toward meeting that goal at the end of 6 months' time. Thus, we needed to formulate specific objectives.

We asked Mr. and Mrs. P. what kinds of things they thought Kyle would do that would tell them that he had changed his perceptions of his skills. How would Kyle act differently if he believed that he would succeed? What activities were both important to him and reflected skills appropriate to his age? We were unable to answer these questions by ourselves; only Mr. and Mrs. P. could fill in the details that would make the goal meaningful and measurable. Mrs. P. indicated that she would know that Kyle felt better about his skills when, at least once a week, he willingly went off to play with other children in the neighborhood who are about his age.

We all recognized this objective might be difficult to meet, but it exemplified how Kyle would act as he began to feel better about himself. Kyle's going off to play with neighborhood children was something that we cared about. Furthermore, objectives are a way of organizing actions; they are predictions, not contracts. If Kyle did not accomplish this objective, we would reexamine it to determine whether it was our predictions that were out of line or our methodology that was ineffective. Because the objective was readily observable by those closest to him, his family would be the ones to determine whether or not it had been met. They needed only to attend carefully to the evidence that he was or was not playing more with his peers.

An Aside about Defining Objectives

The reader may not agree that Kyle's willingly going off with children his own age adequately reflected the goal of developing a belief in success. Objectives, developed to define achievement of a goal established by a team, need not be agreeable to individuals who were not members of that team. However, all members of the team must agree that the objectives reflect the goals (Mager, 1972). Furthermore, all team members should be able to measure the objectives (Mager, 1975).

We need not write objectives for every behavior related to self-concept (or any other function). Rather, targeting a few really meaningful objectives and working toward those collectively is much more critical. We then measure improvement in those areas as representative of the larger goal of improving his beliefs about his skills. Kyle might well make other gains in this area and they may be equally important, but they would not have objectives attached to them.

Improving Kyle's Motor Skills

Both of Kyle's parents expressed a desire that Kyle develop new motor skills that would enable him to complete his schoolwork more easily and enjoy playing the games and activities his peers loved. We agreed that improving Kyle's motor skills was an important general goal. However, once again, we were at a loss to create specific objectives without access to the important information that only Kyle and his parents had. That is, what specific skills did Kyle most need to develop? What should Kyle be able to do better in 6 months that would enable all of us to recognize that he had made progress? And what would it look like if he performed a particular skill better?

We discussed this area for some time. His parents focused on riding his bicycle, pumping a swing, throwing a ball, catching a ball, handwriting, and buttoning. We talked about what seemed to be preventing him from doing each one. We reiterated that we were interested in selecting only the one or two skills that everyone (most importantly, Kyle) thought were most important. We felt certain that if Kyle changed in the ways we specified, he would also develop other skills simultaneously. These would be equally important, but we viewed them as an added bonus.

Mr. and Mrs. P. indicated that Kyle had, on numerous occasions, expressed a desire to be able to make the swing go by himself. That way, he could play on it as long as he wanted, rather than having to stop because his parents were tired of pushing him or had something else to do. Furthermore, Kyle loved swinging, but he was acutely aware that his 5-year-old sister, Laura, had learned some time ago to pump the swing by herself and his 4-year-old brother could nearly do it, too. Thus, we decided that our objective would be that Kyle independently propel a swing by pumping.

Specifying Criteria for Objectives

Readers familiar with the parts of an objective (i.e., learner, behavior, condition, and criterion) will notice that we have not defined a criterion for measuring this objective. That is, we have not specified how well Kyle will have to propel his swing in order for us to say that he has met this objective (e.g., four out of five attempts). In our experience, the issue with pumping a swing is simply learning to do it. After children know what it feels like to work with the swing, they can swing until they tire of it. Thus, we did not believe that the specification of a criterion was necessary. Because no criterion is specified, we assumed that Kyle would be able to do it whenever he wanted. Because that really was our intent, the lack of a criterion did not present a problem.

Mrs. P. also expressed particular concern about Kyle's poor handwriting. She believed that the inordinate difficulty he had writing caused him to be slow and messy in school. This, in turn, resulted in his having to repeat his work or receiving negative feedback from his teacher. Many times, he brought home papers with the word "messy" scrawled across the top.

We agreed that improved handwriting was an appropriate goal for Kyle. Again, we began the process of discovering what exactly Mrs. P. meant by this goal. Should Kyle be able to write faster? If so, how fast? Should he be able to form letters more legibly? And, if so, what would constitute legibility? After discussing this, it became clear that Mrs. P. actually hoped that Kyle would improve in both areas; however, she recognized that he could probably not accomplish both within 6 months' time. We told her that, in our experience, children who wrote quickly could learn to write more legibly. However, children who became overly concerned with legibility often had a particularly difficult time learning to write more quickly. We agreed that the more important immediate objective was for Kyle to complete at least three of four written assignments within the allotted class time.

Improving Kyle's Behavior

Kyle's behavior (i.e., distractibility, increased activity, and tendency to lash out at children who bumped into him) was a major concern for his parents and teacher. Kyle's behavior "got in his way" more obviously than did anything else; it was probably the greatest single reason for the negative feedback he got from those around him. Thus, we all readily agreed that improving Kyle's behavior was an appropriate general goal.

We explored this difficulty more fully with Mr. and Mrs. P. so that we could formulate relevant objectives. We asked them to tell us about circumstances when Kyle's behavior was most problematic (i.e., occurred frequently, were unavoidable, or in which his behavior was especially intolerable). Again, we asked how Kyle would behave differently in the next 6 months if he were making progress.

Mr. and Mrs. P. talked about Kyle's behavior at some length. They mentioned the difficulties they had taking him to restaurants, shopping malls, and their friends' homes. In the end, they concluded that, although all of these created difficulties, they had learned to manage. When they anticipated that the situation would be particularly loud or crowded (e.g., a shopping mall during a holiday season), one of them either stayed home with Kyle (and often one or more of the other children) or they left some or all of the children with a babysitter. They tried to take whole family outings to places where they knew Kyle would not be overstimulated or overwhelmed; they knew many such places.

Kyle's parents were most concerned about his behavior at school. Nearly every week, his teacher called or sent a note home about Kyle's fighting or not paying attention to his work. Thus, we created one objective that Kyle would not hit classmates who bumped into him accidentally.

Creating Criteria

Astute readers will note that the comments pertaining to lack of a specified criterion apply here also. Because we have not specified a criterion, we will assume that when Kyle meets the objec-

tive, he will never hit a classmate who accidentally jostles him. This is precisely the criterion we have in mind. Although Mager (1975) indicated that perfect performance is rarely achievable, we believe that, in this case, it would be nonsensical to write an objective that said that Kyle would only hit a classmate once a month or once a year. Hitting other children because they accidentally bump into you is never acceptable. Furthermore, Kyle does not have a serious problem with violent outbursts; his mother indicated that his fighting occurs about twice a month and is triggered by very predictable occurrences. Therefore, we believe that the objective, as specified, was attainable. We expected that Kyle, like most children, may occasionally "backslide." However, our objective is that he not respond to accidental touch by hitting.

Besides fighting, the other significant aspect of Kyle's behavior at school was inattention to his work. When questioned about what exactly that meant, the parents indicated that Kyle rarely got his work finished on time. We decided that the objective (already specified under the goal to improve his motor skills) that Kyle would complete at least three of four written assignments within the allotted class time also pertained equally well to the goal of improving his behavior. Thus, we also listed it under this goal.

Summary of the Intervention Plan

Together with Mr. and Mrs. P., we formulated four important objectives that guided intervention over the next 6 months. Although this process was difficult and time consuming, it was worth the effort. We all clarified our thinking and made explicit the most desirable outcomes of intervention. Mr. and Mrs. P. said that the process helped them to decide which things to focus on during the next several months. Before our discussion, they had felt guilty if they did not try to teach Kyle each time they interacted with him. Yet at the same time, they felt that he needed time to "just be a kid." They were relieved to talk with someone who understood Kyle and could help them plan.

There is nothing magical about the number four with reference to objectives. However, four is about the maximum number of objectives that should be specified for a short time period (e.g., 6 months). A small number of meaningful objectives forms the basis for a much more cohesive plan than would a large number that reflected a detailed sequence of development.

Two points regarding objectives cannot be emphasized strongly enough. First, objectives belong to the client; unless they are meaningful, they are pointless. Second, intervention is "driven" by objectives. As the Cheshire Cat in *Alice in Wonderland* (Carroll, 1923) reminded us at the beginning of this chapter, if you are not sure where you are going, it does not matter how you get there. If you walk long enough, you are sure to get somewhere, but that place might not be desirable, and surely a lot of time will be wasted. We care both about where we are going and how we are going to get there. We are interested in improving clients' abilities to perform their daily roles and tasks in as effective and efficient a manner as possible. Thus, we must develop and follow meaningful plans.

DETERMINING TYPES OF SERVICE DELIVERY

After formulating the objectives, we went on to determine the types of service (i.e., consultation, direct intervention, monitoring) we would use to meet each objective. We explained that direct service meant that a therapist intervened directly with Kyle in order to change his skills and that consultation meant that a therapist intervened with the parents or the teacher (see Chapter 13). The goals of the consultation were to help his parents and teacher understand Kyle's behavior and needs better and develop more effective strategies for working with him.

In monitoring, we explained, a therapist would teach parents or the teacher a simple procedure that they, in turn, would conduct with Kyle. We also explained that the same therapist could readily serve all three roles in order to meet the objectives in the most effective way.

Kyle was fortunate to be eligible to receive occupational therapy services at school. We recommended that Mr. and Mrs. P. request that the occupational therapist at school serve a primary role as a consultant and a secondary role as a direct service provider (for the times when Kyle needed to practice a new skill at school). We further recommended that Colleen, the clinic's therapist, serve primarily as a direct service provider and secondarily as a consultant to the family and a monitor when she developed a home program. We explained that

Colleen would remain in contact with the school therapist to ensure that the services Kyle received were complementary. We also explained that the therapist at school, along with the special education team, would undoubtedly set some additional objectives. However, we used the objectives we had developed together to demonstrate to Mr. and Mrs. P. how the two therapists would serve complementary roles. The suggestions we presented to Mr. and Mrs. P. are summarized in Table 9–1.

Mr. and Mrs. P. agreed. Kyle's Individualized Education Program (IEP) team meeting was in another week, and Kyle's parents were glad to have had an opportunity to participate in goal setting before that meeting. They planned to take the goals we had established to the meeting and incorporate them into Kyle's IEP.

DEVELOPING PRELIMINARY IDEAS FOR USE IN INTERVENTION

In preparation for Kyle's first intervention session, Colleen, the occupational therapist, thought about three things:

1. Types of activities that would best address his needs
2. The physical layout of the clinic
3. Types of interactions she hoped to have with Kyle

In each case, the therapist wanted to maximize Kyle's participation. Although these aspects of Kyle's direct intervention became inextricably linked in a session, each is important enough to be considered separately. Furthermore, slightly different purposes are associated with each. Therefore, we discuss each briefly before illustrating how they become integrated in intervention.

Selecting Activities

In developing ideas about activities, Colleen considered both the types of enhanced sensation she would incorporate and the adaptive interaction she sought. She planned to address four primary areas; these are italicized in Table 9–1 in the column that describes the methods to be used by the clinic occupational therapist. They included postural stability, BIS, visuomotor skill, and modulation of sensation. Colleen was aware that the more the ac-

■ TABLE 9-1   CONTRIBUTIONS OF CLINIC AND SCHOOL OCCUPATIONAL THERAPISTS TO MEETING KYLE'S OBJECTIVES

Goal	Objective	Clinic OT*	School OT**
Developed belief that he will succeed	At least once a week, willingly play with other children in the neighborhood who are about his age	Work with Kyle's mother to develop strategies for teaching Kyle skills to enter a group of children; work with Kyle's mother to identify activities in which one of Kyle's peers could be included (consider including a peer in clinic sessions)	Work with Kyle's teacher to develop strategies for teaching Kyle skills to enter a group of children; work with Kyle's teacher to develop activities in which Kyle has a partner; work with Kyle to develop particular skills he needs to play with other children
Improve motor skills	Independently propel a swing by pumping	*Improve bilateral integration and ability to plan and produce sequenced projected limb movements;* work on his ability to propel swings in the clinic; point out similarities between clinic swings and playground swings	Encourage Kyle's teacher to help Kyle with this skill
Improve motor skills (handwriting); improve behavior	Complete at least three of four written assignments within the allotted class time	*Improve postural stability so his posture improves at his desk; improve bilateral integration and ability to plan and produce sequenced projected limb movements; improve visuomotor skills, improve ability to modulate incoming sensory information;* design home program specifically addressing handwriting speed	Work with Kyle's teacher to rearrange the classroom so that Kyle's workspace is in a quieter area; work with Kyle's teacher to adapt assignments as needed; provide adaptive equipment as needed
Improve behavior	Not hit classmates who accidentally bump into him	Improve ability to modulate incoming sensory information; explain tactile defensiveness and sensory modulation disorders to Kyle and his parents in terms they can understand; talk to Kyle about strategies he might use when he is feeling overwhelmed; work with Kyle's parents so they can help Kyle develop effective strategies	Explain relationship between Kyle's behavior, tactile defensiveness, and sensory modulation in educational terms; work with Kyle's teacher to rearrange the classroom so Kyle's workspace is in an area with less traffic; work with Kyle's teacher to explore and find alternatives to other circumstances for when fighting is a problem (e.g., while standing in line)

*Primary role: direct intervention; secondary roles: consultant to family, monitoring.
**Primary role: consultant to teacher; secondary role: direct intervention.

tivities "mimicked" Kyle's goals, the more effective and efficient intervention would be.

Sensory integration theory suggests that Kyle's difficulties with postural stability and BIS should be addressed with opportunities for him to take in enhanced vestibular and proprioception sensation. More specifically, the opportunities to take in linear vestibular sensation, along with proprio-

ception, in the context of activities that demanded sustained postural control and coordinated use of both sides of the body would be most appropriate (see Chapter 12).

Although difficulties with visuomotor skill may stem from many sources, Kyle's evaluation suggested that his visual-motor difficulties probably resulted, at least partly, from poor processing of vestibular and proprioceptive sensations. Thus, Colleen planned to build visuomotor demands into intervention activities.

Kyle's difficulties with modulating sensation presented Colleen with a dilemma. Kyle was defensive to tactile and auditory sensation. Sensory integration theory suggested that the most direct approach to remediating his tactile defensiveness was by providing opportunities to take in enhanced deep pressure in the context of activities that required adaptive interactions. Colleen could do this with equipment that provided deep pressure (e.g., net hammock) or by having Kyle rub body surfaces firmly with a textured mitt or a brush. Because poor modulation caused particular difficulty in everyday life, Colleen also considered the Wilbarger protocol (Wilbarger & Wilbarger, 1991), which incorporates a sensory diet and a professionally guided program. This is described more fully in Chapter 14.

The "best solution" for improving sensory modulation has not yet been determined. Colleen made her decision based on what she knew of Kyle and what she had learned from other clients with similar problems. She developed a working hypothesis and created and implemented activities that reflected her hypothesis. She would observe Kyle's behavior and seek information from his parents to determine whether her strategy was successful. If she did not have visible evidence within a few sessions that Kyle's defensiveness was decreasing, she would develop an alternative hypothesis and plan.

Colleen's "hunch" about Kyle's tactile and auditory defensiveness was that it was associated with his generalized overarousal. This belief was based on conversations with his parents and observations of his generally distractible behavior. If this was the case, then she should have been able to change the level of his arousal through the use of enhanced vestibular, proprioceptive, or deep pressure sensation. She decided to see how Kyle's defensiveness would respond to activities that incorporated enhanced linear vestibular sensation combined with proprioception. She would use equipment that also provided deep pressure (e.g., net hammock).

Because Kyle was easily overstimulated, which Colleen related to defensiveness, she considered using activities that would calm him and allow him to focus his attention and engage in meaningful activities. She considered activities that would provide resistance to movement and opportunities to take in enhanced linear vestibular proprioception and deep pressure.

Physical Layout of the Clinic

After considering some activities, Colleen turned to the physical layout of the clinic. She knew that Kyle was easily overstimulated and found it difficult to maintain his attention when there were a lot of distractions. She also knew that Kyle was exceedingly curious. If a lot of equipment was visible, he might run from item to item rather than choose one piece of equipment.

Therefore, Colleen decided to minimize the amount of equipment in the room. Similarly, an important piece of at least two objectives would be to help Kyle's family and teacher create nondistracting environments.

In choosing equipment, Colleen wanted to have some swings that could be suspended by two points because her plan was to incorporate linear movement. Colleen kept out the glider, the bolster swing, the net hammock, and the trapeze for Kyle's first visit.

Anticipating that she might need activities that would help Kyle calm himself down and stay focused, Colleen wanted to ensure that the room was arranged in such a way that it would be easy to create "small spaces" in which almost all distractions were eliminated. Thus, she made sure that a barrel that he could climb into was readily available. She thought about some activities he might enjoy in a confined space that could be used to further the goal of improving fine motor coordination. Colleen thought of blowing and breaking bubbles, fishing with a Velcro fishing rod for Velcro fish, and locating and using a large pair of plastic tweezers to pick up plastic "bedbugs" (i.e., $\frac{1}{2}$-inch diameter, brightly colored, bug-shaped plastic objects that belong to another game).

Thinking about Interactions

Recognizing that their interactions would be an important part of intervention, Colleen wanted to be sure that she had a repertoire of strategies available that she could automatically draw on.

She thought first about providing choices that would give Kyle a sense of control. Colleen wanted to give Kyle opportunities to choose activities that provided just the right challenge but that would not overstimulate him. She had begun to deal with this issue already in deciding which swings to leave in the room. She now began to think about ways for Kyle to make choices while controlling the level of challenge. For example, she could ask Kyle to select the swing and she would choose the activity, or vice versa. She could ask Kyle to select a ball and then choose a bat that would maximize his chances of hitting the ball while still providing an adequate challenge (i.e., a bigger-diameter bat if he chose a small ball, a smaller-diameter bat if he chose a bigger ball).

Colleen also thought about ways to introduce discussion of Kyle's sensory integrative dysfunction to enable Kyle to understand it and develop strategies for minimizing its everyday consequences. Colleen wanted to have these conversations with Kyle when they would be most meaningful, rather than discussing this problem out of context. She knew that some time fairly soon, Kyle was likely to become overstimulated and overly active and she would need to direct him to a situation that would be calming. After he organized himself, they could create plans that he could use at other times when he felt overwhelmed. She might point out that when there was too much going on, he could go to a quiet place because "getting away" might help him concentrate better. Colleen knew that it might take many such conversations before he could actually use this information and that she would have to "check out" any strategies with his parents (and perhaps his teacher). She also thought about engaging Kyle in similar discussions about his poor motor coordination when the opportunities presented themselves.

Colleen recognized that asking a 6-year-old boy to engage in meaningful conversations about sensory integrative dysfunction was likely to be difficult. However, she believed that a very important part of her intervention was to help him understand why he was unable to do some things and to realize that he was neither "bad" nor "dumb" (words he frequently used to refer to himself). Furthermore, she believed that he must develop strategies for dealing with his own difficulties and that these strategies also were an important part of her intervention with him. Colleen knew that Mr. and Mrs. P. planned to spend time talking with Kyle in a similar fashion. She planned to "touch base" with them frequently so that their efforts would be complementary.

PROVIDING INTERVENTION

Now that all of the pieces were in place, Colleen was ready. We describe a number of "snapshots," taken during the first 3 months of intervention. In so doing, we illustrate how the plan was translated into action and how Colleen resolved some of the difficulties she encountered. We demonstrate how Colleen reflected, both in action and on her actions.

The First Direct Intervention Session

During their initial session together, Colleen gave Kyle a tour of the clinic, pointing out several things she thought might interest him. Colleen hung a net hammock from a single point of suspension in the middle of the clinic. After the tour, Colleen suggested that Kyle might like to try "flying" in the net (see Fig. 9–1). She had several thoughts in mind. First, she knew that Kyle, similar to many boys his age, was really into superheroes. Many of Colleen's other clients enjoyed pretending they were Superman while "flying" in the net. Second, Colleen saw the net as a way of providing enhanced vestibular and proprioceptive sensation and also requiring him to maintain extension against gravity. She knew that it would be easy to create activities in the net that required visual-motor skill, bilateral coordination, and the ability to plan and produce projected action sequences.

Kyle was excited about trying the net. Anticipating that he might have difficulty getting into it, Colleen was ready to talk him through it at the first sign of failure. Indeed, on his first attempt, Kyle ended up lying prone over a rolled-up net. Colleen intervened immediately by saying, "I forgot to tell you how hard it was to get in, but I know a trick. Would you like to learn it?" Kyle nodded, and Colleen helped him back into an upright position. She handed him the edge of the net that was farthest from his body and instructed him to use his arms to "stretch it out." Then she told him to put one knee into the side of the net that was closest to him and lie down into it.

The second time, Kyle succeeded. He immediately began to propel himself with his hands, and Colleen encouraged him to see how high he could go. Kyle called out, "I'm flying like Superman!" He seemed delighted with his accomplishment and yelled for his mother (who was observing from behind a one-way mirror) to watch.

However, Colleen noted that, as Kyle reached down to propel himself, he tended to flex his entire body. Because she was looking for extension and Kyle's flexion was becoming more pronounced, Colleen recognized that she must adapt the activity.

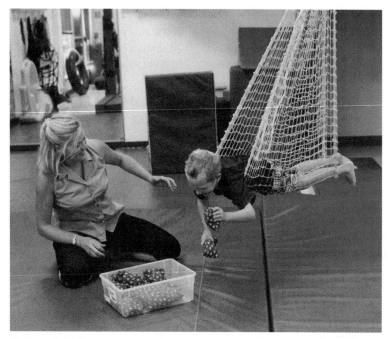

■ FIGURE 9-1 Many young boys enjoy swinging prone in the net hammock. (Photo by Shay McAtee, printed with permission.)

Colleen grabbed a long dowel rod from the shelf behind her, held it at either end between her two outstretched arms, and entered into Kyle's game. "Hey, Superman!" she yelled, "Grab onto this branch and look in this window; I think there's someone who needs your help!" Kyle reached up and grabbed the bar with his arms outstretched. "Hold on," yelled Colleen. "Pull hard so you can come a little closer." As Kyle began to flex his arms, Colleen watched closely to make sure that his body and head remain extended. At the first sign of neck, hip, or knee flexion, she lowered the bar a little to reduce the amount of resistance.

"What do you see?" asked Colleen. Kyle replied, "There's a whole bunch of bad guys in there." Colleen suggested that maybe he had better fly for help because there were too many bad guys to take on alone. Kyle let go of the bar and swung back and forth several times, calling for Batman and Superwoman to come and help him.

Meanwhile, Colleen had pulled a cushion underneath Kyle and laid several beanbags on top of the cushion. She hoped to arrange the beanbags so they were high enough for Kyle to reach down to get them as he flew by, and so that he would do so without using total body flexion. After several more "peeks through the window,"

Colleen suggested that the superheroes might want to use these special "bombs" to throw at the bad guys.

"I know," said Kyle, "let's pretend that clown over there (pointing to an inflatable clown that tipped when hit) is one of the bad guys. I'll hit him with these special bombs."

The game continued with Colleen gradually altering the demands on Kyle and watching his responses. By the time it was over, Kyle was pushing himself with both hands, grabbing a beanbag or two on the way by and throwing them at the inflatable clown. Colleen was impressed with the accuracy of his throw and with the amount of extension he was able to maintain. She cheered as he knocked over the clown. Colleen told Kyle that this game would help him have stronger muscles and that throwing the beanbags was good practice for throwing a ball.

As Kyle grew tired, his throwing accuracy decreased and he began to pull into flexion again. He complained that his neck hurt and that he wanted to sit up to throw the beanbags. Colleen helped him out of the net. It was time for the session to end anyway, and, as Kyle put his shoes and socks back on, Colleen spoke briefly with Mrs. P. Kyle was very excited to tell his mother about everything he had done, even though she had seen it through the mirror.

One Week Later

Having had such a successful first session with Kyle, Colleen looked forward to repeating the same activity in the second session. However, Kyle announced, upon arriving for his second session, that he did not want to lie down to do anything He only wanted to sit on the swing because lying down hurt his neck. Mrs. P. concurred that Kyle had complained about sore neck muscles for 2 days. However, she also said that she had told Kyle that his muscles were sore because they were getting stronger.

Colleen had to think quickly. She had probably demanded too much of Kyle in the first session and she should have had him spend less time in the prone position. However, she believed that he needed to work in the prone position because that was the best position to encourage maintained extension against gravity. Although Colleen planned to create activities for Kyle to do while sitting, she was afraid to create a lot of those activities at this point because it might be difficult to get him to go back to the prone position.

Colleen also knew that when children try throwing from a sitting position in the net, they often come to realize on their own that the prone position is easier. Thus, Colleen decided to follow Kyle's lead. She and Kyle set up the net swing, the cushion with the beanbags, and the clown, in much the same way she had set them up the week before. Kyle sat in the swing and began pushing it with his feet. He soon found that it was difficult to reach the beanbags, and his throwing was very inaccurate because he had to throw around the sides of the net and hold on at the same time. After a few minutes, Kyle told Colleen that he thought it worked better when he was lying down.

Hoping that this would happen, Colleen agreed immediately. Kyle got out of the net and, this time, was able to use the "trick" he'd learned the last time to lie down in it in prone, with very little assistance from Colleen. He seemed pleased with his accomplishment and quickly engaged in "bombing the bad guys."

Colleen could have insisted that Kyle lie prone in the net if he wanted to do the activity. She could have explained to him that it would not work as well while sitting. She also could have helped him to create an activity while sitting, using a different swing, that probably would have been successful. However, Colleen believed it was important to demonstrate Kyle's active role. She wanted him to learn that he could adapt situations to make them turn out better. Colleen knew that Kyle probably would learn on his own that using the prone position was better for doing this particular activity. Although the prone position was, in general, more difficult, Colleen believed that he would choose it because he had enjoyed the activity and the feelings he had when he succeeded.

After Kyle was busily engaged in the activity, Colleen watched the time and his reactions closely. After about 10 minutes, and well before Kyle began to appear fatigued, she suggested that they "bomb the bad guys" from a different swing. This time she helped him to create an activity that he could do well while sitting on the glider.

As Colleen reflected on her sessions with Kyle, she was surprised and pleased by some things. Kyle had been able to focus his attention remarkably well. He did not exhibit much of the distractibility that she had observed during testing and at school. Thus, Colleen learned that, with the undivided attention of an adult and activities he found highly motivating, Kyle was able to pay attention to relevant stimuli. Given the way Colleen had set up the clinic, distractions had been kept to a minimum, but Kyle successfully screened out those that were present. Although Colleen was pleased that this was the case, she was also not fooled into believing that Kyle would necessarily be able to focus his attention in situations that he found more difficult, when he had less adult attention, or when there were more sources of distraction. However, Colleen recognized that this had implications for the way in which she structured the environment. She felt that she might not have to be so careful to be sure that only certain swings remained in the room.

Colleen also knew that she was probably "buying time" with regard to Kyle's willingness to work in a prone position. She hoped she would be able to develop activities that are best done in the prone position that were highly motivating for at least a few more sessions. By then, Kyle might begin to find the prone position easier and be less resistant to it. However, she knew that if he balked, she probably would have to work primarily in sitting for a time and go back to the prone position as his postural stability improved.

Six Weeks Later

After working with Kyle for 6 weeks, as Colleen had anticipated, Kyle had become more familiar with the activities and tried to "steer clear" of those that must be done in the prone position. She had been able to bargain with him a little, but as we entered the clinic, they were engaged in an activity with Kyle seated in the swing. Colleen had created an activity in which she hoped to work on the timing of limb movements and on his ability to flex his neck and upper trunk against gravity. She was also hoping that this activity would carry over into his being able to pump the swing independently.

Kyle was standing on a pile of mats, the net swing slung around him. He was holding on with both hands. Colleen was standing on the floor opposite him, far enough away that she would not get hit as he swung. She was holding a large hula hoop between her outstretched arms. On cue, Kyle jumped off the mats and extended his legs. The goal of the task was to lean back and flex his knees around the hoop. Colleen yelled, "Now!" a fraction of a second before he should bend his knees. After Kyle had successfully "grabbed" the hoop, Colleen pulled him up a little higher, watching to see how far she could move him without his losing control of his head and neck. After she had attained the best possible position, Colleen moved the hoop from side to side and back and forth, making "roaring" noises.

"Let go! Let go!" Colleen said over and over. "You'll never capture me, you mean old monster!" Kyle, fully involved in the activity, did let go after a few seconds, saying, "Okay, just one more chance to be good. But, if you do anything else bad, I'll be back to get you!" As soon as Kyle landed back on his mats, Colleen did something to make Kyle "attack" her again, and the game went on.

After a time, Colleen stopped telling Kyle when to flex his legs in order to grab the hoop because Kyle seemed no longer to require assistance. He continued to be successful at the activity. In fact, Colleen thought that Kyle was doing so well he might be able to shift to pumping the swing. Colleen feigned tiredness. She said to Kyle, "I need a break. Why don't you just swing by yourself for a few minutes?"

He continued to push off the mats, catching himself after each swing. Colleen watched for a while and then suggested he not stop so frequently. "You know," she said, "when Linda [Kyle's older sister] pumps the swing, it's like she's leaning back and reaching out with her legs to catch an imaginary hoop. After she catches it, she pulls it back with her. Then she reaches out for a new hoop. And it just keeps going. Why don't you try that? Pretend I'm still standing there with that hoop."

Kyle thought for a while. Then he tried it once. He leaned back with his trunk as he had when catching the hoop, but he flexed his knees too fast. Knowing that it had not worked, he caught himself on the mats. "Try again," Colleen urged, "but wait until I say 'now' to bend your legs."

Kyle jumped off the mats, and Colleen began to say quietly, "Now," just before he reached the full arc of the swing. At first, Kyle had trouble coordinating his leg and body movements, but gradually he began to coordinate the flexion and extension of his body with the flexion and extension of his legs. He did it very forcefully, and his swinging was jerky, but his timing seemed to be better. "See if I can do it without you telling me when," Kyle said. Colleen followed his lead, and Kyle was able to pump the swing himself, although a little awkwardly. He practiced for a few minutes until it was time for the session to end.

Mrs. P. had been watching from behind the one-way mirror. She was beaming at Kyle as he entered the observation room. "We'll have to hurry home so you can practice before it gets dark. Your father will be very excited when he sees what you've learned," Mrs. P. said.

Two days later, Mrs. P. called to say that Kyle had mastered his first objective. "He's so excited," she said. "He spends every minute on the swing, practicing. His teacher sent a note home yesterday saying that he tried the swing at school for the first time. That's the first positive note we've gotten all year."

Colleen was also excited. She talked for several minutes with Mrs. P., and they decided that the next week, Kyle's individual session would be half as long. Mrs. P. requested that she spend the other half of the session with Colleen so they could begin working out a home program to address Kyle's handwriting problem. Colleen made a note to call the occupational therapist who was seeing Kyle at school

An Aside about Intervention

Intervention activities that "mimic" the demands of a stated objective are the most effective. Thus, in the context of the objective for Kyle to pump the swing independently, it would not be enough for Colleen to create activities to improve Kyle's flexion and bilateral coordination in a general way. Rather, she needed also to create activities that mimicked the actual process of pumping a playground swing.

Another child might have an objective to go up and down stairs quickly and reciprocally. Similar to Kyle's, that child's intervention might also include activities to improve his BIS abilities. However, activities created for this client should involve bilateral movement and projected action sequences *using his feet* (e.g., sitting in the net hammock and pushing off a wall with his feet). At least a portion of those activities should be done in a vertical position, similar to actually climbing stairs. We provide an example of intervention for a child with needs and objectives similar to these in Chapter 1.

Monitoring: Developing a Home Program

When Mrs. P. and Colleen sat down together the next week, Mrs. P. mentioned that she thought she could already see progress in Kyle's handwriting. She had had only one note in the past month from Kyle's teacher indicating that he failed to get his work done on time. Nonetheless, Mrs. P. felt that a home program focusing specifically on handwriting would be helpful.

Colleen explained that the occupational therapist at school was working with the teacher to adapt Kyle's assignments so that he had less written work. She had given Kyle a device to put on his pencil that helped to encourage a better grasp and had given him a slant-top surface to encourage better posture. Also, as a result of the occupational therapist's consultation, the teacher had decided to move Kyle's desk to a rear corner of the classroom, where his classmates rarely went. Both the therapist and teacher were encouraged by the results. However, they also believed that a home program could be beneficial.

Colleen reminded Mrs. P. that Kyle's objective was to write more quickly and get his schoolwork done on time. Thus, the home program would concentrate on speed rather than letter formation. She also told Mrs. P. that a home program should not be just "exercises" that they had to "cram" into their already busy schedules. Mrs. P. agreed. With three other active children, she did not have

time to make sure Kyle did his home program. She continued to express the need to facilitate positive interactions with Kyle rather than setting up situations in which he might need to be reprimanded for his performance.

Colleen wanted Kyle to write without worrying about forming perfect letters. One idea she had was that Kyle could practice quickly writing simple phrases on brown paper bags while he was watching television (Benbow, 1982). Mrs. P. thought Kyle would love that idea. Kyle and his brother and sisters were allowed to watch only a minimum of television; they often protested this rule. If Kyle's home program called for half an hour of television each night, all the children would be delighted.

From the occupational therapist at school, Colleen had obtained lists of the letters that Kyle should already know, those that Kyle was currently working on, and letters that he would be working on in the near future. She and Mrs. P. constructed silly phrases such as "the duck barked" and "the cat flew." The plan was that Kyle would select one of those phrases each night and write it as many times as he could while he watched television. Colleen asked Mrs. P. to remind Kyle that he should "just write" and not pay attention to each letter. He should only need to look down at his paper when he started a new line. It did not matter if he made a mistake; he should just keep going.

When they told Kyle of the plan, he thought it was a "great idea." He wanted to know if he could start that very night. He promised to bring his "bags" in each week to show Colleen.

In selecting an idea for monitoring, Colleen considered that one of Kyle's problems was planning and producing projected action sequences. Writing phrases on a bag (because he was not copying them) involved the ability to plan in advance and write without feedback. As Kyle practiced, Colleen hoped that he would develop a better "feel" for the way to make each letter and that his speed would improve as he did so. Furthermore, she believed that the procedure should be fun and that it should increase the ease with which he wrote. That all the children in the family would be delighted with the "requirements" of Kyle's intervention was an added bonus.

Both Mrs. P. and Colleen believed that the home program was an important part of intervention. Thus, there was no question that they should use some of Kyle's intervention time to develop their ideas for it. In fact, they scheduled a similar time for a month later when they planned to develop strategies for helping Kyle to enter a group of children. They would also talk about having a friend join Kyle and Colleen in some of their sessions.

Although the home program that Colleen created for Kyle was guided by her knowledge of sensory integration theory, it was not a sensory integrative procedure. Rather, Colleen used a type of skills training. She drew from her knowledge of several practice models to create the most effective intervention for Kyle. This "integrated approach" to intervention is discussed more fully in Chapter 15.

After 4 Months

Our final "snapshot" of Kyle and Colleen was taken about 4 months after Kyle began intervention. Kyle had, in fact, made a new friend named Jason. Jason had recently moved next door to Kyle and was in his class at school. Kyle had invited Jason to join him at his "special gym class." This was Jason's first visit to the clinic, and the boys were very excited. Kyle had just completed giving Jason a tour of all the swings. Colleen had asked Kyle what he and Jason would like to do first. Kyle responded that they would like to "fly" in the nets. "It's really cool. You're gonna like it," he told Jason. "It's just like being Superman."

In response to Kyle's request, Colleen hung two nets from single suspension points 8 feet apart. She asked Kyle if he would like to play the "hockey" game that she and Kyle had devised together. Kyle agreed.

The game consisted of both boys swinging prone in the nets. Each had a long stick that they held at both ends. Off to each side, slightly behind each boy, was a stack of cardboard blocks. The object of the game was to use the sticks to hit a large ball that was centered in a small hula-hoop on the floor between them. Each boy tried to use the ball to knock over the other's stacks of blocks. The game continued until one boy's blocks were completely knocked over.

Kyle had played this game with Colleen. Colleen saw it as a means of providing him with enhanced vestibular and proprioceptive sensation while demanding bilateral projected actions. Kyle had gotten to be fairly good at this activity, and he took the lead with Jason, teaching him the rules and showing him how to get the ball into the net.

The two boys were engaged for several minutes in the activity. However, with the competi-tion, Kyle got very excited. He began to swing the stick with one hand and accidentally hit Jason quite hard. Jason was clearly upset and yelled at Kyle, "Hey, that's too hard. We're just playing."

Colleen intervened. She indicated that the boys should get out of the nets and get into a medium-sized box filled with dried lentils. They climbed in. Meanwhile, Colleen turned off the overhead lights and put flashlights in her pockets for each boy. Kyle was still overstimulated. He immediately began to throw lentils. Colleen intervened again before a full-blown lentil fight could develop. "Kyle," she said, "lie down in the corner here, and Jason and I will bury you, all but your head." Colleen knew, from past experience, that this was an activity that Kyle found calming.

Colleen and Jason began dumping containers full of the lentils on top of Kyle. When Kyle moved too much, uncovering a limb, Jason reminded him to be very still. After Kyle was completely covered, Colleen suggested that Jason lie down beside him, and she buried Jason. She talked to the boys in hushed tones, and Kyle calmed down noticeably. Colleen gave each boy a flashlight, and they played a modified game of "I Spy" for a while.

Colleen noticed Kyle's proximity to Jason in the lentil box; his tactile defensiveness was somewhat reduced. Mrs. P. had also observed this. In one of their conversations, Mrs. P. told Colleen that Kyle's fighting at school had been nearly eliminated.

Colleen recognized that being in the lentil box provided a good opportunity to talk with Kyle about developing strategies to use when he felt out of control. She began a discussion with the two boys about what it felt like to be buried under all those lentils. Jason indicated that it made him feel calm, kind of like he felt after he had just taken a bath. Colleen skillfully guided the conversation so that both boys contributed and so Kyle could see that even Jason sometimes felt overwhelmed by "too much stuff going on around him." Seeing that Kyle was very intrigued by this knowledge, Colleen probed a little more. "What do you do when you feel like that?" she asked. Jason answered that sometimes he went to his room to be alone and sometimes he just put his head down on his desk. Kyle did not contribute much to that part of the conversation, but he listened intently.

After a time, Colleen turned the lights back on and dumped some small plastic "bedbugs" into the lentil mixture. The boys spent the last few minutes of the session busily searching for them and picking them up with large plastic tweezers. Colleen had scattered the bedbugs so that they were closer to Kyle. By the end of the session, both boys had found an equal number of bedbugs. They climbed out of the box and got ready to go home, chatting about what they would do together the next time Jason accompanied Kyle to the clinic. They planned that date for 3 weeks later.

SUMMARY AND CONCLUSION

This chapter has demonstrated how one expert therapist took the information she gathered in evaluation and applied that knowledge together with her knowledge of sensory integration theory to the development and implementation of an effective intervention plan. The chapter emphasized the importance of working with clients and caregivers to formulate objectives and described a therapist's reflections in action (Schon, 1983, 1987) and depicted her ability to modify based on her reflections.

This chapter has highlighted the reasoning and roles of a clinical practitioner, performing direct intervention using the principles of sensory integration theory. We have referred only briefly to the complementary roles of the school therapist and to the consultative and monitoring roles of the clinical practitioner. We have done so partly because consultation and the role of the school therapist are emphasized in Chapter 13. We have not done so because we believe that the direct service role of the clinical therapist is any more important than the consultative role of the school therapist.

Direct intervention, conducted by a skilled therapist, is a powerful approach to intervention for individuals who have sensory integrative dysfunction. However, it is only one avenue by which to address the difficulties that these individuals encounter in daily life. Furthermore, intervention based on sensory integration theory alone often is not enough to eliminate these difficulties. We believe that the greatest benefits are attained when a team of individuals pools all of its relevant skills and knowledge, sets meaningful and achievable objectives, and implements an integrated approach to intervention.

References

Ayres, A. J. (1989). *Sensory integration and praxis tests*. Los Angeles: Western Psychological Services.

Benbow, M. (March 1982). Problems with handwriting. Paper presented at Eunice Kennedy Shriver Center, Waltham, MA.

Bundy, A. C. (1995). Assessment and intervention in school-based practice: Answering questions and minimizing discrepancies. *Physical and Occupational Therapy in Pediatrics, 15,* 69–88.

Carroll, L. (1923). *Alice in Wonderland and Through the Looking Glass*. London: John C. Winston.

Dunn, W. (1999). *Sensory profile*. San Antonio: Psychological Corporation.

Mager, R. (1972). *Goal analysis*. Belmont, CA: Fearon.

Mager. R. (1975). *Preparing instructional objectives*. Belmont, CA: Fearon.

Mattingly, C. F., & Fleming, M. H. (1994). *Clinical reasoning: Forms of inquiry in a therapeutic practice*. Philadelphia: F.A. Davis.

Rogers, J. C., & Masagatani, G. (1982). Clinical reasoning of occupational therapists during the initial assessment of physically disabled patients. *Occupational Therapy Journal of Research, 2,* 195–219.

Schön, D. A. (1983). *The reflective practitioner: How professionals think in action*. New York: Basic.

Schön, D. A. (1987). *Educating the reflective practitioner*. San Francisco: Jossey-Bass.

Wilbarger, P., & Wilbarger, J. (1991). *Sensory defensiveness in children aged 2–12: An intervention guide for parents and other caretakers*. Denver, CO: Avanti Educational Programs.

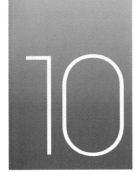

Play Theory and Sensory Integration

Anita C. Bundy, ScD, OTR, FAOTA

> *Doing things for the fun of it constitutes play.*
> *But what is the use of doing things just for fun? What is the use of play? Rather, has it any use? If it had no use, we do not believe a desire for it would have been so firmly planted in our natures, and in the nature of every living thing. . . . The first few years of a child's life . . . seem spent almost wholly in play. Nothing give us more uneasiness than to see a child who does not play. We consider it a sure sign of sickness, either of body or of mind. . . [As a result of playing], the client grows. Growth is the primary use of play.*
>
> —*West, 1888, p. 469*

"I wish you could be my gym teacher," Kimberly, a 10-year-old girl, said as she leapt off a pile of mats, swung forward, grabbed a beanbag, pushed with her feet off a crash mat against the wall, and tossed the beanbag into a container behind her (Fig. 10–1.) When her occupational therapy practitioner, Liza, did not respond, she continued, "I play when I come here. Gym is too much work. Besides, I go to gym more often than I get to come here."

As occupational therapy practitioners and play researchers, we know that Kimberly had paid Liza a very high compliment. Although Kimberly had been actively involved in setting explicit goals for her therapy—goals that were scary and difficult for her (e.g., walking without fear down open stairs)—she still considered her work with Liza to be play. (And recently, Kimberly an-

nounced that she was the first one down the open stairs at a farm her class visited on a field trip.)

The fact that Kimberly considers the time she spends with Liza to be both play and therapy is quite an accomplishment. Kimberly has significant gravitational insecurity and tremendous difficulty with motor planning. In her daily life, she finds most activities that involve movement to be terrifying. Last winter's attempts at ski lessons were pure torture. But in therapy, Kimberly jumps from surfaces more than 4 feet off the ground. She flies through the air in a net hammock, squealing with delight. She turns somersaults over a 4-foot ball. Such is the power of carefully created play!

At present, Kimberly seems like two different people. In real life, gravity is her enemy, and her response is to prefer sedentary activity and quiet games with her mother. When she engages in

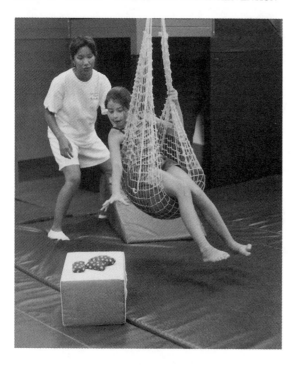

■ FIGURE 10–1 Kimberly challenges herself during a direct intervention session. (Photo by Shay McAtee, printed with permission.)

gross motor activity (often with her father), she is fearful and anxious. In therapy, Kimberly makes friends with her fear and tries things she would never try anywhere else—and she thinks of those things as play.

Of course, the ultimate goal is for Kimberly to experience biking, in-line skating, and soccer, all things she has trouble with in real life, as play. Then her work with Liza will be over. Perhaps Kimberly will stop by occasionally, just to play!

IN CELEBRATION OF PLAY

After many years as a second-class citizen, play has finally come into its own in occupational therapy. We study play openly. We write about it. We discuss it at conferences. We (sometimes, at least) acknowledge that we play with children in the clinic. In short, we are beginning to assume responsibility for understanding play, assessing it, promoting it, and evaluating its effectiveness in intervention.

Play wears many faces; it is perhaps the most complex of the phenomena with which occupational therapy practitioners deal. Play is an important lifelong occupation; it is also a powerful tool for intervention. Finally, playfulness is a style, an approach to daily life events. None of the other primary occupations wears all these faces so easily. We cannot imagine hoping to instill in

someone an "activities of daily living" approach to life. And, although work skills may be a primary target for intervention, one rarely hopes that intervention will be perceived as work. Rather, we hope to make work more like play (Csikszentmihayli, 1975a, 1990, 1993, 1996) and that our clients can develop adaptability as a byproduct of playfulness (Sutton-Smith, 1997).

PURPOSE AND SCOPE

Although play is occupation, medium, and approach, this chapter focuses on a playful approach to intervention. It addresses the creation of play activities within the context of a playful environment. Because this is a text on sensory integration theory, this chapter tailors the discussion to reflect intervention from a sensory integrative perspective. The latter sections of the chapter briefly address play as occupation and the relationship between sensory integrative dysfunction and play.

DEFINING PLAY FOR PLAYFUL INTERVENTION

Play will never be a simple topic (Sutton-Smith, 1997). Perhaps it will never be defined both broadly and narrowly enough to meet all the needs of theorists and researchers in the countless professions that study play. Nonetheless, if we are to create playful interventions, we must accept some general premises about play. The following discussion draws heavily from the work of Neumann (1971), an educator, to develop a working definition of play for use by occupational therapy practitioners attempting to create playful intervention.

Neumann (1971) described three criteria for play: relative internal control, freedom from some constraints of reality, and relative intrinsic motivation. Neumann (1971) considered that any transaction containing all three elements could be considered play. However, she acknowledged that:

> ... rarely does one have total internal control, total intrinsic motivation, or total internal reality. Consequently, play and nonplay must be considered as opposing end-points of a continuum. . . . The degree to which the criteria for play are fulfilled determines where on the continuum the transaction belongs (p. 163).

The consideration of play as a continuum is perhaps the most significant contribution Neumann (1971) has made to the field of occupational therapy, particularly when we use play as a medium to develop other skills and abilities. Neumann cautioned that when play is used as a medium, some-

one other than the player often exerts significant control over the transaction. When that happens, the player is at risk of feeling externally controlled. If relatively high intrinsic motivation or freedom from some of the constraints of reality do not offset the caregiver's control, then the transaction may not actually be play, and the benefits of play will be lost. We have illustrated the contribution of the elements of play (e.g., internal control, intrinsic motivation, and freedom from some constraints of reality) as a playfulness–nonplayfulness continuum in Figure 10–2.

Based on Neumann's (1971) conceptualization, we have proposed the following working definition of play for use by occupational therapy practitioners seeking to create play in intervention. Play is a transaction between an individual and the environment that is:

- Relatively intrinsically motivated
- Relatively internally controlled
- Free of some of the constraints of objective reality

Play transactions represent a continuum of behaviors that are more or less playful, depending on the degree to which the criteria are present (see Fig. 10–2).

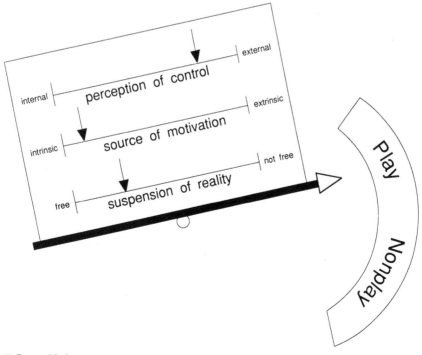

■ FIGURE 10–2 The play-nonplay continuum. A hypothetical balance between perception of control, source of motivation, and suspension of reality.

Because the creation of playful intervention is difficult, we constantly evaluate transactions to determine where on the play–nonplay continuum each falls. When necessary, we adjust aspects of one or more play elements in an attempt to tip the balance toward play. Because each of the play elements provides us with important guidelines for assessing whether or not play is occurring at any given time and because they become intertwined and may be difficult to separate, each requires some additional discussion.

Relative Intrinsic Motivation

Rubin et al. (1983) indicated that intrinsic motivation is almost universally acknowledged as an essential element of play. By this definition, intrinsic motivation refers to the individual engaging in an activity because something about the activity itself is appealing, rather than because someone else told the individual to do it or for some gain outside of the process itself (e.g., winning, admiration).

Other authors (e.g., Berlyne, 1966; Neumann, 1971; Piaget, 1962; White, 1959) have emphasized the link between motivation and the inner drive of the individual. That link is important to occupational therapy practitioners because we usually want to know more than that an individual is intrinsically motivated. We also want to know something about the source of the motivation.

Individuals seek pleasure or other intrinsic benefits from participating in an activity. Many differing benefits and sources of pleasure have been described. For example, although White (1959) associated intrinsic motivation with mastery, Berlyne (1966) linked it with maintaining optimum levels of arousal. Social interaction has been suggested as a common motivator (e.g., Csikszentmihayli, 1975a), as have competition (Caillois, 1979; Csikszentmihayli, 1975a) and pure sensation seeking (Caillois, 1979).

Motivations are likely to differ from person to person, even when they are involved in the same activity (Csikszentimihalyi, 1975a). Because we seek to create activities that our clients will find motivating, it is important to determine what "drives" any particular client and build those things into activity. Thus, the source of a client's intrinsic motivation sets the stage for intervention activities.

Regardless of its source, how do we know intrinsic motivation when we see it? And how can we promote it? To evaluate a transaction for signs of intrinsic motivation, we must be aware of the indicators of its presence. To promote intrinsic motivation, we provide opportunities. However, we must also keep from interfering with or disrupting an individual's motivation.

When individuals are intrinsically motivated, they become totally involved in an activity. Csikszentmihayli (1975a, 1975b, 1979, 1990) referred to this involvement as "flow." Flow occurs in activities that are neither so difficult as to cause worry or anxiety nor so easy as to result in boredom; such an activity represents the "just-right challenge" (Ayres, 1972; Berlyne, 1969; Csikszentmihayli, 1975b, 1979). The relationship among challenge, skills, and flow illustrates one way in which intrinsic motivation depends on internal control.

Other important traits of the flow experience include the opportunity to focus on a limited stimulus field and clear, unambiguous feedback that is a part of the activity. One common trait of activities used in sensory integrative therapy is that they *do* provide clear feedback. Clients know immediately if they have hit a target or jumped to the desired spot. Our running commentaries on the client's performance, even when they are intended to provide support, may do no more than detract from the flow experience because they may draw attention away from the activity (Ayres, 1972).

Persistence and repetition are other signs that a client is motivated to be involved in an activity. Even in the face of significant obstacles or challenges, clients persist with activities they find intrinsically motivating—for the sheer pleasure of doing them. Clients also repeat activities that bring them pleasure. In fact, practitioners must be cognizant of clients' desires to repeat activities. We may feel compelled to carry out several activities within an intervention session, but interrupting an activity in which a client is totally involved can be very disruptive to the flow of the session. Modifying the challenge slightly, within the context of the same activity, can be a more successful way to address goals while maintaining flow. There are no "rules" about how many activities should be done in a session or how long each activity should last. We believe that activities should continue until they are no longer motivating, the client has mastered the challenge, or the session has ended. In fact, one mark of a masterfully created session may be a small number of activities with seamless transitions.

Certain kinds of activities that are intrinsically motivating, especially to children (often gross motor play) also pull for enthusiasm, exuberance, and manifest joy from players. Although manifest joy can be a sign of intrinsic motivation, we prefer to evaluate intrinsic motivation by examining whether or not clients are intensely involved. Often a client is too engrossed to be aware that an activity is fun. After it is over, the client may remark that the activity was fun, but laughing, smiling, or other signs commonly associated with "fun" were notably absent when the activity was in progress. Furthermore, not all activities lend themselves to signs of obvious exuberance. For example, under most circumstances, we would think it very peculiar if a client giggled and squealed with joy as she put together a puzzle. Much can be learned by keeping track of activities in which clients become totally involved or that seem to bring them great joy. Careful analysis of such activities can yield important information about the sources of the particular client's intrinsic motivation.

Although intrinsic motivation is an important part of play and intervention, not all activities are done *only* for the pleasure that the process brings. Many clients are highly motivated by friendly competition with a practitioner or accruing points, which are forms of extrinsic motivation. Although we frequently use some forms of extrinsic motivation, we set those within an activity that the client enjoys for its own sake. Extrinsic motivators are purely an added extra.

Relative Internal Control

Although not always acknowledged as such by play theorists, relative internal control is arguably the most important element of a play transaction (Neumann, 1971). If players are in control, they can act on their motivations by determining who and what to play with and how and where to play. Similarly, players who are in control are free to suspend some of the constraints of reality by transforming objects, themselves, or others into things that they are not or by bending some of the usual rules. Clearly, all the elements of play depend, to some extent, on relative internal control.

Feeling physically and emotionally safe is the most basic aspect of internal control. In therapy, unlike in "real life," Kimberly can joyfully leap off surfaces and swing through the air in a net hammock because she feels safe. Surfaces around and below her are covered in thick foam padding, and she trusts that Liza will keep her from harm.

Safety, in part, comes from a relative match of the challenge with the client's skills. This match enables clients to feel in charge of their actions. Csikszentmihayli (1975a, 1975b, 1990, 1993, 1996, 1997) indicated that individuals become most involved (a reflection of intrinsic motivation) in challenging activities, ones in which they used their best skills and reached just a little beyond their capabilities. Such challenges cannot be met successfully each time they are encountered; clients do not hit a target each time they throw a beanbag! The optimum rate of success is individual, however. Some clients who have sensory integrative dysfunction may initially need a relatively high rate of success if they have experienced significant failure in their lives. However, practitioners must be aware that clients become easily bored when they are too successful.

Unless clients are actively involved, an activity is neither therapeutic nor play. Furthermore, unless an activity results in an adaptive interaction, it is not therapeutic. An adaptive interaction is one that is done just a little better than it has ever been done before. However, "just a little better" may be interpreted as just a little easier or just a little more spontaneous.

When clients feel in control, they help to make some of the decisions about what activities will look like. Clients may contribute to the development of a pretend theme or help select equipment or toys that are a part of a transaction. However, because clients *feel* in control does not mean that they "run the show." Good intervention, even in the context of play, is not chaotic. A practitioner implementing sensory integrative intervention is more than likely to have an explicit real life goal in mind. The more the goal is mimicked in the intervention, the more quickly it will be reached. Thus, the client, who lacks the skills of activity analysis that a practitioner possesses, cannot be expected to create all the components of an activity designed to meet a particular goal.

True feelings of internal control manifest themselves when clients share control, whether with a peer playmate or the practitioner. Clients can share others' ideas for an activity and negotiate to have their own needs met within its context.

Relative Freedom from Some Constraints of Reality

There are at least two important aspects of relative freedom from some constraints of reality:

1. The ability to pretend or to engage in fantasy play (Neumann, 1971; Rubin et al., 1983; Sawyer, 1997)
2. The reduction of consequences that might normally be associated with performing the same activity in "real life" (Vandenberg & Kielhofner, 1982)

In play and in intervention, clients should feel free to transform themselves, and the activity, into anything they desire (Neumann, 1971). One of the "paradoxes of play" (Bateson, 1972) is represented in a client's transformation, for example, of a bolster swing into a bull and himself into a famous rider of bulls. In making both the swing and himself into something that they are not (a bull and a bull rider), the therapeutic activity takes on "real" meaning for the child. This increased level of meaningfulness probably would not have been present if the activity consisted only of the child, as himself, trying to stay on the swing as long as possible while the practitioner shook it.

Relative freedom from some of the constraints of reality involves more than pretend. For clients with sensory integrative dysfunction, objective reality commonly presents many constraints that interfere with play. Not the least among those constraints may be fear of moving or fear of being touched. Gravity also presents an inordinate constraint to clients whose muscle tone or postural responses are not adequate to resist it or who fear falling or being out of an upright position. Complex toys may inhibit a child whose motor planning skills are poor. Practitioners seek to orchestrate an intervention session and environment so that constraints are minimized or eliminated. In creating a safe environment that is free of consequences that have prevented the client from succeeding in "real life," reality is temporarily suspended and both play and therapeutic gain are facilitated.

Most practitioners who routinely work with children are relatively comfortable with and quite skilled at participating in pretend play frames and adjusting the physical environment to minimize the consequences of the child's disability. However, other aspects of freedom from some of the constraints of reality may be less comfortable for practitioners. For example, mischief is a component of the suspension of reality that makes many adults uncomfortable.

Mischief involves breaking the usual rules. For example, squirting a practitioner with a squirt gun, hitting him or her over the head with a pillow, or jumping off a table are not allowed in most situations. Certainly, they would not be allowed in therapy if clients were doing them maliciously. However, we must distinguish between meanness, maliciousness, and true mischief. True mischief requires skill and is done with a gleam in the eye rather than out of wickedness of the heart (Bundy, 2000). Perhaps because clients perceive them as "naughty," mischievous acts can be highly motivating. Furthermore, they provide the perfect opportunity for children to learn that certain behaviors are okay at certain times and under certain circumstances but that they are not okay at other times and in other places.

As beneficial as suspending some of the constraints of reality can be, we need to be aware that not all good occupational therapy involves either play or the alteration of reality. Many individuals may not automatically generalize skills they gain in intervention to their everyday lives. Although play is a powerful tool for gaining skills, practitioners may also have to engage clients in "real-life" tasks to be sure that, after skills have been attained, they can be used. At the very least, we need to follow up on the outcomes of intervention by checking with clients and their families or by observing clients using newly acquired skills in everyday life.

Linda, an occupational therapy student, had been working for a short time with Max, an 8-year-old client who had sensory integrative dysfunction. Linda asked Max how he felt about intervention, to which he responded, "It's fine; it's fun, but I still can't play dodgeball. I cover my eyes when someone throws the ball at me and then it hits me. And I can never hit anybody else with the ball. I aim it, but it just flies off and then the other kids laugh."

For some time, Linda and the supervising practitioner, Jill, aware that Max wanted to get better at dodgeball, had incorporated into Max's sensory integration intervention activities catching and throwing a Nerf ball. His skills seemed to have become much better. Thus, they were a little dismayed by his complaint.

Linda decided to take Max outside and engage

him in a more task-oriented approach with a ball similar to the one he used in gym class. She had him throw the ball repeatedly and practice dodging when she threw it at him. She offered two bits of advice repeatedly, "Keep your eyes on the ball, and throw low."

When Max returned the next week, Jill asked him how it went with the dodgeball. "It was a little better," he replied. "I did what Linda told me and it helped."

"What *did* Linda tell you?" asked Jill.

"Keep my eyes on the ball, and throw low," came the reply.

Although the primary intervention approach used with Max had been based on sensory integration principles, Linda and Jill responded to Max's needs to generalize his developing skills to the "real world" by breaking their typical intervention routine to work on what was bothering Max most at that moment—dodgeball.

For Max, dodgeball was not play; it truly was work (and, at the moment, not very enjoyable work). "Playing" dodgeball, to Max, however motivating it was, meant anxiety and embarrassment, not the typical feelings associated with play. Thus, the session between Linda and Max could not be described as play in any sense. In fact, Max insisted that they search for the appropriate ball so that their "game" would be as close to reality as possible.

Max had already made many improvements in intervention and, in fact, had many of the skills he needed to be able to succeed at dodgeball. However, he did not recognize that the skills he used in intervention were the same skills he needed for dodgeball. Furthermore, he did not seem to understand that he needed to throw low to be successful. When confronted with a real dodgeball sailing toward him, he continued to close his eyes, even though he had long since learned to watch the Nerf ball he caught during intervention activities.

Linda and Jill were implementing good occupational therapy. They left behind both play and sensory integration when they needed to do so. They were not bound by the belief that when Max gained skills in intervention, he would automatically use them in real life. They asked for his assessment of the results of intervention. Furthermore, they felt free to conduct a session in which reality was not suspended. And they made a real difference in the life of their young client.

In summary, the freedom to suspend some constraints of reality by pretending, minimizing con-

sequences, and promoting mischief and related behaviors are powerful tools for therapy. We must be aware, however, that there are times when the demands of real life take precedence.

SETTING UP THE ENVIRONMENT TO SUPPORT PLAY

The environment is an important aspect of play in intervention. When we want play to occur, we try to make certain that particular environmental elements are present. Rubin et al. (1983) included the following:

- An array of familiar peers, toys, or other materials likely to engage children's interest
- An agreement between adults and children, expressed in words or gestures or established by convention, that the children are free to choose from the array whatever they wish to do within whatever limits are required by the setting or the study
- Adult behavior that is minimally intrusive or directive
- A friendly atmosphere designed to make children feel comfortable and safe
- Scheduling that reduces the likelihood of the children's being tired, hungry, ill, or experiencing other types of bodily stress (p. 701)

When all of these factors are present, the chance for play to occur is maximized. However, merely setting up a theoretically playful environment does not ensure that play can, or will, occur. Clearly, practitioners must be vigilant observers to be certain that play is occurring, when such is the intent.

THE POTENTIAL OF PLAY IN THERAPY

When Ayres (1972) wrote about the "art of therapy," she described the skilled practitioner as one who facilitates a child's mastery of the environment. Her terminology is similar to that used by White (1959), who compellingly argued that humans require a long and playful "apprenticeship" in order to become masters of their environments.

If play is the vehicle by which individuals become masters of their environments, then play should be among the most powerful of therapeutic tools. To be able to play with clients is an art, one that few adults possess. When a client acknowledges an occupational therapy practitioner as someone fun to play with, it is a high form of praise.

Play and intervention based on the principles of sensory integration share many common elements. Therapy based on the principles of sensory integration is conducted through activities that incorporate opportunities to take in enhanced sensation, provide the "just-right challenge," and demand an adaptive interaction.

Intervention is most successful when activities are intrinsically motivating and clients are actively involved and in control of at least some aspects of a session. All discussions of sensory integration therapy inevitably describe that clients must be safe from both physical and psychological threat. In other words, at least some of the constraints of objective reality must be kept at bay, including that there should be no adverse consequences to attempting difficult challenges (see Chapter 12).

Although play and intervention share common elements, they are not synonymous. When clients play during occupational therapy based on the principles of sensory integration theory, they play in certain predictable ways. That is, not all kinds of play lend themselves to use in this type of intervention. In intervention based on the principles of sensory integration, clients use their sensorimotor skills to interact with an environment specifically designed to provide opportunities to take in enhanced sensation. They may repeat specific transactions, practicing until they master the challenge. They become totally involved in their play and demonstrate mastery in adaptive transactions. They often transform themselves, the practitioner, and elements of the environment into something that they are not. Thus, intervention based on sensory integration theory, when carried out in the fullest sense, describes a special subset of play transactions in which all activities include enhanced sensation.

Creating playful environments and facilitating the play of individuals with disabling conditions is not easy (Anderson et al., 1987; Rast, 1986). However, play is what practitioners using the principles of sensory integration strive to attain. Play and nonplay reflect a continuum of behaviors, not an either-or situation (Neumann, 1971). If it is necessary for a practitioner to be relatively directive in a session, he or she might compensate by emphasizing activities that are particularly motivating to a client or by supporting a lot of pretending or mischief. Practitioners are aiming

to meet therapeutic objectives within as playful a framework as it is possible for clients and practitioners to create together.

Although clients play in therapy, therapy should not be disguised as play (Rast, 1986). Therapy is driven by real life goals. Most children can be involved in setting those goals. We must help them understand how a particular activity directly helps to meet the goal. For example, Kimberly's goal was to walk down open stairs without fear. Liza helped her understand that pushing off the wall with her feet would give her a better sense of where her feet are and that might make it easier to go down stairs.

Liza strove to provide Kimberly with the sense that she was playing by making available activities that she found intrinsically motivating and that provided challenges that closely matched her skills. However, Liza also orchestrated sessions so they were intervention. That is, she had a plan. Liza incorporated a particular type and amount of enhanced sensation, depending on the adaptive interaction she sought. Liza was prepared to alter activities ever so slightly so that they met the dual purposes of play and therapy, taking her lead from theory, the goal, and Kimberly's responses. Kimberly had the benefit of both play and skilled therapeutic intervention.

Play and playfulness are powerful therapeutic tools. Play promotes competence. The playfulness of the practitioner (and ideally of the client) helps create an atmosphere in which play occurs (Tickle-Degnen & Coster, 1995). When play and playfulness are coupled with skilled therapeutic intervention, they can make a real difference in the lives of clients. Practitioners who use sensory integrative principles in the most skillful manner with children who have disordered central nervous systems strive to create play in intervention.

As powerful as it may be, not all play is good therapy and not all good intervention is play. Intervention based on the principles of sensory integration may be somewhat unique in the amount of latitude it allows for true play to occur. Furthermore, although she rarely used the word "play," Ayres (1972) was a true genius at conceptualizing an approach to intervention that lent itself so readily to play. However, to meet the goals of their everyday life, most clients with sensory integrative dysfunction require more than sensory integrative–based intervention. They also require specific instruction in the tasks they are attempting to master. The story of Max's learning to play dodgeball is one of countless examples of this principle.

Sooner or later, play and intervention based on the principles of sensory integration theory part company. This happens even when the goal of therapy is to improve a client's ability to play. Play is a complex phenomenon. To be a better player requires more than sensory integration and learning to play ball, and performing nearly any daily life task requires more than play. The important point is not to use play or sensory integration but to be clear about the goals and conduct intervention that addresses all the important aspects of those goals.

THE CONTRIBUTION OF SENSORY INTEGRATION TO PLAY

In addition to being a powerful medium for intervention, play is also a primary occupation. Processing sensation effectively and using it to plan and produce efficient interactions enables clients to be in control and sense that they are in charge. Transactions that truly are play are dependent on players' abilities to feel a degree of control (Kooij & Vrijhof, 1981; Neumann, 1971; Rubin et al., 1983). Furthermore, individuals who believe they are more internally than externally controlled may be better players (Kooij & Vrijhof, 1981; Morrison et al., 1991).

This section examines the links between sensory integration and play theory, delving first into the implications for play that can be derived from sensory integration theory and then looking at research that has begun to examine the overlap between play and sensory integration. The section closes by acknowledging shortfalls in our knowledge in both areas.

The Implications of Sensory Integration Theory

It is logical to conclude that some individuals who have sensory integrative dysfunction may also have difficulty playing. Certainly, individuals who are at the mercy of gravity or fear cannot feel in control of many of the activities that characterize play. Lindquist et al. (1982) summed up the theoretical relationship between sensory integrative dysfunction and play:

It is apparent that the relative adequacy of sensory integrative abilities will influence how the client plays. At the sensorimotor level, the child's ability to integrate and organize sensation is of paramount importance in using the body effectively in play. At the constructive level, such end products of sensory integration as praxis, eye-hand coordination, and visual perception will influence the quality of the child's interactions with objects. And at the social level, end products of sensory integration self-esteem and self-confidence may influence the child's willingness and ability to interact, cooperate, and compete with peers in social play. (p. 434)

To play, individuals must believe that they are free to choose what to play with and how to play. They must be able to minimize some of the constraints of reality and be free to interact with people and objects they find intrinsically motivating. They must be able to act on the sources of their motivation. Because sensory integration is one of the foundations for play, sensory integration theory provides practitioners with an *indirect* means of evaluating and instilling *some* of the neurobehavioral antecedents to play. Deficits in sensory integration are most clearly related to individuals' abilities to interact with people and objects and feel as though they are in control. Sensory integrative dysfunction may also affect the types of activities that individuals find to be intrinsically motivating (Clifford & Bundy, 1989).

Deficits in the ability to integrate and organize vestibular and proprioceptive input manifests itself in impaired postural responses, poor bilateral integration and sequencing, gravitational insecurity, or aversive responses to movement. Similarly, deficits in tactile processing may result in poor motor planning or tactile defensiveness. Although some of these manifestations may result in a decreased ability to play, it is a "quantum leap" from poor tactile discrimination to impaired play skills. We must make that leap with care.

Research on Play and Sensory Integration

The premise that sensory integrative dysfunction results in impaired play skills in young children was investigated in a series of studies conducted by Bundy (1987, 1989) and Clifford (now O'Brien) and Bundy (1989). They observed 61 boys (30 typically developing and 31 diagnosed as having sensory integrative dysfunction) during 30 minutes of free play, both indoors and outdoors. They recorded play behaviors on the Preschool Play Scale (Bledsoe & Shepherd, 1982).

The mean scores of the boys with sensory integrative dysfunction were significantly lower than those of the other boys on the overall score of the Preschool Play Scale and on three of its four dimensions: Space Management, Material Management, and Participation. However, further analysis of the data revealed that approximately one third of the boys with sensory integrative dysfunction received scores on the Preschool Play Scale that were no more than 6 months below the norm for their chronological ages and well within the range for the typically developing boys. Thus, sensory integrative dysfunction does not always result in play deficits.

Furthermore, although Bundy (1987) found statistically significant correlations between scores on the Preschool Play Scale and scores on the *Bruininks-Oseretsky Test of Motor Proficiency* (Bruininks, 1978), none of the correlations exceeded $r = 0.40$; most were much lower. Thus, boys with the poorest motor coordination (and theoretically the worst sensory integrative dysfunction) were not necessarily the ones whose play skills were the most impaired and vice versa.

Finally, using the Preschool Play Materials Preference Inventory (Wolfgang & Phelps, 1983) and the Preschool Play Scale (Bledsoe & Shepherd, 1982), Clifford and Bundy (1989) demonstrated that preschool-aged boys, with or without sensory integrative dysfunction, preferred toys that supported sensorimotor play (e.g., swings, slides) over toys that supported construction or symbolic play. However, when the boys' preferences (percentage of toys they selected from each play category) were compared with their actual scores on related Preschool Play Scale domains, many boys had apparently altered their play preferences to match their abilities. Fewer than one-third of the boys with sensory integrative dysfunction expressed strong preference for any domain of play in which their play skills were not age appropriate.

What Sensory Integration Theory and Play Research Do Not (or Cannot) Tell Us

The research conducted to date has indicated that sensory integrative dysfunction does not always result in disruption to play skills and behaviors. However, the research in this area has been limited to preschool-aged boys with heterogeneous types of sensory integrative dysfunction. Furthermore, the assessment tools used to date have captured play skills and play material preferences rather than playfulness. Thus, the research is riddled with unknowns. What consequences does sensory integrative dysfunction have on the play of older children and adults? Are individuals with sensory integrative dysfunction less playful than typically developing individuals? Does sensory integrative dysfunction differentially affect the play of boys and girls? What are the consequences of altering play preferences (particularly in children) to reflect the individual's actual abilities?

Certainly, children who always avoid playing with other children for fear that they will be touched deprive themselves of one of the most important arenas in which to develop the social skills they will need throughout their lives. Is the same true of motor skills? How much motor play is required for individuals to practice the motor behaviors they will need to function adequately in daily life (Clifford & Bundy, 1989)? Vandenberg (1981) suggested that social interaction is more apt to occur in the context of gross motor than fine motor play. If that is true, then clients who avoid gross motor play may inadvertently deprive themselves of the chance to develop and practice social skills. These are only a few of the many questions that remain to be answered through future research.

Although only Bundy and Clifford (Bundy, 1987, 1989; Clifford & Bundy, 1989) have systematically studied the play skills of individuals with sensory integrative dysfunction, a few related studies describing the play (or leisure) of children and adolescents with learning disabilities have been completed (Bryan, 1976, 1978; Levy & Gottlieb, 1984; Margalit, 1984). Although the results of these studies cannot fully answer the questions we have posed, they suggest that the questions are valid and have important implications for intervention.

Margalit (1984) reported that the leisure time of adolescents with learning disabilities was apt to be comprised largely of activities such as television watching. Other researchers (Bryan, 1976, 1978; Levy & Gottlieb, 1984) have concentrated on the sociometric status of children with learning disabilities and on their ability to appropriately enter social situations. Not surprisingly, most of these researchers have found their subjects to be relatively isolated and to lack the skills to initiate and respond to social situations.

If the results of these studies can be extrapolated to individuals with sensory integrative dysfunction (and any extrapolation of this nature certainly must be done with caution), then it is important that we do all we can to facilitate play. In some cases, this may mean working to improve the individual's sensory integration. In other cases, it may mean working directly on play. Most times, it probably means both.

Clearly, the ability to process sensation may influence, in some way, individuals' abilities to play. Thus, sensory integration theory provides practitioners with information that may explain some of a client's problems in play. Likewise, observations of clients in play can provide practitioners with valuable information about their sensory integrative capacities. Finally, play is a critical component of sensory integration intervention. However, sensory integrative theory is not primarily about play; it is a theory about some of the neurobehavioral foundations for play. Play is an extremely complex function (Sutton-Smith, 1997); it is the end product of interaction among a number of inborn traits and acquired skills. Sensory integration is only one of many foundations of play.

PRINCIPLES FOR ASSESSING PLAY AND TREATING PLAY DEFICITS IN CLIENTS WITH SENSORY INTEGRATIVE DYSFUNCTION

The relationship between sensory integration and play is not simple, nor is it clear, either from the theory or the existing research. There are five important points that are related to the play of clients with sensory integrative dysfunction.

First, to find out about how well clients play, watch them play. Watch for signs that sensory integrative dysfunction interferes with skill, but watch for more than that. Watch to see how well they play. Furthermore, it is important to observe individuals playing in a number of different types of environments. A study by Vandenberg (1981) suggested that the playthings available to individuals in various settings had a marked effect on the types of

play in which the children engaged. Vandenberg found that more social interaction occurred in settings that encouraged gross motor play than in settings that encouraged fine motor play. He believed that children engaged in fine motor play had less need to interact with peers because the activities promoted parallel play. This study has important implications for practitioners who have limited time but nevertheless wish to assess the social play skills or playfulness of clients.

Standardized tools such as the Test of Playfulness (Bundy, 2000), the Revised Preschool Play Scale (Knox, 1997), and the Test of Environmental Supportiveness (Bundy, 1999) provide systematic means for observing children's playfulness, the skills they use in play, and the relative supportiveness of the environment for play, respectively. Other assessments such as the Client Behaviors Inventory of Playfulness (Rogers et al, 1998) provide a descriptive assessment of children's playfulness. The assessment is completed by the client's parents or another adult who knows the client well. Standardized tools greatly improve the quality of assessments of play.

Occupational therapy evaluations, especially evaluations of sensory integrative function, are time consuming and costly. Many practitioners believe they cannot justify the expenditure of additional time to observe individuals playing. However, the importance of play to an individual's life cannot be overemphasized. By itself, sensory integrative dysfunction is not a problem to be addressed by occupational therapy; however, sensory integrative dysfunction becomes a problem when it disrupts an individual's ability to perform daily life activity (including play) and assume expected life roles (including the role of player).

Second, if you want to find out whether or not individuals are happy with their play skills, ask them. Ask the child's parents and teacher. Find out who their best friends are and why they like those particular friends. Ask whom they would really like to play with if they could play with anyone, and find out why. Even when clients are very young, find out what they most like to do and what they least like to do, and find out why. Much information, about both individuals and their sensory integrative function and dysfunction, can be gleaned in this way. There may well be important differences between clients who are happy with their play (even if that time is spent doing something very different from their peers) and clients who really want to do what everybody else does but lack the skills. The latter individual is certainly at more risk for impaired self-esteem (Clifford & Bundy, 1989).

Although asking questions directly is certainly one way to get answers, there are also assessment tools that address individual preferences in play. Most of these tools are quite simplistic as well as quick and easy to administer. Some, such as the Pediatric Interest Profiles (Henry, 2000), involve only pointing to pictures of preferred activities or answering questions in a paper and pencil format (for adolescents). The advantage of using a tool to ascertain this information is that it gives individuals a chance to respond to a number of choices. Thus, the practitioner has a more global picture of the child's preferences in play.

Third, do not assume that improving individuals' sensory integrative functioning will automatically improve their play. Play, similar to many of the more well-recognized outcome of sensory integration (e.g., improved motor skills and self-esteem), is a complex phenomenon. Over time, individuals learn what they can and cannot do in play. Often their beliefs about their skills do not change just because their skills or sensory integration improve. Many practitioners have had the experience of suggesting an activity to clients who respond that they "can't do that." Practitioners may be quite sure that the clients could perform the activity. If they are coaxed into trying, they may be quite delighted with their newfound skills. However, the very fact that many clients balk at trying activities at which they previously may have been unsuccessful suggests that self perceptions are not automatically adjusted to reflect improvements in skill or in sensory integrative functioning.

Furthermore, newly developed skills that may be accomplished in a clinic under the vigilant eye and hand of an occupational therapy practitioner may not be generalized automatically to the playground or the home. In observing children, both on an adventure playground and in therapy, Levitt (1975) found that the level of the children's skills was higher in the structured therapy session than on the playground. Apparently, before clients can use a skill spontaneously, that skill must be practiced many times in an environment free of the consequences that would be associated with performing that same skill in "real life." The example of Max learning to play dodgeball is only one of countless such examples we have seen.

Fourth, if the goal is to improve both play and sensory integrative functioning, it is necessary to play with the individual. The individual with deficits in both play and sensory integration needs a role model for good play and assistance to learn how to play (Dunkerley et al., 1997; Lyons, 1984; Tickle-Degnen & Coster, 1995). In fact, Sutton-Smith (1980) suggested that the roles of coach and spectator may be even more important than those of the player in establishing play transactions. Practitioners working with clients who have difficulty playing need to take extra care to be certain that all the elements of play (e.g., relative intrinsic motivation, relative internal control, and freedom from some of the constraints of reality) are present in therapeutic sessions.

Finally, it is necessary to talk to clients and caregivers or significant others about the differences between the way the client perceives the world and the way other people perceive it. Encourage children to bring a friend to therapy. A practitioner can easily schedule intervention that meets the needs of the client but also includes a friend. Parents can be very helpful in assisting children to choose a friend who will participate readily in the therapeutic regimen. The chosen friend usually loves to attend the sessions and, even with older children, the stigma of therapy is thereby easily eliminated. We are not suggesting that intervention based on sensory integrative theory should be conducted with two clients simultaneously. We discuss that issue more fully in Chapter 12. Rather, we are suggesting that conducting intervention with one client and a typically developing friend has many advantages, including the development of social skills and the provision of shared experiences that may form a basis for friendship.

SUMMARY AND CONCLUSION

Play is a powerful tool for intervention. For many clients, the most important byproduct of occupational therapy may be the improved ability to play. If it is carefully planned and conducted, intervention using the principles of sensory integration may be very helpful in facilitating the development of play. Likewise, play, as a part of a well-orchestrated intervention plan, can result in improvements in sensory integration. Although sensory integrative dysfunction may result in disruptions to play, we should not assume that all individuals who have sensory integrative dysfunction also have deficits in play. Clearly, more research is needed in this area.

References

Anderson, J., Hinojosa, J., & Strauch, C. (1987). Integrating play in neurodevelopmental treatment. *American Journal of Occupational Therapy, 41,* 421–426.

Ayres, A. J. (1972). *Sensory integration and learning disorders.* Los Angeles: Western Psychological Services.

Bateson, G. (1972). Toward a theory of play and fantasy. In G. Bateson (Ed.), *Steps to an ecology of the mind* (pp. 177–193). New York: Bantam.

Berlyne, D. E. (1966). Curiosity and exploration. *Science, 153,* 25–33.

Berlyne, D. E. (1969). Laughter, humor and play. In G. Lindzert & E. Aronson (Eds.). *The handbook of social psychology* (Vol 3). Reading, MA: Addison-Wesley.

Bledsoe, N. P., & Shepherd, J. T. (1982). A study of reliability and validity of a preschool play scale. *American Journal of Occupational Therapy, 36,* 783–788.

Bryan, T. (1976). Peer popularity of learning disabled children: A replication. *Journal of Learning Disabilities, 7,* 34–43.

Bryan, T. (1978). Social relationships and verbal interactions of learning disabled children. *Journal of Learning Disabilities, 11,* 107–115.

Bruininks, R. H. (1978). *Bruininks-Oseretsky Test of Motor Proficiency examiner's manual.* Circle Pines, MN: American Guidance Service.

Bundy, A. C. (1987). The play of preschoolers: Its relationship to balance and motor proficiency and the effect of sensory integrative dysfunction. Doctoral dissertation, Boston University.

Bundy, A. C. (1989). A comparison of the play skills of normal boys and boys with sensory integrative dysfunction. *Occupational Therapy Journal of Research, 9,* 84–100.

Bundy, A. C. (1999). *Test of environmental support-iveness (TOES) manual.* Ft. Collins, CO: Colorado State University.

Bundy, A. C. (2000). *Test of playfulness manual* (Version 3). Ft. Collins, CO: Colorado State University.

Caillois, R. (1979). *Man, play, and games.* New York: Schocken.

Clifford, J. M., & Bundy, A. C. (1989). Play preference and play performance in normal boys and boys with sensory integrative dysfunction. *Occupational Therapy Journal of Research, 9,* 202–217.

Csikszentmihayli, M. (1975a). *Beyond boredom and anxiety.* San Francisco: Jossey-Bass.

Csikszentmihayli, M. (1975b). Play and intrinsic rewards. *Humanistic Psychology, 15,* 41–63.

Csikszentmihayli, M. (1979). The concept of flow. In B. Sutton-Smith (Ed.). *Play and learning* (pp. 257–274). New York: Gardner.

Csikszentmihayli, M. (1990). *Flow: The psychology of optimal experience.* New York: Harper-Collins.

Csikszentmihayli, M. (1993). *The evolving self: A psychology for the third millennium.* New York: Harper-Collins.

Csikszentmihayli, M. (1996). *Creativity: Flow and the psychology of discovery and invention.* New York: Harper-Collins.

Csikszentmihayli, M. (1997). *Finding flow: The psychology of engagement with everyday life.* New York: Basic.

Dunkerley, E., Tickle-Degnen, L., & Coster, W. (1997). Therapist-child interaction in the middle minutes of sensory integration treatment. *American Journal of Occupational Therapy, 51,* 799–805.

Henry, A. (2000). *The pediatric interest profiles: Surveys of play for children and adolescents.* San Antonio: Therapy Skill Builders.

Knox, S. (1997). Development and current use of the Knox Preschool Play Scale. In L. D. Parham & L. S. Fazio (Eds.). *Play in occupational therapy for children,* (pp. 35–51). St. Louis: Mosby.

Kooij, R. V., & Vrijhof, H. J. (1981). Play and development. *Topics in Learning and Learning Disabilities, 1,* 57–67.

Levitt, S. (1975). A study of the gross motor skills of cerebral palsied children in an adventure playground for handicapped children. *Client Care, Health and Development, 1,* 29–43.

Levy, L., & Gottlieb, J. (1984). Learning and non-learning disabled children at play. *Remedial and Special Education, 5,* 43–50.

Lindquist, J. E., Mack, W., & Parham, L. D. (1982). A synthesis of occupational behavior and sensory integration concepts in theory and practice, Part 2: Clinical applications. *American Journal of Occupational Therapy, 36,* 433–437.

Lyons, M. (1984). A taxonomy of playfulness for use in occupational therapy. *Australian Occupational Therapy Journal, 4,* 152–156.

Margalit, M. (1984). Leisure activities of learning disabled children as a reflection of their passive life style and prolonged dependency. *Client Psychiatry and Human Development, 15,* 133–141.

Morrison, C. D., Bundy, A. C., & Fisher, A. G. (1991). The contribution of motor skills and play-fulness to play. *American Journal of Occupational Therapy, 45,* 687–694.

Neumann, E. A. (1971). *The elements of play.* New York: MSS Information.

Piaget, J. (1962). *Play, dreams and imitation in child-hood.* New York: Norton.

Rast, M. (1986). Play and therapy, play or therapy? In C. Pehoski (Ed.). *Play: A skill for life* (pp. 29–42). Rockville, MD: American Occupational Therapy Association.

Rogers, C. S., Impara, J. C., Frary, R. B., Harris, T., Meeks, A., Semanic-Lauth, S., & Reynolds, M. R. (1998). Measuring playfulness: Development of the client behaviors inventory of playfulness. In S. Reifel (Ed.). *Play & culture studies* (Vol. 1, pp. 121–136). Greenwich, CT: Ablex.

Rubin, K., Fein, G. G., & Vandenberg, B. (1983). Play. In P. H. Mussen (Ed.). *Handbook of child psychology: Socialization, personality and social development* (4th ed, vol. 4, pp. 693–774). New York: Wiley.

Sawyer, R. K. (1997). *Pretend play as improvisation: Conversation in the preschool classroom*. Mahwah, NJ: Lawrence Erlbaum Associates.

Sutton-Smith, B. (1980). A "sportive" theory of play. In H. Schwartzman (Ed.), *Play and culture* (pp. 10–19). West Point, NY: Leisure.

Sutton-Smith, B. (1997). *The ambiguity of play*. Cambridge, MA: Harvard University.

Tickle-Degnen, L., & Coster, W. (1995). Therapeutic interaction and the management of challenge during the beginning minutes of sensory integration treatment. *Occupational Therapy Journal of Research, 15,* 122–141.

Vandenberg, B. (1981). Environmental and cognitive factors in social play. *Journal of Experimental Psychology, 31,* 169–175.

Vandenberg, B., & Kielhofner, G. (1982). Play in evolution, culture and individual adaptation: Implications for therapy. *American Journal of Occupational Therapy, 36,* 20–28.

West, M. A. (1888). *Childhood: Its care and culture.* New York: Law, King & Law.

White, R. W. (1959). Motivation reconsidered: The concept of competence. *Psychological Review, 66,* 297–323.

Wolfgang, C., & Phelps, P. (1983). Preschool play materials preference inventory. *Early Child Development and Care, 12,* 127–141.

Orchestrating Intervention: The Art of Practice

Anita C. Bundy, ScD, OTR, FAOTA
Jane A. Koomar, PhD, OTR, FAOTA

> *The kind of involvement necessary to achieve the state wherein the child becomes effectively self-directing within the structure set by the therapist cannot be commanded; it must be elicited. Therein lies the art of therapy.*
>
> —Ayres, 1972, p. 259

Occupational therapy has long been defined as an art as well as a science (American Occupational Therapy Council on Standards, 1972; Neistadt & Crepeau, 1998). Whereas science is associated explicitly with knowledge and theory (Mosey, 1981), art is centered on relationships (Peloquin, 1989, 1990, 1998) and the creative and meaningful use of activity (Creighton et al., 1995; Peloquin, 1989, 1998). Science is logical, but our understanding of art seems almost ethereal. Artist Alex Grey (1998) stated, "Art is a communion of one soul to another" (p. 19). "The artist's mission may not ever be reduced to words or rationally understood, but its invisible magnetizing presence will infuse an artist's work completely" (p. 10).

Although a great deal about art is mysterious, Peloquin (1989) indicated that art is the soul of occupational therapy practice. Its benefits are apparent. Art enables practitioners to engender trust, un-

cover and tap motivation, read and respond to cues, and skillfully adjust the challenge and flow of therapeutic activity. "At its best, art . . . inspire[s] and transform[s] us" (Grey, 1998, p. 9). Mosey (1981) claimed that "without art . . . occupational therapy would become the application of scientific knowledge in a sterile vacuum" (Peloquin, 1989, p. 220).

Although the art of practice is critical to occupational therapy, the concept applies equally well across virtually all disciplines. No doubt we have all read or heard stories about a physician who diagnosed a patient's rare disease, a psychotherapist whose work with a client was nothing short of "miraculous," or an architect or landscaper who brilliantly incorporated his or her creation into an existing place, preserving and enhancing its natural beauty. Those practitioners succeeded because of art.

PURPOSE AND SCOPE

Occupational therapy, in general, and intervention based on sensory integration theory, in particular, are about "self-actualization" and enabling clients to do what they need and want to do in their daily lives (Fisher & Murray, 1991; Neistadt & Crepeau, 1998). A number of noteworthy events, decisions, and processes comprise the course of intervention. To advance smoothly, all aspects of the process depend on art. This chapter discusses several important aspects of intervention that depend on art:

- Deciding what to target first
- Therapist–client relationships
- Establishing a safe environment
- Incorporating competition
- Assuming pretend roles
- Voicing praise, feedback, and instructions
- Creating the "just-right" challenge
- Balancing freedom with structure
- Striving to find inner drive
- Modifying or discontinuing activities

Finally, the chapter considers ways in which practitioners can help clients understand sensory integrative dysfunction, bring intervention to a close, and become more artful. Although we cannot provide "rules" regarding the art associated with intervention, we offer stories and practical wisdom garnered through our experience as sources of insight. Because the art of practice is associated closely with playfulness, we also refer readers to Chapter 10.

DECIDING WHAT TO TARGET FIRST

After we have concluded that a client's presenting difficulties can be explained in some meaningful way by sensory integration theory and have set objectives together with clients and caregivers, we must decide what to target first in intervention in order to build a firm foundation for meeting those objectives. For clients with sensory integrative dysfunction, the term "foundation" refers to both the processing of sensation *and* sequelae such as postural competence, praxis, and modulation (see Fig. 1–3). These are some of the important building blocks on which occupational performance is built.

As much as any part of the intervention process, deciding what to target first demands artful reflection. After the decision is made, we act as though it is correct—that is, we plan intervention that directly reflects our decision. However, we are aware that our decision may not be on target, so we constantly look for evidence regarding how accurate it was. When the evidence suggests that we need to change the focus of intervention, we do so. We illustrate the process of deciding what to target first in intervention with two vignettes. In the first, we relate a story in which the evidence suggested that the decision we made was a good one. In the second, we had to change the initial target.

Melanie, a 5-year-old kindergartner, exhibited several problematic classroom behaviors. She frequently reported that other children hit her, although the children said they had just tapped Melanie (e.g., to get her attention) and the teacher had never observed any hitting. Melanie moved around the classroom constantly, rarely sitting for more than a few moments. She continually manipulated objects, her own and other people's. Melanie also became inconsolable when the bell or fire drill sounded.

Melanie had an unusual habit of climbing onto the shelf above the coat rack and jumping off. The teacher was puzzled by this behavior because Melanie did not appear to do it for attention. In fact, she seemed somewhat oblivious to the reactions of her teacher and peers. When asked directly why she did this, Melanie replied, "It feels good to jump."

Melanie experienced significant difficulty in physical education class and on the playground. She had not mastered skipping despite individual sessions with the physical education teacher. Her parents reported that she was unable to pump a swing, a skill most neighborhood children had mastered before their fourth birthdays. She typically ran around aimlessly during recess. She did not seem to judge her position in relation to the swings and was at risk of being hit.

In addition to gross motor and modulation difficulties, Melanie was not interested in coloring or writing the letters of her name. When she was cajoled into writing, her skills were poor. Her lack of interest and poor skills concerned her parents and teacher.

Occupational therapy assessment revealed that Melanie had somatodyspraxia and sensory defensiveness. We used the results of the assessment to explain Melanie's daily life difficulties and contributed to the following goals that became part of her individualized educational program (IEP). Melanie will:

- Not overreact to light touch and loud sounds in the classroom.
- Refrain from inappropriate behaviors (e.g., jumping from unsafe surfaces, manipulating others' possessions).
- Play safely on the playground.
- Be able to skip and to pump a swing.
- Be able to write all the letters and numbers legibly.

To meet these goals, we decided to focus *first* on improving Melanie's sensory modulation. We would determine the effectiveness of intervention (and how good our decision had been) by observing Melanie's response to unexpected touch and noise and her tendency to inappropriately seek sensory input. We hoped that improved *processing* of sensation (of which modulation is a part) would also contribute to improved body schema, postural control, and praxis, thus enabling her to develop the gross and fine motor skills needed for skipping, pumping a swing, and printing. If we found evidence of developing skill, we would conclude that our decision about what to target first had been a good one.

To improve modulation, we provided Melanie with activities that involved movement and resistance to active movement. Melanie especially liked activities that involved swinging prone in the frog swing (Fig. 11–1). We also provided her with enhanced tactile sensation (e.g., hiding her body in the bubble ball bath and finding large objects buried in a box filled with dried beans) (Fig. 11–2).

We focused on improving Melanie's sensory modulation to help her respond more appropriately to daily life events. In improving sensory processing, we also hoped that her body schema, extensor muscle tone, and postural stability would improve because many activities provided resistance to movement and the resulting enhanced proprioception should contribute to those functions.

Although from the beginning Melanie had great difficulty with skipping, pumping the swing, and coloring, we did not begin by training her to do these tasks. Her ability to use sensation and her body seemed inadequate to enable her to benefit from practice of skilled movements. At the same time, we would not focus exclusively on modulating sensation without paying *any* attention to motor skills and abilities.

As Melanie showed signs of improved sensory modulation by demonstrating more appropriate responses in daily life events, we began to work *more directly* on postural stability, praxis, and ultimately skill development. However, we try never to lose sight of the fact that our primary target initially was improved modulation.

After several months, Melanie responded with neutral or positive affect to light touch and a wide variety of noises. Soon thereafter, she was able to retrieve small objects (e.g., pennies, small pegs) from the bean box, suggesting improved tactile dis-

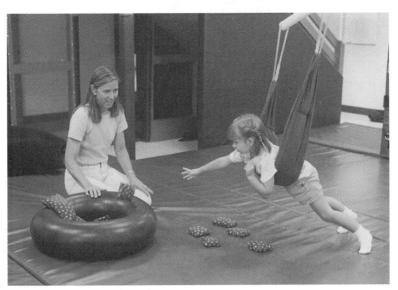

■ Figure 11–1 Swinging prone in the frog swing. (Photo by Shay McAtee, printed with permission.)

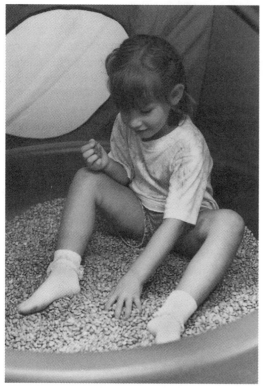

■ FIGURE 11-2 Digging for objects buried in a box filled with dried beans. (Photo by Shay McAtee, printed with permission.)

crimination and fine motor skill. At the same time, her teacher reported that Melanie's inappropriate manipulation of objects in the classroom had lessened greatly. She also began to experiment with painting at an easel and coloring during free play.

After another period of time, Melanie no longer craved intense vestibular proprioception. At the same time, she also stopped jumping from the coat rack.

As her postural control and body schema improved, Melanie was able to use a greater variety of equipment that demands extensor tone and postural adjustments (e.g., glider swing, scooter board). Eventually she developed the bilateral coordination and sequencing abilities necessary to swing while throwing beanbags or balls at a moving target. At the same time, she became interested in pumping a swing and skipping. After practicing repeatedly for a week, she was able to perform these skills well, which was a source of considerable joy for Melanie. Safety was no longer a concern during recess. In addition, Melanie was now writing her name and printing all the letters well.

Deciding where to begin in intervention represents a tremendous challenge to the art of prac-

tice. When modulation is a problem, we generally address it early in the process and hope to simultaneously recognize other gains. However, there are no hard and fast rules about what to target first. Furthermore, some clients experience more than one type of modulation dysfunction. So, how do we decide what to target first?

Jody, a 26-year-old client, experienced significant problems with both sensory defensiveness and gravitational insecurity. She complained that tactile defensiveness, in particular, got in her way both at work and in interpersonal relationships. Thus, it seemed logical to begin intervention by providing enhanced tactile sensation in an attempt to decrease its effects. However, Jody could not tolerate any tactile sensation, even when she administered it to herself. Furthermore, Jody's severe gravitational insecurity presented a particular barrier to the use of a sensory integrative–based approach in intervention. Thus, because we seemed to be making little headway in decreasing Jody's tactile defensiveness (i.e., the decision we made seemed to be wrong), we switched tacks and began to address her gravitational insecurity. Jody engaged in numerous activities that provided resistance to movement (i.e., proprioception) and linear vestibular sensation (see Chapter 12). After some weeks, Jody reacted to movement with far less fear. Although she was pleased with this change, she was far more excited to report that her *tactile defensiveness* had decreased.

Jody's decreased tactile defensiveness was an unexpected benefit. Thus, we attempted to use theory to explain it. We have hypothesized that dysfunction in sensory modulation is a result of poor sensory processing, at least in part within the reticular and limbic systems (see Chapter 2). Apparently, it was possible to improve tactile processing with activity providing enhanced vestibular and proprioceptive sensations. Possibly because both the limbic and reticular structures play a role in integrating sensory input, one form of enhanced sensation may have an effect on the processing of another type of sensation.

In Jody's case, listening to our more artful selves led to a change in how to proceed with intervention, and the results were greater than those we initially sought. We were able to uncover a plausible explanation for the results. Being mindful of unanticipated gains and their theoretical roots contributed to the development of artful practice. Now we no longer assume that the best intervention for tactile defensiveness has a tactile base.

THERAPIST–CLIENT RELATIONSHIPS

Occupational therapy always occurs in the context of interpersonal relationships. Several authors in occupational therapy literature (Ayres, 1972; Creighton et al., 1995; Dunkerley et al., 1997; Mattingly & Fleming, 1994; Mosey, 1981; Peloquin, 1998; Tickle-Degnan & Coster, 1995) have written implicitly or explicitly about the art of practice. Tickle-Degen and Coster (1995) and Dunkerley et al. (1997) wrote specifically about therapist–client interactions in the context of sensory integration-based intervention, finding in general that practitioners and children were playful and worked hard together during the sessions.

In occupational therapy, as in psychotherapy, the relationships between clients and practitioners play an important role in the outcome of intervention (Eltz & Shirk, 1995; Hopkins & Tiffany, 1983; Luborsky et al., 1988; Orlinsky & Howard, 1986; Peloquin, 1990; Shirk & Russell, 1996; Shirk & Saiz, 1992). In fact, Kaplan et al. (1993) suggested that the intense bond that forms between practitioner and client *may be responsible for* changes that occur as a result of intervention based on the principles of sensory integration theory. The therapeutic alliance permeates the intervention process. The art lies in establishing and maintaining the relationship, a process we discuss as it ebbs and flows both within a single session and across the entire program of intervention.

The intervention process begins with a client's or caregiver's initial contact with a therapist, often to inquire about evaluation. The process continues across a number of steps, including assessment and, when indicated, intervention planning, implementation, and discontinuation. We discuss a number of aspects of this process in this chapter, in Chapter 9, and elsewhere (Bundy, 1995). The relationship between the client and practitioner is critical. When the client is a child, forming a therapeutic alliance can be particularly tricky for reasons Shirk and Russell (1996) have elucidated. The art of building a therapeutic relationship lies in the practitioner's ability to become a helper.

The Therapeutic Alliance

Shirk and Russell (1996) used the term *therapeutic alliance* to refer to a type of relationship that enables clients to work purposefully on resolving their difficulties. Thus, shared goals and the sense that the practitioner will help the client to meet those goals are important aspects of the therapeutic alliance. Engaging children, especially young children, in goal setting can be difficult because setting goals implies the willingness and ability of children to acknowledge their limitations. The ability to recognize difficulties and contribute to a plan aimed explicitly at minimizing them requires a certain level of trust as well as cognitive development; it also requires that the practitioner facilitate the process. The problems faced by occupational therapy practitioners in developing the kind of alliance described by Shirk and Russell (1996) are similar to those faced by psychotherapists who treat children. Shirk and Russell described a source of some of the difficulties.

> All too often it seems that the preparatory "relationship building" period [of the intervention process] centers exclusively on the development of positive feelings between child and therapist. Practically, "preparation" is translated to mean that the therapist joins the child as a friendly playmate who does nothing to upset the emerging relationship, for example, by introducing disturbing issues. In turn, the process of therapy often appears to bog down in endless sessions . . . of activities that seem peripheral to the child's difficulties. In fact, the therapy has not "bogged down" but has been shaped by a definition of treatment that omits any reference to therapeutic work. Although one cannot assume that children will orient immediately to the therapist as a helper, equally one cannot expect children to spontaneously discuss their problems and difficulties if the therapist makes no effort to define the relationship as a helping relationship. In other words, the preparatory period of child therapy involves more than development of a positive generic relationship; it involves the development of a positive, *helping* relationship. *The therapist's goal is not simply to be viewed as a positive emotional valence, although this goal can be challenging with some children and is essential for all else in therapy, but instead is to be regarded as [a] person who can be helpful with . . . [minimizing] difficulties* (p. 174) (italics added).

Because activities associated with intervention based on the principles of sensory integration theory can be so much fun, it is easy for practitioners to become "friendly playmates" and neglect their role in helping children recognize their difficulties and collaborate in goal setting and intervention planning. To fail to develop the type of therapeutic alliance to which Shirk and Russell (1996) speak is to undermine both the capacity of the child and the power of intervention. Shirk and Russell, who, in their practice of psychotherapy, have also faced difficulties similar to those encountered by occupational therapists, offered the following:

> This task [of setting goals for intervention] may be one of the most difficult, yet least discussed, problems in child psychotherapy. . . The child's aims may be quite different from the parents'. Whereas the parents may be seeking greater compliance and fewer challenges to their authority, for example, the child may be interested in relief from parental demands. . . . As a starting point in building a working alliance, it can be useful for the therapist to focus on helping the child differentiate his or her own goals for treatment from the goals of referring adults. By offering the child one's best efforts to meet these goals, the therapist is positioned as an ally of the child. This does not mean, however, that the therapist has to accept the child's goals without qualification, particularly if this means joining the child in the denial of obvious problems. Instead the negotiation of a mutually shared definition of a problem is the central task of this phase of therapy. And for the purposes of establishing a working alliance, the initial consensual goals may not be the most important goals for treatment. Instead, the aim, at this point in treatment, is to define the therapy relationship as a working relationship, and this can be facilitated by initially addressing goals that may be somewhat peripheral to the central problems presented by the child. Nevertheless, by forging an alliance around such goals, the therapist's role as a helper . . . becomes clearly defined (p. 175).

The following description illustrates the development of a therapeutic alliance with Christian, a 12-year-old boy with sensory-integrative-based dyspraxia who participated in a 5-day intervention course. Christian and his family met with the occupational therapists to set goals for his intervention. They planned to set only one goal that would logically respond to intervention based on the principles of sensory integrative theory. Predictably, Christian's goals were different from those of his parents. His mother wanted his goal to be "improved running" because peers made fun of the way he ran. Christian, who had both fine motor and gross motor difficulties, wanted to be better at "putting his models together." Wanting to form a therapeutic alliance with Christian but understanding that his goal might not be the highest priority (i.e., his fine motor difficulties did not seem to be causing nearly as many problems as his poor gross motor skills) or the best match for sensory integration, the therapists embraced both goals. Their decision was firmly entrenched in art. The therapists felt confident enough to listen to their intuition and let go of their "assignment" to create only one goal. Perhaps in part because Christian knew that the therapists heard him, he became invested in the therapy and saw the therapists as people who would help him. They forged a true therapeutic alliance.

ESTABLISHING A SAFE ENVIRONMENT

In intervention based on the principles of sensory integration theory, clients are asked to engage in activities that may expose vulnerabilities; this can feel very threatening. For clients to engage fully in the therapeutic process, we must engender their trust—that is, we must provide clients with the sense that they are safe, both physically and emotionally. We remain near enough to be involved in the process and prevent accidents, yet far away enough to promote self-direction and challenge.

A significant portion of promoting emotional safety lies in a therapist's artful ability to give a message that clients will not be asked to do more than they are able. Within the safe space that therapy becomes, they will not experience the negative emotions (e.g., shame, discouragement) that may be common in their day-to-day lives. That, of course, does not mean that clients will never fall down or fail to hit a target. In fact, they would likely become quite bored if every attempt yielded success (Csikszentmihayli, 1975a, 1990, 1993, 1996). Rather, creating a safe environment means that a practitioner carefully matches task demands to a client's abilities and emotional needs, provides support and assistance as needed, and handles a client's successes and failures in a way that promotes growth and safety, including giving honest feedback.

Luke, a 6-year-old boy with significant motor difficulties that stemmed from sensory integrative–based dyspraxia, rarely experienced success on any motor task in his daily life. As he climbed to the top of a jungle gym, the therapist assisted him surreptitiously by helping him to shift his weight to the proper foot each time he came to a corner; this enabled him to smoothly go around the corners. She gave no verbal instruction. When Luke reached the top, both he and the therapist were delighted. "You did it," the therapist exclaimed, and Luke echoed her praise. "Yes, I did!"

Other strategies also give a nonverbal message that therapy is a safe place. For example, young children in particular may need time to observe an activity before they do it. One therapist began a session with a very timid child by putting a stuffed animal in the swing and saying, "My bunny loves to swing. Do you want to push her"? A little later, she asked the child, "Would you like a turn on the swing now"?

Practitioners often become directly involved in therapeutic activities. Our active involvement not only demonstrates that activities are safe but also sends a message about their importance. In addition, it is more fun to do most activities together than alone. We might sit together in a cozy spot while exploring tactile materials. Or we might swing together on a bolster swing, falling off into large cushions, or bat at each other with foam bats as we attempt to balance on inflated inner tubes (Fig. 11–3).

Many children respond positively to a therapist's need for assistance, "Can you help me put the 'meatballs' [medicine balls] in my big bowl of spaghetti [inner tube]? They are so heavy!" When a child is able to provide assistance to an adult, the child usually feels important. Furthermore, some children who feel vulnerable seem to be particularly sensitive to others' needs for assistance.

INCORPORATING COMPETITION

Many clients enjoy competitive games. However, some children are particularly sensitive to failure and unable to deal with true competition. An example of an activity we have used with children who seem particularly sensitive to failure involves throwing "food" (beanbags) to the "baby fish in the pond" (inner tube). When the food goes outside the pond, the big fish in the ocean gladly eat it! Throwing at a target is a common component of competitive games but, in this case, it is not how many points the child obtains or who wins but whether or not the fish eat that becomes the outcome. In activities such as this, there is no competition and little risk of failure.

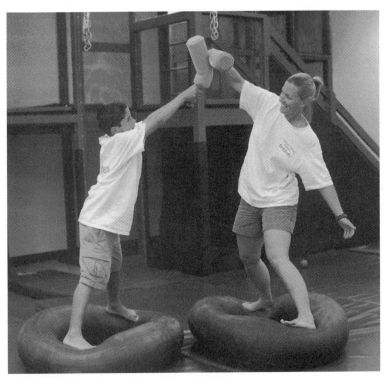

■ FIGURE 11–3 Balancing on a large inner tube while play fighting with Nerf bats. (Photo by Shay McAtee, printed with permission.)

Another activity with minimal competition also involves throwing beanbags or balls into a container. In this activity, each time the client hits a target with the beanbag, the clients get the point; when the client misses the target, we get the point. We design and adapt these activities carefully to ensure that clients hit the target enough of the time to feel successful but not so often that they become bored.

Sometimes activities involve friendly competition. For example, each of us may try to knock over a row of blocks that the other is "defending." Children can sense when we are not trying hard enough or are letting them win. Thus, we should minimize our deliberate failures (e.g., "bad shots"). Instead, we can "handicap" ourselves by increasing the distance to our targets or increasing the number of our targets. Another strategy we have found useful for minimizing the discrepancy between our skill and that of our clients is to change places (and scores) midway through a game (Schaefer & Reid, 1986). In this way, children play from a position of relative advantage gained when they take over the lead. Children usually accept these strategies, especially if we remind them that we have a lot of chance to practice.

ASSUMING PRETEND ROLES

Some children seem to love the feelings of power associated with subduing a "bad guy" or the thrill of being scared (Cohen, 1987). Thus, practitioners may play imaginary adversarial or scary roles as a part of an activity. However, we caution practitioners who get into the habit of playing such roles without an invitation from a child. Many children with sensory integrative dysfunction are particularly vulnerable and become overly frightened. With vulnerable children, we prefer to play assistive roles. Instead of being a bad guy, we join the "good team" and together with the child go after the bad guys. We relegate adversarial or scary roles to a punching bag or other inanimate object.

Creating a funny situation involving pretend play often can draw children into an activity without their realizing it. Will, a 4-year-old boy who had gravitational insecurity and dyspraxia, typically refused any new activities. His therapist stuck large therapy balls inside a Spandex hammock hung low to the ground. She told him the balls were friendly space aliens stuck on Earth or Winnie-the-Pooh and Tigger stuck in Pooh's spilled honey and engaged him in a drama. "My goodness, what has happened here?" she asked. When the therapist created voices for the characters and kept repeating their mishaps, Will responded with laughter and became readily engaged as the rescuer, a role that enabled him to expand on his movement and practic abilities.

When practitioners cast themselves as clowns, children seem naturally to become teachers, directors, or leaders (Wipfler, 1990). Being in charge can enhance children's sense of competency and control. As children take on leadership roles, they also may take new risks and try new skills.

VOICING PRAISE, FEEDBACK, AND INSTRUCTIONS

Skillful provision of verbal feedback is another reflection of artful practice. Ayres (1972) believed that it was not always necessary to provide verbal praise. She believed that the expression on a practitioner's face often was sufficient and that clients' own knowledge of success was the most important reinforcement. However, verbal feedback can be very important, particularly for children who have difficulty reading body language and other social cues. Luke's story is one example; the art was in deciding what and how much to say.

Clients use practitioners' verbal feedback in a number of ways. We believe that it is important for feedback to be accurate. To tell children they have done a good job when they have not is to be less than honest. Children know when we have not been honest and they may become unsure about when they actually can trust our words. Or worse, they may trust our words initially and later feel deceived. For example, rather than, "You did it!" Luke's occupational therapist might have said, "You're really great at the jungle gym!" If Luke took her words at face value, he might later have tried climbing on the jungle gym at school without the occupational therapist, only to be disappointed and frustrated.

Many clients use practitioners' verbal feedback as a basis for modifying inaccurate perceptions of movement and body position. For example, one client believed that she was falling each time her muscles contracted in response to movement. The practitioner's verbal feedback helped her understand that those contractions were equilibrium reactions that *prevented* her from falling.

Some clients seem unable to use feedback from their bodies to recognize their accomplishments.

They rely on the practitioner's verbal feedback, especially during early stages of intervention, to learn about their movements. When 12-year-old Kerry completed her first forward flip on a trapeze bar, the therapist cheered. Kerry appeared pleased, but then asked, "What did I do?" When the therapist demonstrated, Kerry was able to repeat her success.

Finally, sometimes we use verbal instruction to modify clients' behaviors (e.g., help a child discontinue an undesirable action). Positive instructions often are more successful than negative commands. For example, "Put your foot here" often works better than "Stop kicking" (Ayres, 1985). Luria (1961) indicated that children younger than age 5 years routinely have difficulty discontinuing an action in response to a verbal command. Children who have delayed language are likely to be much older before they can respond reliably to verbal commands to stop an action. Similarly, children with poor self-esteem generally respond more positively when we focus on actions that they *can* do rather than on ones they *should not* do. Sometimes we craft verbal feedback to reprimand gently and give simultaneous encouragement. For example, if a child rushes into an activity, fails, and then stops trying, we might say, " I'm going to help you do it better."

CREATING THE JUST-RIGHT CHALLENGE

Occupational therapy practitioners have long believed that the just-right challenge represents an important key to intervention (Ayres, 1972). When we speak of the just-right challenge, we refer to activities that prompt clients to stretch a little beyond their current abilities but are not so difficult as to generate frustration. Csikszentmihayli (1975a, 1990, 1993, 1996) used the term "flow" to describe the experience that accompanied the just-right challenge. He suggested that individuals in flow were totally involved in what they were doing and oblivious to events or people outside of the activity. As a just-right challenge unfolds into success, a client suddenly begins to work with, not against, equipment, becoming intensely committed to mastering the challenge. The look of delight all over the face of a tired but successful client can light up a whole room.

How do practitioners achieve the just-right challenge? Tickle-Degnen and Coster (1995) and Dunkerley et al. (1997) named scaffolding as an impor-

tant tool (Rogoff, 1990; Rogoff & Gardner, 1984; Wood et al., 1976).

> Through scaffolding, the therapist adjusts and controls task elements that are just beyond the child's current skills. This allows the child to focus on the elements that are within his or her abilities and to achieve success in completing a task that he or she would be unable to complete without assistance. The therapist also models and demonstrates while scaffolding, encouraging the child's interest and active participation (Dunkerley et al., 1997, p.799).

Interestingly, Dunkerley et al. (1997) described children involved in the just-right challenge as "working" rather than "playing." They also observed that the children appeared "somewhat anxious" (p. 804). By way of explanation, Koomar (1997) drew on the work of Neiss (1988), who indicated that a certain level of anxiety is needed to perform at peak.

Shaping the just-right challenge for a client sometimes represents a formidable task. Without detracting from its importance, Dunkerley et al. (1997) offered respite to practitioners who may feel pressured by theorists or managed care mandates to provide the just-right challenge throughout an entire intervention session (Koomar, 1997).

> It is possible that the optimum-for-growth moment (Ayres, 1972) is a culminating moment that must be embedded within moments of fun and moments of failure. Overchallenges would allow the child to experience failure without dire consequences, underchallenges would allow the child to experience playful respite and relaxation, and just-right challenges would allow the child to experience mastery (Dunkerley et al., p. 805).

The art lies in knowing how much and when.

BALANCING FREEDOM WITH STRUCTURE

Ayres (1972) indicated that "It is the child who must change within himself [*sic*]; the therapist can only promote and guide" (p. 265). Thus, another significant challenge to the art of practice lies in the balance between structuring a session and allowing clients (children, in particular) freedom to explore, initiate, and choose activities. Ayres continued:

> A balance of freedom and structure that maximizes constructive exploration is not easily achieved. . . .

Free play does not inevitably, in itself, further sensory integration, but too rigid structure will inhibit the manifestation of potential. . . . Structure may push the child further toward the therapeutic objective than he can reach alone but too much will defeat its purpose (p. 259).

Although clients who have a strong inner drive may select appropriate activities independently, usually we need to impose enough structure to ensure that the activities are safe and promote increasingly complex adaptive behaviors. We may need to intervene with physical or verbal prompts or with slight alterations to a client-selected activity (Ayres, 1972). For clients with more severe dysfunction, we may set up activities and model ideas. The art is in the balance.

Jason, a 9-year-old gifted child who had sensory integrative-based dyspraxia, nearly always voiced the same greeting when he arrived for therapy. "I have a great idea of what we should do today!" Although happy about Jason's enthusiasm, his occupational therapist learned the hard way that Jason's ideas were not always good ones. Once when Jason arrived with a "great idea," he laid several pieces of equipment in a row on the floor, seemingly to form an obstacle course. The first piece of equipment in the line was a barrel, thankfully padded on the edges. Jason sat in front of the barrel, hit himself on the head with a Nerf bat, and slammed himself backward into the barrel. Even though the barrel was padded, he sustained a bump on the head. Apparently, Jason's body schema was so poor that he was unable to judge the distance from the barrel. The occupational therapist needed to be both a vigilant observer and sensitive to Jason's desire to be actively involved in planning his intervention.

Although some clients need structure, others need greater freedom to act on their own motivations. Emily, a 7-year-old girl, showed signs of tactile defensiveness, especially with regard to clothing. Nonetheless, her overall arousal level generally seemed quite low. Wanting to make Emily's intervention as efficient as possible, her therapist created activities that provided a lot of enhanced tactile sensation. Emily dug in a ball pit, crawled through a large stockinette tunnel, and played in shaving cream with her hands and feet. Emily was extremely compliant; she did anything her therapist asked. However, even though her mother indicated that Emily always wanted to go to therapy, Emily never showed any signs that she had fun while there. There was no laughing or giggling, even in activities that called for exuberance. She answered the therapist's queries but rarely initiated conversation or made any requests. When her therapist decided to take another tack and follow Emily's lead, things changed dramatically. Emily chose to stand on the glider. The therapist created a "storm" and gave Emily a rough ride. Periodically, "whales" (i.e., therapy balls) swam underneath the swing, causing it to move in unexpected ways. The level of Emily's arousal increased. She became more animated, directing the therapist and altering the activity in subtle ways. Emily blossomed with less structure and a helper/playmate attuned to her needs.

STRIVING TO FIND INNER DRIVE

"The ultimate goal of sensory integrative treatment is a being which wants to, can, and will direct himself [*sic*] meaningfully and with satisfaction in response to the environmental demands" (Ayres, 1972, p. 257). Because activities reflecting sensory integration theory are fun and seem to tap a common source of motivation, children generally engage in them readily. However, occasionally, a child balks, either at a particular activity or at activities in general that involve movement and enhanced sensation. Then we endeavor to find that child's inner drive.

Apparent lack of motivation may take several forms. Some children say they do not want to do an activity because it is "boring" or "babyish." Some try to divert our attention with conversation or another activity. Others withdraw to a protected space (e.g., inside a stack of inner tubes or a barrel). Still others become increasingly anxious, overly active, or disorganized. When clients express, either verbally or nonverbally, the idea that they are not interested in an activity, we seek to discern the reason because the cause suggests a remedy. In our experience, a child's "lack of motivation" usually means one of several things, including:

- The activity is too difficult.
- The child *believes* the activity is too difficult.
- The child's level of arousal is not optimal.
- The theme of the activity is too juvenile.
- The activity lacks meaning for the child.

The art is in uncovering the cause. When an activity is too difficult, we modify the demands until they match the child's skills more closely or give the child support to accomplish it. If it is necessary to discontinue an activity because it cannot be adapted to meet the needs of the child, we take the responsibility for the "mistake" so that clients do not have additional reasons to believe that their skills have, once again, caused an activity to fail. It is easy enough to say, "This really is too hard. Let's do something different. I made a mistake."

Many adults and older children indicate reliably when they are ready to discontinue an activity; younger children or clients who have cognitive impairments may not. For all ages, if the activity is too hard and we do not respond quickly enough, clients can become frustrated, and it may be difficult to reengage them, even in subsequent sessions.

If the activity is *not* too difficult but a child believes it is, we choose between modifying the activity and enticing the child to try. The latter is a way of showing children that they possess skills of which they seem to be unaware.

The decision to modify, support, or entice depends on which best fits the practitioner's style and the child's needs and how adamantly the child is refusing. If we decide to entice a child into attempting a task, we should not enter into a "power struggle." The primary purpose of therapeutic activity is to help clients discover new skills, not to force them to do something. If a child cannot be easily convinced to try a task, we must change the plan and move on to another activity.

If children are "unmotivated" because their level of arousal is not optimal, we must try to respect their needs and assist them to enter a more optimal arousal state. We express our understanding of their needs verbally and nonverbally. If children move to a protected space, we gradually move closer and offer calming sensation (e.g., deep pressure, oral motor activities, or music). We allow the child to remain in a protected area as long as necessary (see the Matrix Model in Chapter 12).

Sometimes clients express a desire to "go home." Asking to terminate a session may represent an adaptive behavior, especially in response to overarousal. We try to identify the source of the problem (often frustration encountered before or during therapy). Usually we can assist the child to enter a more optimal state and continue. However, if we do terminate a session, we must do it in a nonpunitive fashion.

Some children seem to need intense sensation to attain an optimal level of arousal. Emily, who was previously described, was such a child. When she was engaged in activity that provided intense vestibular and proprioceptive sensation, she came "alive."

Sometimes children balk at activities they perceive to be too juvenile. Jeff, a 12-year-old boy, found the Harry Potter Quidditch game that his therapist created to be "babyish." Although many children his age would have loved that theme, Jeff was more motivated by his muscles' getting stronger and his aim more accurate when he threw beanbags at a target while prone in the net.

Similarly, some activities designed to meet a particular goal may be contrived and seem purposeless to a child. Aimee, an 8-year-old girl, had difficulty crossing the midline. Her occupational therapist created an activity in which Aimee straddled a barrel and moved beanbags from one side to a container on the other side. Aimee, however, found no real reason to cross the midline. The activity was contrived; Aimee had to cross the midline simply because the occupational therapy practitioner had instructed her to, not because the activity itself really demanded it. In contrast, when Aimee swung on the moon swing (see Fig. 12–15), she had to hold on tight with one arm. Thus, she had to cross the midline when using a squirt gun to hit a stationary clown.

> The inner drive toward sensory integration exists in most, if not all, young children who come to the attention of a therapist. It often lies buried beneath many other needs which interfere. Enabling the child to gain contact with that drive is difficult, but necessary for maximum response to treatment (Ayres, 1972, p. 257).

TO MODIFY OR DISCONTINUE: WHEN THE PRACTITIONER WANTS A CHANGE

Some therapeutic activities simply come to a logical ending recognized by both client and practitioner; then the two simply move to the next activity or the session ends. However, at times, the client may seem more invested than the practitioner in an activity, making the two "out of sync." Should the activity be discontinued or not? That is the question; that is the art.

In short, we believe that it is desirable to remain with a given activity as long as clients demonstrate active involvement and increasingly adaptive interactions. When clients remain totally involved in therapeutic activity, they are usually benefiting. Certainly, we should not discontinue an activity because *we* are bored or because we are fearful that a particular session lacks variety. At times clients, simply need to repeat an activity in order to master it or develop a skill.

While prone in a net swing, 11-year-old Don attempted to propel himself forward to hit a suspended punching bag (Fig. 11–4). He had great difficulty sequencing the steps of pushing off the mat and getting his hands in position to strike the punching bag at the optimal instant. When we tried making subtle modifications to the activity, they disrupted his efforts. When we allowed him to continue working independently for 5 minutes, he was able to figure out how to propel himself forward and hit the punching bag consistently. Any of a number of factors may have enabled Don to succeed, including enhanced vestibular and proprioceptive sensation, repetition, and feedback from his body. Although the reason for his success was unclear, after Don established the sequence and could strike the punching bag, he engaged eagerly in the activity for an additional 15 minutes. If we had stopped the activity too soon, we would not have allowed him to meet a challenge of which he was capable. At times, the most art-

ful intervention means remaining observant and not interfering.

Although sometimes practitioners simply need to be patient and allow the client time to master a challenge, there are other times when the practitioner's feeling that the activity should either be changed or discontinued is right on target. When it can be done readily, modification or scaffolding is generally preferable to discontinuing an activity because it usually is less disruptive to the flow of the session. We periodically shift elements of an activity to alter the challenge, but we need to be ready to abandon the adaptation if the client rejects it. A good session is achieved when a client feels both challenged and successful. When art is evident in therapy, a practitioner and client flow from one activity to another similar to skilled dancers responding to changing pieces of music. At certain times, we take the lead and modify, scaffold, or initiate a new activity. At other times, we follow the client's lead and surreptitiously incorporate challenges.

Jerry, a 10-year-old boy who had significant motor planning problems, frequently requested activities that allowed him to use his relatively strong postural extensor muscles rather than activities that challenged his weak flexor muscles. During one session, he asked to play a game in which he rode prone on a scooter board down a ramp in order to "steal jewels from the queen's castle while she slept" (Fig. 11–5). We wanted to involve Jerry in an activity that encouraged movement into flexion.

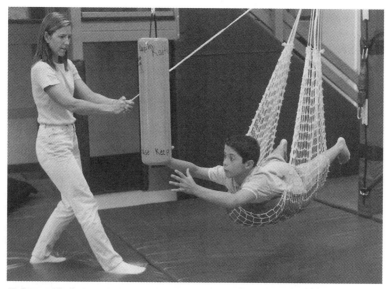

■ FIGURE 11–4 Hitting a punching bag while swinging requires careful sequencing of a number of movements. (Photo by Shay McAtee, printed with permission.)

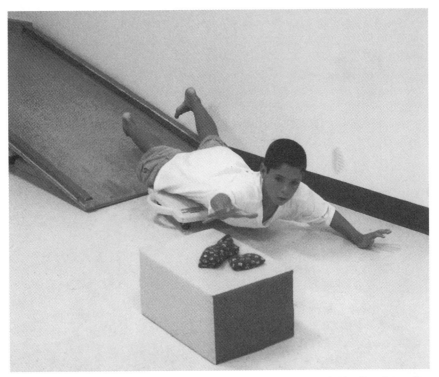

■ FIGURE 11-5   Riding prone on a scooter board down a ramp in order to "steal jewels from the queen's castle." (Photo by Shay McAtee, printed with permission.)

Our task with Jerry, as with many clients who seem fearful of failure, was to capture his motivation and invest it in a slightly more challenging activity.

After a few minutes of riding down the ramp, we announced that the queen had decided to find a better way to protect her jewels because Jerry was too good at stealing them. She decided to put them in a moat filled with alligators that could only be reached with a "helicopter" (the T-swing) (Fig. 11–6). Moving Jerry's story into a new activity allowed us to maintain his interest and enthusiasm while providing a greater challenge to flexion.

Of course, sometimes it is necessary to discontinue an activity that is not going well. Often this occurs when the task lacks flexibility—that is, it does not inherently allow for modification either by varying the position of the client or the desired outcome. For example, although a Sit 'N' Spin (Fig. 11–7) may be fun, it is not readily adaptable. A child can do only a limited number of things on it. Active involvement with this piece of equipment may provide brief, intense fun, and then the practitioner needs to facilitate the transition to another activity.

Activities that are far too easy do not challenge clients; their primary value, therefore, is for playful respite and relaxation (Dunkerley et al., 1997). Furthermore, clients may benefit emotionally from performing activities they have mastered, particularly if peers or family members value the activity. Beginning with activities a child can perform easily can also be beneficial for establishing rapport. However, although an emotional boost and a certain amount of rest are important parts of intervention, most clients become bored with very easy activities (Csikszentmihayli, 1975, 1990, 1993, 1996).

Moving fluidly from one activity to another results in a session that looks and feels playful. To the untrained observer, the most skillful intervention may appear unstructured. Parents and teachers sometimes misinterpret the playful nature of the interactions and question their validity (e.g., "Can anything that much fun really be doing any good?" or "Why isn't he doing what you tell him?") Thus, it is important to express the purpose of activities and the benefits of playful, fluid interactions (see Chapter 10).

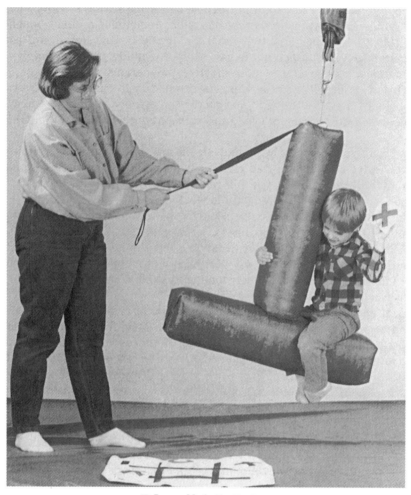

■ FIGURE 11-6 The T-swing.

HELPING CLIENTS UNDERSTAND SENSORY INTEGRATIVE DYSFUNCTION

An important part of intervention is helping clients and caregivers understand sensory integrative dysfunction and the purpose of intervention so that they can develop strategies to adapt to—and compensate for—dysfunction. By the time they reach age 6 or 7 years (and often earlier), most children with sensory integrative dysfunction are aware that they are somehow different from other children. They usually notice that they are unable to perform activities and skills that come easily to other children or that they get into trouble more often. Although many individuals with sensory integrative dysfunction already are trying as hard as they can,

they often have received feedback that they could do better if they tried harder. In response, they develop "explanations" for their failures. Having never heard of sensory integration theory, they may come to believe that the reason they cannot do certain things well is because they are "bad," "lazy," or "dumb."

Many clients experience immense relief when they learn about sensory integration theory. One mother reported that it was as though someone had taken a huge weight off her 7-year-old son's shoulders. "He's like a different kid," she said. "I guess I never realized how much he worried about not being able to do things as well as the other kids."

As a part of the evaluation process, we elicit clients' *explanations* of why they have difficulty with particular things. In this way, we open the door for teaching about sensory integration theory. We ask children if they have ever talked to their

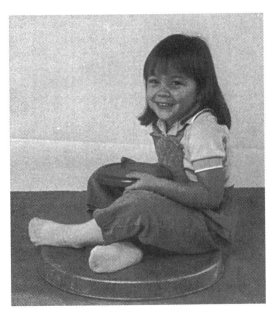

■ FIGURE 11-7   The Sit 'N' Spin™.

parents or teachers about why some things are difficult and, if so, how these adults explained the child's difficulties. When necessary, we reframe the explanations using sensory integration theory selecting carefully chosen words that clients understand. We continue to discuss sensory integration theory as opportunities are presented throughout the intervention process. In so doing, we hope to help clients and caregivers understand sensory integrative dysfunction and its impact on daily life.

Anna was an 11-year-old girl with gravitational insecurity and sensory integrative-based dyspraxia, which caused her significant difficulty in gym class and prevented her from participating in activities such as in-line skating and riding a scooter. Despite her parents' efforts, Anna's self concept suffered; she believed she was "stupid."

The occupational therapy practitioner wanted to help Anna reframe her difficulties. One day, as Anna swung gently on a bolster swing, the occupational therapy practitioner drew pictures on a chalkboard to illustrate sensory integrative dysfunction (Fig. 11–8). First she drew a crude brain and probed to learn what Anna knew about its functions. She made sure Anna understood that the brain did a number of things. One was to help her learn, and another was to tell her muscles how to move; there were many more. The occupational therapist explained that a person could have difficulty with one brain function while the others were okay.

Next the occupational therapist asked Anna what she knew about the senses. Anna listed several: vision, hearing, smell, taste, and touch. As Anna spoke, the occupational therapist drew crude representations of the senses. Then the occupational therapist explained about the vestibular system (i.e., "It comes from your inner ear and it tells you about movement") and proprioception (i.e., "It comes from the muscles and tells you about how hard you're pushing or pulling") and drew figures representing them. The occupational therapist drew arrows from the senses to the brain and explained that they provide information to the brain, which it processes in order to tell a person how to move next.

Finally the occupational therapy practitioner drew a picture of a person running and drew a line between the brain and the person. She explained that when a brain did not do a good job of putting together all the information that came from the senses, the person might have trouble with coordination. But that same person could be very smart. She could know exactly what she wanted to do but would have trouble doing it (see Fig. 11–8).

The occupational therapy practitioner went on: "When you come to therapy, we do things that give your brain a lot of sensation. We think that will help it process better. When it processes better, in-line skating and riding your scooter will be easier because your brain will be sending better messages to your muscles, telling them what to do." Although Anna made little comment, her mother remarked that she seemed less frustrated and less apt to refer to herself as "stupid."

MAKING EVERYDAY LIFE EASIER

Developing strategies to minimize the impact of sensory integrative dysfunction and make daily life easier is an important part of intervention. Although we contribute to the creation of strategies, we do so *with* clients and caregivers. We help them to be as actively involved as possible. When the client is a child, at the very least we check to be certain parents and teachers understand and embrace a strategy *before* asking them to implement it. The art lies in helping clients and caregivers solve their own problems as much as possible without leaving them feeling that they alone must come up with all the answers.

One situation we encounter commonly is deal-

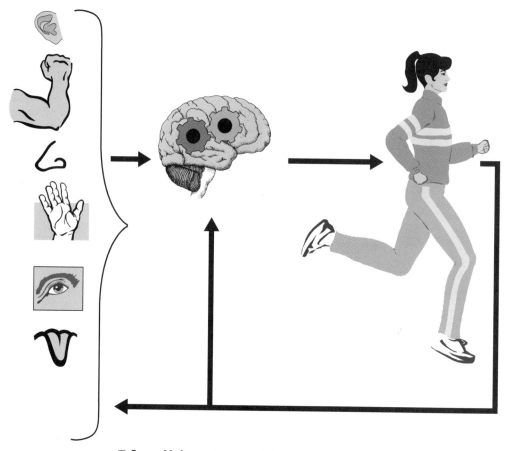

■ Figure 11–8 Simple representation of sensory integration.

ing with children who become overly stimulated. As we work with them, we make a point of saying, "When you feel like this, it is a good time to go into a quiet place." We then create a safe, enclosed space, such as underneath a large cushion or inside a carpeted barrel. Thus, we try to teach children that an appropriate way to deal with too much stimulation is to go to a place where it is minimized. When children have attained a more optimal state of arousal, we talk to them about the difficulty of concentrating when too much is happening. We explain that it is easier to concentrate in an enclosed space because not so many things are happening at the same time (see also Chapter 12 for a description of "womb space").

Of course, some children become overly active and distractible when their level of arousal is *too low*. Thus, they seem to be moving in order to keep themselves awake. Those children require strategies that provide *enhanced* sensation. When we suspect that clients' behavior (e.g., increased activity, twisting hair or chewing on shirt collars) is for the purpose of seeking sensation, we might suggest that they chew bubble gum or engage in other activities that provide proprioceptive input (e.g., jumping on a mini-trampoline). Some clients find that pulling on both ends of a piece of rubber tubing or Theraband that they carry in a pocket can replace the need to move. Wilbarger and Wilbarger (1991) referred to sensory-based strategies for altering level of arousal as a sensory diet (see also the appendix to Chapter 13 for commonly used strategies and Chapter 14 for more on sensory diets).

Using simple terminology, Williams and Shellenberger (1994) developed an extensive program to enable clients to become aware of their ability to focus at any given time. Likening the central nervous system to an engine, these authors' program also helps clients use strategies to adjust the engine speed for optimal performance (see also Chapter 14 for further discussion of the engine program).

We believe it is very important that clients with sensory integrative dysfunction become able to explain their difficulties and alter their environments

to minimize the impact of those difficulties. Billy, a 4-year-old boy with tactile defensiveness, demonstrated an unusual ability to generalize his understanding of his difficulties and the purpose of his intervention. Billy found deep pressure followed by joint compression (i.e., part of the Wilbarger protocol) to be calming. One day, Billy asked his father why he did not wear his wedding ring. When his father responded that he did not like the feeling of things on his hands, Billy promptly produced his brush and told his father that if he used the brush on his hands he might be able to wear his ring.

DISCONTINUING INTERVENTION

The decision to terminate intervention often becomes more a matter of art than science. When clients have reached their objectives and many of the day-to-day interferences of sensory integrative dysfunction have been minimized or eliminated, intervention is discontinued, at least temporarily. We are interested in clients' abilities to function adequately and more easily in their roles and routine daily tasks. The extent to which sensory integrative dysfunction interferes with functional abilities is the critical factor in deciding to discontinue intervention. Although our decisions must be justifiable and substantiated, we often are guided by "gut" reactions.

Often it is difficult to predict the total duration of intervention. When children receive therapy once a week, the minimum duration of intervention usually is 6 months or approximately 25 sessions; in our experience, clients most commonly receive intervention for 1 to 2 years. A few clients may continue to benefit from intervention for 3 or more years. Short-term intensive intervention may be particularly effective for meeting specific goals with children who experience either modulation or praxis problems. Ideally, clients receive intervention as long as they continue to benefit in a meaningful way.

When a child is nearing the time for discharge, frequently a parent reports that, for the first time the child wanted to stay at home and play with a friend or sibling rather than come to therapy. We are always pleased to hear this because it signals that our work has been effective and the child is getting ready to function without our support.

To help with making decisions about the duration of intervention, we recommend that clients be reevaluated every 3 to 6 months to determine the amount of progress that has been made toward meeting the objectives and to specify any new objectives that may have emerged. More formal assessments of progress, using standardized instruments, may also be periodically warranted.

During the course of intervention, a client's progress may plateau for several weeks, followed by periods of significant progress. This may reflect a time when clients are consolidating, or integrating, gains they have made. Although currently there is no research examining the discontinuation of intervention during plateaus, it provides an interesting hypothesis. We have had some success with this strategy.

As we consider discontinuing intervention, we must remember that clients can generally use skills in the clinic before being able to use them in other settings. They may not yet be able to use their new skills without assistance or they may not recognize that they have acquired them. Skills are of little use unless clients can use them at home, in school, and at work. In some instances, clients need assistance to transfer skills from the therapy setting into daily life.

Before we discontinue intervention, we prepare clients and caregivers for the possibility that evidence of dysfunction may again become prominent with stress (e.g., when learning a new or complex skill or during activities that provide strong sensation). Scott had been receiving extensive intervention for severe gravitational insecurity and had shown tremendous gains, particularly in play. Now, at the age of 8 years, he could climb the jungle gym, descend the slide, ride a two-wheeled bike, roughhouse with his parents, and tumble with other children effortlessly and without fear. However, when his parents took him sledding for the first time, he was more fearful than his younger siblings of a moderately steep hill. In this case, Scott's day-to-day functioning was adequate for most play and social activities. However, in an unfamiliar situation in which he believed that he had little control, some of his gravitational insecurity resurfaced.

Because of our ongoing consultation with Scott and his parents, they understood this reaction. We had discussed the reasons that he was afraid of certain activities and helped them develop strategies to minimize that stress. Because Scott really wanted to go sledding, he and his father went to a smaller hill to "get warmed up." Later they returned to the bigger hill, and one of his parents rode with Scott on a two-person sled until he developed a sense of control over the movement.

Scott did not need further direct intervention. When an activity resulted in fear, Scott and his family evaluated the importance of the activity. If it was important, they worked together to grade the activity so Scott could master it.

When intervention is discontinued, it always is with the understanding that clients may contact the occupational therapy practitioner if new problems arise. Although consultation is the best solution for some difficulties, clients occasionally choose to reenter direct intervention.

In some cases, because of the support and caring they receive in the intervention process, parents, caregivers, or adult clients find it difficult to end routine visits with an occupational therapy practitioner. The role of the practitioner then may be to help the adults make the transition to a psychotherapist, a support group, or other activities in which they can continue to receive assistance with family issues and the impact of remaining dysfunction. Directing families toward outside resources can prevent *their* needs from interfering with timely and appropriate discharge of a client. Talking about discharge from the beginning of the intervention process may also help.

BECOMING AN ARTIST

Artful practice reflects a balance of competence and caring (Peloquin, 1990, 1993, 1998). Without technical skill, a practitioner lacks the ability to tie theory to practice, minimize clients' underlying difficulties, and enhance occupational performance. Thus technical skill is critical to good intervention, and the only way to develop it is "to work and work, studying and perfecting the craft. . . . Well crafted work . . . requires discipline" (Grey, 1998, p. 19). However, in the current health-care climate, competence often overshadows caring. When that happens, the would-be healer becomes simply a technician (Peloquin, 1990, 1993, 1998). That may be what happened initially with Emily's therapist, described in this chapter, who learned that following Emily's lead resulted in more effective intervention.

Art must be built upon technical skill, but technique is just one ingredient (Grey, 1998). "The art of practice . . . is a process of making connections and finding meaning" (Peloquin, 1998, p. 105). Art

in practice enables the recognition of possibilities. Quoting Rodin, Grey (1998, p. 205) indicated that, "The artist reveals spiritual riches until then unknown, and gives people new reasons for loving life, new inner lights to guide them." Clearly, art is shrouded in mystery.

Artful practice is the practice of a master clinician; it is what we all seek for ourselves. How, then, does a practitioner become an artist? "An . . . artistic vision is both acquired from the surrounding culture and attained through a depth of personal experience and introspection" (Grey, 1998, p. 8).

Several authors have offered practical suggestions for developing art. Acknowledging the lack of nurturance for art that exists in the current health-care system, Peloquin (1990) proposed that therapists reflect on phenomenological accounts of illness and disability in order to learn the value of caring. Earlier, Peloquin (1989) proposed that fictional accounts of occupational therapy practitioners may serve a similar purpose. Literature can be approached in both an aesthetic and a moral fashion. In the aesthetic approach, readers have the opportunity to scrutinize relationships. In the moral approach, practitioners reflect on "life either as it is being lived or as one hopes to live it" (p. 221).

Apprenticeship is another approach suggested to those who seek to become artists. Writing about learning the art of using therapeutic activity, Creighton et al. (1995) quoted one practitioner:

> I don't know if you can verbally instruct somebody in why, and how you know, and what to look for. . . . Looking at an activity and figuring out why it doesn't work and how you could move it over here, move it over there, pick it up in a different way—the student really has to watch me (p. 316).

We have also found the mentoring role to be successful in helping inexperienced practitioners become masters. Watching and reflecting with a mentor are often worth more than years of reading and didactic instruction.

Finally, some particularly insightful authors (Grey, 1998; Mosey, 1981; Palmer, 1998) have offered difficult but cogent advice on becoming an artist: *know yourself.*

> The individual who strives to bring art into practice must be able to engage in the often uncomfortable process of learning more about one's

self, changing one's self, and gaining knowledge about how one's values and expectations differ from those of others (Mosey, 1981, p. 25).

How does a practitioner come to know the self? Palmer (1998, pp. 31–32) answered, "I have no particular methods to suggest, other than the familiar ones: solitude and silence, meditative reading and walking in the woods, keeping a journal, finding a friend who will listen." Grey (1998, p. 24) offered simply "by entering the studio [of the] heart."

SUMMARY AND CONCLUSIONS

The art of therapy is a multifaceted phenomenon. Much of the success of direct intervention depends on the artistic ability of the practitioner. Although the art of practice is a somewhat mysterious entity and is difficult to grasp in its entirety, this chapter has discussed many aspects. Effective intervention is characterized by a partnership between art and science. As in all good partnerships, the relationship between art and science is fluid. One may predominate for a time, but both make equal contributions to the effectiveness of a session and the long-term outcomes of intervention. Effective intervention involves much more than designing a sequence of activities; art holds it all together.

How does a practitioner become an artist? As a preface, Margaret Short (personal communication, March 26, 2001), an occupational therapist, offered:

I become more and more aware that we have two brains—the one inside our skulls that is excellent at associative work and then, the other, the visceral, enteric "brain." Some authors have actually written about this "gut" brain—the one [that is involved when we make . . .] "gut judgements." This is the thing computers cannot yet do but that is the hallmark of excellent clinicians. Perhaps that is some of the "art" of therapy—letting the logical brain get out of the way—once it has been rehearsed enough.

With that introduction, Short addressed the means for becoming an artful clinician:

You learn the basics of art and science. You practice (i.e., you develop skills). You become confident. You begin to trust your judgments. Then you begin to know more and more that there is

something you can let go. Now it is at this place that great practice occurs and art emerges.

References

American Occupational Therapy Council on Standards. (1972). Occupational therapy: Its definitions and functions. *American Journal of Occupational Therapy, 26,* 204–205.

Ayres, A. J. (1972). *Sensory integration and learning disorders.* Los Angeles: Western Psychological Services.

Ayres, A. J. (1985). *Developmental dyspraxia and adult onset apraxia.* Torrance, CA: Sensory Integration International.

Bundy, A. C. (1995). Assessment and intervention in school-based practice: Answering questions and minimizing discrepancies. In I. R. McEwen (Ed.), *Occupational and physical therapy in educational environments.* New York: Haworth.

Cohen, D. (1987). *The development of play.* New York: New York University Press.

Creighton, C., Dijkers, M., Bennett, N., & Brown, K. (1995). Reasoning and the art of therapy for spinal cord injury. *American Journal of Occupational Therapy, 49,* 311–317.

Csikszentmihayli, M. (1975a). *Beyond boredom and anxiety.* San Francisco: Jossey-Bass.

Csikszentmihayli, M. (1990). *Flow: The psychology of optimal experience.* New York: Harper-Collins.

Csikszentmihayli, M. (1993). *The evolving self: A psychology for the third millennium.* New York: Harper-Collins.

Csikszentmihayli, M. (1996). *Creativity: Flow and the psychology of discovery and invention.* New York: Harper-Collins.

Dunkerley, E., Tickle-Degnen, L., & Coster, W. (1997). Therapist-child interaction in the middle minutes of sensory integration treatment. *American Journal of Occupational Therapy, 51,* 799–805.

Eltz, M. J., & Shirk, S. R. (1995). Alliance formation and treatment outcome among maltreated adolescents. *Child Abuse and Neglect, 19,* 419–431.

Fisher, A. G., & Murray, E. A. (1991). Introduction to sensory integration theory. In A. G. Fisher, E. A. Murray, A. C. Bundy (Eds.), *Sensory integration: Theory and practice* (pp. 3–29). Philadelphia: F. A. Davis.

Grey, A. (1998). *The mission of art.* Boston: Shambhala.

Hopkins, H. L., & Tiffany, E. G. (1983). Occupational therapy—A problem-solving process. In H. L. Hopkins & H. D. Smith (Eds.), *Willard & Spackman's occupational therapy* (Ed. 6, pp. 89–100). Philadelphia: J. B. Lippincott.

Kaplan, B. J., Polatajko, H. J., Wilson, B. N., & Faris, P. D. (1993). Reexamination of sensory integration treatment: A combination of two efficacy studies. *Journal of Learning Disabilities, 26,* 342–347.

Koomar, J. (1997). Clinical interpretation of "therapist-child interaction in the middle minutes of sensory integration treatment." *American Journal of Occupational Therapy, 51,* 806–807.

Luborsky, L., Crits-Cristoph, J., Mintz, J., & Auerbach, A. (1988). *Who will benefit from psychotherapy: Predicting therapeutic outcomes.* New York: Basic.

Luria, A. (1961). *The role of speech in the regulation of normal and abnormal behavior.* New York: Liveright.

Mattingly, C. F., & Fleming, M. H. (1994). *Clinical reasoning: Forms of inquiry in a therapeutic practice.* Philadelphia: F. A. Davis.

Mosey, A. C. (1981). *Occupational therapy: Configuration of a profession.* New York: Raven.

Neiss, R. (1988). Reconceptualizing arousal: Psychobiological stress in motor performance. *Psychological Bulletin, 103,* 345–366.

Neistadt, M. E., & Crepeau, E. B. (1998). *Willard & Spackman's Occupational Therapy* (9th ed.). Philadelphia: Lippincott, Williams, & Williams.

Orlinsky, D. E., & Howard, K. I. (1986). Process and outcome in psychotherapy. In S. L. Garfield & A. E. Bergin (Eds.), *Handbook of psychotherapy and behavior change* (3rd ed., pp. 311–381). New York: Wiley.

Palmer, P. J. (1998). *The courage to teach: Exploring the inner landscape of a teacher's life.* San Francisco: Jossey-Bass.

Peloquin, S. M. (1989). Sustaining the art of practice in occupational therapy. *American Journal of Occupational Therapy, 43,* 219–226.

Peloquin, S. M. (1990). The patient-therapist relationship in occupational therapy: Understanding visions and images. *American Journal of Occupational Therapy, 44,* 13–21.

Peloquin, S. M. (1993). The patient-therapist relationship: Beliefs that shape care. *American Journal of Occupational Therapy, 47,* 935–942.

Peloquin, S. M. (1998). The therapeutic relationship.

In M. E. Neistadt & E. B. Crepeau (Eds.), *Willard & Spackman's Occupational Therapy* (9th ed., pp. 105–119). Philadelphia: Lippincott, Williams & Wilkins.

Rogoff, B. (1990). *Apprenticeship in thinking.* New York: Oxford University Press.

Rogoff, B., & Gardner, W. (1984). Adult guidance of cognitive development. In B. Rogoff & J. Lare (Eds.), *Everyday cognition: Its development in social context* (pp. 95–116). Cambridge, MA: Harvard University Press.

Schaefer, C.E., & Reid, S.E. (1986). *Game play: Therapeutic use of childhood games.* New York: John Wiley & Sons.

Shirk, S. R., & Russell, R. L. (1996). *Change processes in child psychotherapy,* New York: Guilford.

Shirk, S. R., & Saiz, C. (1992). Clinical, empirical, and developmental perspectives on the therapeutic relationship in child psychotherapy. *Development and Psychopathology, 4,* 713–728.

Tickle-Degnen, L., & Coster, W. (1995). Therapeutic interaction and the management of challenge during the beginning minutes of sensory integration treatment. *Occupational Therapy Journal of Research, 15,* 122–141.

Wilbarger, P., & Wilbarger, J. (1991). *Sensory defensiveness in children aged 2–12: An intervention guide for parents and other caregivers.* Denver, CO: Avanti Educational Programs.

Williams, M. S., & Shellenberger, S. (1994). *How does your engine run?: A leader's guide to the alert program for self-regulation.* Albuquerque, NM: TherapyWorks.

Wipfler, P. (1990). *Listening to children: Play listening.* Palo Alto, CA: Parents Leadership Institute.

Wood, D., Bruner, J. S., & Ross, G. (1976). The role of tutoring in problem solving. *Journal of Child Psychology and Psychiatry, 17,* 89–100.

12

Creating Direct Intervention from Theory

Jane A. Koomar, PhD, OTR, FAOTA
Anita C. Bundy, ScD, OTR, FAOTA

The child's sense of fulfillment radiates as he experiences himself [sic] interacting with the world of objects, as he pits himself against gravity and finds that it is not quite the ruthless master it was a short time before, or as he finds his body bringing him satisfying sensation. He is no longer the impotent organism shoved about by environmental forces; he can act effectively on the world. He is more of a whole being.
—A. Jean Ayres (1972, p. 262)

Intervene: To come between as an influencing force.

—Webster's New World Dictionary

PURPOSE AND SCOPE

Chapter 11 discussed the art of intervention, the use of one's unique self to orchestrate intervention. This chapter describes therapeutic activities and programs drawn from sensory integration theory that we have used successfully in direct intervention. Clearly, we cannot describe every activity a practitioner might develop in any given area. Rather, our goal has been to provide readers with ideas for activities and a systematic method for evaluating them in order to determine what they might be used to accomplish.

Rarely does any therapeutic activity meet only one objective. The difficulty is in determining which, of all the possible uses an activity might have, is most appropriate for this particular client at this particular point in intervention. Because we frequently alter activities during a session, we must have a clear idea of what we hope to achieve to alter it appropriately. As much as possible, this chapter points out some of the multiple uses for the therapeutic activities discussed.

The chapter begins by discussing activities that can be used to provide enhanced sensation. It then moves on to a discussion of intervention for a number of manifestations of sensory integrative dysfunction. These include dysfunction in:

• Sensory modulation

- Sensory discrimination
- Posture
- Praxis

Before we present activities, however, we note that direct intervention is only one way to deliver occupational therapy. Consultation with clients, caregivers (e.g., parents, teachers), and other professionals also is a very powerful approach to intervention. In consultation, we offer sensory integration theory as a new "frame" through which to view a client's behaviors. Based on a new understanding, clients and therapists work together to develop strategies for solving problems. Chapter 13 discusses consultation.

ACTIVITIES THAT OFFER ENHANCED SENSATION

The ability to create effective intervention based on sensory integration theory depends, in part, on knowledge of the sensory systems (see Chapter 2). Although the vestibular, proprioceptive, and tactile systems continue to be cornerstones of sensory integration theory, some therapists are also exploring the effects of combining enhanced auditory or visual sensation with vestibular, proprioceptive, and tactile sensations. (See Chapter 14.)

This chapter begins with a discussion of creating activities that provide enhanced vestibular, proprioceptive, and tactile sensation. Then this information is applied to improving central nervous system (CNS) processing of sensation.

All of the comments should be prefaced by a word of caution: *Whenever we incorporate enhanced sensation in activity, we must be vigilant observers of clients' responses.* Much is known about what we can expect from various types of sensation. Therefore, with clear goals in mind, we create activities in a logical fashion, based on accepted principles of sensory integration theory. However, much is also *unknown* about the use of enhanced sensation. Furthermore, we know that clients' responses to sensation are individually determined. Thus, "accepted principles" serve only as guidelines; they can never replace the knowledge gained from observing and listening to clients.

Enhanced Vestibular and Proprioceptive Sensation

The vestibular system is a specialized proprioceptor—that is, it provides us with valuable information about the position and movement of the head relative to the body, gravity, and the world around us. Therefore, any time we create activities that involve movement; we are providing proprioception. However, for simplicity, we will refer to the sensation that accompanies whole body movement and position as *vestibular* and reserve the term *proprioception* for sensation detected by receptors in muscles and, to a lesser extent, joints. The muscle spindles are the primary receptors of proprioception. They are particularly receptive to activation by resistance to movement (see Chapter 2).

Three aspects of active movement yield vestibular and proprioceptive sensation into therapeutic activities:

1. Type of movement (i.e., linear vs. angular)
2. Speed of movement (i.e., slow vs. fast)
3. Resistance to active movement

Enhanced vestibular and proprioceptive sensation almost always involves *active* movement. The otolith organs of the vestibular system detect slow or linear movements in any direction and position. The semicircular canals detect fast or angular movements. The muscle spindles detect resistance to movement. One additional source of proprioception is the information "fed forward" in the CNS *before* a movement occurs (see Chapter 3).

Because different receptors are particularly sensitive to different kinds of sensation, activities can emphasize input to specific receptors. This enables us to facilitate desired behavioral responses. For example, swinging very slowly while prone in a net swing stimulates primarily the otolith organs and facilitates tonic postural responses. Spinning rapidly in the net swing stimulates primarily the semicircular canals and facilitates phasic postural responses, such as equilibrium.

Most activities provide multiple sources of sensation. For example, pulling on an elastic cord to swing oneself rapidly back and forth in a net swing provides stimulation to the semicircular canals, the otolith organs, and the muscle spindles. Although many activities stimulate more than one type of receptor, a client pulling on an elastic cord to swing back and forth in a net swing is having a very different kind of sensory experience than a client who is spinning in it. The behavioral responses to the two activities is also very different.

Enhanced Tactile Sensation

When we create activities incorporating enhanced tactile sensation, we consider the characteristics of the touch as well as clients' responses to it and the reasons for providing it. Are we interested in effecting change in sensory modulation, sensory discrimination, or both? When we are addressing sensory modulation dysfunction, we use deep pressure, which is typically calming, and we avoid light or unexpected touch, which is often interpreted as noxious or painful (see Chapter 4). When trying to enhance the ability to detect the spatiotemporal characteristics of touch (i.e., sensory discrimination), we provide tactile experiences that are rich in many qualities.

SENSORY MODULATION DYSFUNCTION

Sensory modulation deficits result in consistent responses that are disproportionate to the magnitude of the sensation experienced. Evidence of deficits in sensory modulation can occur in any sensory system. This section discusses intervention for poor sensory modulation in general and then for four specific types:

1. Sensory defensiveness
2. Underresponsiveness
3. Gravitational insecurity
4. Aversive responses to movement

Sensory Defensiveness

Sensory defensiveness is the most common sensory modulation deficit. Clients who experience sensory defensiveness have a tendency to respond negatively to sensation that is considered by most people to be harmless or nonirritating (Wilbarger & Wilbarger, 1991). Frequently, this includes hyperresponsiveness to light or unexpected touch, high-frequency noises, certain visual stimuli, or certain smells and tastes.

A variety of behavioral and emotional responses are associated with sensory defensiveness. These behaviors generally reflect flight, fright, or fight in response to noxious sensations (Oetter et al., 1993). Individuals may have particular difficulty with transitions or exhibit mood swings. Flight, fright, or fight behaviors may be more pronounced in the presence of stress that results from motor, cognitive, or social demands.

Examples of *flight* behaviors include increased activity, gaze aversion, moving or pulling away, distractibility, clowning, redirecting others' attention, or verbalizations (e.g., "this is babyish," "bor-

ing," or "stupid," "I'm tired and I want to leave"). Examples of *fright* behaviors include the reluctance to separate, reluctance to try new things, crying or whining, clinging, verbalizations (e.g., "I can't," "I don't like this!"). Examples of *fight* behaviors include expressions of rage, aggression toward the self or others, explosiveness, or verbalizations (e.g., "I won't!" " No!" "You can't make me!"). Although the presence of any of these behaviors can be challenging for a practitioner, they provide feedback to alter the activity.

Underresponsiveness to Sensation

Some individuals appear underresponsive to sensory events and pain. Although some actually seem to have diminished awareness of sensation, others may actually be *overly* responsive. Their paradoxical reaction may be a means of protecting themselves. Commonly, practitioners describe such a client as "shut down." Some clients who underrespond as part of a protective response appear to become overly responsive (i.e., defensive) part way into intervention, causing caregivers to wonder if intervention has caused a new problem. However, we interpret the appearance of defensiveness as a sign of *improvement*. Although the clients' responses continue to be out of proportion, they are now in the expected direction—that is, an individual who is overly sensitive is now overresponsive rather than failing to respond. (The mechanism [or mechanisms] that underlie these observations remain to be delineated.)

We have found that individuals who seemingly fail to notice sensation are more often protecting themselves from sensory defensiveness than actually underresponsive. Therefore, when evaluating or intervening with a client who appears lethargic, we generally assume that the client is extremely defensive and proceed accordingly.

Individuals who are truly underresponsive appear lethargic or apathetic and may fail to become alert even in the presence of intense sensation. They often take a long time to do simple tasks (e.g., dress or eat), which can be annoying to others. Their lethargy may be mistaken for laziness or lack of motivation. Individuals who are hyporesponders may benefit from frequent opportunities to take in enhanced sensation in order to be alert enough to engage in everyday activities.

Some individuals move rapidly between underresponsiveness and defensiveness. Their ability to sustain optimal alertness and responsiveness is very limited. This seems particularly common in individuals with fragile X syndrome (Miller et al., 1999).

The section that follows does not include intervention for underresponsiveness to sensation because it closely resembles that for sensory discrimination described below. Rather, it discusses various approaches to *overresponsiveness* to sensation. We have divided these into two categories according to whether they include the provision of enhanced sensation.

Although the subject of this chapter is direct intervention, education to increase clients' and caregivers' knowledge of sensory modulation dysfunction (i.e., reframing) and alteration of the environment to minimize its effects and assist clients to attain an optimal level of arousal are critical aspects of intervention. (See Chapter 13 and the discussion of sensory diet in Chapter 14.)

Sensory-Based Interventions

There are a number of approaches to decreasing sensory defensiveness or increasing responsiveness to sensation. Ayres (1972) was the first to promote the idea of providing clients with enhanced sensation that was calming and organizing. She focused on tactile defensiveness and on interventions that used deep pressure. More recently, however, others (e.g., Frick, 2000; Oetter, Laurel & Cool, 1991; Richter & Oetter, 1990; Wilbarger & Wilbarger, 1991) who have considered tactile defensiveness to be a part of a broader modulation disorder, *sensory defensiveness,* have developed strategies that address multiple sensory systems and behavioral sequelae (see also Chapter 14).

Even though views of defensiveness have changed considerably, many of Ayres' ideas for intervention continue to fit the newer views. Thus, we review Ayres' approach as well as some other sensory and non–sensory-based approaches not described in Chapter 14.

Qualities of Enhanced Sensation: Intensity, Frequency, Duration, and Rhythm

One sensory-based approach to poor modulation involves assessing the qualities as well as the types of sensation that influence state of arousal (Oetter et al., 1991). Clients' needs change with changing environmental demands, and thus this approach to intervention involves constant monitoring of both need and demand.

Oetter et al.'s (1991) approach focuses on monitoring both the type and qualities of enhanced sensation used during intervention. After the type of enhanced sensation most appropriate for a specific client is identified (typically deep pressure, proprioception, vestibular, or auditory sensation), the qualities are specified. Oetter et al. recommended assessing benefits of sensation by varying intensity, duration, frequency, and rhythm. Frequency and duration of enhanced sensation usually are related to intensity. The effects of intense sensation may be quick and relatively long lasting and, thus, intense input may need to be available only in infrequent, short bursts.

Oetter et al. (1991) cautioned practitioners against evaluating the intensity of sensation by their own reactions. Sensations that most adults find mildly pleasurable (e.g., rocking in a rocking chair) may be much too intense for some clients. Conversely, sensations that many adults find overwhelming (e.g., spinning on an amusement park ride) may be barely satisfying and leave a client asking for more. The following case helps to illustrate the interplay of intensity, frequency, duration, and rhythm.

Case Study

When Adam, a 6-year-old boy with Asperger's syndrome and attention deficit disorder (ADD), began intervention, he ran around the therapy room and had a difficult time focusing on any purposeful activity. We tried having him use a mini-trampoline and a bolster swing. However, the postural and bilateral demands were too great for him. Thus, we tried sitting with him on a therapy ball and bouncing. After 5 minutes of bouncing, he could sustain his focus for 1 or 2 minutes. After 40 minutes of bouncing, he could sustain his focus for 30 minutes. However, this left little of the 45-minute session for other activities. On the other hand, swinging in a spandex hammock (Fig. 12–1) provided both maximal support and intense sensation. Adam was able to swing for the first 15 to 20 minutes of each session and then move to more demanding activities.

Six months later, Adam's teacher reported that after Adam sat for 15 to 20 minutes of a group ac-

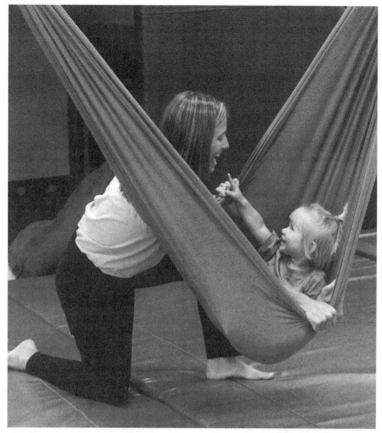

■ Figure 12-1 The spandex hammock. (Photo courtesy of Shay McAtee, printed with permission.)

tivity, he needed 3- to 4-minute movement breaks, during which he paced in the back of the classroom. Drawing from our previous experience with intensity and duration and knowing that Adam now had improved postural skills, we suggested that Adam jump on a mini-trampoline (Fig. 12–2) in the back of his classroom. The teacher reported that Adam jumped for approximately 2 minutes every 30 to 40 minutes. Initially, the teacher had been concerned that jumping on a mini-trampoline would be disruptive to the other children. However, she found that, after the novelty had worn off, the trampoline was less disruptive than Adam's pacing because Adam left the group less often and was absent from the group for less time.

Although there are some guidelines based on findings in neuroscience for how long certain types of sensation may affect the nervous system, most effects depend on the individual's response. Therefore, it is essential to monitor each client's responses carefully to provide optimal intervention.

Activities Providing Enhanced Tactile Sensation (deep pressure) and Proprioception

In developing intervention to decrease tactile defensiveness, Ayres (1972) found clients generally responded best to deep pressure as well as proprioception. Deep pressure and proprioception continue to be important therapeutic tools in intervention to decrease tactile and other forms of sensory defensiveness. Deep pressure and proprioception can be provided through a number of media. We have listed activities below with those that involve primarily deep touch pressure first, then those that provide combined tactile and proprioception, and finally activities that provide primarily proprioception.

- Textured coverings (e.g., carpeting, corduroy, and sheepskin) on equipment
- Wide paint brushes or textured mitts for brushing or scrubbing large areas of skin (Fig. 12–3)

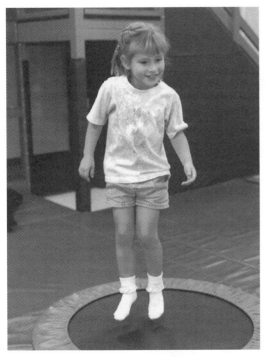

■ FIGURE 12-2 The mini-trampoline. (Photo courtesy of Shay McAtee, printed with permission.)

- Ace bandages wrapped around extremities
- Large containers of plastic bubble balls, in which clients submerge themselves and move around (Fig. 12–4)
- Boxes filled with dried lentils, beans, or rice, in which young clients can sit and older clients can submerge their arms and hands while searching for hidden objects (see Fig. 11–2)
- Large pillows and mats for burrowing (Fig. 12–5)
- Large therapy balls that a practitioner can roll firmly over a client's back and legs or that the client can push against while the therapist pushes as well
- The Wilbarger protocol (see Chapter 14)
- Wearing weighted vests, backpacks, or hats
- Heavy objects for pushing or pulling (e.g., large beanbags on the end of a rope, barrels, the therapist on a piece of equipment)
- Resistive substances for sucking through a straw (sour substances seem particularly organizing)

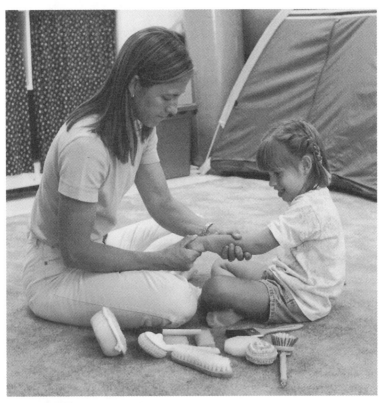

■ FIGURE 12-3 Brushes, textured mitts, and joint compression. (Photo courtesy of Shay McAtee, printed with permission.)

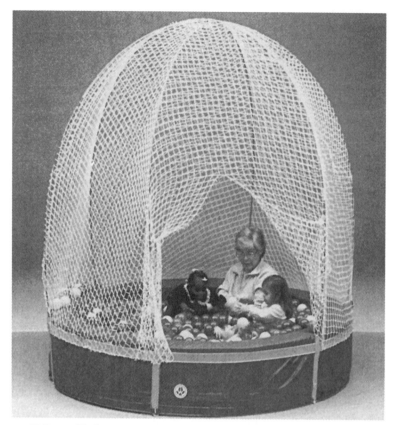

■ FIGURE 12-4   Bubble ball bath. (Photo courtesy of Southpaw Enterprises.)

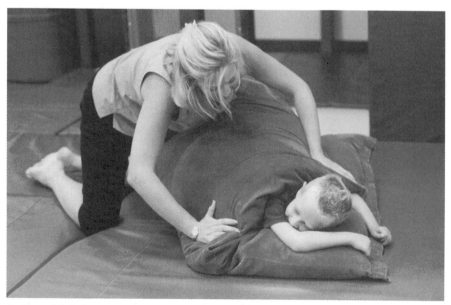

■ FIGURE 12-5   Large pillow for burrowing or "smooshing." (Photo courtesy of Shay McAtee, printed with permission.)

- Toys, objects, food, or gum appropriate for chewing
- Equipment that enables jumping, bouncing, or pulling (e.g., rope or rubber strip) while swinging
- Vibrators applied to the arms and legs

Shaving cream, powder, or lotion rubbed onto the skin may provide deep pressure. However, light touch often accompanies their application. Thus, their use may be more appropriate when defensiveness has begun to decrease.

General Guidelines for Providing Tactile and Proprioceptive Experiences

This section presents six guidelines for enhanced tactile and proprioceptive sensation. Practitioners can judge the effectiveness of enhanced sensation by evaluating whether clients concentrate better, behave in a more organized fashion, and enjoy social interactions to a greater degree, indicating that their defensiveness has decreased.

First, we recommend that clients administer enhanced tactile or proprioceptive sensation to themselves. Thus, they select the areas, relative pressure, and length of time it will be applied. However, we are working with increasing numbers of clients whose impairments prohibit them from administering their own enhanced input. Many of these clients are nonverbal. When we administer sensation, it is crucial that we recognize signs of hyperalertness, overactivity, or autonomic nervous system indicators of stress (e.g., sweating, pallor). An individual's behavior may appear organized and focused one moment, but it can become disorganized very quickly.

Second, although maintained, deep pressure is the type of enhanced tactile sensation most commonly recommended for decreasing tactile defensiveness, some clients prefer light touch or rapidly moving stimulation. Ayres (1972) hypothesized that some clients actually perceive light touch as deep pressure. Thus, it is important to experiment with different types of sensation to determine which is the most effective.

Third, it usually is not necessary to provide enhanced tactile or proprioceptive sensation to the whole body. Applying input to the arms and legs is usually sufficient to decrease tactile defensiveness. Ayres (1972) postulated that deep pressure and proprioception have a central inhibitory effect. Therefore, although the input is applied to specific body areas, it may have a more generalized effect. Our clients usually find enhanced tactile and proprioceptive sensation to be most acceptable when it is applied to the arms, legs, and back rather than to the face or other body areas. Furthermore, although it is not necessary to apply sensation to the entire body, simply dipping the hands or fingers into textured media is probably not sufficient to consider the sensation "enhanced." For the sensation to be considered enhanced, it must be more than one gets in daily life.

Fourth, clients seem to find tactile sensation more tolerable if it is applied in the direction of hair growth. Moving against the hairs often seems to result in hyper-alertness and overactivity. However, for some individuals, lifting the brush repeatedly to avoid going against the hair may be very irritating.

Fifth, clients often find that quiet enclosed spaces (e.g., a large empty box lined with pillows, a tent, a "clubhouse") are the best places to use scrub mitts and paint brushes for administering enhanced tactile sensation. They may prefer enclosed spaces because other forms of sensation, particularly threats of unexpected touch, are minimized.

Sixth, proprioception is generally the most organizing type of sensation; clients are rarely sensitive to it. When a client appears to be bothered by tactile sensation, substituting proprioception, or combining deep pressure with proprioception is often successful.

If sensory defensiveness is not decreased as a result of intervention, the intervention should be modified. Practitioners are advised that negative effects of enhanced sensation may not appear immediately after an activity. In fact, the effects may be delayed for several hours (Fisher & Bundy, 1989). We must communicate regularly with clients and caregivers about responses that occur up to several hours after a therapy session to be certain that intervention is having the desired effects.

We have observed that auditory defensiveness seems particularly resistant to change from traditional intervention based on the principles of sensory integration theory. Thus, it may be that the auditory system must be addressed specifically before auditory defensiveness can be significantly diminished. In Chapter 6, Burleigh et al. offer considerable insight into the nature of central auditory processing deficits and intervention. In Chapter 14, Frick describes the use of therapeutic listening, a technique to address sensory integration problems, including sensory defensiveness, through the auditory system.

Special Notes on Vibration

Vibration is a form of deep pressure that activates proprioceptors. All of the guidelines specified in this chapter for enhanced tactile sensation also apply to vibration. However, because it is requested so often and because it is so potent, vibration warrants a little further discussion.

We have found vibration from a battery-operated or electric body massager to be a particular favorite for some clients who have tactile defensiveness. Sometimes a client wants to put the vibrator in his or her mouth or on his or her ears. Because these areas of the body are so sensitive, we interpret this as a desire for unusually powerful or intense stimulation. Most clients who seek vibration administer it for a short time and then put down the vibrator in favor of some other activity, suggesting that they have had enough. We never encourage them to continue. However, some clients seem to be unaware or unable to indicate that they have had enough. With clients who may not reliably discontinue vibration, a practitioner may allow its use briefly and make careful observations regarding behavioral changes afterwards.

Special Notes on Activity Directed at the Mouth and Face

When a client's mouth or face is particularly hypersensitive, deep pressure administered directly to these areas can be beneficial. There are a number of ways to provide stimulation to the mouth. For infants and young children, deep pressure may be provided to the roof of the mouth or gums with the therapist's fingers or another soft, rounded object, such as the Nuk toothbrush. Older children and adults can be taught to provide deep pressure to their own mouths. Clients sometimes seem to enjoy a variety of types of whistles for this purpose. As clients maneuver the whistles in the mouth, they provide themselves with deep pressure. Some clients like to bite on knotted rubber tubing as a means of providing deep pressure and proprioception to oral structures. Another favorite activity is to blow into a rubber strip that is stretched across the mouth, thus creating "raspberries." This activity provides vibration to the lips and face.

Non–Sensory-Based Programs

Oetter and her colleagues (Oetter et al., 1993; Richter & Oetter, 1990) have developed two additional interventions to address problems commonly associated with sensory modulation dysfunction. Although both of these programs are combined with enhanced sensation, enhancing sensation is not the focus of the programs.

Sucking, Swallowing, and Breathing

In the first of these non–sensory-based programs, Oetter et al. (1993) described ways to assess difficulties with respiration, including shallow and arrhythmic breathing and difficulty coordinating breathing with sucking and swallowing. Although coordinated sucking, swallowing, and breathing are the first skills of a newborn, many of our clients have difficulty with these skills. Oetter et al. believed that coordination of sucking, swallowing, and breathing formed a foundation for regulating arousal and developing postural-ocular skills and praxis. They believed it was important to assess these skills in all individuals with sensory integrative dysfunction, not only those with frank oral motor issues (e.g., poor articulation and feeding difficulties).

Intervention to improve sucking, swallowing, and breathing begins, when possible, with resistive sucking through a straw or piece of aquarium tubing. When a client cannot suck through a tube, sucking is graded (e.g., the client may begin by sucking food from a finger). Blowing is the next target of intervention. Similar to sucking, blowing is graded (e.g., blowing through a straw into water with soapsuds, whistles, balloons) (Fig. 12–6). The next intervention includes biting, crunching, and chewing (e.g., biting and tugging on tubing, a washcloth, pieces of licorice, dried beef, or fruit; chewing crunchy foods such as chips and crackers, carrot sticks, bagels, or apples). Finally, licking activities (e.g., licking lollipops, ice cream, peanut butter on a spoon) are introduced because they require the most fine-tuned oral skill. Although we have listed this approach as non–sensory based, it frequently involves various smells and tastes. Furthermore, many of the activ-

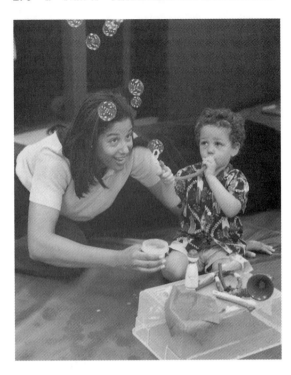

■ FIGURE 12–6 Blowing bubbles through a long straw. (Photo courtesy of Shay McAtee, printed with permission.)

ities provide enhanced proprioceptive and tactile sensation to the mouth. In *M.O.R.E.—Integrating the Mouth with Sensory and Postural Functions,* Oetter et al. (1993) present a useful grading system for oral motor activities.

The Matrix Model

In a second non–sensory-based program, the Matrix Model, Richter and Oetter (1990) adapted and expanded Pearce's (1963) ideas to address difficulties associated with sensory modulation dysfunction. Using the Matrix Model, practitioners classify interactions on a matrix with axes representing task and environment. Four types of task and environment interactions are named: womb, mother, kid power, and brain power.

Womb interactions take place in small, protected environments that are separate from the world at large and invoke feelings of security and safety. An individual may receive constant physical contact from another person or deep pressure from a large pillow or blanket. Very few demands are placed on the client. *Mother interactions* occur in close proximity (typically 8 to 10 inches away) to an adult who gives intermittent physical or eye contact. The adult may bend toward or sit at the child's level. Verbal input is typically in short, rhythmic utterances. Mother interactions provide safe, nurturing

environments to support risk taking. *Kid power* involves mastery of the earth and gravity. Children develop a sense of physical and personal competence through demands to praxis. Intervention based on the principles of sensory integration typically focuses on developing kid power. *Brain power* represents the final position on the matrix; it involves problem solving, cognitive challenge, and complex practic and verbal demands.

The four types of interactions described by the matrix represent a developmental progression. However, regardless of age, clients may have times when they want or need to retreat to womb or mother space briefly before beginning or returning to kid or brain power activities. In addition, some kid and brain power tasks may be completed more competently in spaces that provide womb or mother space. Application of the Matrix Model ensures that the therapeutic environment offers safe places and comfortable demands along with the more challenging demands of kid and brain power interactions.

For example, in all of our therapy rooms, there is at least one readily available womb space (e.g., tunnel, clubhouse). We also have spandex or blankets and clothespins or clips to enclose suspended equipment and create additional womb spaces. We may turn off the lights and hum softly or play soothing instrumental music to create womb spaces. Clients with sensory modulation dysfunction often retreat to womb space. Occasionally, clients are so overwhelmed by sensation and so active that they cannot move by themselves into a womb space even though it might prove to be beneficial. Thus, we sometimes move clients into these spaces. Although we may not believe that time spent in womb space is a cost-effective intervention, respecting clients' needs to have quiet time may be the only way we can move forward effectively. When we move children from womb space to other spaces represented on the matrix, we must go slowly, observing and responding to the child's' reactions.

We also routinely create opportunities for clients to engage in mother space interactions. Placing ourselves close to a client creates such a space. Clubhouses or lofts big enough for two facilitate mother space. (Although the term "mother" is used, fathers, therapists, and other caretakers, male or female, can create the same type of interaction.) Time spent in mother space allows children to develop trust that ultimately allows them to master kid and then brain power activities.

The following case example is used to illustrate implementation of two of the non–sensory-based interventions discussed above. Here we share a description of a session in which the three programs developed by Oetter et al. (1991, 1993) and Richter and Oetter (1990) to address problems associated with sensory modulation dysfunction are combined.

Case Study

Amalia, a 4½-year-old girl who experienced sensory modulation as well as praxis difficulties, was transferred to a new therapy practitioner. Amalia was particularly defensive to tactile, auditory, and visual sensation. The previous therapist felt that Amalia was ready to engage in activities to promote more mature hand skills and pre-writing abilities but found it difficult to engage Amalia in such activities.

Amalia appeared anxious about the transition, stating that she did not want to come into the room. When she did enter, she darted around, avoiding eye contact. She seemed unable to become involved in any purposeful activity. Although she was typically able to work in a room with other children and therapists, on this day she seemed unable to tolerate the activity and verbalizations of

others. The therapist was able to move her into a room where the two could be alone. They turned off the lights, illuminating the room with only natural light from a window. Amalia got into a net swing with a long, soft pillow inside. She curled up on her back and asked for a blanket on top of her, which helped to create a womb space. The therapist swung Amalia slowly and sang a lullaby, providing her with rhythmical movement, deep pressure, and neutral warmth from the blanket. Amalia calmed noticeably.

After several minutes, the therapist began pushing Amalia by her feet to introduce more deep pressure and create mother space. Amalia did not withdraw, and whenever the therapist stopped, Amalia pushed on the therapist's hands with her feet. Amalia also indicated that she was enjoying the song. The therapist sang several nursery rhyme songs and then gave Amalia a whistle so that she could join in when she desired. Amalia was asked if *she* had a song. Amalia suggested several songs and ultimately sang to the therapist (a kid power task). The breath support to sustain blowing the whistle—and, later, the songs—required that Amalia slow and deepen her breathing, which, in turn, seemed to calm her further. Amalia initiated teaching songs to the therapist, who purposefully made some errors. Amalia took great delight in helping the therapist sing the songs correctly.

Providing the opportunity for Amalia to begin in the womb space with a vocal activity that required breath support calmed her and allowed her to prepare herself for other activities. After 20 minutes in the net swing, Amalia announced that she was ready to get out and do something else. She moved onto a sitting position on a dual swing that continued to provide enhanced vestibular and proprioceptive sensation and challenged her to remain stable by using both her flexor and extensor muscles. This activity also required that Amalia time her movements so that she did not crash into the therapist. After this activity, Amalia was able to make the transition to a fine motor task, successfully turning the knobs on small wind-up toys.

Ayres (1972) focused primarily on deep touch pressure as an intervention for decreasing tactile defensiveness. Over the past 30 years, many sensory and non–sensory-based interventions have been developed to address defensiveness that involves all sensory systems. We have described a few programs. Readers are also referred to Chapter 14.

INTERVENTION FOR GRAVITATIONAL INSECURITY

Gravitational insecurity is described as a "primal fear" response to changes in head position or disturbances to the base of support (May, 1988); it is one of the most devastating types of sensory integrative dysfunction. Although it is commonly understood that gravity is a pervasive phenomenon, unless one has difficulty in processing information from the vestibular receptors in the inner ear, it is easy to forget that every moment of our lives is influenced by our relationship to gravity. When clients are terrified by every change in position, they can become easily "paralyzed" by the demands of daily life.

Gravitational insecurity may result from difficulty processing sensation typically received by the otolith organs of the vestibular system (Fisher & Bundy, 1989; see also Chapter 4). Fisher (1991) speculated that gravitational insecurity was associated with poor development of the body scheme and inability to resolve sensory conflict. Certainly, in our experience, gravitational insecurity is accompanied by a perceptual disorder. Clients who are afraid of moving or having their heads out of an upright position often perceive very small movements to be larger than they actually are. Furthermore, although a swing appears to be moving in a straight line, clients who have gravitational insecurity may perceive an imperceptible arc as "going around in circles." Thus, gravitational insecurity may be a problem of discrimination as well as of modulation.

Regardless of the cause, intervention for gravitational insecurity centers on activities that provide enhanced proprioceptive and linear vestibular sensation. The client's active participation in intervention is important for the development of body schema as well as the discrimination of sensation related to movement and position. Thus, we alter therapeutic activities so they do not elicit the fear response we are trying to eliminate.

General Guidelines

Clients who have gravitational insecurity need a lot of support and encouragement. They must trust a therapy practitioner implicitly, and the practitioner must earn that trust. We have found two strategies that have been particularly helpful for developing the trust of clients with gravitational insecurity. First, the client should always be involved, at least initially, in activities in which the feet are on or near the ground. That way, the client can immediately stop the activity. Stopping the activity is usually most easily accomplished if the client is sitting.

After clients have worked through some of their fear of moving the head out of an upright position, we create activities done in prone (e.g., swinging prone over a suspended inner tube or frog swing). Clients control the movement of a swing when they are prone and very close to the mat. Some clients feel safest when using a therapist's outstretched hands to swing themselves. Using handles or elastic ropes offers another alternative that allows clients to propel themselves.

Secondly, in our experience, clients who have gravitational insecurity especially fear movements into backward space, in part because they cannot see where they are going. Of course, all swings move backward half the time. We have found that stacking cardboard blocks (or other lightweight objects that are easily knocked over) behind the swing at a distance that the client approves often helps the client to overcome some of the initial fear. Perhaps having previous knowledge of an endpoint for the backward movement helps resolve some of the sensory conflict. The target gives both the client and the therapist a measure of improvement and may enable intervention to progress at a more rapid rate.

Many clients who have gravitational insecurity also have poor body flexion and difficulty with eye convergence. Part of their fear of falling may be caused by difficulty assuming a safe and protected position; some of their difficulty dealing with objects coming toward them (e.g., balls) may be related to poor eye convergence. However, by definition, gravitational insecurity is fear of movement (vestibular input) that is out of proportion to that which could be accounted for by poor posture or ocular movements alone.

Suggested Activities

Some young children who experience severe gravitational insecurity may not be able to tolerate moving equipment. For them, walking up and down a ramp (Fig. 12–7) may provide the just-right challenge. Bouncing up and down on a mini-trampoline, pad, therapy ball, or whale (Fig. 12–8) provides enhanced vestibular and proprioceptive sensation without the need to move into backward space. Clients who cannot bounce independently may enjoy bouncing on the whale or a therapy ball together with a therapist. For clients who can tolerate swings and moving equipment, we recommend several as sources of enhanced vestibular and proprioceptive sensation. These can all be used in prone as well as sitting; they include:

- The frog swing
- The square platform swing (with an inner tube atop to sit in) (Fig. 12–9)
- The platform glider
- The bolster swing
- The dual swing
- Scooter boards

Platform gliders or bolster swings should be suspended from two points to promote linear movement and minimize rotational movements that often induce fear. If it is not possible for a client's feet to be on the ground (e.g., on a platform swing with an inner tube on top), a beanbag chair or cushion should be placed under the swing to slow it down.

Although most clients with gravitational insecurity prefer equipment that provides maximum stability and support, we have occasionally seen clients who prefer equipment such as the dual swing, which provides little support to the trunk and limbs but gives pressure to the shoulder and hip joints when the client is prone. This activity seems to be most enjoyable when the straps of the swing are made from rubber inner tubes.

Beth, a 7-year old first-grade student, initially responded to many kinds of movement by keeping her body rigid and complaining that she was afraid. She avoided swings, slides, and climbers and refused to participate in physical education. After watching Beth, we believed that her responses were caused by gravitational insecurity. We gradually introduced activities that incorporated linear motion and resistance to movement into intervention, creating increasingly greater challenges for Beth.

Beth was initially willing only to sit on the platform swing or bounce and swing back and forth in the frog swing. The platform swing offered a firm base of support, and the frog swing allowed her to place her feet on the floor. The course of intervention was very gradual; it was crucial that Beth feel safe. She needed to develop a trusting relationship with the therapist before she could be challenged by activities that required more movement.

As Beth became more willing to try new challenges, she and her therapist rode together on a plastic mat down a ramp. After several sessions, Beth was able to slide alone. The therapist eventually introduced a scooter board for the ramp. Beth performed this activity cautiously at first. Gradu-

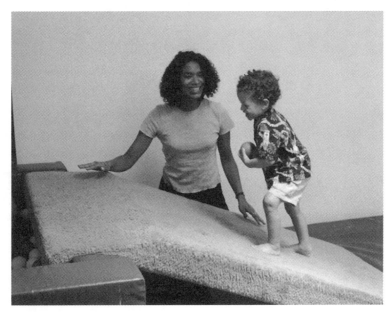

■ FIGURE 12-7   Walking up a ramp. (Photo courtesy of Shay McAtee, printed with permission.)

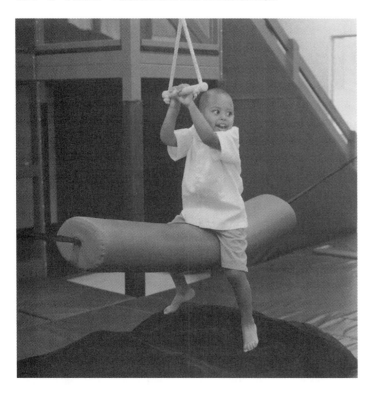

■ FIGURE 12–8 Bouncing up and down on a whale. (Photo courtesy of Shay McAtee, printed with permission.)

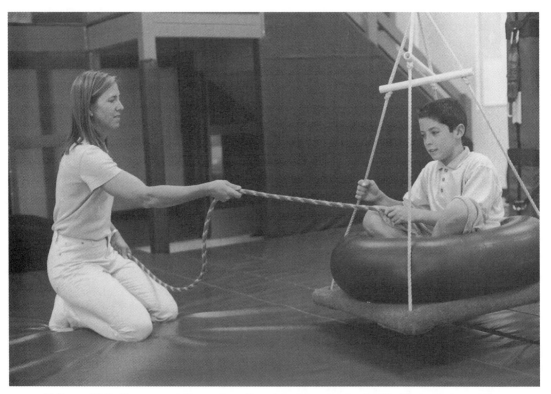

■ FIGURE 12–9 The square platform swing with an inner tube atop for stability. (Photo courtesy of Shay McAtee, printed with permission).

ally, she began to ride down the ramp freely and express her enjoyment.

Beth progressed to riding on equipment that moved less predictably. She liked lying prone on the bolster swing and hugging it and then falling off onto a "crash pad" underneath (Fig. 12–10). Later she began to release her hold on the bolster while being swung side to side. As her flexion improved, her desire to experiment with falling increased. She enjoyed falling backwards into the ball pit. She began to seek out opportunities to jump off surfaces that were 3 feet high. As her gravitational insecurity diminished, she sought more movement experiences on playground equipment and in gym class. She began to enjoy gross motor play. Her parents reported they had a better sense of her "true personality" now that she felt more secure moving. Beth seemed more outgoing and increasingly self-confident.

With the advent of the Therapeutic Listening Program (TL) (see Frick's contribution to Chapter 14), which is thought to enhance auditory spatial processing, we have another tool to add to our intervention planning for individuals with gravitational insecurity. In TL, specially designed music that involves nature sounds has been reported to assist some clients with gravitational insecurity. This music was recorded outdoors so one can hear sounds that were close by as well as at varying distances from the recorder. The music is thought to help individuals with gravitational insecurity gain an increased sense of their position in space.

INTERVENTION FOR AVERSIVE RESPONSES TO MOVEMENT

Intolerance of or aversive response to vestibular input is another modulation problem that is based in poor vestibular processing. Aversive responses to movement are hypothesized to relate to poor processing of sensation within the semicircular canals (Fisher & Bundy, 1989). Fisher (1991) speculated that aversive responses might be related to impaired use of vestibular and proprioceptive sensation to resolve sensory conflicts. Previc (1993) hypothesized that the two parts of the vestibular system have differential effects on the autonomic nervous system. He suggested that aversive responses might be related to the otolith receptors, resulting in sympathetic hypofunction and parasympathetic activation. Aversive responses are manifested as vertigo (i.e., sensation of self-movement), sweating, pallor, nausea, or vomiting in response to movement that most individuals readily tolerate. Avoidance of angular movement or an increase in restlessness after movement

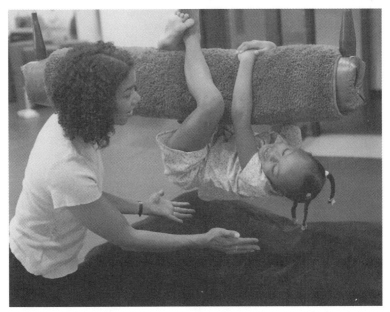

■ FIGURE 12–10   Hugging the bolster swing while preparing to fall into a pillow. (Photo courtesy of Shay McAtee, printed with permission.)

may also suggest mild aversive responses.

Activities that provide linear movement (vestibular) and resistance to active movement (proprioception) help to minimize aversive responses. If aversive responses are caused by difficulty processing information from the otolith organs as Previc (1993) hypothesized, then linear movement should be the most effective form of enhanced sensation for its remediation. Thus, many of the activities described above for intervention for gravitational insecurity can also be used to address aversive responses to movement. Initially, swings that are hung from two suspension points (e.g., platform glider, bolster swing) are recommended to decrease the likelihood of rotation. Later swings hung from one point of suspension (e.g., frog swing, net swing) can be introduced as long as they allow clients to maintain control over the movements. Suspending a swing so that it is low to the ground increases control. Lying prone enhances proprioception because of the need to resist gravity to hold the head and legs up.

A goal of intervention is to help clients tolerate common movement experiences (e.g., bending over to tie one's shoes, riding in a car or on a swing) without feeling sick or dizzy. The goal is *not* to help clients tolerate spinning or other rotary movement. Clients with aversive responses to movement that prevent them from participating in daily life activities and impede their progress in intervention sometimes respond positively to two non-sensory integrative intervention techniques known as vestibular habituation training (Fisher & Bundy, 1989) and vestibular rehabilitation (Cohen, 1992, 2000; Cohen et al., 1995). Both techniques are prescribed and carefully monitored programs of desensitization to movement.

INTERVENTION FOR POOR SENSORY DISCRIMINATION

Poor sensory discrimination is a decreased ability to interpret the spatial or temporal qualities of touch, movement, or body position; it is thought to underlie body schema, which, in turn, contributes to praxis (see Chapter 3). Unlike poor sensory modulation, in which symptoms fluctuate from day to day or even hour to hour, deficits of sensory discrimination remain relatively stable without intervention. Poor sensory discrimination is identified most commonly in conjunction with poor praxis.

Typically, individuals with poor sensory discrimination have a meaningful cluster of indicators of diminished vestibular or proprioceptive processing (seen as deficits in postural skills) or depressed scores on a constellation of tests of tactile discrimination. In older clients, evidence of diminished tactile discrimination may be heard in such complaints as, "I can't tell a penny from a dime in my pocket without looking" or, "I only know up from down by knowing where my head is." We also expect to see depressed scores associated with practic deficits.

Many individuals who have decreased sensory discrimination seem to crave enhanced sensation. However, craving and need are not synonymous, and not all clients who have decreased sensory discrimination crave sensations they do not process effectively. Furthermore, craving is not necessarily a sign that enhanced sensation will be therapeutic, although it may suggest a need.

Decreased Discrimination of Vestibular and Proprioceptive Sensation

Clients who have difficulty recognizing the characteristics of sensation received by the *otolith organs* have trouble determining the spatial orientation of the head (e.g., upright from upside down). Clients who have difficulty with discrimination of sensation received by *muscle receptors* have trouble determining relative position or movements of body parts; they have difficulty judging the amount of force needed for a task. Clients with either of these discrimination deficits often have poor body schema. Clients who have difficulty discerning characteristics of sensation received by the *semicircular canals* have trouble distinguishing small, rapid movements. For that reason, they have poor equilibrium because equilibrium reactions occur in response to small, rapid movements. Clients with poor discrimination of sensation detected by the semicircular canals also may have diminished postrotary nystagmus.

When addressing poor discrimination of movement or body position, we create activities that provide movement and resistance to movement. As with all interventions based on sensory integration theory, active participation in meaningful tasks is crucial. We discuss interventions for each of the manifestations of decreased discrimination of vestibular and proprioceptive sensations.

Targeting Processing Related to the Otolith Organs

For clients who have difficulty distinguishing head orientation, we emphasize activities that provide linear movement. Many activities are similar to those described for gravitational insecurity and aversive responses to movement. However, unless clients also have a modulation dysfunction, we usually are able to incorporate more movement and larger excursions.

Although it is relatively rare for an individual to not intuit the difference between his or her head being upright compared with upside down, such individuals do exist. Furthermore, we believe that difficulty discriminating orientation of the head and body occurs in more subtle forms. Feeling the orientation of the head and body is an important foundation for movement; thus, when a client has difficulty, we address it in an initial phase of intervention. Activities usually involve suspended equipment and should be done in a variety of positions (e.g., prone, sitting). Because linear movement is desired, swings are generally suspended from two points. We try to provide opportunities for vertical and upside down movements because of the less common occurrence of those types of movement in day-to-day life. Equipment such as a trampoline or a whale provides vertical movement. Scooter boards also provide opportunities for linear movement in the horizontal plane. Horizontal movements, such as those generated while prone or sitting in a swing are the easiest to incorporate into activities that involve throwing or catching.

Targeting Processing Related to Muscle Receptors

For clients who have difficulty distinguishing relative position or movement of body parts or judging the appropriate amount of muscle force to exert, we emphasize activities that provide resistance to active movement. The weight of the body against gravity ensures that many activities that involve swings, scooter boards, or trampolines provide resistance to body movements. Resistance to movement, rather than joint compression, provides the most critical source of proprioception when jumping on a trampoline (see Chapter 2). Active movement against resistance, whether clients are using squirt guns or jumping on a trampoline, pro-

vides the enhanced proprioception needed to calibrate force or judge extent of movement.

Targeting Processing Related to Semicircular Canals

For clients who have difficulty distinguishing rapid or small movements or who have depressed duration of postrotary nystagmus, we emphasize activities that provide rapid or angular (i.e., rotary) movements. However, we do this with caution because angular movement is extremely powerful (see precautions below). Although depressed duration of postrotary nystagmus is part of the assessment of a client with a vestibular problem, increased duration of nystagmus is not an objective of intervention. Therefore, we do not measure gains in this area by reassessing duration of nystagmus. Rather, we assess functional areas influenced by the vestibular system.

Angular movement is generated most readily when swings are hung from a single suspension point. We have successfully used a variety of swings in this way, including the net swing, dual swing (Fig. 12–11), T-swing, bolster swing, platform swing, frog swing, and others that are commercially available (see Appendix 12–A for a list of vendors). Swings suspended from two points also provide input to semicircular canals when swings do not travel in a straight line or activities incorporate relatively fast swinging. Because the hair cells of the semicircular canals are stimulated during acceleration and deceleration, activities should include frequent *starts and stops, changes in direction,* and *changes in speed.*

Activities that involve picking up beanbags or balls from a mat or batting or throwing at suspended objects while swinging also inherently involve varying head positions. In turn, input to the vestibular mechanism is varied when stopping or changing direction. Activities of this type also challenge clients' bilateral and oculomotor skills and abilities to perform projected action sequences.

We provide input specifically to the less often stimulated anterior and posterior canals by having clients spin around the body's anterior-posterior axis while lying on one side and rotating the head approximately 45 degrees. This can be done on a platform swing or while curled around a disc swing with a pillow under the head to keep it in line with the body. Such input is extremely powerful; it is important to observe clients at all times

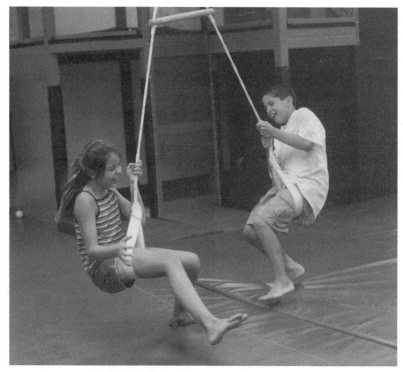

■ Figure 12-11 The dual swing. (Photo courtesy of Shay McAtee, printed with permission.)

and make necessary changes as quickly as possible if the vestibular sensation becomes disorganizing. Over time, the need for such powerful input usually lessens. Clients also like to experiment with head position on various pieces of equipment. Presumably, they are "playing with" vestibular sensation (Fig. 12–12).

When Clients Seem Not to Respond to But Crave Input

Many clients who have little or no response to spinning (e.g., diminished duration of postrotary nystagmus, absence of dizziness) crave fast, rotary movement. Often a mother will say, "He never gets tired of swinging. The other kids have left the playground long ago and he just wants to stay and swing." In therapy, the child often expresses preference for spinning or for swings that "go hard and fast." What he appears to be craving, in fact, may reflect an absence of the normal response that would ordinarily limit an individual's tolerance.

As clients begin to respond more typically to sensation, they usually show less craving for the input. However, they may not readily interpret body signs that they have enough stimulation and should stop. Some clients express displeasure when they get dizzy after spinning. They viewed their "increased tolerance" as an accomplishment and now need reassurance that it is normal to get dizzy.

Precautions

Negative reactions to vestibular sensation (i.e., sensory overload or sensory disorientation) may not be apparent for several hours (Fisher & Bundy, 1989) and may occur even though clients enjoyed a session and had no negative reaction during or immediately afterwards. Individuals who have difficulty responding to movement may also have difficulty recognizing when they have had enough. Again, we emphasize the need to communicate regularly with clients and caregivers.

If sensory overload (e.g., pupil dilation, sweaty palms, changes in rate of respiration, flushing or pallor) or sensory disorientation (i.e., distortions of body schema) occur, we alter the amount and type of sensation clients receive. We emphasize activities that incorporate slow—and primarily linear—movement and that provide considerable resis-

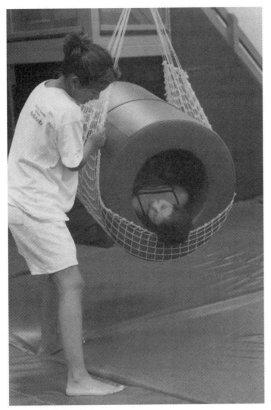

■ FIGURE 12-12 Lying supine with the head tilted to provide unique input to the semicircular canals. (Photo courtesy of Shay McAtee, printed with permission.)

tance to movement. Clients who have experienced sensory disorientation have indicated that deep pressure helps to lessen some of the symptoms.

Although we proceed cautiously, enhanced sensation is a critical element of intervention. Many clients spend the majority of a session engaged in activity that provides strong vestibular and proprioceptive sensation without any ill effects. Furthermore, they appear to benefit from enhanced sensation, as noted by their development of skills the vestibular system influences (e.g., increased extensor tone, improved equilibrium).

Decreased Discrimination of Tactile Sensation

Some individuals with sensory integrative dysfunction have a decreased ability to process the spatial or temporal aspects of information gained through touch. These individuals have difficulty knowing both the precise locations of touch and the properties of objects they have touched. They may also

constantly—and seemingly unconsciously—manipulate nearby objects.

Tactile discrimination is thought to underlie praxis (Ayres, 1972). Most often poor tactile discrimination is discovered in the context of evaluation of praxis. In addition, many clients with poor tactile discrimination also have deficits in vestibular and proprioceptive processing. Intervention for poor tactile discrimination is usually done in conjunction with intervention for dyspraxia.

Activities that provide tactile sensation rich in temporal and spatial qualities generally are used to improve tactile discrimination. Furthermore, deep pressure is important throughout intervention. Although tactile discrimination is thought to underlie body schema and thus affect the client's ability to use the entire body, it seems to have considerable influence on fine motor development (i.e., hand and oral skill). Hence, we create activities that provide deep pressure to large areas of the body, but we pay particular attention to the hands and mouth. As with intervention for tactile defensiveness, activities may involve:

- Brushing or rubbing the skin with various textures
- Using a vibrator
- Hiding body parts under balls in a bubble ball bath, heavy cushions, or a mixture of dried rice and beans

As clients become better able to process tactile sensation, we challenge their discrimination abilities by having them search for objects in mixtures of dried macaroni, beans, corn, lentils, or rice. Finally, clients can identify objects of different shapes, sizes, or textures without looking.

Nathan, a 6-year-old boy with significant difficulty in tactile discrimination, constantly manipulated objects and ran his hand along the walls as he walked down halls. Nathan also had poor hand skill development and other problems associated with somatodyspraxia. Initially, he showed great pleasure when he played in the bean mixture. He shoved his hands in deep and poured it over his arms. We placed 3-inch long plastic animals into the mixture for him to find. Although he was allowed to look, he often had difficulty locating the animals. When he finally could find them without looking, he was at first unable to describe an animal in his hand despite more than adequate verbal skills.

After several months of intervention, Nathan was able to identify animals and other similarly sized shapes. Eventually, he was able to find small objects (e.g., pennies and Monopoly game pieces) in a box of dried rice, peas, and popcorn. This required finer tactile discrimination and improved ability to manipulate objects in his hands, and we interpreted his developing abilities as improvements in both. Nathan's teacher reported that Nathan no longer inappropriately touched and manipulated objects. Most importantly, he exhibited an increased willingness to engage in handwriting and art projects and was able to independently manipulate fasteners (e.g., buttons, snaps, and zippers).

Multiple Processing Problems

Some clients have evidence of more than one type of sensory processing dysfunction. For example, when beginning therapy at age 4 years, Emilio had severe gravitational insecurity. During his initial evaluation, he refused to participate in the Postrotary Nystagmus Test. After 6 months of intervention emphasizing enhanced proprioception and linear movement, his gravitational insecurity seemed greatly diminished. He readily climbed onto equipment 4 or 5 feet off the ground and jumped onto mats below. He enjoyed performing somersaults and other activities that require change of head position and angular movement. He began to express a craving for angular movement; he spun himself happily on the Sit 'n' Spin at home and on swings in the clinic. When he was able to tolerate the Postrotary Nystagmus Test, he showed decreased nystagmus (reflective of poor sensory discrimination). Initially, his gravitational insecurity made it impossible to detect this difficulty.

Similar to multiple processing problems within the vestibular system, clients may also have more than one manifestation of poor tactile processing. Many clients have evidence of both defensiveness and poor tactile discrimination. In addition, poor sensory processing can occur across modalities. For example, clients might have tactile defensiveness and gravitational insecurity.

Balancing Intervention for Modulation and Discrimination Difficulties

Distinguishing between difficulties with discrimination and modulation is not always easy, especially for individuals who appear to have low arousal or poor discrimination. Furthermore, needs of clients who crave certain sensations are not always easy to interpret. Some may crave certain sensations to gain increased information for discrimination and improved body schema. Others may seek sensation as a way to improve modulation and alter their arousal level. For some clients, both may be true.

Some clients crave and seem to need enhanced vestibular sensation to improve discrimination, but they may exhibit outbursts of boisterous behavior that reflect poor sensory modulation and CNS overarousal. These individuals may need to engage in activities that provide enhanced sensation followed by activities that are calming, all within the same session. Otherwise, they could become so overly active that their behavior deteriorates. Other clients have increased craving and frequent bursts of boisterous behavior when involved in "calming" activities. They may run around to keep themselves alert. When calming activities threaten their alertness, they compensate by becoming increasingly active. For these clients, enhanced sensation may increase alertness and thereby diminish the need for increased activity.

INTERVENTION FOR IMPROVING POSTURE

In order to act effectively on the environment, an individual must be able to assume and maintain stable positions, move in and out of positions without losing balance, and have adequate postural control to support limb movement. Individuals with vestibular and proprioceptive dysfunction often have postural deficits, including a meaningful cluster of the following:

- Low tone in extensor muscles
- Poor postural stability
- Poor equilibrium reactions
- Difficulty assuming and maintaining prone extension
- Poor tonic flexion in the neck muscles

One adult client stated that each time she dropped a pencil, she had to get out of her chair, turn around, bend down, pick up the pencil, and then reverse the procedure to return to her chair. She lacked the postural control to remain seated and retrieve her pencil. When clients demonstrate a meaningful cluster of postural difficulties, we hypothesize that they have difficulty processing vestibular and proprioceptive sensation. In intervention, we emphasize activities that provide enhanced vestibular and proprioceptive sensation and that simultaneously challenge posture.

We discuss intervention to develop five aspects of postural control, including:

- Tonic postural extension
- Tonic flexion
- Postural stability (balancing flexion and extension)
- Weight shifting, lateral flexion, and rotation
- Righting and equilibrium reactions
- Oculomotor control

Developing Tonic Postural Extension

In developing extension against gravity, we emphasize activities that provide linear movement in either the horizontal plane (e.g., swinging on a platform glider swing) or the vertical plane (e.g., jumping on a trampoline). Although activities can be done in any position, the prone position demands the greatest amount of extension. To enhance proprioception, we create activities that involve movement against resistance, including the resistance of gravity; we carefully grade resistance so clients are able to perform activities successfully. We may begin with an individual bouncing

up and down while prone in a frog swing, where proprioceptive input is strong to the neck from lifting the head and neck against gravity. Furthermore, although activities done in the prone position may emphasize extension, good posture (i.e., with chin tucked and back straight) demands the use of both the flexor and the extensor muscles.

For clients with low muscle tone, we begin with activities that primarily challenge their neck and upper back stability (e.g., swinging prone over a frog swing or working in prone on elbows) without demanding total extension of the body. For example, a client assumes a prone-on-elbows position on a swinging glider and blows cotton balls off raised mats in front of the glider. We watch carefully to be sure the client maintains good posture, which includes:

- The neck is *not* hyperextended (i.e., chin is tucked).
- The upper chest is raised off the surface.
- The upper arms are perpendicular to the surface.

Activities (e.g., throwing at a target) that require weight shifting while in a prone position on the elbows are slightly harder. Activities that require weight bearing on the extended arms (e.g., lying prone on a barrel and "walking" it forward to place objects on a magnetic board) (Fig. 12–13)

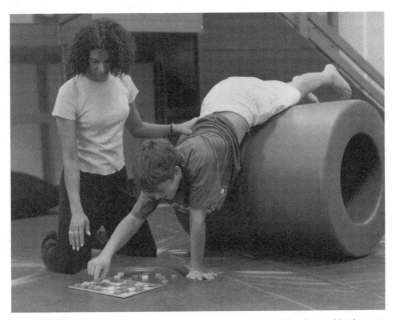

■ FIGURE 12–13 "Walking" forward while prone on a barrel to place objects on a magnetic surface. (Photo courtesy of Shay McAtee, printed with permission.)

or that demand prone extension (e.g., riding prone in a net while catching a beach ball) provide even greater challenges.

Finally, activities that require both prone extension and supporting full body weight with the arms (e.g., lying in the dual swing while climbing hand over hand up a rope) provide the greatest challenge to tonic postural extensor muscles. Another example of an activity that demands considerable extension against gravity is "net basketball." In this activity, a therapy practitioner (or another client) and a client are prone in nets suspended at least 5 feet apart. Each player attempts to throw beanbags onto the back of the other. This activity also provides deep pressure from the weight of the beanbags.

Developing Tonic Flexion

When promoting the development of tonic flexion, we create activities that provide resistance to movement into flexion or that require sustained flexion. As with extension, we carefully grade the amount of flexion and resistance. For clients who have low flexor tone (especially of the neck and abdominal muscles), we begin with activities that require flexion of only the head and upper trunk rather than a full antigravity position. In one such activity, a client lies supine on a wedge, flexing the neck to blow bubbles from a wand held in position by the practitioner. The practitioner can facilitate the client's moving into flexion by placing a hand on the client's upper chest and exerting gentle pressure in a caudal direction.

Many activities simultaneously incorporate enhanced vestibular and proprioceptive sensation with the demand to flex the neck against gravity. In the course of those activities, "chaining responses" (Peiper, 1963) may assist clients to bring the rest of the body into positions of antigravity flexion. Similarly, activities that initially require flexion only of the legs and lower trunk seem to facilitate flexion of the neck. One activity requires clients to lie supine on the glider or the floor with a small wedge under the head. The therapist throws a large lightweight ball to the client who flexes the knees and hips and kicks it back. Initially, the head may be fully supported. However, as the activity continues, clients usually lift the head spontaneously in order to see the ball.

Swings suspended from a vertical stimulation device (i.e., several lengths of bungee cord) are particularly useful for facilitating flexion. The bungee cord allows a therapy practitioner to vigorously bounce the swing, essentially creating a situation in which the client must hold on tightly in order not to be thrown off the swing. Riding on a disc swing (Fig. 12–14), which provides a stable base of support while simultaneously requiring flexion of limbs around a central post, may be enough to challenge a client who has low flexor tone. Gradually, as the client develops sufficient flexion to withstand greater resistance, swings such as the T-swing may be used. Because the T-swing has a smaller base of support than the disc swing, it provides a greater challenge to flexion. Activities such as sitting and swinging in a dual swing and using two feet to kick a ball suspended at an appropriate height or holding onto a moon swing (Fig. 12–15) while swinging into or throwing at a target provide the next level of challenge.

As flexion improves, activities such as "holding on to a hotdog" (i.e., lying prone on top of a bolster swing while a therapist swings it back and forth) or going for a rough ride on a large suspended inner tube offer greater challenges to flexion. Although activities such as the hotdog game

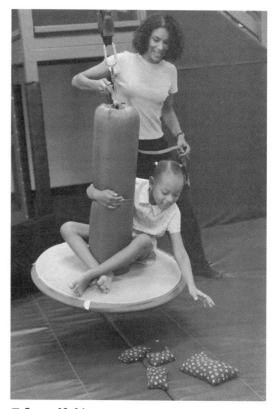

■ Figure 12-14 The disc swing. (Photo courtesy of Shay McAtee, printed with permission.)

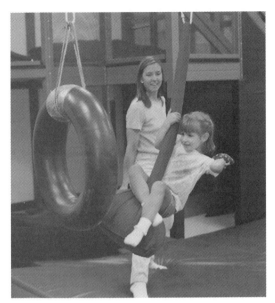

■ FIGURE 12-15 Moon swing. (Photo courtesy of Shay McAtee, printed with permission.)

require fairly constant force from the flexors, both the bolster and large inner tube can be used in such a way as to require subtle adjustments to flexion. Some of the most popular activities on the bolster and inner tube are games such as Bronco Billy at the rodeo or riding a boat through rough seas. They require individuals to adjust their hold and slide around to the side of, and then underneath, the piece of equipment as it swings or the therapist shakes it (Fig. 12–16).

The greatest challenges to postural flexion are provided in activities that require clients to maintain flexion against resistance *and* the full force of gravity. Activities of this type include lying in supine flexion on a scooter board and pulling along a rope suspended from both walls, approximately 2 feet above the floor. Activities on a trapeze that require maintained flexion while swinging over obstacles also provide significant challenges to flexion.

Ayres (1977) found that after clients developed adequate flexion, they enjoyed activities that included falling (e.g., releasing the bolster swing and falling onto crash pads below). In activities in which falling is involved, clients use flexion to pull themselves into a protected position. Ayres believed there was considerable affect and enthusiasm associated with the development of flexion against gravity.

Jeanne, an 11-year-old girl, was unable to as-

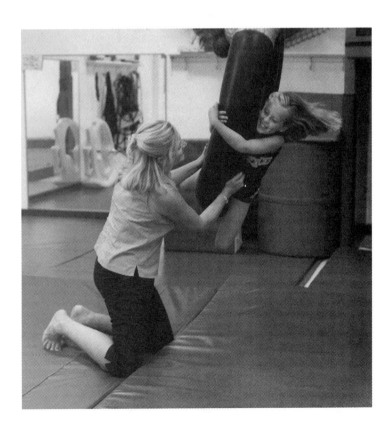

■ FIGURE 12-16 A rough ride on an inner tube swing. (Photo courtesy of Shay McAtee, printed with permission.)

sume supine flexion until she mastered hanging on underneath the bolster swing. Although she had mastered many challenges during 2 years of intervention, none was as salient as postural flexion. Mastering antigravity flexion allowed her to easily move herself into a protected position when falling and gave her the foundation she needed to further development in other postural, ocular, and praxis areas.

Combining Flexion and Extension: Developing Lateral Flexion and Rotation

As antigravity flexion and extension develop, lateral flexion, rotation, and weight shifting also emerge. Rotation and weight shifting, in particular, allow clients to move in ways that are efficient and that look smooth and fluid. Clients who have postural deficits frequently move with little rotation; rotation depends on weight shifting. Thus, creating activities to promote weight shifting and rotation assist clients to move more efficiently.

Unlike the development of postural flexion and extension, which are facilitated by engaging in activities that require symmetrical movements, the development of lateral flexion, weight shifting, and rotation require movement into asymmetrical patterns. Perhaps the simplest means of encouraging rotation is an activity that involves

rolling in a barrel (Fig. 12–17). Many children enjoy flattening letters or shapes created from Theraplast or Silly Putty by "steamrolling." Lateral flexion, weight shifting, and rotation can also be elicited by having a client who is swinging while seated in a dual swing or net swing reach for beanbags on the mat and then sit up and throw them at a target (see Fig. 9–1).

Another activity that encourages weight shifting and rotation involves swinging on a trapeze from one landing pad to another and then turning around to swing back while continuing to hold the trapeze with both hands. A variation involves suspending two ropes from the ceiling approximately 6 feet apart. A client seated on a scooter board in line with and facing the ropes pulls on one rope to move toward the second rope. The client then lets go of the first rope, grabs the second, and uses it to turn around. The client then pulls on the second rope to move back to the first one. If the client maintains contact with both hands on the rope, rotation happens during the turning.

Balancing Flexion and Extension: Developing Alternating Movements

As flexion and extension develop, we create activities that involve alternating flexion and extension (e.g., pumping a swing). When pumping a

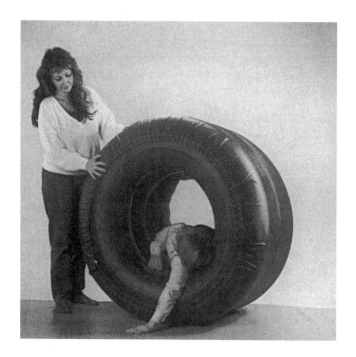

▪ FIGURE 12–17 Rolling in an inflatable barrel to encourage rotation. (Photo courtesy of Southpaw Enterprises.)

swing, the desired response is flexion of neck, arms, trunk, and legs followed by relative extension of all those body parts. However, it is possible to do most activities without using the desired motor response. Thus, if a response is not the desired one, we adapt the activity so that it serves the intended purpose.

Developing Righting and Equilibrium Reactions

Equilibrium (i.e., balance) reactions enable the maintenance of positions that have been threatened by body or support surface perturbations through compensatory movements of head, trunk, and limbs (Weisz, 1938). Most equilibrium responses are very subtle and occur in response to relatively small changes in position. Sensory integration theory offers us little description of equilibrium per se. Therefore we rely on explicit descriptions of equilibrium reactions available elsewhere (Bly, 1994; Bobath, 1985; Boehme, 1988; Fisher, 1989; Howison, 1988; Weisz, 1938). Equilibrium is the most complex of the postural responses described in this chapter and is one of the first to be compromised by CNS dysfunction. Thus, clients with postural deficits almost always have impaired equilibrium.

When equilibrium is delayed, we develop activities to elicit subtle reactions in various positions (i.e., prone, sitting, quadruped, kneeling, and standing). This can be accomplished using any piece of equipment that moves or any activity that involves reaching. Our goal is to create activities that challenge equilibrium but that can be accomplished with automatic, fluid responses.

Ari, a 5-year-old boy, had significant postural difficulties. He was first able to maintain his balance in the prone position against significant resistance when riding on a "boat" (glider) with "whales" (therapy balls) swimming underneath (Fig. 12–18). The whales caused the swing to tilt. Ari yelled with delight that he was not going in for a swim. He pumped the swing and maintained his position. Occasionally, bigger whales swam under his boat, requiring him to work against greater resistance to generate a full-blown equilibrium response. Periodically, he lost his balance and fell into the "water," enjoying a playful and calming moment with the whales as we rolled the therapy balls over his back and legs. This activity provided Ari with enhanced vestibular and proprioceptive sensation and facilitated a balance of extension and flexion, lateral flexion, and equilibrium reactions. In addition, the activity provided periodic deep pressure to address his sensory defensiveness, allowed him to rest, and prevented

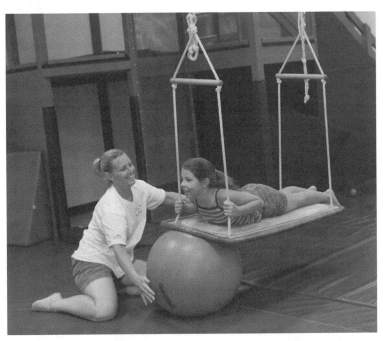

■ FIGURE 12–18   The glider becomes a boat and the therapy ball a whale. (Photo courtesy of Shay McAtee, printed with permission.)

him from becoming overly aroused by the excitement of the game.

Developing Oculomotor Control

Compensatory eye movements, controlled by the vestibular system, and eye movements used for following moving objects (smooth pursuits) or looking around the room (saccades) that are under the control of the visual system represent very different ocular processes. Clients who have sensory integrative dysfunction often have difficulty dissociating movements of the head and eyes. They move the head in response to visual stimuli rather than moving only their eyes, which they find very difficult.

Sensory integration theory has offered very little regarding assessment or treatment of visually controlled eye movements. Chapter 14 presents techniques for improving oculomotor control. Working in this area requires advanced training. In the course of intervention based on the principles of sensory integration theory, we develop many activities that challenge the ability to produce visually controlled ocular movements (e.g., smooth pursuits and quick localization) and to separate head and eye movements. Throwing beanbags at a moving target (e.g., a plastic bottle disguised as an "alien spaceship") is an example. However, some clients with poor oculomotor control may benefit from a more systematic approach designed by or in conjunction with a developmental optometrist who specializes in oculomotor training.

INTERVENTION FOR PRACTIC DISORDERS

Ayres (1985) identified three processes that are a part of praxis:

1. Conceptualizing (i.e., ideation)
2. Planning and programming
3. Executing the action

She described planning as the primary problem in sensory integrative-based dyspraxia. Movements appeared awkward because they were poorly planned rather than because of a primary problem with execution. We have described two manifestations of practic dysfunction, deficits in bilateral integration and sequencing (BIS) and somatodyspraxia.

Individuals with BIS have difficulty with bilateral coordination and anticipatory, or feedforward-dependent, actions. Individuals with somatodyspraxia have difficulty with both feedforward- *and* feedback-dependent tasks. Whereas BIS is generally associated with vestibular-proprioceptive processing deficits, somatodyspraxia has been associated with polymodal (i.e., tactile, vestibular, proprioceptive) sensory processing. We have proposed that deficits in BIS and somatodyspraxia represent levels of practic dysfunction (see also Chapters 1 and 3).

Ayres (1985) seemed to suggest that *ideation* was a primary problem only for clients with the most severe impairments. However, more recently, May-Benson (2001) found that poor ideation was a far greater problem than Ayres originally thought. May-Benson suggested that poor ideation can accompany all levels of practic dysfunction and that individuals without other practic deficits sometimes show evidence of poor ideation (see also Chapter 3).

The section on improving practic deficits begins by addressing difficulties with ideation. Then we described activities to address planning deficits. Activities are divided into three categories:

1. Activities that require bilateral coordination
2. Feedforward-dependent projected action sequences
3. Feedback-dependent movements

Developing Ideation

Clients who have poor ideation may not be capable of self-directed or self-initiated actions because of difficulty knowing what they can do with objects (Ayres, 1985); they do not appear to recognize *possibilities*. Clients with poor ideation may explore objects (i.e., try to find out what objects do) rather than play with them (May-Benson, 2001). They use a limited repertoire of interactions, which they apply to all objects (e.g., throwing).

Some equipment may be so novel that certain clients cannot figure out how to use it. Thus, initially we select objects that are very familiar or have familiar properties (e.g., rolls) and that are responsive to clients' slightest actions. For Peter, a 4-year-old boy, figuring out that he could walk up and down a carpeted incline was an appropriate initial challenge to ideation. To generate new ideas, clients may need equipment that is quite similar to playground swings or familiar riding toys. As Ayres (1985) indicated, "If the child leaves a task with a feeling of failure, he or she will probably not want to return to it" (pp. 67–68).

We take a cognitive approach to helping clients see possibilities in objects. We follow activities with identification of the idea. Clients may be able to identify what they *have* done before they can describe what they *plan* to do. We provide sufficient cues that they can generate their own ideas. Asking questions (e.g., how many ways can you think of to use this swing?) invites clients to think of novel ideas. The more they generate new ideas, the more likely they will be to produce future plans.

Wehman (1977) described an instructional hierarchy to be used with clients who have poor ideation and impaired cognition. Early on, we provide physical guidance. As soon as we can, we withdraw physical cues and model activities. When less modeling is needed, we provide specific instructions (as long as a clients' verbal receptive ability is adequate). We then fade those full instructions into partial prompts or cues.

As clients gain the ability to formulate ideas for using objects, they may begin to act more spontaneously in carefully arranged, familiar environments or do what is familiar to them in novel environments. Only later do clients act spontaneously with novel objects in less familiar environments. Some clients with significant deficits in ideation may never be able to act totally spontaneously. We need to help them generalize new skills to home and school.

Developing Coordinated Use of Two Sides of the Body

There is scant research that describes the development of coordinated limb usage. The ability to use a lead hand and an assisting hand together when acting on objects in any spatial orientation with respect to the body is the culmination of the development of bilateral motor coordination (Keogh & Sugden, 1985; Williams, 1983). The newborn infant, who does not consistently bring two hands to midline, must develop considerable skill and strength before learning using the two sides of the body to draw, cut, or open a jar.

We have confined our discussion to bilateral limb use. However, bilateral coordination refers to the use of two *sides* of the body, including the trunk. Furthermore, many tasks that require bilateral coordination also require the ability to plan and produce projected action sequences (e.g., catching

a ball with two hands). Individuals must adjust their actions to meet future conditions. We discuss feed-forward-dependent actions in the next section.

Keogh and Sugden (1985) and Williams (1983) have provided important information regarding the development of bilateral coordination. We have summarized their findings below. However, there remain significant gaps in knowledge about the development of bilateral motor coordination. For example, little is known about the ages by which various aspects of bilateral performance are usually mastered.

When we test clients using the Bilateral Motor Coordination test of the Sensory Integration and Praxis Tests (SIPT) (Ayres, 1989), we test only the ability to produce alternating arm or foot movements. Although we may learn that clients have difficulty with bilateral motor coordination, we have little knowledge of where on the developmental continuum they first experience difficulty. We often begin intervention with developmentally early bilateral tasks. We observe clients' abilities and grade the bilateral demands of tasks accordingly.

Discrete versus Sequenced Bilateral Movements

Children seem to develop control of discrete bilateral movements before they develop the ability to produce sequences of bilateral movements. Short sequences of bilateral movements clearly are easier to perform than long sequences.

Symmetrical versus Alternating Bilateral Movements

Sequences of movements performed symmetrically are easier than sequences of alternating movements; however, clients do not master symmetrical movements before they begin to perform alternating movements. Building on this knowledge, we have proposed that the activities shown in Table 12–1 form two hierarchical sequences from easiest to hardest. The first sequence refers to the development of bilateral symmetrical movements, and the second to the development of bilateral alternating movements.

Coordinated Bilateral Use of Arms and Legs

Coordinated use of two arms develops before coordinated movements of two legs (Williams,

---

■ TABLE 12–1 **TWO PROPOSED HIERARCHIES OF DIFFICULTY WITH BILATERAL ACTIVITIES**

Task Requirements	Activity Examples
Bilateral Symmetrical	
Hold on, move passively forward and backward with swing	Client prone on glider; therapist pushes glider back and forth while client looks for pretend obstacles up ahead; client's arms move passively into flexion and extension as the ropes move
Hold on, actively move equipment forward and backward using ropes that suspend the swing	Client prone on glider; client actively moves glider back and forth by alternately flexing and extending arms
Hold on, actively propel self forward and backward using a stable object	Client prone in net; therapist holds stick or hula hoop between outstretched hands; client places hands between therapist's on stick and actively flexes arms to pull self closer to stick, then lets go and swings
Hold on, actively propel self forward and backward using an unstable object	Client prone in net; two ropes with handles are suspended from the wall opposite the client (6 feet away); client holds handles and pulls rhythmically on them to propel self back and forth
Bilateral Alernating	
Hold on, move passively with equipment side to side	Client seated on platform swing; therapist pushes swing side to side while client looks for pretend obstacles on either side; client's arms move passively into alternating flexion and extension as the ropes move
Hold on, actively propel self using ropes that suspend the swing	Client seated sideways on glider, holding on to glider ropes; client actively propels self side to side by alternately flexing first one arm, then the other
Hold on, actively propel self side to side using an unstable object	Client seated in large inner tube suspended from the ceiling; two handles are suspended freely by ropes from the ceiling on either side of the tube; client grasps handles and pulls self side to side

---

1983). Thus, from a purely bilateral perspective, kicking a ball suspended from the ceiling with two feet while swinging in a net is harder than pushing the same ball away with both hands while swinging in the net.

Although coordinated bilateral upper extremity movements are generally easier than bilateral lower extremity movements, certain aspects of upper extremity movements are relatively difficult. One such aspect is bilateral symmetrical release (Keogh & Sugden, 1985). Letting go of a trapeze or zip line (Fig. 12–19) simultaneously with both hands is especially challenging. Similarly, letting go with both arms and legs when falling off a bolster swing onto a crash pad is also difficult. Clearly, coordinated, simultaneous use of all four limbs is more difficult than using either arms or legs separately (Williams, 1983).

Simultaneously flexing the arms and extending the legs, or vice versa, also seems to be a particularly difficult aspect of bilateral coordination. Activities done on the trapeze often demand this skill. For example, one might swing from a trapeze to jump through an inner tube suspended from the ceiling (Fig. 12–20) or maintain upper extremity flexion while extending the lower extremities to kick a suspended ball.

Although very different from a sensory integrative–based approach, we have recently found that the Interactive Metronome, a computer-based training program, is helpful for improving bilateral coordination. The Interactive Metronome involves matching bilateral movements to auditory cues given through headphones (Shaffer et al., 2001). This training is also helpful for improving timing, rhythm, and planning and sequencing of movements and, therefore addresses many aspects of praxis (Koomar et al., 2001). The Interactive Metronome may be most beneficial after a client has participated in sensory integrative–based intervention.

Inhibition of Movement

Inhibition of movement in one or more extremities seems to develop relatively later than do many other aspects of coordinated limb usage. In fact, movements of body parts not involved in an activity, such as the tongue or the opposite hand (i.e., associated movements), are commonly ob-

or squirting a squirt gun at a target while seated in the net or dual swing. Because the swing is suspended from one point, it generally rotates, eliciting weight shifting, trunk rotation, and midline crossing when clients aim at specific targets. Squirt guns, however messy, are highly motivating. The plastic mat from the game of Twister provides several "mess-reducing" targets, as do chalkboards or white boards, on which several targets can be drawn.

Activities to promote weight shifting, trunk rotation, and crossing the midline should not be contrived. Movements should be inherent to activities rather than occurring because a practitioner instructed a client to perform the task in a particular way. Unless the movements are natural, it is very unlikely that they will generalize to everyday use. Of course, some young children may need to be reminded to use the preferred hand to throw or shoot the squirt gun. Using the preferred hand should make the activity more successful.

Projected Action Sequences

Virtually all clients who have sensory integrative-based practic deficits have difficulty planning and producing projected action sequences (see Chapter 3). They cannot plan and initiate effective movements in response to a changing environment or events that have not yet happened. These difficulties are seen in such activities as catching or kicking a ball, riding a bicycle around obstacles, jumping rope, or walking through a room crowded with people. That the disorder is so common is not surprising because, as Keogh and Sugden (1985) indicated, "Children first must have sufficient control of their own movements before they can move in relation to external environmental conditions" (p.101).

Many activities require planning of projected action sequences. For example, in order to kick a ball, clients must anticipate the point at which the foot will intercept the ball and move the foot to that point *before* the ball arrives. Because they require anticipation, projected action sequences are more feedforward than feedback dependent. Of course, this is a relative statement because feedforward and feedback may be considered as different points of a spectrum representing the sensory control of movement. As depicted in Figure 12–21, the extent and speed of movement of both the client and the target

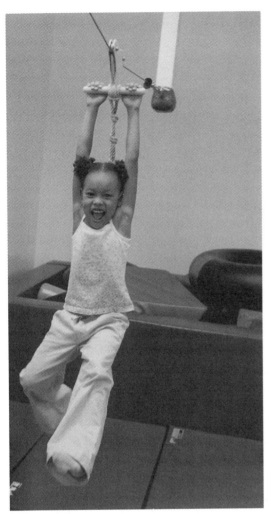

■ FIGURE 12-19 The zip line. (Photo courtesy of Shay McAtee, printed with permission.)

served when typically developing adolescents are involved in difficult activities (Keogh & Sugden, 1985).

Crossing the Midline

Crossing the midline, an important part of bilateral coordination, often occurs in conjunction with weight shifting and trunk rotation. The combination allows individuals to perform several kinds of actions efficiently. Some examples include picking up objects placed to one side and throwing or kicking with a mature pattern (Keogh & Sugden, 1985; Williams, 1983).

Activities designed to address difficulties with weight shifting, trunk rotation, and crossing the midline include throwing beanbags, kicking balls,

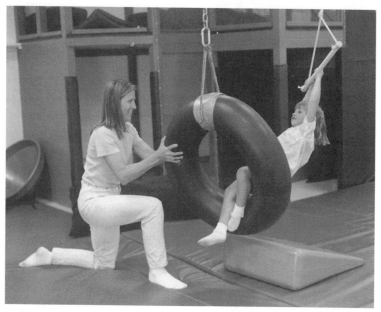

■ FIGURE 12-20 Swinging by a trapeze to jump through an inner tube. (Photo courtesy of Shay McAtee, printed with permission.)

determine the relative contributions of feedback and feedforward control. This information is important because feedforward- and feedback-dependent movements are associated with different types of sensory integrative dysfunction. Whereas clients who have BIS deficits primarily have difficulty with feedforward-dependent movements, clients with somatodyspraxia generally have difficulty with both feedback- and feedforward-dependent movements.

Clients who have BIS deficits may be able to perform quite well when both they and the target are relatively stationary (e.g., when throwing a ball at a target). They usually have greater difficulty when they are either moving (e.g., letting go of a swinging trapeze to land in a pile of pillows) or the target is moving (e.g., catching a ball). When both the client and the target are moving (e.g., running to kick a rolling ball), the challenge is even greater. Activities performed when client, target, or both are moving have spatial and temporal requirements. In response to spatiotemporal demands, clients must time the initiation of the movement and adjust its force and direction (Henderson & Sugden, 1992; Keogh & Sugden, 1985).

Keogh and Sugden (1985) indicated that by age 6 years, most children are well on their way toward mastering the spatial requirements of play-game skills (e.g., batting, throwing). They listed five general movement problems that we can observe and address through intervention. These include:

- Simultaneously controlling limb movements and posture
- Moving a limb along a path to contact an object or reach the desired release point
- Coordinating the sequence of limb segment movements to finish at the time of contact or release
- Modulating the force generated in limb movement and imparted to an object
- Navigating in relation to stationary objects or other persons

Temporal accuracy means, "coinciding the self with objects and other people to stay in unison or to intercept or avoid them" (Keogh & Sugden, 1985, p. 111). Requirements for temporal accuracy arise when a target moves or the client moves rapidly.

Figure 12–21 lists a number of activities according to whether client and target are stationary or moving when the activity is performed. As was the case with feedforward and feedback, "stationary" and "moving" represent points on a spectrum. Clients who are moving very slowly, over very small distances, or with only one body part are relatively stable. Also depicted in Figure 12–21 are the relative spatial and temporal demands of these activities.

CLIENT

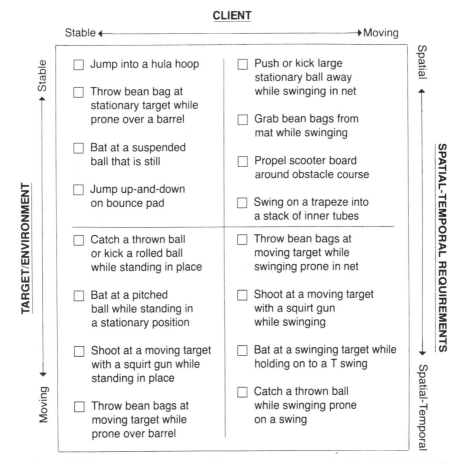

■ Figure 12–21   Common treatment activities, by category, according to their spatial-temporal requirements. (Adapted from Keogh and Sugden, 1985.)

Sensory integration theory suggests that difficulty with planning and producing projected action sequences is one sequela to poor processing of vestibular and proprioceptive input. Thus, we typically create activities that are designed both to provide enhanced vestibular and proprioceptive sensation and to improve clients' abilities to plan and produce projected action sequences. If the need arises, we adapt activities by modifying their spatial and temporal demands.

Micah, a 5-year-old boy, had extraordinary difficulty planning projected action sequences. His problems were similar to those of Melanie, whose case is presented in Chapter 11. We use the story of Micah's intervention to illustrate how we modified the spatiotemporal demands of activities to alter the challenge.

Early in his intervention, while Micah was swinging prone in the frog swing, we asked him to "feed the fish" by throwing "fish food" (beanbags) into the "fish pond" (inner tube). This activity re-

quired a relatively simple response. Because the inner tube was stationary, the only temporal requirement was that Micah release the beanbag at the proper time. Because the inner tube was large, even the spatial requirement was not great. However, Micah refused.

We modified the activity to require a simpler response. Micah simply had to use both hands to push a stationary "boulder" (large therapy ball) out of his way as he swung past it. Because the boulder was large and directly in the path of the swing, this activity made even fewer spatial demands and essentially no temporal demands. However, Micah also refused this activity, saying, "I just want to swing!"

We complied with Micah's request, interpreting his refusals as a statement that even the simplest projected action sequence presented too great a challenge. For the rest of that session and several subsequent sessions, we emphasized, separately, activities that provided enhanced vestibular and proprioceptive sensation (e.g., just swinging in the frog) and activities that involved limb movements that he did while stationary (e.g., tossing weighted balls at a large stationary target).

Several sessions later, we reintroduced the "boulder" game. This time, Micah eagerly pushed the ball. Apparently, at this point, it represented the just-right challenge. Either his ability or his perception of his ability had improved. After several more sessions, Micah was able to meet the challenge of repeatedly throwing beanbags into the inner tube, delightedly "feeding the fish."

An endless number of activities can be created to address planning and producing projected action sequences. Simple modifications make activities more or less challenging. We can vary the speed and extent of movement of the client, the target, or both; we can vary the size of objects used or the target. One activity that we have found to be highly motivating to young clients is a game of "bumper cars" (Fig. 12–22). We suspend two large tractor inner tubes vertically from the ceiling, 6 feet apart. The client and the therapist each straddle one of the tubes and pull them as far apart as the ropes allow, preparing to smash into one another. The object of the game is to bump the opponent out of his or her tube. Be-

cause both the client and the therapist (target) are moving, this game has both temporal and spatial requirements. If the bump is to be hard enough to knock the therapist out of the tube, the client's movements must be timed, sequenced, and directed precisely. Bumper cars can be made more challenging by suspending the tubes high enough off the ground that feet do not touch and propelling the tubes with handles at the ends of suspended ropes. These modifications increase the postural demands of the activity.

We sometimes play a more challenging game of "tag" that is set up similarly to bumper cars. The object of this game, as in conventional tag, is to not be caught. For this game, the practitioner and the client are each seated in net swings suspended 6 to 8 feet apart. A tractor inner tube with a large therapy ball inside it lies between the nets. The therapist and the client brace their feet against the tube. They push off, and whoever is "it" tries to tag the opponent. The opponents must time, sequence, and direct movement in order not to get caught. The person who is "it" must also time, sequence, and direct movements to catch the opponent. The tire is a free space, but players can remain there for only 10 seconds at a time. Tag is both challenging and

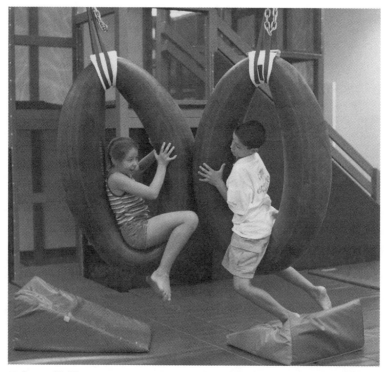

■ FIGURE 12–22 "Bumper cars." (Photo courtesy of Shay McAtee, printed with permission.)

highly motivating for older clients, but we recommend that it not be played by two clients together because at least one player must be skillful enough that neither gets hurt.

A more commonly used activity that also has significant spatial and temporal demand consists of having two clients, both in seated positions, orbit one another in a dual swing. The two clients must begin moving at the same time and at the same speed. They run for a few steps and then, on cue, simultaneously lift their feet and orbit.

Activities to Promote Sequencing

When the term *sequencing* is used in sensory integration theory, it refers to projected action sequences. However, practitioners commonly misinterpret the term and address sequencing problems with obstacle courses. Obstacle courses, because they usually contain several activities, represent sequences of sequences. Therefore, they can be quite difficult. The best type of obstacle course for addressing difficulties with sequencing requires smooth transitions between several different kinds of projected action sequences. For example, an obstacle course may include the following:

- Swinging by a trapeze from a raised surface
- Jumping off through a moving suspended inner tube onto a mat
- Leaning down to pick up beanbags
- Turning around and throwing the beanbags through the swinging tube
- Running back to the raised surface through a maze of plastic cones
- Catching the trapeze
- Beginning again

Addressing Somatodyspraxia

In addition to problems associated with BIS, clients with somatodyspraxia have difficulty planning and producing feedback-dependent movements. Thus, although the activities we presented for developing bilateral integration and projected action sequences also apply to intervention for clients with somatodyspraxia, many of them initially present too great a challenge.

For clients with somatodyspraxia, we often focus on whole-body actions. Going down a ramp on a scooter board and knocking down a tower of foam blocks, hugging a bolster swing tightly with both arms and legs, or jumping into and climbing out of a ball bath can be particularly useful. Another activity requiring a simple motor plan is riding a train (i.e., a glider) and getting on and off at each stop to retrieve or deliver a "package" (i.e., large, heavy beanbags or containers).

With some clients, we use simple cause-and-effect tasks (e.g., blowing a whistle or jumping from a raised surface onto a mat). Gradually, we increase the complexity of activities. We might have clients blow a whistle to indicate that they are stopping, starting, or changing the speed of a swing.

We grade activities from:

- Simple, discrete movements to complex movement sequences
- Whole-body movements to movement of specific body parts and inhibition of others
- Feedback- to feedforward-dependent actions

Because clients with somatodyspraxia frequently have poor proprioceptive processing, we emphasize active movement against resistance to develop improved body schema that serves as foundation for improved motor planning.

Many children use singing and counting to organize themselves. This ability to verbally mediate movement may not occur naturally for children with somatodyspraxia. Thus, we sometimes say "one, two, three, go" to help children initiate actions or use songs or rhymes to help them maintain rhythm. In some cases, we label clients' movements as they occur. Much learning of new skills happens cortically. Only when a skill is mastered does it become automatic. Sometimes clients pause before initiating a movement as though they were planning it. We try not to distract them. We give brief instructions and feedback, trying not to talk too much.

Verbalizing a plan can also be helpful for organizing and understanding it. At times, however, clients can verbalize a plan but are unable to execute it. P.J., a 7-year-old with somatodyspraxia, described a complicated sequence of movements needed for an obstacle course involving four pieces of suspended equipment. When asked to demonstrate the plan, he walked to each piece of equipment and pushed it while verbally describing the actions he would have liked to do. He was unable to figure out how to make his body do what his mind conceptualized. Clients such as P.J., at least initially, may benefit more from instruction and physical cues than from verbalizing a plan.

Because somatodyspraxia is characterized by difficulty learning new motor skills (Ayres, 1972, 1979, 1985; Cermak, 1985), intervention involves novel tasks or tasks that clients have not yet mastered. However, we also provide ample time for practice. An activity has not been mastered until a client can perform it automatically and without conscious effort. For clients with somatodyspraxia, mastery may require considerable practice (see also Chapter 3).

Many tasks that incorporate catching or kicking remain novel for a long time because they continually require new motor responses. Furthermore, altering the way a familiar piece of equipment is used can also produce novelty. For example, suspending a glider from one rather than two points changes the required postural adjustments.

Clients who have somatodyspraxia usually have difficulty generalizing a motor plan. We help clients generalize skills in at least two ways. First, we create new activities that require movements similar to those of familiar activities. For example, a client may jump off a pile of mats into an inner tube during one session and onto pillows during another session. The child might jump from the rungs of a jungle gym into the inner tube in a subsequent session.

Second, we point out similarities between the requirements of a current activity and those of activities that have been mastered or that must be done in daily life. For example, clients use similar movements when they sit in a net swing and propel it by pumping with their legs and trunk and when they propel a playground swing.

INTERVENTION WITH CLIENTS WHO HAVE AUTISM

This section addresses some of the needs of clients with autism because of the unique features of this population and because so many practitioners apply sensory integration theory to intervention with clients who have autism. However, readers are strongly encouraged to seek other sources for greater detail regarding intervention with these clients (Mailloux, 2001; Miller-Kuhanek, 2001) and those with other diagnostic conditions (Spitzer & Smith Roley, 2001).

Many individuals with autism have limited social and language skills and significant sensory modulation dysfunction, as well as problems with sensory discrimination and praxis. Ayres (1979) postulated that clients with autism often appeared to have dysfunction in neural substrates for sensory perception and attachment of meaning. Some lack initiation of purposeful action, have limited ideation, and have impaired planning of new actions. However, after a new motor task is mastered, they often become very proficient in that task (Mailloux, 2001).

We set up environments so they are likely to invite interaction. We may work alone with clients who are defensive in spaces with natural or dim lighting. We may work in rooms painted a dark color (e.g., Wedgewood blue) to minimize light bouncing off walls that can be very bothersome to an individual who experiences visual defensiveness. We may simplify the environment by putting away extra equipment.

Next we provide opportunities for meaningful sensory experiences that can elicit adaptive interactions. Sensory activities are selected based on clients' needs. Clients who have autism often need to experiment with the intensity, duration, frequency, and rhythm of sensations. Because many individuals cannot communicate verbally, observation is the key to the success of intervention (Ayres & Tickle, 1980). For example, a client with autism who had poor vestibular and proprioceptive processing did not derive pleasure from being pushed gently on a swing, leading the practitioner to question whether swinging was an appropriate activity. However, careful observation indicated that pushing the same client higher elicited smiles and sounds of pleasure, indicating that more intense input was needed to create a meaningful experience.

Levels of an Adaptive Response

Ayres (Spitzer & Smith Roley, 2001) described several levels of an adaptive response. We find it helpful to determine the level at which a client performs most consistently, the highest level he or she can achieve, and the lowest level at which he or she becomes overstimulated or excessively challenged. Although they are helpful with all clients, we have found Ayres' levels to be particularly useful for evaluation of clients who are autistic or whose difficulties preclude formal testing. The levels of the adaptive response are as follows:

1. Responds to passive stimuli
2. Holds on and stays put
3. Alternately contracts and relaxes muscle groups (e.g., pushing, pumping)
4. Initiates an activity requiring familiar, typically simple movements but does not sustain it
5. Initiates and sustains an activity requiring familiar, often simple movements (e.g., gets on and off a swing independently)
6. Initiates and sustains a simple two- or three-step activity requiring unfamiliar, often complex movements (e.g., swinging from a trapeze onto an inner tube)
7. Initiates and executes a complex activity requiring unfamiliar, typically complex movements, timing, or multiple adaptations (e.g., a multistep obstacle course)

Case Study

When intervention began for Justin, a 4-year-old boy with pervasive developmental disorder, he could not respond consistently to passive sensation, and his focus on activities varied widely. He sometimes enjoyed the tactile sensation derived from pouring beans over his hands and legs as he sat in a box full of beans. If others were involved in boisterous play nearby, he responded defensively and became overly active. After 6 months of intervention once a week, he could perform consistently at the second level of Ayres' hierarchy: holding on and staying put. Justin was able to stay on suspended equipment that did not require a lot of postural control (e.g., frog swing). He could propel simple swings but became easily frustrated by his inability to sustain the rhythm of the swing. Occasionally he was able to initiate an activity (e.g., lying prone across a frog swing or swinging the frog back and forth), but he usually needed assistance to complete it. He generally did not remain involved unless activities provided intense vestibular and proprioceptive or tactile sensation.

Over time, Justin became better able to meet challenges representing higher levels of adaptive responses across a variety of settings. When on the frog swing, he enjoyed activities that require projected actions (e.g., pushing a therapy ball away from him). This activity was at the adaptive response level of initiating and sustaining an activity requiring simple motions.

Eventually, Justin developed the bilateral coordination and sequencing abilities necessary to swing while throwing beanbags or balls at a moving target, reflecting a new-found ability to initiate and sustain simple two- or three-step activities that require complex movements. At the same time, he became interested in riding a small bicycle with training wheels. After practicing repeatedly for a week, he was able to perform this skill well. Justin's story provides an example of how various adaptive responses elicited during intervention sessions and then generalized to activities at school and home reflect the progression Ayres described (Spitzer & Smith Roley, 2001)

Even in an ideal environment, many clients do not interact readily with people or equipment. In these instances, in addition to using Ayres' levels of adaptive interaction to guide therapy, we reflect on Greenspan' s (1992) developmental stages:

1. Regulation and interest in the world
2. Forming relationships
3. Intentional two-way communication
4. Development of a complex sense of self, involving behavioral organization and elaboration
5. Development of emotional ideas and emotional thinking

Greenspan (1992) developed an approach called Floor Time that may assist families to look beyond the symptoms of autism. He encouraged caregivers to tie affect and meaning to everything that they do with children in order to develop communication.

Using a Floor Time model, we attempt to enter clients' activities in such a manner that they must respond. The focus of the Floor Time model is opening and closing an increasing number of "circles of communication."

When 6-year-old Alex was uninterested in therapy equipment and ran back and forth across the room, the therapy practitioner pretended that his running was intentional. She stated that it was time to go to the next part of the running race where he needed to run around or jump over obstacles (e.g., pillows and bolsters). Because Alex was very interested in Winnie-the-Pooh and Pooh's friends, the practitioner began talking like Tigger ("I love to bounce. Oh boy, a running, bouncing, jumping game!") as she modeled what Alex was to do. This caused Alex to shift his attention to the pillows and bolsters, but he continued to run back and forth. The practitioner continued to play the part of Tigger and began pretending that Alex was Pooh. "Oh, Pooh, this is so much fun! You are such a good runner! What else can you do?" When Alex accidentally bumped into one of the bolsters, she said in an exaggerated way, "Oh, Pooh, you are so good at bumping into things!" The practitioner continued in this manner, until Alex attempted to jump onto a pillow. Next Alex burrowed under a large pillow. The practitioner asked, "Are you Rabbit now? You are burrowing just like Rabbit." This provided an avenue for a new circle of communication. Combining Floor Time and sensory integrative approaches often enhances clients' participation.

Clients with a diagnosis along the autism spectrum frequently respond best to dramatic interactions with a practitioner. At times, it seems that a practitioner's actions are not meaningful unless they are highly enthusiastic, if not exaggerated. This may be because of limbic system involvement suspected in clients with autism (Bauman & Kemper, 1994).

Because of their social and communication difficulties, we often take a more active role in selecting sensory experiences for clients with autism than for clients with other diagnoses (Mailloux, 2001). We offer activities they will likely enjoy after they get past the automatic "no" to disruptions in their established routine. If demonstrating and verbally prompting clients to engage in new activities does not prove effective, we may physically assist them.

PRACTICAL CONSIDERATIONS FOR PROVIDING SAFE AND EFFECTIVE INTERVENTION

As we plan intervention and make recommendations to clients and caregivers, we continually confront important issues, such as:

- Age of the client
- Frequency and duration of intervention
- Whether intervention can be effective with groups of clients

Similarly, when we decide to provide intervention based on the principles of sensory integration theory, that decision has important implications for resources. These include:

- Space
- Equipment
- Reimbursement

Client's Age

Because she believed that the plasticity of the CNS decreased after age 9 years, Ayres (1972) believed that young children would respond more readily to intervention than older children or adults. This statement has been misinterpreted to mean that clients older than 9 years will not benefit from intervention. However, there is increasing evidence that plasticity exists even in mature organisms (Elman et al., 1998). Clinically, a number of adults have reported intervention to be highly beneficial. They have developed greater ease with motor skills and felt better about themselves. They, thus, are better able to interact effectively in social situations. Older children and adults who have suffered a great deal as a result of sensory integrative dysfunction are usually highly motivated to engage in intervention. A key to success seems to be a belief that intervention can make their lives easier. Paul, a 12-year-old boy, wistfully stated that he had dreamed of a place like our clinic since he was 5 years old. His strong inner drive to be involved in intervention was manifested in hard work.

Direct Intervention: How Long and How Often

Another important element of direct intervention is the length of each session. From our experience, individual sessions between 45 and 60 minutes in length seem to be more beneficial than short sessions, even when shorter sessions occur more frequently and the total intervention time each week is the same. This seems to be particularly true for older clients and those who need periodic breaks to become calmer or more organized. In longer sessions, activities unfold logically and come to a natural conclusion.

Ayres (personal communication, April 14, 1984) recommended that children receive direct intervention at least two or three times per week. However, such intensive intervention is rarely possible. Nonetheless, some children who receive intervention once a week need services for 2 to 3 years. During that time, they may develop secondary problems. Thus, it might be more effective to provide more frequent intervention over 1 year than to provide the same total amount of intervention over 2 to 3 years. Although this idea has intuitive appeal, research is needed to examine whether increased frequency of intervention, over a shorter period of time, is actually as effective or more effective than intervention provided less often over a longer period of time. Thus far, the limited research in this area has not supported the premise of increased frequency with any intervention approach used in pediatric occupational or physical therapy (Harris, 1988).

In the past several years, we have been experimenting with short bursts of intensive intervention (i.e., four 1-hour individual sessions) in the context of intervention courses. Before beginning intervention, children were assessed and therapist–participants met with parents to agree on functional objectives; older children were also included in the planning. We most commonly addressed goals that reflected improved praxis, although more recently we experimented with consultation and goals reflecting sensory modulation. Some common objectives included bicycle riding and reciprocal stair climbing. After the objectives were set, therapist-participants analyzed the objective and observed the child's performance, hypothesized about ways that sensory integrative dysfunction interfered with task performance, and created intervention plans.

In accordance with sensory integration theory, activities were meaningful, provided enhanced sensation, and involved numerous repetitions of particular movement patterns inherent to the goal. We also sometimes included skills training.

One participant was a 7-year-old boy, Erik, whose goal was to ride his bicycle. He was not yet able to get on the bike independently. He could not balance while holding on and lifting his leg over the bar. His sensory integrative assessment suggested difficulties with BIS based on poor processing of vestibular and proprioceptive sensation. The therapist used a bolster swing to create activities that interspersed swinging with getting on and off the swing (e.g., to deliver packages). The therapist pointed out the similarity between the movements used to get on and off the bolster swing and the bicycle. At the end of the four sessions, Erik was able to get on the bicycle independently and without fear. He was able to ride down the hospital corridors with minimal assistance from his mother, who intermittently held a bar the therapist had mounted to the back of the bicycle seat.

There is nothing magical about conducting four sessions per week. That number simply allows for maximum interaction between clients and therapists in the context of intervention courses. As noted with Erik, we have experienced success in attaining goals using this intervention paradigm.

Therapist-to-Client Ratio

A therapist attempting to provide direct intervention to more than one client at a time can have a difficult time because all activities must be appropriate for all clients. This may greatly limit the number and scope of activities. Furthermore, two clients double the demands for observation and adaptation. Sometimes adaptations required by one client are not appropriate for the other. Children who have previously experienced repeated rejection may also develop unhealthy competition for a therapist's attention.

Although it is quite difficult for a practitioner to work with more than one child at a time, it can be beneficial to have several practitioners, each working with one child, sharing a large space. The interactions among children may result in improved social skills and the development of friendships. Furthermore, both children and practitioners are exposed to new activities that the practitioner therapist can modify as needed and that each practitioner-client team is free to alter.

Groups definitely have their place in intervention, and children with sensory integrative dysfunction may have needs that are met best in groups that target play, social skills, or specific functional skills such as handwriting. Groups can also be excellent settings to teach sensory diet ideas to older children and adolescents. We encourage practitioners to consider the range of services they can provide to clients and be cognizant of the primary purpose of the particular intervention they are conducting. Intervention that targets development of play skills would probably look quite different from intervention that targets improvements in sensory integration.

Designing Adequate Space and Suspension Systems

Sensory integration-based intervention requires suspended equipment and sufficient space to engage in therapeutic activity that yields enhanced sensation and provides a variety of postural and practic challenges. An adequate suspension system is critical (Bonder & Fisher, 1989; Koomar, 1990; Parham & Mailloux, 2001). To ensure that clients will be safe,

- The suspension system must be installed correctly.
- There must be adequate space to use the suspended equipment.
- The floor beneath the suspended equipment must be covered fully by mats.

To use suspended equipment safely, the room must be a minimum of 12 feet square. We prefer rooms that are at least 14 feet square, and 14 by 20 feet is ideal. A large room allows full orbits on equipment without danger of crashing into a wall with some space remaining for equipment not in use.

Many pieces of equipment (e.g., bolster swing, platform glider) are generally hung from two points of suspension. We believe that at least three successive points of suspension, centered in the ceiling and spaced 2.5 to 3 feet apart, are optimal. These enable practitioners to combine equipment and provide progressively greater challenges (e.g., swinging on a trapeze to jump through two suspended inner tubes).

Suspension systems must sustain a minimum working load of 1000 pounds. Although many clients are children who weigh less than 100 pounds, when they bounce and swing on a piece of suspended equipment; the shearing forces on the suspension system are tremendous.

All suspended systems must be installed properly. Southpaw Enterprises publishes the *Ceiling Support Manual,* which illustrates a number of safe ways to install a suspension system (see Appendix 12–A for a list of vendors). When installing a suspension system, use a structural engineer or contractor with a background in design. Even then, it is necessary to clearly explain the necessity of having a system that supports such a large working load. Consultants frequently incorrectly assume that a structure similar to an outdoor swing set is sufficient.

Forged steel eyebolts (indicated by the lack of any opening in the circular part of the eyebolt) or similar hardware installed through support beams must be locked securely with nuts and washers. *Never put bolts directly into the ceiling, even if the bolts are lag bolts or bolts that expand as they are tightened.* Only bolts that go all the way

through a part of the ceiling structure (through-bolts) and are locked on the other side can safely support the strong shearing forces generated by suspended equipment. In addition, rotational devices should be used with any piece of equipment that will be used with equipment that rotates to minimize the torque on the ceiling suspension point from which it is hung.

In places where a ceiling system cannot be installed, commercially available, freestanding suspension systems may be used. Large, heavy, nonportable systems with a working load of 1000 pounds are preferred (Koomar, 1990). Many lightweight, portable systems have a working load less than 1000 pounds. These systems are limited as far as the types of activity that can be done on them.

ESTABLISHING INTERVENTION PROGRAMS BASED ON SENSORY INTEGRATION THEORY

Occupational therapy practitioners work in a variety of settings, including hospitals, clinics, schools, private practices, and homes. Each setting presents different challenges related to initiating and implementing new programs. Private practices may be the easiest settings in which to develop programs based on the principles of sensory integration theory. Practitioners are free to rent, buy, or build a clinic with the necessary space, equipment, and ceiling structure for a suspension system. Practitioners with experience developing such a practice are often the best sources of assistance to others beginning such a venture (Koomar, et al., 1996).

Generally, it is easier and more appropriate to develop a program based in sensory integration theory in a hospital than in a school, where direct intervention must explicitly reflect educational goals. A wide variety of technical equipment is standard in hospitals. However, the cost of establishing programs necessitates significant *a priori* negotiations, especially in the current health-care climate. Such negotiations occur at multiple levels. Practitioners first must gain approval from their immediate supervisors. When the immediate supervisor has approved the program, permission must be sought from agency administrators. The following information applies to negotiation with administrators at all levels.

In-service training can provide administrators with information on anticipated numbers of clients as well as an understanding of sensory integration theory and its benefits. The former should be based on a thorough needs assessment (Witkin & Altschuld, 1995). Therapists who hit roadblocks because administrators have reservations about sensory integration theory must be prepared to discuss current research that both supports and refutes such practice. Sometimes therapists need to provide several in-services over months or years before administrators are willing to support the development of a program.

In rare cases, administrators may support a program if therapists are willing to conduct research to measure its effectiveness. Single-case or small-group design studies seem to be the most feasible in these cases. Providing research results along with anecdotal reports from parents, teachers, or other staff members can be a powerful impetus for continuing and further developing a program. However, in our zeal to begin a new program, we should not promise more than we can deliver. Research requires time and resources. Furthermore, although negative results in a study may suggest that the procedures are ineffective, they may also mean that we failed to measure the proper constructs or to measure them in an appropriate way (Bundy, 1990). The results of one study neither prove nor disprove a theory or the effectiveness of the procedures associated with it. The bottom line is that tying the establishment of a program to the outcomes of studies that have yet to be planned or implemented may be unwise.

Along with support for program development, we need funds for design and installation of a suspension system and equipment. In hospitals, the approval of funds is often tied to whether or not therapists can logically project that the program will make a profit. We discuss third-party reimbursement below. Again, a thorough needs assessment should be done. Therapists who have begun similar programs can provide estimates of start-up costs and help to project the rate of income growth.

In schools, the approval of funds is very likely tied to availability of money. School personnel work on very tight budgets, and the incidence of students who will receive the services is often low in proportion to the total population of special education students.

THIRD-PARTY REIMBURSEMENT FOR SERVICES

Reimbursement for service always is a concern when establishing programs, especially in a hospital or private practice. Third-party reimbursement for occupational and physical therapy varies greatly from state to state. In general, hospitals are more frequently reimbursed than are private practices.

When seeking reimbursement, it is important to use the proper code on documentation. The International Classification of Disease code (US Department of Health and Human Services, 1998) is useful for establishing diagnoses. Two codes appropriate for clients with sensory integrative dysfunction who do not have any other medical diagnosis are Dyspraxia Syndrome (315.4) and Coordination Disturbance (781.3). The latter includes apraxia as a subcategory.

The Physician's Current Procedural Terminology (CPT-4) (American Medical Association, 1998) provides codes for evaluation and intervention. We have found the following codes to be most useful for evaluation:

- Developmental Testing Limited (96110)
- Extended Evaluation (96111).

The following codes are used to address elements of sensory integrative intervention:

- Development of Cognitive Skills and/or Sensory Integration Activities (97770)
- Therapeutic Exercise (97110)
- Functional Activities (97530); ADL-Not Diversional (97535)
- Neuromuscular Re-Education (97112)

Always use the most current version of the diagnostic code and procedural terminology codes for billing. These manuals are revised periodically.

For some insurance companies, it is useful to specify that sensory integrative procedures are being used, especially with insurance companies that provide reimbursement only when specialized evaluation or intervention procedures are documented. For these companies, the Sensory Integration Code (97770) can be most useful. However, we always describe the goals of intervention functionally (e.g., specific improvement in activities of daily living). Because this code covers cognitive skills as well as sensory integration, some confusion exists. In the future, these codes may be split. For other insurance companies that prefer practitioners to focus on occupational or physical therapy rather than specialized procedures, the most commonly used codes are a combination of Therapeutic Exercise (97110) and Functional Activities (97530).

When insurance companies are reimbursing for intervention, it is important to use a format for daily notes that provides measurable data and is understandable to claim agents. We have developed a format (Appendix 12–B) that includes numerical ratings as well as short comments; this format provides a concrete way to measure progress. A system such as this is potentially useful for internal quality assurance programs and for research. In addition, we have developed a numerical rating system that is used at the beginning of intervention and again when a client is discharged to measure gains (Appendix 12–B).

CONTINUING EDUCATION

Sensory integrative theory is complex and continually evolving. To provide effective, state-of-the-art intervention, it is important to acquire a sound understanding of the theory and update knowledge continually. Professional journals are one excellent source of current research and reports of theory development. Several Websites are available that address various aspects of sensory integration function and dysfunction. As with any Website, readers should make themselves aware of the quality of material that is posted. The Sensory Integration Resource Center Home Page (http://www.sinetwork.org) is an excellent site for obtaining educational materials geared toward parents, educators, therapists, and children as well as links to many other related sites.

The staff at Sensory Integration International (SII) (1987/1988), a private, not-for-profit organization whose mission is to promote sensory integration theory and practice, suggests that therapists have a minimum of 3 months' supervision from a therapist knowledgeable in sensory integration theory and experienced with intervention. In addition, they recommend ongoing participation in continuing education courses that specifically address recent advances in sensory integration theory and practice and neurobiological

theory. SII offers many continuing education courses throughout the year.

More recently, Western Psychological Services (WPS), the publisher of the SIPT (Ayres, 1989), has joined with the Department of Occupational Therapy at the University of Southern California (USC) to provide courses related to sensory integration theory, SIPT administration and interpretation, and intervention for sensory integrative dysfunction. Although similar in concept to the SII courses, the WPS/USC teaching faculty emphasizes the relationship between occupation and sensory integration.

SUMMARY AND CONCLUSIONS

Intervention based on sensory integration theory is both complex and exciting. To be effective, therapists must be able to combine a working knowledge of sensory integration theory with an intuitive ability to engender a client's trust and create the just-right challenge.

The ultimate goals of intervention are development, self-actualization, and improvements in occupational performance. Several elements are critical to optimal intervention. First, intervention should always be set in the context of specific objectives. What will improved development, self-actualization, or occupational performance look like for *this* client?

Second, based on observation, interaction, and assessment, practitioners should create environments that invite client interactions and provide realistic challenges. The environment includes both the physical layout of the space, including the equipment, and interactions between client and therapist.

Third, intervention is based on knowledge of sensory integration theory, understanding of clients' needs and interests, and objectives that the client and practitioner have established together. The practitioner and client create activities that:

- Capture the client's motivation
- Provide enhanced sensation
- Invite active participation in the just-right challenge
- Demand an adaptive interaction

Fourth, practitioners observe clients' responses to intervention and adapt to attain maximum benefit. Practitioners:

- Anticipate the results of an activity.
- Vigilantly observe clients' responses.
- Alter activities without disruption to the overall flow.
- Communicate regularly with clients and caregivers to learn about undesirable or unexpected responses.

Practitioners also help clients and caregivers understand the daily life effects of sensory integrative dysfunction and develop strategies to minimize negative effects.

Finally, practitioners, together with clients and caregivers, monitor progress toward meeting objectives and the degree to which intervention has helped clients meet daily life demands. An important part of this monitoring is discovering whether or not clients have generalized skills and abilities to everyday life. Based on the result of these assessments, the practitioner adapts the intervention and recommends a time when intervention should be discontinued.

This chapter has focused on direct intervention based on the principles of sensory integration theory. It has outlined activities for clients who have a number of different characteristics of sensory integrative dysfunction. The chapter has also discussed practical considerations related to direct intervention with individual clients and for developing programs within occupational therapy departments in a number of different kinds of settings.

Direct intervention based on the principles of sensory integration theory is a powerful tool for effecting change in clients' lives. Because direct intervention is complex and difficult, we have devoted this entire chapter to discussing its provision. However, we wish to emphasize two points. First, direct intervention *is only one means* for providing intervention to individuals who have sensory integrative dysfunction. Direct intervention should be provided concurrently with consultation to caregivers. Second, intervention based on sensory integration theory is never used in isolation. Because clients have a variety of needs, an integrated approach to intervention generally is both the most effective and efficient.

References

American Medical Association (1998). *Physician's current procedural terminology* (4th ed.). Chicago: Author.

Ayres, A. J. (1972). *Sensory integration and learning disorders*. Los Angeles: Western Psychological Services.

Ayres, A. J. (March 1977). Developmental dyspraxia. Symposium conducted in Dayton, Ohio.

Ayres, A. J. (1979). *Sensory integration and the child.* Los Angeles: Western Psychological Services.

Ayres, A. J. (1985). *Developmental dyspraxia and adult-onset apraxia.* Torrance, CA: Sensory Integration International.

Ayres, A. J. (1989). *Sensory Integration and Praxis Tests.* Los Angeles: Western Psychological Services.

Ayres, A. J., & Tickle, L. S. (1980). Hyper-responsivity to touch and vestibular stimuli as a predictor of positive response to sensory integration procedures by autistic children. *American Journal of Occupational Therapy, 34,* 375–381.

Bauman, M. L., & Kemper, T. L. (1994). Neuroanatomic observations of the brain in autism. In M. L. Bauman & T. L. Kemper (Eds.), *The neurobiology of autism* (pp. 119–145). Baltimore: Johns Hopkins University Press.

Bly, L. (1994). *Motor skills acquisition in the first year.* San Antonio: Therapy Skill Builders

Bobath, B. (1985). *Abnormal postural reflex activity caused by brain lesions* (Ed. 3). Rockville, MD: Aspen Systems.

Boehme, R. (1988). *Improving upper body control.* Tucson, AZ: Therapy Skill Builders.

Bonder, B. R., & Fisher, A. G (1989). Sensory integration and treatment of the elderly. *Gerontology special interest section news, 12,* 2–4.

Bundy, A. C. (1990). The challenge of functional outcomes: Framing the problem. *Neuro-Developmental Treatment Association Newsletter.*

Cermak, S. A. (1985). Developmental dyspraxia. In E. A. Roy (Ed.), *Neuropsychological studies of apraxia and related disorders* (pp. 225–250). New York: Elsevier.

Cohen, H. (1992). Vestibular rehabilitation reduces functional disability. *Otolaryngology—Head and Neck Surgery, 107,* 638–643.

Cohen, H. S. (February 14, 2000). Vertigo and balance disorders: Vestibular rehabilitation. *OT Practice, 5,* 14–18.

Cohen, H., Kane-Wineland, M., Miller, L. V., & Hatfield, C. L. (1995). Occupation and vestibular/vestibular interaction in vestibular rehabilitation. *Otolaryngology—Head and Neck Surgery, 112,* 526–532.

Elman, J. L., Bates, E. A., Johnson, M. H., Karmiloff-Smith, A., Parisi, D., & Plunkett, K. (1998). *Rethinking innateness.* Cambridge, MA: MIT.

Fisher, A. G. (1989). Objective assessment of the quality of response during two equilibrium tests. *Physical and Occupational Therapy in Pediatrics, 9,* 57–78.

Fisher, A. G. (1991). Vestibular-proprioceptive processing and bilateral integration and sequencing deficits. In A. G. Fisher, E. A. Murray, & A. C. Bundy, (Eds.), *Sensory integration: Theory and practice* (pp. 69–107). Philadelphia: F. A. Davis.

Fisher, A. G., & Bundy, A. C. (1989). Vestibular stimulation in the treatment of postural and related disorders. In O. D. Payton, R. P. DiFabio, S.V . Paris, E. J. Protas. & A. G. Van Sant (Eds.), *Manual of physical therapy techniques* (pp. 239–258). New York: Churchill Livingstone.

Frick, S. (2000). An overview of auditory interventions. *Sensory Integration Quarterly,* Spring/Summer.

Greenspan, S. (1992). *Infancy and early childhood.* Madison, CT: International Universities Press.

Harris, S. R. (1988). Early Intervention: Does developmental therapy make a difference? *Topics in Early Childhood Special Education, 7,* 20–32.

Henderson, S. E., & Sugden, D. A. (1992). *Movement Assessment Battery for Children manual.* New York: Psychological Corporation.

Howison, M. V. (1988). Cerebral palsy. In H. L. Hopkins, & H. D. Smith (Eds.), *Willard and Spackman's occupational therapy* (Ed. 7, pp. 675–706). Philadelphia: J. B. Lippincott.

Keogh, J., & Sugden, D. (1985). *Movement skill development.* New York: Macmillan.

Koomar, J. (1990). Providing sensory integration therapy as an itinerant therapist. *Environment: Implications for occupational therapy practice.* Rockville, MD: American Occupational Therapy Association.

Koomar, J., Burpee, J., DeJean, V., Frick, S., Kawar, M., & Fischer, D. M. (2001). Theoretical and clinical perspectives on the Interactive Metronome™: A view from Occupational Therapy Practice. *The American Journal of Occupational Therapy, 55,* 163–166.

Koomar, J., Palmstrom, L., Szklut, S., Carley, K., Raredon, M., Dobbin, M. Rossettie, J., & Capanna, P. (1996). *Plan for success: A business workbook for OTs in private practice.* San Antonio, Texas: Therapy Skill Builders.

Mailloux, Z. (2001). Sensory integrative principles in intervention with children with autistic disorder. In S. Smith Roley, E. I. Blanche, & R. Schaaf (Eds.), *Understanding the nature of sensory integration with diverse populations* (pp. 365–384). San Antonio: Therapy Skill Builders.

May, T. (1988). *Identifying gravitational insecurity in children with sensory integrative dysfunction.* Unpublished master's thesis, Boston University, Boston.

May-Benson, T. (2001). A theoretical model of ideation in praxis. In S. Smith Roley, E. I. Blanche, & R. Schaaf (Eds.), *Understanding the nature of sensory integration with diverse populations* (pp. 163–182). San Antonio: Therapy Skill Builders.

Miller-Kuhanek, H. (2001). *Autism: A comprehensive occupational therapy approach.* Bethesda, MD: American Occupational Therapy Association.

Miller, L. J., Mcintosh, D. N., McGrath, J., Shyu, V., Lampe, M., Taylor, A. S., Tassone, F., Neitzel, K., Stackhouse, T., & Hagerman, R. (1999). Electro-dermal responses to sensory stimuli in individuals with fragile X syndrome: A preliminary report. *American Journal of Medical Genetics, 83,* 268–279.

Oetter, P., Laurel, M., & Cool, S. (1991). Sensori-motor foundations of communication. In C. B. Royeen (Ed.), *Neuroscience foundations of human performance.* Rockville, MD: American Occupational Therapy Association.

Oetter, P., Richter, E., & Frick, S. (1993). *M.O.R.E— Integrating the Mouth with Sensory and Postural Functions* (2nd ed.), Hugo, MN: PDP.

Parham, L. D., & Mailloux, Z. (2001). Sensory integration. In J. Case-Smith (Ed.), *Occupational therapy for children* (4th ed., pp. 329–381). St. Louis: C. V. Mosby.

Pearce, A. (1963). *The magical child.* New York: Bantam Books

Peiper, A. (1963) *Cerebral function in infancy and childhood.* New York: Consultant's Bureau.

Previc, F. (1993). Do organs of the labyrinth differentially influence the sympathetic and para-sympathetic systems? *Neuroscience and Biobehavioral Reviews, 17,* 397–404.

Richter, E., & Oetter, P. (1990). Environmental matrices for sensory integrative treatment. *Environment—Implications for occupational therapy practice, a sensory integrative perspective.* Rockville, MD: American Occupational Therapy Association.

Shaffer, R., Jacokes, L., Cassily, J., Greenspan, S., Tuchman, R., & Stemmer, P. (2001). Effect of Interactive Metronome™ training on children with ADHD. *The American Journal of Occupational Therapy, 55,* 155–162.

Spitzer, S., & Smith Roley, S. (2001). Sensory integration revisited: A philosophy of practice. In S. Smith Roley, E. Blanche, & R. Schaaf (Eds.), *Understanding the nature of sensory integration with diverse populations* (pp. 3–28). San Antonio: Therapy Skill Builders.

US Department of Health and Human Services (1998). *The international classification of diseases* (Rev. 9). *Clinical Modification.* DHS No. (PHS) 89–1260. Washington, DC: U.S. Government Printing Office.

Wehman, P. (1977). *Helping the mentally retarded acquire play skills: A behavioral approach.* Springfield, IL: Charles C. Thomas.

Weisz, S. (1938). Studies in equilibrium reactions. *Journal of Nervous and Mental Disease.* 88, 150–162.

Wilbarger, P., & Wilbarger, J. (1991). *Sensory Defensiveness in Children Aged 2–12,* Santa Barbara, CA: Avanti Educational Programs.

Williams, H. G. (1983). *Perceptual and motor development.* Englewood Cliffs, NJ: Prentice Hall.

Witkin, B. R., & Altschuld, J. W. (1995). *Planning and conducting the needs assessments: A practical guide.* Thousand Oaks, CA: Sage.

■■ Appendix 12–A
List of Vendors by Type of Equipment

Floor Equipment

Air Mattress
Flagouse, Southpaw

Balance Beams/Boards
Achievement Products, Childcraft, Constructive Playthings, Flaghouse, Sammons Preston

Balance Stools
Equipment Shop, Flaghouse, Sammons Preston

Balls
Achievement Products, Childcraft, Equipment Shop, Flaghouse, PDP Products, Sammons Preston, Southpaw

Ball Baths
Flaghouse, Sammons Preston

Body Socks
Southpaw

Bounce Pads
Southpaw

Climbing Structures
Childcraft, Constructive Playthings, Southpaw

Equilibrium Boards/Boats
Achievement Products, Constructive Playthings, Flaghouse, Southpaw

Foam Play Pools
Southpaw

Foam Ramps
Childcraft, Constructive Playthings, Flaghouse, Southpaw

Foam Steps
Achievement Products

Inner Tubes (Stackable)
Southpaw

Large Pillows
Southpaw

Mats
Childcraft, Constructive Playthings, Equipment Shop, Flaghouse, Sammons Preston

Nested Benches/Stools
Southpaw, Tramble

Pom Pon Balls
Equipment Shop, Flaghouse, Sammons Preston, Southpaw, Tramble

Sensory Shaker
Southpaw

Tractor Crawler
Flaghouse

Trampolines
Achievement Products, Flaghouse

Vestibular Bowls/Discs
Childcraft, Equipment Shop, Flaghouse, Southpaw

Wheeled Floor Equipment

Roller Racer
Childcraft

Scooter Boards
Achievement Products, Constructive Playthings, Equipment Shop, Flaghouse, Sammons Preston, Southpaw, Tramble

Sit 'N' Spin
Southpaw

Tilt 'N' Whirl
Whiz Wheel

Obstacle Course Equipment

Barrels
Flaghouse, Sammons Preston, Southpaw

Bolsters
Best Priced Products, Flaghouse, Sammons Preston, Southpaw, Therapy Skill Builders

Foam Blocks
Childcraft, Southpaw

Tunnels
Achievement Products, Childcraft, Flaghouse, Southpaw

Wedges
Childcraft, Flaghouse, Sammons Preston, Southpaw

Suspended Equipment

Air Walker
Southpaw

Bolster Swings
Flaghouse, Southpaw

Dual Swings
Flaghouse, Southpaw

Flexion Disc
Flaghouse, Sammons Preston, Southpaw

Frog Swings
Southpaw

Gliders
Childcraft, Southpaw

Inner Tube Swings
Southpaw

Ladders
Southpaw

Nets and Net Swings
Achievement Products, Flaghouse, Sammons Preston, Southpaw

Surfboard
Flaghouse, Southpaw

Tire Swings
Southpaw

Trapeze
Southpaw

Miscellaneous Equipment

Audiotapes and Books
Southpaw, Sensory Comfort, Bell Curve, Sensory Integration International

Ceiling Supports
Southpaw

Clothing and Equipment for Sensory Defensive Clients
Sensory Comfort

Fine Motor/Visual Supplies
Pocket Full of Therapy

Free-standing Supports
Sammons Preston, Southpaw

Helmets
Flaghouse, Sammons Preston, Southpaw

Inflators and Air Pumps
Equipment Shop, Flaghouse, Sammons Preston, Southpaw

Oral Motor Activity Supplies
PDP Products, Southpaw

Shock or Bungee Cord
Airport or boat supply stores

Stopwatches
Meylan, Western Psychological

Tactile Activity Supplies
Sammons Preston, PDP Products, Pocket Full of Therapy, Therapro

Weighted Vests and Other Vests
Southpaw, Jump-In

Sources

Achievement Products
PO Box 9033
Canton, OH 44711
1-800-373-4699
fax: 330-453-0222
achievepro@aol.com

Belle Curve Records, Inc.
PO Box 18387
Boulder, CO 80308
303-546-6211

Childcraft
PO Box 3239
Lancaster, PA 17604
1-800-637-5652
fax: 1-888-532-4453
www.Childcrafteducation.com

Constructive Playthings
13201 Arrington Rd
Grandview, MO 64030-2886
1-800-448-4115
fax: 1-816-761-9295
www.cptoys.com

The Equipment Shop
PO Box 33
Bedford, MA 01730
781-275-7681
1-800-525-7681
fax: 781-275-4094

Flaghouse
601 Flaghouse Dr.
Hasbrouck Heights, NJ 07604-3116
1-800-793-7900
fax: 1-800-793-7922
sales@flaghouse.com

Jump-In
10315 Moon Lake Court
Pinckney, MI 48169
734-878-0166
fax: 734-878-0169
www.jump-in-products.com

Meylan Corporation
264 West 40th Street
New York, NY 10018
212-391-9150

PDP Products
PO Box 2009
Stillwater, MN 55082-2009
651-439-8865
fax: 651-439-0421
www.pdppro.com

Pocket Full of Therapy
PO Box 174
Morganville, NJ 07751
732-411-0404
www.pfot.com

Sammons Preston
PO Box 5071
Bolingbrook, IL 60440-5071
1-800-323-5547
fax: 1-800-547-4333

Sensory Comfort
Jeremiah Hart House
The Hill
Portsmouth, NH 03801
603-436-8797
fax: 603-436-8422

Sensory Integration International
1602 Cabrillo Ave.
Torrance, CA 90501
310-320-9986
fax: 310-320-9964

Southpaw Enterprises
PO Box 1047
Dayton, OH 45401-1047
1-800-228-1698

Therapro
225 Arlington Street
Framingham, MA 01702-8723
508-872-9494
800-257-5376
fax: 508-875-2062
fax: 888-860-6254

Western Psychological Services
12031 Wilshire Blvd.
Los Angeles, CA 90025
800-222-2670

■■ Appendix 12–B

EVALUATION COMPLETION FORM/THERAPY PROFILE/DISCHARGE SUMMARY

Client Name: _____ Date of Birth: _____ Age: _____ Parent Names: _____

Eval Therapist: _____ Date of Eval: _____ Diag: _____ Home#: _____

Evaluation Given: _____SIPT _____SIM _____MAP _____Other _____Hand Eval

Outcome of Conference (Check Below)
_____Desires TX   _____May want TX   _____No TX Recommended
_____# Sessions Per Week   _____Needs to Ck Insurance   _____Getting It Write
Available Days and Times: _____Ck for School Coverage   _____Oral Motor Group
_____   _____Will Receive TX Elsewhere

Therapist Comments: _____

Rate and Describe Difficulty: Key: 1. Definite Difficulty 2. Moderate Difficulty 3. No Problem or Difficulty or not expected for this age.

Date of first rating: _____ Therapist's Initials _____   Date of second rating: _____ Therapist's Initials _____

Sensory Modulation Problems		Ocular Control		Adaptive Responses	
1 2 3 General State of Arousal	1 2 3	1 2 3 Separating Head & Eyes	1 2 3	1 2 3 Respond to passive stimuli	1 2 3
1 2 3 Tactile	1 2 3	1 2 3 Quick Localization	1 2 3	1 2 3 Holds on and stays put	1 2 3
1 2 3 Vestibular	1 2 3	1 2 3 Pursuits	1 2 3	1 2 3 Pushes, propels, or pumps	1 2 3
1 2 3 Auditory	1 2 3	1 2 3 Convergence	1 2 3	1 2 3 Initiate activity, not	1 2 3
1 2 3 Visual	1 2 3	1 2 3 CXML with eyes	1 2 3	complete independently	
1 2 3 Multiple Inputs	1 2 3			1 2 3 Moving independently/	1 2 3
		Bilateral Control		somewhat familiar manner	
Sensory Discrimination Problems		1 2 3 Establishing Dominance	1 2 3	1 2 3 Moving through environ.	1 2 3
1 2 3 Tactile	1 2 3	1 2 3 Crossing Midline	1 2 3	in unfamiliar way	
1 2 3 Vestibular	1 2 3	1 2 3 UE Bilateral Coordination	1 2 3	1 2 3 Perform complicated acts	1 2 3
1 2 3 Proprioceptive	1 2 3	1 2 3 LE Bilateral Coordination	1 2 3	w/ unfamiliar ways of	
1 2 3 GI	1 2 3			moving	
1 2 3 Vest/vis/prop interaction	1 2 3	**Praxis/Motor Planning**			
1 2 3 _____	1 2 3	1 2 3 Oral Praxis	1 2 3	**Hand/Visual Perception Skills:**	
1 2 3 _____	1 2 3	1 2 3 Fine Motor Praxis	1 2 3	1 2 3 Pencil/Grasp Patterns	1 2 3
		1 2 3 Total Body Coordination	1 2 3	1 2 3 Grip Strength	1 2 3
Postural Problems		1 2 3 Feed Forward	1 2 3	1 2 3 Distal Finger Control	1 2 3
1 2 3 Muscle Tone	1 2 3	1 2 3 Ideation/Initiation	1 2 3	1 2 3 VMI/Handwriting	1 2 3
1 2 3 Shoulder Stability	1 2 3	1 2 3 Imitation	1 2 3		
1 2 3 Trunk Stability	1 2 3	1 2 3 Plan/Sequence	1 2 3	**Functional Problems**	
1 2 3 Strength	1 2 3	1 2 3 Variation/Adaptation	1 2 3	1 2 3 Feeding	1 2 3
1 2 3 Extension	1 2 3	1 2 3 Problem Solving Organization	1 2 3	1 2 3 Self-care/Dressing	1 2 3
1 2 3 Flexion	1 2 3			1 2 3 Sleeping	1 2 3
1 2 3 Weight Shift/Rotation	1 2 3	**Projected Action Sequences**		1 2 3 Toileting	1 2 3
1 2 3 Balance Righting/Equil	1 2 3	1 2 3 Client stationary/Target	1 2 3	1 2 3 Play Skills	1 2 3
1 2 3 PI (Postural Insecurity)	1 2 3	stationary		1 2 3 Social Interaction	1 2 3
		1 2 3 Client moving/Target	1 2 3	1 2 3 Coping	1 2 3
		stationary		1 2 3 Language	1 2 3
		1 2 3 Client stationary/Target	1 2 3		
		moving		_____ Profile Total _____	
		1 2 3 Client moving/Target moving	1 2 3		

Comments:

Date of Discharge: _____   Are 80% of the goals achieved? Y / N
Therapist Signature: _____ Why or why not?
_____

HISTORY OF THERAPIST CALL BACKS

Date	Initials	Notes

Clinical Master #4
Assessment Forms: Eval Completion_DC Form
04/19/01

Occupational Therapy Associates - Watertown, P.C.
Therapy Notes

Client's Name: _____   Therapy Frequency: _____

Key to Progress: 1 = slight,   2 = moderate,   3 = definite,   NC = no change,   -1 = regression,   NA = not applicable

Key for # 14. Adaptive Response: A. Respond to passive stimulus   B. Hold on/Stay put   C. Contract/Relax Muscles
     D. Initiate/Not Complete Ind.   E. Independent/Familiar   F. Independent/Unfamiliar   G. Complex/Unfamiliar

Goal Areas	Date:	Date:
1. Sensory Regulation/ Arousal Level		
2. Force/Body-Scheme Awareness		
3. Temporal/ Spatial Awareness		
4. Movement Security		
5. Oral/ Respiratory		
6. Postural Control/ Strength		
7. Balance		
8. Bilateral Coordination		
9. Ideation/ Initiation		
10. Plan/Sequence		
11. Variation/Adaptation		
12. Problem Solving/ Organization		
13. Projected Action		
14. Adaptive Response Levels		
15. Fine Manipulation		
16. Visual Perception		
17. Visual Motor/ Handwriting		
18. Feeding		
19. Self-Care/ Dressing		
20. Toileting		
21. Sleeping		
22. Safety Awareness		
23. Play Skills		
24. Social Interaction		
25. Coping Skills		

Comments:

Therapist Signature: _____

13

Using Sensory Integration Theory in Schools: Sensory Integration and Consultation

Anita C. Bundy, ScD, OTR, FAOTA

> *Collaborative problem solving takes time. Giving advice is easy—usually wrong but fast and easy.*
>
> —*DeBoer, 1995, p. 63*

For about 25 years, federal law has mandated that occupational therapy practitioners provide intervention for children who require it to benefit fully from special education. That intervention is provided in a number of different ways, according to the needs of the individual student (i.e., direct service, monitoring, consultation) (American Occupational Therapy Association, 1989) in the least restrictive environment (Individuals with Disabilities Education Act [IDEA] Amendments of 1997).

Sensory integration theory is commonly used by occupational therapists working in schools (Case-Smith, 1997). Until relatively recently, intervention based on sensory integration theory has taken the form of direct intervention. Therapists worked directly with students in an area equipped with swings, a suspension system, and other equipment that could be used to create opportunities for enhanced sensation and adaptive behaviors. Usually that space was outside the student's classroom.

In recent years, however, a number of theorists and researchers (Bundy, 1995; Dunn, 1990, 1992; Hanft & Place, 1996) have expressed the value of consultation for enabling students to succeed in the educational environment *despite* limitations imposed by sensory integrative (or other types of) dysfunction. Consultation in schools generally is case-centered and collaborative (collegial) (Hanft & Place, 1996; Jaffe & Epstein, 1992), although certainly other types occur (e.g., educational, program, administrative, process) (Rourk, 1992; Schein, 1999; Spencer, 1992; Weiss, 1992).

PURPOSE AND SCOPE

This chapter defines educational relevance as it applies to occupational therapy. It also describes three types of service delivery that are viable in schools—direct intervention, consultation, and monitoring—and the outcomes expected from each. Finally, the chapter discusses consultation, its stages, and the resources required for implementing it successfully. In an extensive appendix, the text offers strategies germane to consultation for children with sensory integrative dysfunction.

DETERMINING EDUCATIONAL RELEVANCE

Occupational therapy services in school must be educationally relevant—that is, they must be necessary to enable students to meet objectives specified in the Individualized Educational Program (IEP). Bundy (1995) argued that there are four broad areas in which students can have difficulty in school:

1. Learning (acquiring information)
2. Expressing learning
3. Assuming the student role
4. Self-care and mobility

Each of these represents a continuum from "little ability" to "no problem" (See Fig. 13–1). Occupational therapy practitioners have particular expertise in the last three and can act as effective consultants in the first one, helping teachers to develop new strategies within their own particular area of expertise (i.e., teaching). None of these areas represents an *exclusive* area of expertise of occupational therapy practitioners. Although they may approach objectives in a different way, other professionals also have expertise in all these areas. When students' explicit objectives fall in an area of expertise for occupational therapy *and* when occupational therapy practitioners are the best qualified and most logical professional to provide the intervention, then their services can be argued to be educationally relevant.

DETERMINING APPROPRIATE SERVICE DELIVERY

The service delivery models that practitioners use are dependent on the nature of a student's objectives (i.e., the outcome sought). In the best of all worlds, the educational team makes that decision. However, an occupational therapy practitioner may well provide recommendations to the team. More than one service delivery model must often be used to meet the varying needs of a student.

In *direct intervention,* an occupational therapist practitioner works directly with a student to change something about that student's performance (Dunn, 1992), including helping the student develop explicit skills (Bundy, 1995). Direct intervention can be implemented within or outside the classroom. Although IDEA-97 emphasizes the least restrictive environment, which some teams have interpreted as meaning that intervention should occur in the classroom, it is generally difficult to implement direct intervention based on sensory integration theory in a classroom. Appropriate equipment and space generally is lacking, and the whole experience would likely be very disruptive to other students in the classroom.

In direct intervention, practitioners are responsible for determining how to solve a problem. In contrast, in consultation, practitioners work with teachers, other professionals, parents, or older students to enable them to solve problems that prevent them from carrying out their own roles in the most effective way. In consultation, the client owns both the problem and the solution. The major role of the consultant is to help the client define the problem and create workable solutions (Schein, 1999). Consultation is defined in various ways. Jaffe and Epstein (1992) indicated that,

> inherent in any definition of consultation is the concept of an interactive process and a relationship perceived as egalitarian, with give-and-take in an atmosphere of mutual respect. The difference between other interprofessional activities and consultation activities is that the consultant operates *within other people's perspectives,* working with the consultee rather than directly with the problem. The consultant does not assume responsibility for the decisions, but enables the person receiving the help to work more effectively by improving skills, widening perspectives, and changing attitudes, without the consultant taking over their work (p. 18).

Consultation can be extremely powerful. We believe it should be the *primary* type of service delivery used by practitioners working in schools. What little research there is in this area (Dunn,

1990; Giangreco, 1986; Miller & Sabatino, 1978; Schulte et al., 1990) has supported that view and suggested that consultation is either as effective or more effective for meeting student objectives than is direct service. In fact, we have found no published evidence to the contrary.

Several myths surround the use of consultation in schools. These often become barriers to its effective use. Hanft (1996) described three such myths. First, because it requires less time, therapists can dramatically increase their caseloads through consultation. Second, through consultation, therapists train teachers to implement therapy. Finally, consultation can always substitute for direct intervention.

One reality is that consultation requires considerable time (Dunn, 1992; Hanft, 1996). To be effective, consultants must meet regularly with clients, sometimes over an entire school year. However, because they come to understand students' needs in more compelling ways, teachers and parents learn to generalize principles and apply them to new situations and with new students with little assistance from a therapist. Thus, many other students, with or without disabilities, may benefit from consultation directed at the difficulties of teaching and parenting one particular student. When older students are the consulting partners, they learn to identify and solve problems associated with their disabilities. Thus, consultation promotes independence and empowerment.

Consultation is not the same as either monitoring or direct intervention. Different outcomes are associated with each. With monitoring, parents or teachers learn to implement procedures typically done by therapists; however, their principal roles do not change. They may implement a procedure because they believe that frequent repetition will be beneficial to the student, but they do not become the student's therapists.

Students who need direct intervention to establish a new pattern of performance or acquire a new skill do not achieve the same outcome from consultation. Consultation seeks to enable parents, teachers, or older students to assume their own roles more effectively.

Despite its power, or perhaps *because* of it, consultation can be extremely complicated, and many practitioners have not been prepared well in the knowledge and skills necessary to perform it effectively. Thus, consultation requires considerably more discussion, so most of the rest of this chapter is devoted to examples and theory related to consultation.

In contrast, *monitoring* (or indirect service) is a type of service delivery in which occupational therapy practitioners teach skills for managing students' daily needs to caregivers (i.e., parents, professionals, and paraprofessionals). Practitioners most commonly teach skills related to positioning, handling, feeding, toileting, or use of adaptive equipment. Students with sensory integrative dysfunction are less likely than students with more significant disabilities to require monitoring. However, monitoring *is* indicated when programs such as the Wilbarger protocol (Wilbarger & Wilbarger, 1991) are implemented in school to reach a specific objective or when a student needs to practice a particular program daily (e.g., a handwriting program prescribed by the occupational therapist).

CONSULTATION IN SCHOOLS

Consultants help clients reframe students' behavior or difficulties (Bundy, 1995; Niehues et al., 1991) and serve as catalysts to enable them to solve their own problems (Schein, 1999). Consultants may suggest or provide specific activities or materials; however, their primary role is to enable clients to solve their own problems.

Reframing

Reframing behavior is the process of enabling others to understand a student's behavior in a different way or to view behaviors from a new perspective. We speak of *reframing,* rather than "setting the frame" (Schön, 1983, 1987) because almost invariably, teachers, parents, and students already have set a frame for the student's behavior. Setting the frame is only necessary when they have no prior view or interpretation of the student's behavior. Moreover, in the case of students with sensory integrative dysfunction, often the frame that teachers or parents have set is negative (Case-Smith, 1997).

Parents and teachers may view a student as poorly disciplined, immature, destructive, careless, rigid, or overreactive. The frame teachers and parents have for viewing a student's behavior determines how they react to that behavior (i.e., the strategies they will use in teaching or parenting). By using sensory integration theory to change the frame, we provide teachers or parents with the basis for developing different strategies for interacting with students. In turn, these strategies often result in a dramatic lessening of problem behaviors because situations or activities that are apt to be difficult for the student can be avoided or made easier.

Rebecca was a 5-year-old child with sensory integrative dysfunction. She exhibited extreme hypersensitivity to touch and minor pain. However, Rebecca's reaction to pain was delayed; often 5 or more minutes pass after a minor incident, such as bumping her elbow, before she erupted in tears and screams of agony: "This is gonna hurt me forever!" Rebecca's parents and teacher viewed Rebecca's reactions as melodramatic. "After all, if she really were hurt, wouldn't she begin to cry immediately?" they asked. Believing that Rebecca was only "acting" to get attention, her parents and teacher tried ignoring her wails and telling her that she was not hurt and was "acting silly." However, both responses only resulted in Rebecca's screaming more loudly.

During a conference after Rebecca's evaluation, we told her parents and teacher about the extent of Rebecca's difficulties processing sensation. They discussed her reactions to pain, and we helped them see how this behavior might be explained by sensory integrative dysfunction. "Perhaps," we reasoned, "Rebecca's sensory integrative dysfunction results in its taking longer for her to process sensory information. When she does process it, Rebecca interprets stimuli that others would consider nonaversive as painful."

The result was that Rebecca's parents and teacher came to view this very problematic behavior in a different way. Rather than seeing her behavior as melodramatic, they understood that Rebecca's intense, but delayed, reaction to pain was the result of her difficulty processing sensory information. The frame was changed.

Developing New Strategies

Reframing is one of the therapist–consultant's most important tools (Case-Smith, 1997; Niehues et al., 1991). However, the role of a consultant usually does not end with reframing. Rather, reframing provides the basis on which further consultation is built. After a new frame has been established, the consultant helps the parents, teachers, or older students develop new strategies for solving their own problems.

The story of Rebecca provides a good example of successful strategies built on a new frame. With our help, Rebecca's parents and teacher used their new-found knowledge to develop different strategies for responding to her outbursts. They began to acknowledge that what Rebecca felt was pain and that they understood that she believed as though it would "hurt her forever." They asked to see the hurt place and applied deep touch pressure and firm rubbing to the area. Using these strategies, they found that Rebecca was much easier to console. Although her reaction to minor pain remained intense and delayed, she screamed less and was more easily distracted from her pain.

Rebecca's parents and teacher also felt better. As they became more skilled at using their new strategies, her parents no longer dreaded taking Rebecca to their friends' homes. They stopped believing that they had to apologize for Rebecca's "overreactions." When it seemed appropriate, they explained the source of Rebecca's discomfort. Otherwise, they used their new strategies to avert disaster and behaved as though nothing out of the ordinary had occurred. Other adults picked up on this new strategy and also began to implement it. The result was that everyone became more comfortable with Rebecca, including herself.

With the story of Rebecca, we have illustrated an example of effective consultation with parents. However, consultation in schools happens even more frequently with teachers than with parents. For example, a teacher may believe that a student constantly gets into fistfights while standing in line because he is poorly disciplined. This teacher is more likely to behave differently toward that student than another teacher who understands the student's tactile defensiveness and knows that the student was probably jostled accidentally from behind. In the latter case, the student may be allowed to stand at the back of the line where he or she can avoid unexpected touch. In the former case, the child is likely to be kept near the front of the line, under the teacher's watchful eye, but also an easy target for more accidental jostling. The likely result is more fistfights. Thus, the child is apt to be punished repeatedly for circumstances beyond his or her control. Because the teacher does not understand the basis of the problem, the solution is likely to make the problem worse.

Consultation also might happen with an older student. Shaw, a student in 7th grade, had significant difficulty with organization. When Elizabeth, his occupational therapist, served as a direct service provider with Shaw, she developed and implemented solutions to Shaw's organizational difficulties. For example, she installed dividers in his locker and arranged for him to have a second set of books at home to use for completing assignments. Such strategies were moderately successful. However, when Elizabeth assumed the role of consultant to Shaw rather than direct service provider, she no longer assumed that she was the expert on Shaw's difficulties. Rather, *Shaw* became the expert. Elizabeth helped him to identify the things he would like to change. Elizabeth was surprised when Shaw indicated that his inability to keep track of his schedule was most troubling to him. After that was identified, however, Shaw was able to develop a strategy for solving the problem. He made a schedule and fastened it permanently to his backpack. This strategy worked much better when Shaw developed it than it would have if it had been Elizabeth's idea. Furthermore, because the schedule had been his idea, Shaw felt empowered to alter it to fit his needs and did so without assistance from Elizabeth. The concept of consultation is deceptively simple. The process, however, may prove much more difficult.

Consultation with a Teacher: A Case Example

The following case example illustrates the consultation process that occurred between an occupational therapist consultant and a teacher during the course of a school year. The case is then used as the basis for a discussion of stages of consultation.

Duncan was an 8-year-old boy of average intelligence who had learning disabilities. He was a second grade student in a combined first and second grade classroom. His teacher, Ms. R., having attempted unsuccessfully for the past year to teach handwriting to Duncan, had reached her "level of tolerance." She referred Duncan to Lily, the occupational therapist, for evaluation and possible intervention.

Upon questioning Ms. R. about the instructional methods she had tried with Duncan, Lily learned that Ms. R. had attempted numerous strategies and that she was currently using a "multisensory approach" to teach handwriting. When asked to describe the multisensory approach, Ms. R. indicated that she showed Duncan a letter and then asked him to practice making that letter in, or with, various media. These media included sand, rice, fingerpaint, chalk, markers, and other items.

When asked about the problems that Duncan had reproducing letters with a pen or pencil, Ms. R. showed Lily copies of some of Duncan's papers. The letters were poorly formed and so light that they were barely legible.

Lily spent some time in the classroom watching Duncan form letters with the various media his teacher had described. As she watched, Lily noted that the letters Duncan made looked different in each medium; he did not have a consistent pattern for forming each letter. She realized that, rather than practicing the same letter formation over and over, Duncan was actually performing new motor patterns as he moved from one medium to another. When he formed the letter in fingerprint, he used finger motions; but when he wrote on the chalkboard, he used whole arm movements. Both of these were different from the motor patterns he used when he attempted to write the letter on paper with a pencil. Although most individuals would create letters that looked essentially the same no matter whether they used arm or finger movements, that was not the case with Duncan.

In addition to observation of Duncan in his classroom and interviews with his teacher, Lily's evaluation consisted of clinical observations of neuromotor behavior, the tactile tests of the Southern California Sensory Integration Tests (Ayres, 1972), and the Bruininks-Oseretsky Test of Motor Proficiency (Bruininks, 1978). Duncan had deficits on all of these measures. After gathering all the data, Lily concluded that Duncan was dyspraxic; his dyspraxia seemed to stem from decreased processing of tactile, vestibular, and proprioceptive sensations. Additionally, Duncan's dyspraxia seemed to be interfering with his ability to learn cursive handwriting skills.

Having determined that much, Lily was faced with the important decision of what type of intervention to recommend to the educational team. Lily believed that Duncan would probably benefit from occupational therapy. However, rather than recommending direct intervention, Lily suggested to the team that she provide consultation to Ms. R.

This recommendation was based on a number of factors. First, Duncan's inability to learn to write seemed to be caused by dyspraxia. However, Lily reasoned that it would take months, perhaps years, of direct intervention before his deficits could be remediated sufficiently for him to learn handwriting through the methods Ms. R. was using. If Ms. R. was to succeed, she needed Lily's help.

Second, Duncan's primary difficulty in his classroom seemed to be with learning handwriting. Ms. R. was instructing Duncan daily in handwriting. Although Lily could have developed a direct intervention program that targeted improvements in handwriting, she could only have provided intervention once or twice a week. Furthermore, Lily knew very little about teaching proper letter formation, but that was one of Ms. R's areas of expertise.

Third, although he was of average intelligence and despite of his good auditory learning skills, Duncan had difficulty keeping up in school. If he heard information and instructions, he could remember them, but it was difficult for him to learn by reading. Therefore, it was important that Duncan be present for and attend to his teacher's instructions. He could not afford time out of class for occupational therapy because he would probably fall further behind in school. Even if Lily elected to provide direct intervention in his classroom, it was very likely that Duncan would miss some important information during that time.

Finally, Ms. R.'s openness to working with Lily was an important factor in her recommendation for consultation. Ms. R. was a skilled teacher who had invested a lot of time and effort in trying to teach Duncan to write. However, nothing she tried had worked. She knew that his problems required the input of another professional, and she was eager to accept help from someone who could explain Duncan's problems. Although Ms. R. was a master teacher and had taught letter formation for years, her knowledge of dyspraxia was limited. As a result, she unknowingly developed a method to teach Duncan to form letters that "played to his weaknesses." This method, although creative and motivating for Duncan, resulted in his having to formulate several different motor responses for each new letter he learned. Because forming new motor responses was his greatest deficit, Duncan had not learned to write by this method.

When Lily presented her recommendation to Duncan's education team, including his parents and teachers, they agreed with Lily's recommendation for consultation. In fact, Lily's presentation of Duncan's motor planning difficulties and the benefits of consultation was so clear and convincing that the physical education teacher also requested consultation with her.

Lily began consulting with Ms. R. by listening carefully to her concerns and offering a new frame for the problem. Lily again explained about Duncan's extraordinary difficulty with planning new movements. She told Ms. R. that Duncan's difficulties were the result of poor feedback he received from his body when he moved. She also showed Ms. R. that each of the media Duncan was using to learn letter formation resulted in his planning a new way of moving.

That simple reframing was all that Ms. R. needed to help her to understand the problem. She had already known that Duncan was poorly coordinated and that he seemed not to know how his body moved. Therefore, she had reasoned that providing him with a lot of sensation might help him learn to write better. However, she had not recognized that, with each new medium, Duncan had to formulate a new plan for moving.

"I guess that means that I should pick one medium and stick with it," Ms. R. stated. Lily agreed. Ms. R. and Lily concluded that Duncan needed to concentrate on learning to write with a pen or pencil. They discussed Duncan's difficulties with forming letters and pressing hard enough that they could be seen. Lily knew that Duncan was not getting adequate feedback from his body as he wrote with his pencil, and she believed that the deficit in feedback was contributing to his poor letter formation. She suggested that Duncan write with a grease pencil because its increased resistance would provide him with more feedback. Ms. R. agreed that the grease pencil might work. She and Lily made arrangements to meet again the next week to discuss Duncan's progress.

The next week, Ms. R. reported that the grease pencil did not seem to be working; Duncan still did not press hard enough to make his handwriting legible. Lily and Ms. R. then devised a plan for Duncan to use carbon paper between two sheets of paper. Ms. R. taught Duncan to lift the carbon periodically to see whether or not he had been pressing down hard enough for his writing to come through.

Duncan responded very well to the carbon paper. Within a few weeks, he learned to write much more legibly and to press harder with his pencil. After about 6 weeks, Ms. R. and Lily decided that the carbon paper might no longer be necessary. Ms. R. prepared Duncan for the change by trying to make him conscious of the amount of pressure he used when he wrote successfully using the carbon paper. She gradually withdrew the carbon paper by giving him more papers each day that did not have carbon paper attached to them.

An important part of consultation was that Lily continued to meet regularly with Ms. R. They worked together to solve a number of difficulties that Duncan had in the classroom. As Ms. R. came to understand Duncan's difficulties with formulating new motor programs, she began to devise her own alternative strategies for teaching Duncan. Initially, she liked to discuss her plans with Lily before implementing them to be sure she was on the right track. However, as she began to succeed, she needed less input from Lily. During one of their sessions, about 3 months into the consultation process, Ms. R. remarked to Lily, "You know, this all was once so new to me; now it seems so logical. I know that I will look at other students' problems differently from now on."

Lily did a similar type of consultation with the physical education teacher that was also highly successful. Duncan's physical education class focused on physical fitness. The students spent the majority of their time doing calisthenics. Mr. S., the physical education teacher, led the students in various routines composed of jumping jacks, push-ups, sit-ups, running in place, and other basic skills. Although the exercises were always the same, he varied their order. Duncan's coordination was not very good, but if he concentrated intensely, he could perform some of the exercises passably. However, this required inordinate effort on his part, and he often chose to stand and watch the others rather than to participate. When Lily talked with Mr. S., she learned that it was Duncan's "standing around" that bothered Mr. S. the most.

In her consultation with Mr. S., Lily recommended some very simple adaptations to the way the class was run, which resulted in Duncan's participating more frequently and more effectively. Lily explained that Duncan would be able to do the exercises better if there were set routines. He could then memorize them and would not have to think so hard about what was coming next. Furthermore, she explained that Duncan's strongest channel for learning was auditory. Thus, she suggested, it might be helpful if Mr. S. always called out the next exercise shortly before it changed and again at the time of the change. Lily also recommended that Mr. S. stand near Duncan and perform the exercises with the class. In that way, Duncan would always hear the instructions and also have a visual model.

Lily was able to use her knowledge of sensory integrative theory to help Ms. R. and Mr. S. understand Duncan's motor planning difficulties. In doing so, she helped them see why their teaching methods had failed and helped them develop new strategies that worked. When Ms. R.'s knowledge of proper letter formation was combined with Lily's cognizance of Duncan's motor planning deficits, the result was the development of strategies that allowed Duncan to learn cursive writing. Initially, Duncan did not participate in Mr. S.'s physical education class. With a few simple modifications, however, Duncan became an active member of the class. None of these professionals could have accomplished their goals alone in such a short time period; together they succeeded.

STAGES OF CONSULTATION

The general goals that guide consultation are to use practice theories to reframe a student's behavior for our clients and, based on that reframing, to help our clients develop new and more effective strategies for interacting and working with students. However, consultation is complicated, and a consultant cannot simply move into the situation, reframe the problem, provide strategies, and exit. Effective consultation occurs in stages. A number of authors (e.g., Hanft & Place, 1996; Jaffe & Epstein, 1992) have described various stages to consultation. All have common elements, including the need to establish an egalitarian relationship.

When we think of consultation, we think of four stages:

1. Formulating expectations
2. Establishing the partnership
3. Planning strategies
4. Implementing and assessing the plan

The relationship of these stages to one another is shown schematically in Figure 13–2.

Each of the four stages is equally important to the process. In certain instances (and in all of the examples we have used), some of the stages seem to be accomplished very easily, almost automatically, and the consultant and client are able to make rapid progress. Thus, an observer to this process might have been unaware that some of the stages had occurred. In instances in which the process does not go so smoothly, we attempt to

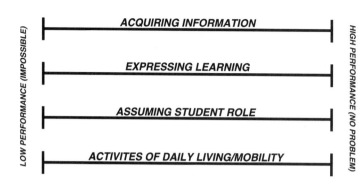

■ FIGURE 13-1 Four Continua for describing a student's performance in school and curricular expectations.

trace backward through the stages to find out where the process went awry. In doing so, we are able to determine where to begin again to facilitate the consultation process.

The consultant and client participate as equals in all four stages of the process. However, it is the therapist's responsibility to facilitate and examine the process and to change its course if the process does not seem to be working.

We will use the case of Lily and Ms. R. to illustrate how partners pass through these stages. We will also describe one therapist's attempt at developing a consultative partnership that did not begin smoothly. We will discuss some strategies that therapists used to facilitate the development of the relationship. Although parents (such as Rebecca's parents) and older children are frequently our partners in the consultative process, the discussion in the next section is simplified by referring to the client as the teacher.

Stage I: Formulating Expectations

This first stage occurs before the consultant and teacher have begun to work together. In preparation for beginning the process, both the teacher and the consultant, consciously or unconsciously, formulate expectations of what will happen during, and as a result of, intervention.

Mattingly and Fleming (1994) suggested that these expectations take the form of real or imagined stories created using information from a number of sources. These sources may include information that the teacher and therapist have because they have worked together before, information shared with one of them by a colleague or the student's parent, past experiences that they have had working with or observing other therapists or teachers, or their own imaginations. The creation of expectations enables therapists to prepare for

intervention. When we understand that we begin the process with expectations that may be based in falsehoods, we are prepared to seek new information and to alter the stories we have created in response to our actual situation as we begin working with the teacher.

In instances in which the teacher and the consultant have worked together before, as with Ms. R. and Lily, the stories or expectations that the two create may be very similar to what actually happens when they begin working together. However, in situations in which a consultant and teacher have not worked together, one or both of them may have created stories or set expectations that impede the development of the relationship.

Stage II: Establishing a Partnership

This second stage of the process is composed of four very important phases (Fig. 13–2). Because it is a preliminary stage (in that the partners are not yet ready to develop strategies), we may minimize its importance and "gloss over" it in favor of moving on to the "more important business" that lies ahead. However, if we move on too quickly and attempt to offer solutions or strategies before we have established an equal partnership, we may give the impression that we "know all the answers" and are not interested in the teacher's contributions to the process. Clearly, perceived inequality in the relationship will hamper both the development of a partnership and the effectiveness of the process. This is particularly true when consultant–client teams have not worked together before or when one team member has considerably less experience than the other. Thus, it is not surprising that consultative relationships that go awry often do so at this stage.

Of course, the need to develop a partnership does not mean we never offer solutions early in the process. Sometimes a simple suggestion can go a long way toward gaining a teacher's interest in the process. However, we must guard against being perceived as the expert rather than as a conduit.

There are many valid reasons why a teacher may be hesitant to enter into a consultative partnership. The teacher may believe the consultant is "invading" or interrupting the important business of the classroom. The teacher may think that because teaching is a full-time job, taking on additional work just is not possible. The teacher may never before have worked with a therapist who was interested in consulting. Based on past experience, the teacher may perceive that intervention is a somewhat mysterious process carried on somewhere other than the classroom. Some teachers may feel threatened, fearing the therapist will judge their teaching ability.

We must be prepared for whatever reaction a teacher has. There are real reasons for the reaction. Furthermore, we enter the process knowing that intervention is most successful when teachers are willing and able to add their valuable knowledge and skills to the process. We do what it takes to facilitate the development of a consultative partnership with the teacher. Above all, we must realize that the formation of this relationship can take a great deal of time. However, the benefits to the stu-

dent and to future students in the teacher's classroom are well worth the time and energy invested.

Therapists, also, are sometimes hesitant to enter into a true consultative partnership. Many have said that they believe that being a consultant requires that they be experts in a particular problem area and that they do not feel like experts. Others have felt that teaching is the teacher's business and that they have a separate role—to provide intervention. Others have expressed that "real intervention" involves "putting their hands on a student" and that working with teachers, although it is important, is a secondary concern (Niehues et al., 1991). Still others have become confused by their perceptions that particular parents or teachers are demanding that a child's intervention be provided as direct intervention.

We believe that many of these fears and beliefs arise from therapists' misconceptions about consultation. Historically, occupational therapy practitioners have not been trained as consultants. Furthermore, very little literature exists in our field to assist us in developing these skills. Because we have neither understood consultation clearly nor envisioned ourselves in a primary role as consultants, we have not been able to effectively explain the benefits of consultation to parents and teachers with whom we work. As we have said earlier, we believe that the importance of the outcomes asso-

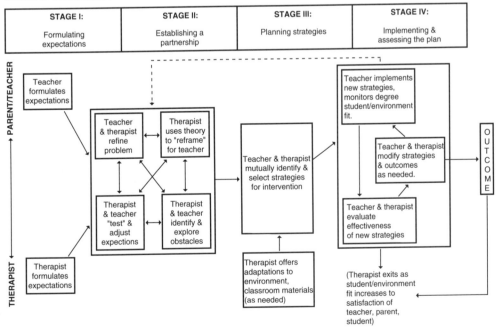

■ FIGURE 13-2 Stages of consultation.

ciated with consultation necessitates that we develop our skills in this area and that we take a proactive stance with regard to consultation.

The phases of stage II are somewhat circular. There is no particular order in which they must be accomplished. Rather, each "feeds into" the others. For the sake of simplicity, we begin with the phase in Figure 13–2 labeled "teacher and therapist test and adjust expectations." We will discuss each phase as it appears in Figure 13–2, moving in a clockwise fashion.

Testing and Adjusting Expectations

When teachers and consultants begin working together, they "test" and adjust their expectations of one another. They compare the stories they have created about the other individual with the "real" individual they encounter. Expectations often are created about the person with whom we will work, the form the intervention will take, or the anticipated outcomes.

As much as possible, we try to uncover teachers' expectations as they enter into the consultation process. We use our skills to elicit teachers' expectations in a nonthreatening manner, and we share some of our own expectations (DeBoer, 1995; Schein, 1999).

Although learning about teachers' expectations for consultation and the partnership, we listen and observe carefully to discern their preferred styles of thinking and interacting. We remain cognizant of our own typical styles and alter them as needed (DeBoer, 1995).

If the style and expectations of a teacher are somewhat similar to our own, we move forward in building our relationship. However, what happens when, for example, the teacher's expectations for intervention do not include any relationship between the teacher and the therapist? In the following story, that is precisely what happened. Unlike Lily's experiences with Ms. R. and Mr. S., Lynn, the therapist in this story, never really felt that she was able to develop a true consultative relationship with Ms. M., the teacher. Although Lynn did not attempt to pressure Ms. M. into receiving consultation, Lynn used several strategies that resulted in Ms. M.'s seeking consultation the next year.

Kelly was a 7-year-old girl with sensory integrative–based dyspraxia and significant visual-spatial deficits; she was included in a first grade classroom. Because she had extreme difficulty with any classroom task that required motor output, Kelly qualified for occupational therapy services at school.

Kelly's IEP called for her to receive occupational therapy twice a week; it did not specify the type of service delivery. Lynn was new to the district. When she met Ms. M. for the first time, Lynn indicated that she would like to spend one session each week consulting with Ms. M. Ms. M. responded immediately that she had understood that Lynn would remove Kelly from the classroom for both periods. Ms. M.'s "story" of therapy did not include any interaction between herself and the therapist. She had not realized she would have to participate in any way. She did not leave Lynn with many choices.

Lynn decided to move very slowly; she responded by providing direct intervention to Kelly twice a week. However, each time she arrived at the classroom, she asked Ms. M. what Kelly was having trouble with that she might include in intervention. She frequently took math papers to work on, adapting them so that Kelly could figure out where to place the answers. Each time she returned with Kelly, Lynn spent a few minutes telling Ms. M. what they had accomplished and sharing the adaptations she that enabled Kelly to complete a particular assignment.

One day when Lynn arrived, Ms. M. handed her a math assignment and told her she would like to have it done when Kelly came back. Lynn responded by telling Ms. M., again, that she did not feel qualified to teach math. Ms. M. seemed a little offended, but the next time Lynn arrived, Ms. M. shared with her that Kelly was having a lot of trouble with phonics. She asked if Lynn could incorporate phonics into her occupational therapy activities. Lynn said that she could. She and Kelly spent time doing an activity in which Kelly used a magnetized fishing pole to "fish" for different letter sounds. When she and Kelly returned to the classroom, they both excitedly told Ms. M. about what they had done.

Ms. M. began to think of other concepts that could be incorporated into Kelly's intervention. Gradually, she began to ask Lynn's advice about various classroom activities, such as cutting with scissors. This was the breakthrough for which Lynn had been hoping. She responded by coming into the classroom during several art activities. She took the opportunity to work with Kelly, but she also adapted the task for several other students who seemed to be having difficulty.

The next school year, Lynn worked with another student in Ms. M.'s class. When Lynn approached Ms. M. about the schedule, Ms. M. suggested that maybe a part of the time could be spent consulting with her.

Clearly, Ms. M.'s expectations of occupational therapy changed because of her interactions with Lynn. The process of changing those expectations took considerable time, but by the beginning of the second year, Ms. M. and Lynn were well on the way to establishing a real partnership. Initially, Lynn recognized that she could not implement the consulting program she had envisioned. However, she still devoted a few minutes each week to telling Ms. M. about occupational therapy as it related to Kelly. Lynn went out of her way to find out how she might tailor her intervention to meet Kelly's needs in the classroom. By viewing the situation as a challenge and being assertive, she influenced Ms. M.'s beliefs. Ms. M. learned a great deal about occupational therapy. She gained new respect for Lynn and learned something about how Lynn's training could help her to change the classroom so that it better met the needs of her students.

Refining the Problem

Another important part of stage II involves eliciting as much detail as we can about the problem the teacher is experiencing in teaching a student in order to refine the problem. We ask questions and make observations until the teacher pinpoints a solvable problem. We find out as much as we can about how students' difficulties are affecting their teachers' ability to teach them and, thus, their ability to benefit fully from the educational experience. We also try to learn which strategies have been tried and how well they have worked. The teacher and consultant also explore which resources they will need.

Refining the problem is a particularly important step. There might have been any number of reasons why Mr. S., the physical education teacher, sought Lily's assistance. However, what was really bothering Mr. S. was Duncan's failure to participate. The approach to solving the problem would have been entirely different if Mr. S. had been most bothered by Duncan's poor coordination. When refining the problem, we use caution not to assume that we already know what the problem is (Schein, 1999). We are mindful of the fact that the client is the expert on the problem.

Reframing the Problem

In this stage, the consultant uses sensory integration (or another) theory to reframe the problem that the teacher has described. We have described reframing in some detail above. However, to reiterate, it is important that we listen carefully to the difficulties the teacher is describing and address these difficulties. The client is the expert on the problem.

In the example of Lily and Ms. R., Lily listened carefully to Ms. R.'s problem teaching handwriting to Duncan. She observed Duncan in his classroom and interpreted the results of his testing in light of what she saw and heard. Lily explained Duncan's dyspraxia as it applied to handwriting. She did not attempt to explain the neuroanatomy of the tactile, vestibular, or proprioceptive systems. Rather, she made it clear that there is a hypothesized causal relationship between sensory feedback from the body and the ability to learn new motor tasks. She told Ms. R. that the tests Duncan took revealed that he had difficulty processing information about touch and body movement. Lily then went on to show Ms. R. that the teaching method she had devised was unintentionally making the task of learning handwriting more difficult. With the frame shifted in this way, Ms. R. understood Duncan's problems differently. This new frame also suggested possible strategies for Ms. R.

Identifying Obstacles

The final phase of the second stage of consultation requires that a teacher and consultant identify obstacles that may interfere with effecting a change. A commonly encountered obstacle is scheduling sufficient time to meet together when a teacher is not worried about what is going on in the classroom or the therapist thinking about traveling to the next school (Hanft & Place, 1996). When the decision to provide consultation is a team decision, the team has responsibility for providing resources. Thus, we must ask for the resources we need.

If it is not possible to schedule uninterrupted time before or after school or during breaks, it may be necessary for the principal or some other adult to take responsibility for a teacher's class during consultation. This is the strategy Lily and Ms. R. used when they found that it was impossible to be free at the same time. Lily explained to the school principal what she hoped to accomplish and why she needed a particular block of time. The principal agreed that he or another adult would be free during that time period or that they would hire a regular substitute.

After the principal was informed of the problem, he was willing to provide support to Ms. R. and Lily. If Lily had not talked with him, he probably would have remained unaware that there was a problem, and Lily and Ms. R. might have needlessly compromised their plans for consultation. Furthermore, it was Lily's, rather than Ms. R.'s, responsibility to approach the principal because the consultant secures the necessary resources to conduct intervention. Lily did so, however, with Ms. R.'s knowledge and approval.

Bundy et al. (1989) reported the results of a large national survey of special education administrators. When asked what one thing therapists could do to improve their effectiveness in public schools, these administrators commonly answered, "Be more assertive." We should not take this suggestion lightly. To provide high-quality consultation, we need the support of the educational team and the administration. Unless we make our needs known, they will not be met.

The formation of the consultative partnership is the most crucial phase in the consultation process. To be effective, we must demonstrate our respect for our clients' knowledge and skills, our willingness to respect the constraints of their positions, our ability to listen, and our ability to share what we know in a way that is meaningful (Bundy et al., 1989). Sometimes this stage flows so smoothly that we are hardly aware that we have passed through it. However, when we become aware that consultation feels uncomfortable or is not yielding effective strategies, we should examine the phases associated with this stage to determine where the process went awry.

Stage III: Planning Strategies

In stage III of the consultation process, the consulting partners use the new frame to examine and select strategies for the teacher to use with the student. If the underlying problems have been identified correctly and the partnership has been firmly established, it should be relatively easy to develop strategies to address the difficulties, provided the therapist has access to a repertoire of possibilities. As much as possible, the client is responsible for developing the strategies. The con-

sultant primarily helps the client figure out what will work (DeBoer, 1995; Schein, 1999).

Having explained that Duncan was not getting adequate feedback from his body, Lily suggested a different kind of writing implement. When the problem of Duncan's not pressing hard enough on the paper persisted, Lily and Ms. R. decided he should use carbon paper. Without the carbon paper, Duncan did not seem to be able to determine how hard was "hard enough." With the carbon paper, "hard enough" became defined as hard enough to make marks appear on the paper underneath. This was the kind of feedback from which Duncan could benefit. He was able to lift the carbon paper periodically to make sure that he was writing hard enough. Consequently, Ms. R. was freed from having to stand over him and give him verbal feedback.

This mutually developed strategy was agreeable to everyone. Ideally, all strategies are mutually developed and agreeable to both consultants and clients. However, we keep in mind that *clients* are the ones primarily responsible for identifying problems that interfere with their ability to meet the responsibilities of their roles. Moreover, clients are the ones who implement the strategies. Clients are the experts on the problems *and* the solutions (Schein, 1999).

Although developing strategies may be *relatively* easier than establishing and maintaining the partnership, it is not easy to develop strategies in all situations. One important benefit of consultation *to the therapist* is the acquisition of a repertoire of strategies that have worked in similar situations. Appendix 13–A presents a list of strategies contributed by occupational therapy students and practitioners from many locations in the United States. These strategies are divided into groups. One group is composed of activities that students do commonly during the school day and that provide enhanced sensation. The second group is made up of strategies to solve problems commonly encountered by students with sensory integrative dysfunction but that do not incorporate enhanced sensation.

As part of her role in the partnership, Lily provided alternative writing utensils and paper. These materials were not really "adaptive equipment" per se. However, we may find that one important role we play in the planning stage is to provide teachers and students with adaptive or alternative devices and materials. This is an important tool of consultation and a way of modifying the environment so that it better fits the needs of students with sensory integrative dysfunction.

Stage IV: Implementing and Assessing the Plan

In the final stage, the teacher implements the plan and the teacher and consultant mutually evaluate its effectiveness, modifying it as necessary. This stage is fairly self-explanatory. However, as in the previous stage, it is important to recognize that the teacher is responsible for implementing the plan; therefore, no matter how well the occupational therapist thinks something is working, the plan must be modified if the teacher is not comfortable with it.

There are many reasons why a strategy may not feel comfortable to particular teachers. Perhaps it does not reflect the teacher's teaching styles or values. Perhaps the teacher just needs to practice a strategy until it becomes more his or her "own." Some teachers may need to see someone "model" the strategy before implementing it themselves. Some strategies just are not practical. When a strategy feels wrong, the teacher and consultant try to uncover the source of the teacher's discomfort so that the appropriate changes can be made. The solution to the problem when a teacher needs a model is very different from the solution when the problem is that the teacher just needs practice. We need to be careful not to give up on a strategy because it does not work the first time. However, we also need to work with teachers to modify strategies when they clearly are not working.

RESOURCES REQUIRED FOR CONSULTATION

All service provision requires resources. Consultation is no exception. Without the proper resources, consultation cannot be effective. Thus, to some extent, a discussion of the required resources also describes some of the limitations of consultation.

The success of consultation centers on the ability to build a partnership and on the partners' skills, commitment, and time. Because consultation requires a relationship of equals, the skills needed to build and maintain it are particularly important. Each participant must respect the other's skills and knowledge and openly demonstrate that respect. Participants must communicate regularly, and the

therapist must listen actively to the problems the client is experiencing (DeBoer, 1995). The partners must believe that between them they have the skills and commitment to solve the problem. Both participants must feel comfortable with their own skills and professional identities; they must feel free to admit when they do not know an answer (Niehues et al., 1991). Each must be willing to take risks and to credit the other for the contributions toward improving the student's performance (Case-Smith, 1997). In addition, the consultant must be willing to ask for and obtain administrative support.

If, as happens on rare occasions, it is impossible to form a partnership, then consultation cannot be effective and should not be implemented. However, we believe that this rarely occurs. Good consultation is designed to resolve problems that the client, not the consultant, is facing. Consultants may need to invest considerable time and energy to establish and maintain consultative partnerships, but usually it can be done.

SUMMARY AND CONCLUSIONS

In consultation, we offer others (e.g., parents, teachers) access to sensory integration (or another) theory as a way of understanding students' behaviors. After students' behaviors have been "reframed," consultants can assist parents, teachers, or older students to develop new strategies for solving their own problems.

The expected outcome of consultation is that the human and nonhuman environment changes such that it more closely reflects students' needs. In other words, consultation enables students to succeed in the environment *despite* their limitations.

Students with sensory integrative dysfunction confront many difficulties in daily school life. Furthermore, their actions may be confusing to parents and teachers, who may find it difficult to assume their own roles effectively with the student. The combined difficulties of students and professionals seeking to instruct and interact with them often lead to students' referral to occupational therapy. Thus, sensory integration theory is an important tool used by occupational therapists working in schools.

Sensory integration theory lends itself to many types of service delivery. The service delivery selected for each student depends on that student's needs. Direct intervention is most effective for establishing new patterns of performance, including skill acquisition. Monitoring is most effective for teaching professionals and parents skills typically performed by a therapist and for programs established by the therapist that require frequent repetition. Consultation, on the other hand, enables other professionals and parents to reframe students' actions and develop more effective strategies for teaching and parenting. Because students spend the majority of the day with parents and teachers, we have argued that consultation should be the primary type of service delivery in schools. Except under very extraordinary circumstances, all students who qualify for occupational therapy services should receive consultation. When necessary, direct intervention or monitoring may be provided above and beyond the consultation. Although consultation can be extremely powerful, it is also very complicated. Consultation is composed of a number of stages, the most important of which involve establishing an egalitarian relationship.

References

American Occupational Therapy Association (1989). *Guidelines for occupational therapy services in school systems* (Ed. 2). Rockville, MD: Author.

Ayres, A. J. (1972). *Southern California Sensory Integration Tests*. Los Angeles: Western Psychological Services.

Bruininks, R. H. (1978). *Bruininks-Oseretsky Test of Motor Proficiency manual*. Circle Pines, MN: American Guidance Services

Bundy, A. C. (1995). Assessment and intervention in school-based practice: Answering questions and minimizing discrepancies. In I. R. McEwen (Ed.), *Occupational and physical therapy in educational environments*. New York: Haworth.

Bundy, A. C., Lawlor, M. C., Kielhofner, G., & Knecht, H. (April 1989). Educational and therapeutic perceptions of school system practice. Paper presented at the Annual Conference of the American Occupational Therapy Association, Baltimore, MD.

Case-Smith, J. (1997). Variables related to successful school-based practice. *Occupational Therapy Journal of Research, 17,* 133–153.

DeBoer, A. L. (1995). *Working together: The art of consulting*. Longmont, CO: Sopris.

Dunn, W. (1992). Occupational therapy collaborative consultation in schools. In E. G. Jaffe & C. F. Epstein (Eds.), *Occupational therapy consultation: Theory, principles, and practice* (pp. 210–236). St. Louis: Mosby.

Dunn, W. (1990). A comparison of service provision models in school-based occupational therapy services: A pilot study. *Occupational Therapy Journal of Research, 10,* 300–320.

Giangreco, M. (1986). Effects of integrated therapy: A pilot study. *Journal of the Association for Persons with Severe Handicaps, 6,* 15–21.

Hanft, B. E., & Place, P.A. (1996). *The consulting therapist: A guide for OTs and PTs in schools*. San Antonio: Therapy Skill Builders.

Individuals with Disabilities Education Act Amendments of 1997, 40 U.S.C. § 1400 *et seq.*

Jaffe, E. G., & Epstein, C. F. (1992). *Occupational therapy consultation: Theory, principles, and practice*. St. Louis: Mosby.

Mattingly, C. F., & Fleming, M. H. (1994). Clinical reasoning: Forms of inquiry in a therapeutic practice. Philadelphia: F. A. Davis.

Miller, T., & Sabatino, D. (1978). An evaluation of the teacher consultation model as an approach to mainstreaming. *Exceptional Children, 45,* 86–91.

Niehues, A. N., Bundy, A. C., Mattingly, C. F., & Lawlor, M. C. (1991). Making a difference: Occupational therapy in public schools. *Occupational Therapy Journal of Research, 11,* 195–209.

Rourk, J. D. (1992). The occupational therapist as a state education agency consultant. In E. G. Jaffe & C. F. Epstein (Eds.), *Occupational therapy consultation: Theory, principles, and practice* (pp. 195–209). St. Louis: Mosby.

Schein, E. H. (1999). *Process consultation revisited: Building a helping relationship*. Menlo Park, CA: Addison-Wesley.

Schön, D. (1983). *The reflective practitioner: How professionals think in action*. New York: Basic Books.

Schön, D. (1987). *Educating the reflective practitioner*. San Francisco: Jossey-Bass.

Schulte, A., Osborne, S., & McKinney, J. (1990). Academic outcomes for students with learning disabilities in consultation and resource programs. *Exceptional Children, 57,* 162–172.

Spencer, K. C. (1992). Transition program planning in the public education system. In E. G. Jaffe & C. F. Epstein (Eds.), *Occupational therapy consultation: Theory, principles, and practice* (pp. 244–251). St. Louis: Mosby.

Weiss, D. (1992). Program development consultation for the classroom. In E. G. Jaffe & C. F. Epstein (Eds.), *Occupational therapy consultation: Theory, principles, and practice* (pp. 237–243). St. Louis: Mosby.

Wilbarger, P. & Wilbarger, J. (1991). *Sensory defensiveness in children aged 2–12: An intervention guide for parents and other caretakers*. Denver, CO: Avanti Educational Programs.

Appendix 13-A

Part I: Strategies and Activities for Addressing Common School Problems

*Ideas created by occupational therapy students,
Colorado State University, Fall, 1995, and by participants in
Sensory Integration Theory and School Consultation,
sponsored by Sensory Integration International, 1996;
compiled by Carol Kurtzweil, OTR; edited by Anita Bundy, ScD, OTR*

The following pages contain a number of activities and strategies to address school problems commonly experienced by children with sensory integrative (and other types of) dysfunction. These activities by no means represent an exhaustive list. In each case, a problem is listed along with its possible relationship (if any) to sensory integration theory. Of course, all the difficulties that children with sensory integrative dysfunction experience are not caused by the sensory integration dysfunction.

For all problems, one or more "direct" strategies are provided. With these strategies, we approach the problem in the most direct manner. You will note that these strategies are not usually drawn from sensory integration theory.

In cases in which a problem does have a logical sensory integrative basis, additional categories of activities and strategies are suggested; these activities either provide a particular type of enhanced sensory input or require a particular type of response. Activities related to sensory integration theory are found in Part II: Selected Activities to Address Underlying Aspects of Sensory Integrative Dysfunction.

The problems addressed in Part I have been grouped together into categories. The categories, in the order in which they appear, are as follows:

I.   Clothing
II.   Writing
III.   Art and Construction
IV.   Lunches and Snacks
V.   Homework
VI.   Distractibility
VII.   Social Behavior
VIII. Lockers and Desks
IX.   Posture
X.   Miscellaneous

	Problem	Possible Cause (Relation to Sensory Integration Theory)	Possible Strategies
I. CLOTHING	Child cannot manage fasteners on clothing.	Poor fine motor coordination, possibly secondary to poor tactile or proprioceptive discrimination.	Clothing with elastic waist bands: Velcro fasteners.
II. WRITING	Child has a "death grip" on pencil.	Poor proprioception resulting in poor modulation of force.	Have child use any of a variety of pencil grips. Wrap the pencil or pen in stiff clay and instruct the child that, if the clay is misshapen, the child is gripping too hard.

continued

Problem	Possible Cause (Relation to Sensory Integration Theory)	Possible Strategies
Child erases hard and puts holes in paper.	Poor proprioception resulting in modulation of force.	Provide several animal erasers and tell child that the animal likes to eat only pencil marks and that paper makes him sick. Have child use soft (gum) erasers. Do not allow the student to use eraser; draw single line through error and turn the mistake into part of the assignment.
Child erases hard and puts holes in paper.	Poor posture encourages child to slump over desk and work in excessive flexion; poor posture, by itself, is unlikely to result in a child's using too much force; however, poor perception of muscle proprioception and vestibular input are often seen together.	Tilt the writing table to improve positioning; prevents child from working in a lot of flexion, thus decreasing chances he or she will use too much force.
Child uses so little pressure on pen that writing is almost illegible.	Poor proprioception resulting in poor modulation of force.	Have child use carbon paper underneath and encourage pressing through all layers. Have child use pencil with soft lead or felt tip marker.
Child can't copy accurately from blackboard.	Poor oculomotor control; child has particular difficulty switching planes (vertical to horizontal) when copying.	Have child copy assignment from a book or paper at his or her desk instead of from the blackboard. Provide slant-top surface; this decreases the angle of change with which the child must cope.
Child can't keep columns lined on arithmetic papers, so he or she always gets the wrong answer.	This problem may have many causes, including decreased organization skills or poor oculomotor control. The relationship to sensory integration theory is not always clear.	Provide child with grid or graph paper in which only one digit is allowed per space. Teacher could line up the math problems for child. Use a black marker to divide the student's numbers into columns for better tracking.
Child has difficulty forming letters or shapes.	Decreased awareness of what letters look like or poor form and space skills; form and space are endproducts of sensory integration; however, sensory integration dysfunction is only one reason why a child might have difficulties with letter formation or form and space.	Place a piece of clear plexiglass in a stand; an adult sitting behind the plexiglass can draw letters (backwards), which the child traces on his or her side; when the child is finished, the adult can erase the lines, leaving only the child's work. A Magnadoodle can be used in a similar way; after the child traces the outline, the adult's marking can be erased.
Child runs out of space on paper; seems not to recognize boundaries of paper.	Decreased visuomotor skill secondary to poor processing of proprioceptive information.	Use paper with raised lines (often available for partially sighted children).

continued

	Problem	Possible Cause (Relation to Sensory Integration Theory)	Possible Strategies
III. ART AND CONSTRUCTION	Child refuses to use paste because he or she can't stand the feel of it drying on his or her skin.	Tactile defensiveness.	Have child use glue stick, glue in a squeeze bottle, rubber cement, stapler, or Scotch tape instead of paste. Use Popsicle stick instead of fingers to spread paste. Give child wet paper towel to wipe fingers off right away. If the task is to glue correct answer to paper, use another method of demonstrating knowledge (e.g., writing the correct answer).
	Child cannot cut with regular scissors.	Poor fine motor coordination, possibly secondary to poor tactile or proprioceptive discrimination.	Have child use alternative types of scissors (e.g., Fiskar soft touch scissors that evenly distribute pressure across the fingers and palm, loop scissors, self-opening scissors adapted to open only to midrange). Have child cut thick paper (e.g., file folder weight) which gives a bit more resistance and is easier to cut.
	Child cannot cut with regular scissors.	Poor bilateral integration.	Fasten loop scissors to a scissors to a small board and fasten that to the top of the child's desk; child can cut by pushing down with one hand and then turning and moving the paper with the other; this significantly reduces the bilateral demand.
IV. LUNCHES AND SNACKS	Child cannot open milk carton.	Decreased bilateral coordination.	Allow child to stabilize the carton by setting it in a drawer and leaning gently against it while opening carton; this alleviates the problem with stabilizing.
	Child cannot open milk carton.	Poor proprioception resulting in poor modulation of force (may be coupled with above bilateral coordination).	Instruct child on ways of breaking the seal such as using a fork. Provide milk or juice cartons that come with perforated openings for straws. To draw attention away from children who cannot open cartons, provide special paper cups for all children; every day, opening cartons can be the job of a couple of children who are good at it. Create an atmosphere in which asking for and giving help are the norm.
	Child is distracted in the lunchroom and eats only a small part of his or her food and then gets hungry half way through the afternoon.	When distractibility is associated with increased sensory input, it may be a result of sensory defensiveness.	Child brings a couple of wrapped snacks (e.g. granola bars) for afternoon; he or she might place them in a fanny pack so they are nearby. Child and a few of her friends could sit at a "special" table

continued

Problem	Possible Cause (Relation to Sensory Integration Theory)	Possible Strategies
		in a quieter area in or outside of lunchroom.
		Be sure parents know child is not always eating lunch; perhaps trying to include many favorite foods at lunch would decrease the problem, or they may have some other solutions.
V. HOMEWORK Child cannot do homework because he or she forgets to take needed books home at night.	Many children, including children with sensory integrative dysfunction, fail to remember things; although there are many causes for this problem, none is DIRECTLY related to any aspect of sensory integration theory.	Laminate individual pictures of textbooks and create magnets or other manipulables; during the day as an assignment is received, child can attach the relevant book icon to his or her backpack or side of desk; at the end of the day, magnets remind the child which books to take home.
		Similarly, a blank piece of paper can be taped to desk; during the day as each assignment is received, child writes down the needed books; at the end of each period, the student takes needed books directly to the backpack.
		Student keeps a second full set of books at home.
		Each afternoon before child leaves the classroom, he or she must show his teacher that he has his books in the backpack.
		Teacher or designated student creates an ongoing assignment list on the chalkboard.
Child cannot remember homework assignments.	Although many children with sensory integrative dysfunction fail to remember assignments, this is not clearly related to any particular aspect of sensory integration theory.	Child will write homework assignments down in a homework notebook as they are given; teacher will check it at the end of the day.
		Send a list of weekly homework assignments home to the parents.
		Assign "homework pals"; pair up children to remind each other of homework and have them exchange phone numbers to assist each other after school hours.
		Teacher writes all homework assignments on chalkboard as they are given; at the end of each day, teacher routinely asks, "Who can tell me what your homework assignments are for tonight?" to reinforce for all children what is due the next day.
		Consequences for forgetting

continued

Problem	Possible Cause (Relation to Sensory Integration Theory)	Possible Strategies
		homework for the entire class (e.g., each child who fails to turn in homework has to get up in front of class and sing a solo of their choice).
Child forgets to take notices and report cards home from school, so parents don't know when events are happening.	Again, although many children with sensory integrative dysfunction fail to remember, this problem has not been associated with any aspect of sensory integration theory.	All children have a special folder that they must take home every day; as notices are distributed, the teacher reminds children to place them in the folder; the teacher can spot check folders.
		Safety pin notes, report card to children's jacket or shirt.
		Have all of the children in the class put reminders and reports in their backpacks as they are handed out.
		Child could have a special pocket sewn on backpack and notices would be placed there; parents would be instructed to check this pocket.
VI. DISTRACTIBILITY		
Child follows instructions given to every child in the classroom because he or she is unable to screen out stimuli.	Distractibility secondary to sensory defensiveness (of course, there are many other causes of distractibility).	Have child sit in the least distracting area of the classroom, probably in a back corner.
		Provide child with written directions as well as verbal; make him or her responsible for checking instructions himself.
		Provide an area in the classroom, such as a loft or quiet space (e.g., refrigerator box lined with carpet) where children can go when they feel they need a quiet place to work.
		Some children find that wearing headsets helps cut down the amount of auditory stimulation coming in; also, some children find the weight of the headset to be calming.
Child wanders around and disrupts classmates when he or she gets overstimulated or tired.	Distractibility secondary to sensory defensiveness (of course, there are many other causes of distractibility).	Reduce amount of stimuli.
		Place child's desk in the part of the class where there is the least noise and activity, usually a back corner.
		Help child to organize his workspace so he does not have to expend a lot of energy finding things.
		Decrease bright lights, clutter, and provide a "cove" for child's desk or a quiet space where the child can go to regroup.
Child wanders around and disrupts classmates when he	Some children who have motor planning problems	Build in many opportunities for child to get up and

continued

Problem	Possible Cause (Relation to Sensory Integration Theory)	Possible Strategies
	or she gets overstimulated or tired.	fatigue easily with the motor demands of school; they may also wander aimlessly when tired.	move around during the day. Have the child help out with "chores" around the classroom; if these provide increased proprioception through resistance to movement, all the better (e.g., banging erasers, washing the blackboard, carrying books to the office). Provide the child with clay or "fidget toys" to use at desk; this will give the child something to do but help keep him or her from disrupting others.
VII. SOCIAL BEHAVIOR	Child pushes other children who come too close to his or her desk.	Fight-or-flight reaction secondary to sensory defensiveness.	Put child's desk in the area of the classroom where there is the least amount of activity (usually a back corner) and provide a quiet space in the classroom where all children can go when they need to be alone (e.g., refrigerator box, loft). See description of desktop box in discussion of child who has a tactile defensive reaction to paste. At the appropriate time, discuss the problem with the child; help the child understand that he or she reacts differently than other kids to touch and noise; ask for the child's ideas and solutions and give alternative explanations for the other children's behavior (e.g., "Other children often come very close to you because they are your friends and feel comfortable with you."). Help the child develop strategies for acceptable replacement behaviors to be used when he or she wants to hit (e.g., pull on a bungee cord attached to a belt loop or the desk). Teach the whole class about the importance of respecting others' personal space and individual differences about comfort level in being close to others.
	Child gets too close to other children when he or she is playing and during circle time.	This problem, which sometimes seems related to knowledge of the boundaries of the body, is not usually seen in children with sensory integrative dysfunction; however, it is a complicated	Because the problem seems related to a lack of internal sense of boundaries, provide the child with external guides to help him or her stay out of others' personal space.

continued

Problem	Possible Cause (Relation to Sensory Integration Theory)	Possible Strategies
	problem and not clearly associated with any aspect of sensory integration theory.	During circle time, allow the child to choose a stuffed animal that he or she is responsible for; the animal requires being held firmly throughout the circle time activity. Begin circle time by explaining that everyone needs to be at arm's length away from each other; after the correct distance is established, provide carpet squares or hula hoops for children to sit on or in; the hook side of Velcro can also be used to form a stationary, but readily removed, square. During playtime, engage the child in games that promote being in contact with other classmates such as steamroller; point out that this game is intended for being close but that most other games are not.
Child needs help to be able to enter groups of children with whom he or she wants to play.	This problem is very common among children, including those with sensory integrative dysfunction; however, it is not associated with any particular aspect of sensory integration theory.	Teach child the strategy of finding something very enticing with which to play that will draw other children to help him or her identify a role for him- or herself in the game and then just assume it without asking permission; the latter is the single most effective strategy for entering a group successfully; the least effective strategies are asking to join and being disruptive.
VIII. LOCKERS AND DESKS Child's locker or cubby is so disorganized that he or she cannot find anything.	Disorganization is common to many children, including those with sensory integrative dysfunction; however, it is not clearly associated with any particular aspect of sensory integration theory.	Color code all supplies to match color coding placed in locker or cubby. Match the color of child's folders with the color of the child's book cover so that they know what to bring to each class. Provide time in the class in which all students clean their cubbies so child does not feel singled out.
Child's desk is so disorganized that he or she cannot find anything.	Disorganization is common to many children, including those with sensory integrative dysfunction; however, it is not clearly associated with any particular aspect of sensory integration theory.	Line the child's desk with butcher paper; outline and label the places where the folders, pens, books, and so on should go. Attach small boxes to the desk floor for various objects. Give the child a colored folder for each subject; require that the child take

continued

Problem	Possible Cause (Relation to Sensory Integration Theory)	Possible Strategies
		time after a subject is completed to put supplies away before the next subject is started.
		If the child feels rushed and then stuffs things into the desk, give the child a timer to set or give verbal reminders so he or she can anticipate when an activity will end and can put thins away properly
IX. POSTURE Child slouches in seat or falls out of seat.	Decreased postural control secondary to poor processing of vestibular-proprioceptive information; this problem is often accompanied by poor ability to cross the midline while doing desk work; child moves nearer to the edge of the chair and is at risk for falling, especially if he or she does not have a good sense of the vertical.	Allow the child or class to lie or sit on the floor during some activities; wedges, pillows, and beanbag chairs can make this more appealing. Slanting the table surface makes it easier for the child to maintain good posture and may decrease incidences of falling. Some therapists have been successful having children sit on t-stools; they believe that the children must pay closer attention to their posture and, therefore, remain more erect. Make sure the child's feet touch the floor; if they do not, a footrest slanted toward the child may help. Apply a nonslip surface to seat of the chair (e.g., Dycem, bathtub decals).
X. MISCELLANEOUS Student misses recess because he or she can't complete assignments on time; the child really needs recess to "let off steam."	There are many reasons why a child may fail to finish work on time; two that are related to sensory integration theory are distractibility secondary to sensory defensiveness (which makes it difficult to focus) and poor motor planning (which makes it difficult to get large quantities of work done); in either case, periodic opportunities to be active can help the child get more done.	Provide as many opportunities as possible for active work during the day; for example, instead of sitting at desk while doing math, have child do math problems on the board. For a child who is distractible, reduce the number of distractions; see above strategies for child who follows directions meant for others and who wanders and disrupts classmates. If the problem is with the quantity of work, see if the teacher would consider shortening in-class assignments; for example, how many problems does the child have to do correctly to demonstrate that he or she has mastered the concept of adding two-place numbers? Break assignments into two parts and allow child to work on them in smaller segments.

continued

Problem	Possible Cause (Relation to Sensory Integration Theory)	Possible Strategies
Child chews collars of clothing or hair when stressed, which is frequently; he or she is ruining clothes and smells bad much of the time.	Stress is not unusual among children who have sensory integrative dysfunction, but it is not associated with any aspect of sensory integration theory.	Teach stress reduction strategies to the whole class (e.g., pet a stuffed animal, listen to rain on a personal stereo, find a safe space to regroup). Provide replacements for hair or clothing (e.g., a length of knotted tubing, and object at the end of pencil, sugar-free gum); some children seem to thrive on oral stimulation; rather than (or in addition to) chewing, they might enjoy blowing on whistles (with the noise maker removed) or blowing into dental dam stretched tight across the face to produce a "raspberry" noise.
Student gets lost going from the classroom to other destinations in school.	A poor sense of real space is common to many children, some of whom have sensory integrative dysfunction; however, this problem has not been clearly tied to any aspect of sensory integration theory.	Have the child take a buddy with him or her. Create colored lines along the walls going to common destinations (e.g., office, bathroom, lunchroom).

Part II: Selected Activities to Address Underlying Aspects of Sensory Integrative Dysfunction

NOTE: The activities listed below are different from those in Part I in that they are meant to address aspects of the underlying problem which prevents a child from accomplishing certain school tasks. This is by no means an exhaustive list of activities. Be aware that the more the activity clearly seems related to a particular school problem, the more likely a teacher is to incorporate it into the day's routine.

ACTIVITIES THAT PROVIDE ENHANCED PROPRIOCEPTION

- Use vibrating pen that changes oscillations as pressure on pen changes.
- Do graphite or crayon "rubbings" of three-dimensional objects (e.g., leaves).

- Use media that encourage the child to pull and work hands and fingers such as putty, play dough, clay, or rubberbands.
- Use activities that encourage child to push, pull, or carry heavy loads such as stacking chairs, carrying books to the office, or collecting all the blocks on the floor into a large box.
- Allow child to lie supine under small table and write against the underneath surface of the table. Some children even enjoy bracing their feet against the bottom of the table surface. Of course, that probably means someone will have to sit on the table to keep it from going up in the air.
- Provide child with balloon filled with flour or gel to fidget with as he listens. Hearthsong of California (1-800-325-2502) makes stress balls shaped like animals for squeezing.

ACTIVITIES THAT PROVIDE ENHANCED TACTILE SENSATION (especially deep pressure)

- Fill tub with beans or rice and child will search for familiar object by touch.
- Fasten textured substance (e.g., carpet square or object such as a surgical brush) on top of or underneath desk surface. Encourage child to rub hands briskly across it before engaging in activity.
- Techniques such as wrapping child tightly in a blanket and also rocking or sitting on teacher's lap during story time (as tolerated) can provide deep pressure under certain circumstances.

ACTIVITIES THAT PROVIDE ENHANCED VESTIBULAR SENSATION

- Use movement activities, especially activities that involve swinging or jumping, and many playground activities.
- Encourage child to rock in rocking chair before a new activity is started or during the activity.
- Some children work well sitting on a gymnastic ball or other surface on which they can bounce and move around. Stabilize the ball in a cardboard box or small square wooden frame.

ACTIVITIES THAT REQUIRE MODULATION OF FORCE

- Use the Hungry-Hippo game. Requires correct amount of pressure to shoot objects into correct spot.
- Pick up small objects with tweezers. For example, collect pretend "poisonous" insects. This requires deft prehension and modulation of force.
- Play the Operation game; this requires proper pressure on the tweezers to get object in correctly.
- Do the egg, water balloon, or shaving cream ball toss. Catching, especially, requires modulation of force so as not to break object.

SUGGESTIONS FOR TACTILE DEFENSIVENESS

- Do activities that provide light, unexpected, or noxious touch when a child is relatively calm.
- Provide a quiet place for the child to engage in tactile activities.
- Create loft areas or refrigerator boxes placed in a corner of the room where any child can go when he or she feels a need to be in a quiet place.
- Have a child prepare for an activity by having a little quiet time.
- Provide a child with a box to sit on his or her desk into which he or she can insert his or her head. The box is painted a dark color on the inside and the outside and has a curtain across the open side. Glow-in-the-dark stars can be attached to the inside walls of the box. The child uses a flashlight to illuminate the stars and is then allowed to stay in the box until the stars stop glowing.
- Any activity that provides deep pressure input may be useful before engaging in an activity that may "aggravate" a child's tactile defensiveness.

14

Alternative and Complementary Programs for Intervention

Complement: Something that completes or makes perfect.
—*Random House Webster's College Dictionary (Ed. 2)*

We invited several occupational therapists who are well known for their contributions to professional development and the creation or implementation of innovative alternative and complementary programs to contribute to this chapter. Giving voice and venue to these professionals offers readers an opportunity to evaluate some of the alternative and complementary programs that hold a relationship to sensory integration theory. All are in need of empirical research.

Included in this chapter are programs that form a subset or expansion of sensory integration principles, others that fall outside the constructs that underlie sensory integration, and still others that have features of sensory integrative intervention along with features that fall outside the realm of sensory integration. We defined intervention based on the principles of sensory integration as containing both:

- Opportunities for *enhanced* sensation
- Active involvement in meaningful activity

that demands an adaptive response from the client

Programs represent a *subset* of intervention based on the principles of sensory integration when they illustrate techniques or principles for intervening with a type of dysfunction that has traditionally been described in sensory integration theory (e.g., poor sensory modulation). Programs represent an *expansion* of intervention based on the principles of sensory integration when they illustrate techniques for intervening with a difficulty typically experienced by individuals with sensory integrative dysfunction but not previously described explicitly (e.g., improving oculomotor control). Programs fall *outside* the construct of sensory integration when they do not involve enhanced sensation, active participation, *and* meaningful activity or when goals commonly addressed do not reflect areas of need typical of individuals with sensory integrative dysfunction (e.g., decreasing spasticity). Finally, programs *overlap* with intervention based on the principles of sensory integration when some aspects fall *within* the construct of sensory integration but other aspects are outside of it.

This chapter does not provide an exhaustive review of alternative and complementary interventions available to clients; readers should explore additional interventions on their own. Furthermore, although not all the programs described fall within the construct of sensory integration, all may be beneficial to certain individuals with sensory integrative dysfunction.

Occupational therapy is about occupation. We have embraced a definition of occupation that includes the tasks clients need or want to do and the roles they assume in daily life. Intervention programs are *directly* related to occupation when they involve daily life tasks and roles. Programs are *indirectly* related to occupation when their primary emphasis is on improving performance components (e.g., strength, range of motion [ROM]) that may enable clients to more easily perform tasks and assume roles in their daily lives.

Occupation is a much larger construct than sensory integration. In fact, sensory integration is, itself, a performance component. When intervention is aimed at improving performance components, we must make certain that the client is able to use newfound skills and abilities in daily life.

We asked contributors to this chapter to describe their programs and to indicate:

- The population for which the program was intended
- The rationale for its development
- Its relationship to sensory integration theory and occupation
- Training recommended or required to implement the program
- Recommended readings

In some cases, the rationale provided or terminology used by the authors is in contrast with information or terminology used elsewhere in this book. We have attempted to preserve the authors' terminology. Readers are asked to weigh conflicting information carefully, evaluating what is most useful for particular clients. Sensory integration represents a *theory;* the theory will grow only as a result of discussion among knowledgeable clinicians and theorists. Certainly, Ayres would have wanted her theory to grow.

The Wilbarger Approach to Treating Sensory Defensiveness

Julia Wilbarger, MA, MS, OTR

Patricia Wilbarger, MEd, OTR, FAOTA

BACKGROUND

Sensory defensiveness is a constellation of symptoms that involve avoidance reactions to sensation from any sensory modality (Wilbarger & Wilbarger, 1991). Sensory defensiveness can constrain adaptability and performance in all areas of function. In fact, Wilbarger has argued that sensory defensiveness is so disruptive to an individual's life that it should be a primary concern in intervention (Wilbarger & Wilbarger, 1991).

The Wilbarger approach to treating sensory defensiveness involves a comprehensive, intensive, and individualized program (Wilbarger & Wilbarger, 1991). It is based on the belief that certain sensory experiences repeated frequently over a short period of time can effectively reduce sensory defensive symptoms. Wilbarger was strongly influenced by Ayres (1972, 1979), but this intervention strategy has also evolved over the past four decades guided by the study of functional neurology, collaboration with colleagues, and experience in clinical practice.

RATIONALE

Many of the symptoms of sensory defensiveness suggest a disruption in a central nervous system (CNS) process that evaluates incoming stimuli for positive or negative valence (LeDoux, 1996; Pri-

bram, 1991). This process has been referred to by a number of names such as the "protocritic system" or "low route" processing. In general, it is responsible for the rapid, automatic, and subconscious evaluation of the affective qualities of stimuli. This evaluative process also affects and is affected by CNS structures related to emotions, memory, autonomic arousal, and adaptation to stress. As a result, sensory defensive responses lead to changes in arousal, affective tone, and stress.

Certain types of sensory experiences are thought to be effective for reducing sensory defensive responses (Ayres, 1972, 1979; Wilbarger & Wilbarger, 1991). These include deep pressure, proprioception (i.e., muscle resistance, joint traction, and compression), and vestibular input (Ayres, 1972, 1979). These types of sensation are believed to influence the adaptation to and modulation of environmental sensory input along with the resultant physiologic responses (Fields, 1998; Ornstien & Sobel, 1987; Pribram, 1991). Presumably, the ultimate effectiveness is caused by the global integrative effects these inputs have on the CNS.

Current research has pointed to the power of somatosensory input for improving health and reducing stress and pain (Fields, 1998; Melzack, 1995). Repeated application of sensory input is believed to facilitate homeostasis and regulation of behavior in much the same way that intense subpainful somatosensory-based interventions (e.g., transcutaneous electrical nerve stimulation [TENS] and acupuncture) reduce chronic pain (Melzack, 1995). Long-term adaptation takes place at the biochemical, cellular, and behavioral levels (Fields, 1998, Pert, 1997; Wall & Melzack, 1995).

DESCRIPTION

Patients with sensory defensiveness are difficult to treat. The Wilbarger approach to treating sensory defensiveness involves a specific, individualized intervention program. The approach incorporates three essential components:

1. Education of the client and caregivers to promote awareness of the presence and impact of symptoms of sensory defensiveness
2. A sensory diet that incorporates sensory-based activities into daily routines
3. A professionally guided program that may involve the application of deep pressure and proprioception

The latter is sometimes called the Wilbarger protocol. (This procedure also has been referred to as "brushing," but this term does not accurately convey the intent of the technique and is misleading.)

Although the scope of this section does not allow for a complete description of this program, we will highlight the essential benefits and procedures associated with each of the three components.

EDUCATION AND THE PROMOTION OF AWARENESS

Education can provide an explanation for and awareness of previously incomprehensible reactions and feelings. It allows clients and their caregivers to reinterpret sensory defensive behaviors and recognize how they disrupt an individual's life. This awareness is, by itself, therapeutic. Both knowledge and awareness come from conducting a detailed assessment consisting primarily of a structured clinical interview about responses to sensation in daily life and individual coping styles. The assessment should result in a relatively comprehensive, prioritized list of behaviors related to sensory defensiveness. The "problem list" is the basis for intervention planning, monitoring, and assessment of outcomes.

SENSORY DIET

A sensory diet is a treatment plan that involves the therapeutic use of sensation in the context of daily activities (Wilbarger, 1993) and is used to treat sensory defensiveness in two different ways. First, activities with sensory qualities most likely to reduce defensive behaviors are identified and implemented in the course of daily life routines. Sensory-based activities provided at regular intervals are the cornerstone of the sensory diet. The activities are chosen to emphasize sensory inputs such as deep pressure, proprioception, and movement (Ayres, 1972, 1979; Wilbarger & Wilbarger, 1991). Other types of activities (e.g., oral and respiratory) also can be used, particularly for gaining and maintaining regulation of arousal states (Oetter et al., 1995; Williams & Shellenberger, 1994). One must keep in mind the power of a particular activity to produce adaptation and how long it may be expected to influence behavior. Activities can be brief and provide a specific type of sensory input or adaptation can be achieved by engaging in play, leisure, or work activities.

Second, the sensory diet includes adaptations to the environment to promote optimum functioning and reduce disruption. For instance, adaptations frequently are made to daily routines (e.g., dressing, bathing, and transitions) to reduce the distress and the discomfort that often accompany them. Suggestions may include preparatory sensory activities or simply altering the way in which routines are done. In addition, caregivers are informed about ways to reduce some sources of sensation in the environment (e.g., sounds, smells, visual distraction) and ways to develop consistent routines and predictability. These suggestions must be customized to match the challenges unique to each individual.

PROFESSIONALLY GUIDED INTERVENTION

Professionally guided intervention involves assessment, development of goals and objectives, and formation of an intervention plan in collaboration with clients and their caregivers. Furthermore, the program requires frequent (sometimes daily) evaluation of effectiveness. Modification and continuation of the plan are informed by the changing needs of the client. There is no specific time frame for the duration of intervention.

The professionally guided intervention program may include the therapeutic use of deep pressure and proprioception. This protocol should be considered an adjunct to direct intervention and never used in isolation. It involves the use of a specific densely bristled brush which, when used correctly, can deliver deep pressure without friction, tickle, or scratch. The authors recommend only one brush for this program. It is manufactured by Clipper Mills (San Francisco, CA) specifically for this purpose and is available through multiple vendors of sensory integration materials and equipment.

Deep pressure is applied to the hands, arms, back, legs, and feet. The tactile input is never applied to the stomach, groin, buttocks, head, or face. Deep pressure is always followed by compression or approximation of a number of joints in the trunk, arms, and legs. The provision of deep pressure and proprioception seems deceptively simple. However, the procedure cannot be conveyed adequately in written form. The authors' experience with training professionals and caregivers in this technique has revealed many misinterpretations of its application, particularly in the amount of pressure needed. Anyone executing the deep pressure and proprioceptive procedure described by Wilbarger should have specialized training or direct supervision from someone with such training.

This procedure must be repeated frequently. Ideally, deep pressure and joint compression are administered every 90 minutes to 2 hours. However, frequency and timing depend on the daily routines and unique needs of the client. Clinical experience has shown that lack of appropriate pressure or less frequent application not only reduces efficacy but may be detrimental. The duration and modification of the treatment plan is based on the client's progress.

Other intervention procedures may include techniques for reducing oral defensiveness, postural problems, or disruptions in the suck-swallow-breathe synchrony. Referrals to other professionals, such as a psychologist, may be necessary to address social and emotional issues related to sensory defensiveness.

Individuals with sensory defensiveness exhibit unique behaviors that complicate the use of sensory-based intervention. Because of sensory defensiveness, these individuals often avoid sensory experiences in general and novel activities in particular. Involving a client in a novel sensory experience

(such as the Wilbarger protocol) requires skill and good clinical reasoning. One must approach a client with sensory defensiveness positively and create as little anticipatory anxiety as possible. Care must be taken to use the procedures correctly and appropriately.

RELATIONSHIP TO SENSORY INTEGRATION AND OCCUPATION

The treatment of patients with sensory defensiveness draws on principles of both sensory integration theory and occupational therapy. It capitalizes on the use of enhanced sensation in order to achieve better adaptation to sensory experiences. The concept behind a sensory diet reflects the use of enhanced sensory experience in self-selected or preferred activities in the context of daily routines. Thus, the sensory diet can be considered to represent a *subset* of activities that reflect the principles of sensory integration theory. Programs such as the Wilbarger approach are directed toward helping the client achieve internal adaptation, which eventually results in overall improved overt adaptive responses and thus improved occupational and role performance.

POPULATIONS FOR WHICH THE WILBARGER APPROACH IS APPROPRIATE

The Wilbarger approach was developed specifically to address sensory defensiveness. In most cases, it is not appropriate for use with individuals who have other behavioral or health problems. The deep pressure and joint compression techniques should not be used on infants younger than age 2 months (when age has been corrected for prematurity) or with individuals with autonomic, physiologic, or CNS instability. Medical histories, psychological status, and appropriate individual precautions should be considered in all cases.

Intervention to reduce sensory defensiveness must always occur within the context of a more comprehensive intervention plan that considers all aspects of the individuals' life. Individuals with sensory defensiveness, without other significant problem areas, who are treated with the comprehensive application of all three components and consistently adhere to the program are likely to show the most improvement.

Clinical reports suggest the Wilbarger approach is remarkably successful at reducing sensory defensive responses in some people. Because there has been limited systematic research on the efficacy of this approach, the information presented here is based on the clinical experience of the authors and other clinicians using this approach. In general, expectations for effectiveness depend on the complexity of the individual's clinical picture, confounding problems, adequacy of the program, and faithful adherence to the program.

No one program will be effective with all people. Intervention must be appropriate to the client's age, level of disability, context, and available social support systems. Furthermore, intervention to reduce sensory defensiveness is not limited to the Wilbarger approach. Occupational therapists have been treating sensory defensiveness for decades using the principles of sensory integration theory (Ayres, 1972, 1979). When sensory defensiveness co-occurs with other disorders or complications, additional or alternative approaches should be considered.

TRAINING RECOMMENDED OR REQUIRED

Intervention for and management of sensory defensiveness require expertise gained by specific training through continuing education, mentoring, and advanced knowledge of sensory processing and sensory integrative theories. The deep pressure and joint compression techniques described here should not be used without direct training. The Wilbargers offer continuing education courses on intervention for sensory defensiveness using this approach. These are commonly advertised through occupational therapy newsletters and magazines. It is also recommended that therapists complete courses in sensory integration theory.

SUMMARY

The Wilbarger approach to the intervention of sensory defensiveness includes the development of specific, individualized intervention plans that include three components: awareness, a sensory diet, and professionally guided intervention. The appropriate application of deep pressure and proprioception as described by Wilbarger requires advanced training and knowledge. Solid clinical reasoning must be used to develop and modify intervention plans based on assessment data. Although we believe that this program can be applied to a wide range of individuals, therapists must use clinical judgment when working with their own clients. Although to date there has been little research on the effectiveness of this approach, when it is used appropriately, we believe the Wilbarger approach has promise to be beneficial in reducing sensory defensiveness in many people.

Clinical Application of the Sensory Diet

Julia Wilbarger, MA, MS, OTR

Patricia Wilbarger, MEd, OTR, FAOTA

BACKGROUND

A sensory diet is not a specific intervention technique; rather, it is a strategy for developing individualized home programs that are practical, carefully scheduled, and based on the concept that controlled sensory input can affect functional abilities. The unique feature of these home programs is the emphasis on systematic use of sensory-based activity to address developmental goals.

Patricia Wilbarger (1984) coined the term "sensory diet" to explain how certain sensory experiences can be used to enhance occupational performance in any individual as well as contribute to the remediation of developmental and sensory processing disruptions. She originally developed the sensory diet concept for use with families of infant graduates from neonatal intensive care units. The original concept has been expanded to encompass a wide range of persons, regardless of age or context, for the promotion of health and optimal functioning (Wilbarger, 1995).

RATIONALE

The sensory diet is based on the principle that individuals require a certain quality and quantity of sensory experiences to be skillful, adaptive, and organized in their daily lives (Wilbarger, 1995; Zuckerman, 1994). Sensory integration and sensory processing theories indicate the ways in which various *types* of sensation can be used for the promotion of adaptive functioning. The *timing, intensity,* and *duration* of sensory-based activities also are critical in promoting adaptation and optimal performance. Wilbarger (1995) uniquely

melded types, timing, and intensity of sensory input with daily life routines to form the sensory diet concept.

A large body of research (Kandel et al., 1991; Ornstien & Sobel, 1987) supports the idea that specific sensory experiences influence the function, structure, and neurochemistry of the brain. Repeated or sustained input has been shown to result in lasting changes in brain function (Field, 1995; Greenough et al., 1987; Greenough & Black, 1992; Morgan, 1997; Schanberg & Field, 1988).

Most people naturally choose activities and experiences to meet their individual needs and preferences. For example, Zuckerman (1994) has differentiated "high sensation seekers" from "low sensation seekers." These two different types of individuals have distinctly different activity patterns and preferences. However, some individuals lack the capacity or environmental support to attain the proper sensory diet without intervention.

A mismatch between an individual's needs and his or her sensory diet can have wide-ranging effects. For example, prolonged or severe deprivation can result in impaired cognitive, social, and emotional development (Cermak & Daunhauer, 1997; Goldberger, 1993). Conversely, exposure to selectively applied and enriched sensory input has been shown to have beneficial effects on development and health (Field, 1995, 1998). For example, Field and colleagues (Field, 1998; Schanberg & Field, 1988) demonstrated that premature infants receiving controlled tactile and kinesthetic stimulation gained weight faster, spent fewer days in the hospital, and had better developmental outcomes than matched controls.

Sensory processing theories described by Ayres,

Rood, and others influenced the development of the sensory diet. Ayres (1972, 1979) highlighted the important functions that somatosensory and vestibular processes serve in development, skill, states of alertness, and adaptation. Sensation can affect specific behavior such as motor skill, or more global adaptation such as changes in arousal states (Kandel et al., 1991; Wilbarger & Wilbarger, 1991). Rood (1962) described the importance of timing on the application of sensation. She conceptualized sensation as having "latency effects" (i.e., influencing the nervous system for a certain period of time). Activities or sensory experiences may need to be repeated frequently, particularly if a level of adaptation, or state, must be maintained over time. In other cases, such as the promotion of specific skills, enhanced sensation can be used as preparation (i.e., before) or support (i.e., during) a task.

The sensory diet involves the therapeutic use of sensation in the context of activities embedded within the daily routine. Preferably, the activities are self-selected, self-initiated, and self-organized (Wilbarger, 1995). Sensory integration theory suggests that sensory experiences are most effective when they are incorporated into self-selected, meaningful activity that demands an adaptive response (Ayres, 1972). In the context of meaningful activity, short-term changes in arousal, body awareness, or muscle activity may lead to more lasting adaptive capacities. This important principle has been confirmed through basic research on postnatal brain and behavioral development (Greenough & Black, 1992).

DESCRIPTION

When used therapeutically, a sensory diet is not a recipe. Rather, it is a carefully constructed activity plan designed to meet the individual needs of each client. The specific sensory diet varies according to an individual's goals, preferences, resources, and limitations.

Careful planning is the key to a successful sensory diet. To construct an effective sensory diet, the therapist must understand the nature of the client's sensorimotor or modulation difficulties and how they interfere with his or her daily life. Thus, the sensory diet is based on evaluation data. Sensory histories and structured interviews regarding daily events yield information about the sequence and sensory qualities of daily experiences and identify challenging tasks or times of day. Priorities and clear objectives emerge from the evaluation data.

Caregivers must understand how deficits in sensory integration disrupt a client's ability to function. Thus, an important part of the sensory diet is education about the principles of sensory integration and the sensory diet. Use of family- or client-centered principles enhances the effectiveness of intervention based on the sensory diet. Setting goals and selecting and scheduling activities is done in collaboration with the client, family, or both. Activities must be compatible with an individual's or family's beliefs and fit easily into their routines. The plan should contain only a few well-chosen activities and suggestions rather than a long list of ideas.

Activities are chosen because they are particularly effective for meeting specific goals. Because of the type and intensity of sensation used, some activities have a greater effect on behavior or skill development than others. Vestibular input, whole body muscle activity or resistance, and respiration are thought to be particularly powerful. Timing and duration of the activities are also important. For example, activities could be used to enhance body schema before tasks demanding motor coordination and planning are done. Another common example is the use of oral motor activity in preparation for eating (Oetter et al., 1995). For children with difficulties in organization of behavior, one may suggest specific activities that promote focused attention for use before or during tasks (Williams & Shellenberger, 1994). For people with sensory defensiveness, activities to reduce defensive or avoidant responses should be repeated at regular intervals throughout the day to help the individual maintain an optimal level of arousal and adaptation (Wilbarger & Wilbarger, 1991). (See next section for more detail.)

Other suggestions for sensory diets include adaptation of the daily routine, changes to the environment, modification of social interactions, and suggestions for appropriate leisure and play activities. The sensory diet activities and adaptations should be applied to all relevant settings such as school, work, home, and community. As noted earlier, these suggestions should be concrete, specific to the individual, and easily incorporated into the daily routine of the individual or family.

RELATIONSHIP TO SENSORY INTEGRATION AND OCCUPATION

Many of the principles of the sensory diet were drawn from sensory integration theory. When properly constructed, the activities that comprise the diet include enhanced sensory input and active involvement in meaningful activity with the daily routine. Ideally, activities are self-selected and intrinsically motivating. The overriding goal of the sensory diet is to enable individuals to succeed in their daily life tasks and roles. Thus, the *effect* of carefully constructed sensory diets should be to improve occupational and role performance.

POPULATION FOR WHOM THE SENSORY DIET IS INTENDED

A sensory diet plan can be developed for any individual across a range of ages and stages of development. The outcomes of the intervention vary by severity of dysfunction, focus of the goals, and adherence to the program. Any suggestion should take into account precautions particular to the individual.

BENEFITS OF THE SENSORY DIET

A number of goals can be addressed using sensory diets. These include improved postural functions, enhanced body schema (for motor coordination and praxis), improved self-regulation, and reductions in sensory defensiveness. Specific objectives, however, focus on the improvement of functional skills such as competent participation in play, self-care, social interactions, and productive behaviors. Although the sensory diet often is used as an adjunct to direct occupational therapy, it also can be used independently such as to:

- Address self-regulation problems of children in a school setting (Williams & Shellenberger, 1994)
- Reduce sensory deprivation, self-stimulatory behavior, or sensory overload in adults with cognitive limitations living or working in institutional environments (Sime,1991)
- Decrease sensory defensiveness (Wilbarger & Wilbarger, 1991)

TRAINING RECOMMENDED OR REQUIRED

In order to develop effective sensory diets, a therapist must have a thorough understanding of sensory integration theory and its foundations in neuroscience. Advanced clinical reasoning and knowledge of the principles of family- and client-centered intervention are also necessary to design effective sensory diets. Most therapists benefit from specific training and education in the application of sensory diets. Continuing education opportunities on the use of the sensory diet are advertised in occupational therapy newsletters and magazines. Some sensory processing disruptions require more extensive assessment and greater expertise on the part of the therapist. For example, factors such as disruption in the suck-swallow-breathe synchrony, sensory defensiveness, and medical complications require unique considerations and advanced training.

SUMMARY

A sensory diet can be a useful tool in the treatment of individuals with sensory integrative disorders. The sensory diet is based on the principle that enhanced sensation can have a profound effect on adaptive functioning. The fact that it is principle based rather than task based makes it applicable to a wide range of persons across multiple settings. Therapists must have an understanding of the therapeutic use of sensory-based activity and artfully incorporate those activities into the daily lives of their clients.

"How Does Your Engine Run?": The Alert Program for Self-Regulation

Sherry Shellenberger, OTR/L
Mary Sue Williams, OTR/L

BACKGROUND

"If your body is like a car engine, sometimes it runs on high, sometimes it runs on low, and sometimes it runs just right." These simple words were used first when I (MSW) began working with one of my finest teachers, an 11-year-old girl.

The child entered each occupational therapy session in a low arousal state and appeared to be lethargic, disinterested, and resistant to activities or interactions. After a short period of active play using sensory integrative techniques, she became alert, communicative, confident, energetic, and enthusiastic (i.e., in an optimal arousal state). Despite this dramatic change during therapy, the child then returned for subsequent sessions in the same low arousal state and, reportedly, there was little carryover to home or school.

Clearly, the child needed to understand her own arousal states in order to generalize the effects of therapy. I began to explain arousal states to the child by observing and naming her "engine levels" (arousal states): "Oh, it looks like your engine is low right now. Let's go play on the swings." Then as the child's arousal state changed, I would comment, "Now your engine is running 'just right.' It's easier for you to think up games and play with me." Similarly, if the child went into a high state of arousal, I would comment in a neutral tone of voice that her engine was at a high level.

In subsequent therapy sessions, the child and I played together and shared our inner experience of arousal states through the framework of the engine vocabulary. I continued to benefit from the guidance that the child offered in learning about self-regulation. Through the interactions with this client and the many clients that followed, Sherry Shellenberger and I developed the Alert Program. We summarized our experiences with hundreds of children in the book "*How Does Your Engine Run?*" *A Leader's Guide to the Alert Program for Self-Regulation* (Williams & Shellenberger, 1994). Many therapists and clients now use these simple engine words to recognize how self-regulation influences all daily living skills.

RATIONALE

To attend, concentrate, and perform tasks in a manner suitable to the situation, one must be in an optimal state of arousal for the particular task. When difficulties in self-regulation occur, individuals have trouble changing their levels of alertness, which in turn compromises their ability to function.

We believe that self-regulation affects all kinds of learning. For example, if an occupational therapist or parent is helping a child button a shirt, the child must be in an optimal state of arousal to best learn the task. If a speech and language pathologist is helping a client to articulate the "r" sound, the client should be prepared and ready for learning. If a teacher is supporting a student to type a story on a computer, the student's mind and body need to be alert and attentive to facilitate the most accurate keyboarding.

DESCRIPTION

The Alert Program is a step-by-step method by which adults (preferably a team) determine which sensory strategies support children's optimal performance and identify sensory hypersensitivities that hinder their performance (Stevens Dominguez et al., 1996). The Alert Program is designed to improve awareness of self-regulation through charts, worksheets, and activities. Adults guide children to recognize the ways in which hypersensitivities affect alertness and help them learn strategies to change their levels of alertness or arousal. Few adults or children are conscious of what they do to remain attentive while completing a task. The Alert Program helps children realize that their "engines" (i.e., nervous systems) need the proper amount and kind of sensory information to function optimally. Although the program was originally intended to increase awareness of self-regulation for children, many adults have come to understand the importance of sensory strategies to their own functioning. The engine vocabulary leads to effective problem solving by avoiding professional jargon among team members.

The Alert Program also increases the individual's repertoire of strategies for changing levels of alertness. Children with self-regulation difficulties often have a limited number of strategies to draw on to change how alert they feel. These children frequently have difficulty transitioning between activities, coping with changes in routines, and generally adapting to the challenges of real life. Through the program, children and adults together determine the strategies that support optimal functioning. For example, children learn what to do if their engines are running on high when they need to sit down and concentrate on their homework. Teachers learn what they can do in their classrooms between reading and math to support students in "waking up their engines and their minds" so they will be ready to learn the next subject material. Parents learn that if their toddlers are in an optimal arousal state, practicing eating with a utensil will be much more successful. Through the program, individuals enhance their abilities to learn, interact with others, and work or play. As an added bonus, when

children learn to monitor their levels of alertness, they often experience concomitant improvements in self-esteem and self-confidence.

The Alert Program assists children who have learning disabilities and attention deficits (as well as typically developing children) to apply basic principles of sensory integration theory related to arousal states. The goal of the program is not to teach children how to get their "engines to run just right" and remain there throughout the day but, rather, to learn how to *change* their levels of alertness to meet situational demands.

After years of working with public school systems, we have found that it is important for adults to understand their own self-regulation needs and strategies to appreciate children's self-regulation needs. Thus, before initiating the Alert Program, adults observe themselves and their own strategies for remaining alert. Adults are asked to fill out the Sensory Motor Preference Checklist (Williams & Shellenberger, 1994), which helps them identify sensorimotor strategies they use to self-regulate. The form lists five ways to change engine levels: put something in your mouth (oral motor input), move (vestibular input), touch (tactile input), look (visual input), and listen (auditory input). As adults fill out the form, they come to realize that "chewing" on a pencil, tapping their feet, fidgeting with jewelry, watching the sparks of a campfire, or listening to classical music all can be ways to self-regulate. Invariably, adults find that they use both strategies that are "socially acceptable" and some that may be labeled "idiosyncratic." The same self-regulation strategies in children are labeled inappropriate and called a "problem."

Children often need sensorimotor strategies that are bigger, louder, longer, faster, harder, and stronger than those used by adults. Through the Alert Program, adults and children come to understand that every "body" has an engine that runs at its own speed and that there are many ways to alter engine speed. They learn about their own needs and develop strategies for changing their alertness to meet the demands of different activities.

After the adults recognize what strategies they use (by filling out the checklist), they teach children that these same five sensory categories guide their choices in determining their own sensory diets (Wilbarger & Wilbarger, 1991). The children learn that if their engines are running on high or low and they want to get to "just right," they can "put something in their mouth, move, touch, look, or listen" to change how alert they feel. Movement and manipulation of objects are important parts of the program. In fact, we originally had some concern about publishing our program, fearing that our methods would become a "ditto program"; children would sit at desks, fill out charts, and try to learn how alert they felt without moving.

The program also involves teaching the basics of self-regulation and sensory integration theory (through experiential learning) to the parents, teachers, and other team members. By using the engine analogy and emphasizing the importance of self-regulation, team members are taught to disseminate the basics of sensory integration theory to others. Educating as many adults as possible in a child's life about the theory behind self-regulation strategies is a crucial part of the program. For example, if a principal looks into a classroom and exclaims, "I'm concerned your students are not sitting still and paying attention," the teacher will be able to explain quickly and concisely why her students can *either* sit still *or* pay attention. A parent will be able to deal effectively with a grandparent who says, "Your son just needs discipline. Then he would not have such tantrums." The parent can explain why her son with sensory processing difficulties does not need stricter discipline but instead needs an awareness of what affects his engine and more strategies to change his own engine level at school and at home.

RELATIONSHIP TO SENSORY INTEGRATION AND OCCUPATION

The Alert Program was drawn directly from sensory integration theory; it is a unique adaptation of the theory specifically addressing self-regulation. The Alert Program meets the criteria proposed for assessment and intervention based on the principles of sensory integration *that pertain to arousal and state maintenance*. Ideally, a child who participates in the program receives a full occupational therapy evaluation, including a sensory history interview with parents, classroom observation or report from the student's teacher (or teachers), and standardized testing. During assessment, information is gathered regarding the effect of various types and amounts of sensory input on an individual's level of alertness. The results of the initial assessment become

the basis for the "detective work" to determine what supports the child's function and what compromises his or her function (Stevens Dominguez et al., 1996).

The Alert Program is intended to be an adjunct to intervention based on the principles of sensory integration theory. After the evaluation is completed, the team determines whether the child needs direct, indirect, or consultative intervention. If the Alert Program is deemed appropriate, one of the team members (a teacher, parent, or therapist) becomes the "leader" of the program. If the leader is not familiar with sensory integration theory, it is recommended that an occupational therapist be consulted, especially to support the development of the sensory diet and to do the "detective work."

At school, home, or in the therapy clinic, individuals learn strategies to alter alertness in order to complete necessary tasks. The strategies involve the provision of controlled sensation. The leader of the program guides a child or groups of children to find their own sensory-motor preferences, determining together what best supports optimal functioning. Thus, the program meets the important criterion of meaningfulness. In addition, the Alert Program focuses on developing practical ways to improve performance in everyday life directly influencing occupational performance.

POPULATION FOR WHOM THE ALERT PROGRAM IS APPROPRIATE

Although initially designed for children ages 8 to 12 years, the Alert Program has been adapted for preschool through high school students and for adults; it has been implemented successfully in a variety of settings, including classrooms, homes, private practice clinics, and camps. If children are intellectually challenged or developmentally younger than age 8 years, parents and other adult team members can use the program's concepts to facilitate the child's optimal functioning. In such cases, the adults become the "detectives," identifying and providing the types of sensorimotor input that best support the child's self-regulation and performance.

The program's success with children who are developing typically or atypically and with adults suggests that all can benefit from greater awareness of self-regulation. Even children who are diagnosed with attention deficit disorder and are taking medication benefit from use of the program. Through the program's charts and worksheets, children become aware of and learn to describe their engine levels more accurately. While medication dosages are being monitored, children become a part of the team, using the engine vocabulary to report to the physician. This information supplements information provided through traditional observation checklists.

TRAINING RECOMMENDED OR REQUIRED

Because the Alert Program is based in sensory integration theory, we believe it is important that at least one team member have special knowledge of this theory. The program itself is contained in *"How Does Your Engine Run?": A Leader's Guide to the Alert Program for Self-Regulation.*

The Leader's Guide, an introductory booklet, and an audiotape are available from TherapyWorks, Inc., 4901 Butte Place, NW, Albuquerque, NM 87120; (505) 897–3478. We also offer courses in the implementation of the Alert Program. Information about these courses can be obtained by contacting us directly at TherapyWorks or visiting our Website at *www.alertprogram.com.*

SUMMARY

Each individual's formula for self-regulation is unique. Through the Alert Program, children learn that simple changes to their daily routine (e.g., taking a brisk walk to the bus before school, packing extra crunchy food in the lunch box, or jumping on a trampoline before homework time) is all that is needed to maximize their ability to function and keep their engines running "just right." Empowering children to discover their own answers to the question, "How does your engine run?" is a joyous adventure.

Water-Based Intervention

Gudrun Gjesing

BACKGROUND

Throughout history, water has been associated with life and health. In ancient times, the Romans and Incas built baths. People of all times have flocked to places with healing springs. Today, we relax in bathtubs, hot tubs, and at SPAs (SPA is an acronym for sane per aqua, which means "health through water.")

All of us began life in water. Before birth, children grow and frisk about in "aqua vitae," the water of life. In this element, the embryo moves. At birth, all of us face a world in which gravity predominates, making us "disabled," until we mature and master our bodies in this new environment. Most people—children and adults, with or without disabilities—enjoy water activities. Water invites movement and promotes play. Thus, occupational and physical therapy practitioners often draw on the power of water when designing intervention programs.

RATIONALE

Water-based intervention combines swimming (a desirable and motivating recreation activity) with simultaneous involvement in a variety of therapeutic activities. In the water, we perform active movements in an ever-changing context. Because of buoyancy, it may be easier to move freely in water than on land. Water-based activities can be fun and, thus, highly motivating. In short, water-based intervention programs provide "a means of widening experience—physically, developmentally, cognitively, and psychologically" (Campion, 1991, p. 12).

DESCRIPTION

At present, I conduct two or three water intervention groups weekly in a local public swimming pool. The water temperature is approximately 84°F (or 28°C), and the depth of the water varies from 3 to 12 feet (1 to 4 meters). The children range in age from 6 months to 10 years. The groups are divided according to the children's ability in water rather than their diagnoses, age, or difficulties on land. We work one-on-one with six to eight children. [Editors' note: Although this author works at present with children, this description also applies to adults.] Until clients have developed full independence in water, an aide assists them. The aide may be a parent, a relative, or a caregiver. I supervise the aides at all times.

Aides give clients both physical and psychological support. They use their hands to facilitate clients' balance reactions, so it is essential that they know the correct handling of people in water. This may be quite different from the correct handling of the same person on land. In order to not disturb the client's balance, the aid supports the client at the body's center of balance, which is about waist level.

As with intervention on land, the instructor often motivates children (and adults) with play. With children, we use a lot of action songs and rhymes. We also use colorful, plastic playthings (e.g., balls, rings, and water pistols) to promote children's understanding of different tasks (Fig. 14–1). These activities provide useful feedback and knowledge of the results of their movements.

Instructors primarily design group games and

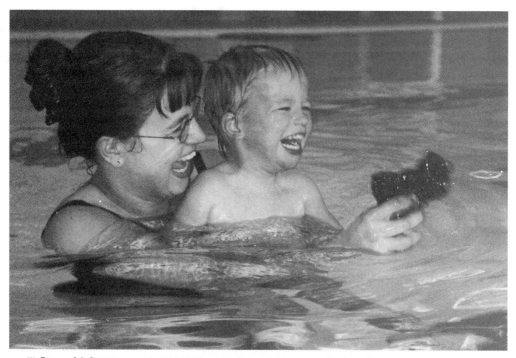

■ FIGURE 14–1 Using a water pistol in the swimming pool increases the fun. (Photo courtesy of Gudrun Gjesing.)

learning situations. Games need groups, and groups need games! Some of the activities have goals that apply to all the clients. For example, clients learn to anticipate movements associated with different songs, rhymes, and playthings. Later, these movements are incorporated into specific purposeful "water skills" (e.g., stability, rotational control, mobility, and swimming strokes). Other activities have goals that are more specific to an individual. We place markers along the edge of the pool with playthings and instructions (written or drawn) for tasks that may be done by particular clients in specific ways, depending on their abilities and needs.

RELATIONSHIP TO SENSORY INTEGRATION AND OCCUPATION

Water activities potentially provide clients with a number of benefits related to sensory integration. The provision of enhanced sensation is inherent to water-based intervention. Furthermore, active involvement and the demand for an adaptive behavior also are a part of water-based intervention. Thus, when carefully conducted, water-based activities may be viewed as *overlapping* with intervention that reflects the principles of sensory integration.

However, the goals addressed and the activities used with a particular swimmer frequently cause water-based therapy to fall *outside the traditional construct of SI*. For example, activities designed to reduce muscle tone and improve passive range of motion with a swimmer who has cerebral palsy would fall outside the construct of SI. Similarly, activities designed to maintain muscle strength in a swimmer with muscular dystrophy would not be considered to be sensory integrative in nature.

Water-based intervention may also reflect occupation. Swimming is a valued leisure or recreation activity that can be shared with friends and family. Water-based intervention programs often lead to participants' attending swimming clubs or going with family or friends to public pools. Such recreation is fun for the whole family and capitalizes on clients' abilities rather than emphasizing their disabilities. Water activities provide satisfying experiences that lead to increased self-esteem and opportunities to develop valued interpersonal relationships. These are certainly as important as, if not more important than, the sensorimotor and fitness goals also achieved in water.

Water programs provide an opportunity for the mastery of numerous other occupational performance–based goals. Undressing and dressing, toileting, showering, and using public transportation are a few of the many tasks individuals may perform when involved in a therapeutic water-based program. In my program, we spend a long time in the changing room and the shower (as well as the sauna). Caregivers are taught not to help children with tasks they have mastered, to assist with tasks the children are practicing, and to do only what the children are not yet able to do. Children readily understand the relevance of these skills in the context of a meaningful activity for which they are required

POPULATIONS FOR WHOM WATER-BASED INTERVENTION IS APPROPRIATE

In more than 20 years of experience, I have found that people of all ages and with nearly all kinds of disabilities benefit from intervention in water. I have worked successfully in water with children and adults who have emotional disorders (e.g., from sexual abuse or neglect), behavior disorders, learning difficulties, speech deficits, visual and hearing impairments, sensory integrative dysfunction, congenital abnormalities, cerebral palsy, cognitive impairments, muscular dystrophy, spina bifida and hydrocephalus, and arthritis. Persons with different disabilities often work well in groups in which their abilities and needs in water are similar.

SENSORY INPUT

Water provides many different kinds of sensory information. Because movement of water is felt differently than how air is felt, the tactile system receives a great deal of stimulation. In a pool with a lot of people moving around, the water also moves in continually new ways. This may result in lack of habituation by the tactile receptors. Water invites movement in a number of positions, including the vertical and horizontal planes.

Because of buoyancy, rotations of the body also are common. Movement in a number of planes provides enhanced information to the vestibular system. In water, you cannot always compensate for poor processing of vestibular information by using vision because you cannot see your body well and, therefore, cannot use it as a visual reference. When clients move against the resistance of water, their proprioceptors receive input. However, because of buoyancy or upthrust, the proprioceptors receive different stimulation in water than on land, where gravity or downthrust dominates. Therefore, it is difficult to tell exactly the effect of proprioceptive stimulation received in water. However, I believe that the increased tactile input provided by the water may make up for the changes in proprioceptive input.

BENEFITS OF WATER-BASED INTERVENTION

Water can be a powerful and highly motivating therapeutic medium. A number of physical and psychosocial benefits have been associated with water-based intervention.

Physical and Psychosocial Benefits

Improvement in many performance components can be addressed in the water. These include (but are not limited to) respiration and breath control, stability and mobility, rhythmicity and coordination, fitness, playfulness, activities of daily living, self-esteem, and social and emotional development. In the water, alertness also is enhanced, and clients may become more aware of their bodies and surroundings. Clients with sensory defensiveness also react positively to the kind of tactile stimulation water offers. Furthermore, clients may develop abilities in self-care and instrumental activities of daily living activities as well as important leisure interests and skills.

TRAINING RECOMMENDED OR REQUIRED

An instructor must be specifically trained in both hydromechanical principles and water safety instruction in order to conduct water-based intervention. If the instructor is not a physical or occupational therapy practitioner, a therapist can be an important consultant and help to tailor goals and activities to the needs of the clients.

Client's abilities in water are different from their abilities (and disabilities) on land. Although intervention in water and on land share many traits, in water we use different strategies to promote movement and stability. Instructors must learn the hydromechanical principles of control for posture and movement using The Halliwick Concept (Association of Swimming Therapy, 1992; Campion, 1985). To create appropriate intervention plans, therapists must do qualitative assessments of each client's abilities in the water. In addition, they must do continuous evaluation of each client's development and learning in order to adjust goals and plans appropriately. The Halliwick Concept inspires what we do in water, why, and how we do it. In short, it requires more than a swimsuit and a pool for a therapist to be qualified as an instructor in the water! [Editors' note: In the United States, swimming instructors must be certified in water safety instruction. This certification is available from the American Red Cross.]

AN EXAMPLE: "THE ALARM CLOCK"

"Come on, now we are going to do the Alarm Clock!" I say. All the children and their aides immediately know exactly what is going to happen, and they begin to prepare. They form a circle around me, the children in vertical position facing me, with the aides supporting them, according to their needs, from behind. I then say: "Now you are going to sleep, all of you, with your eyes closed!" The children lie supine by bending their heads backward into the water and allowing their legs to float upward. (Fig. 14–2). (The goals of this part of the activity are concentration, trusting in their own ability, and being able to move from one stable position into another by changing only head position.)

Then I move around the circle, touching each child's feet and saying his or her name. "Now I know that you are all fast asleep!" (The goal of this part is to have supine stability with eyes closed.) "Ding-a-ling-a-ling!" I yell until all children move into a vertical position by flexing the neck and hips and stretching their arms forward. As they move into a vertical position, their mouths go under water, and they begin to blow bubbles. (The goals of this part are being able to move from one stable po-

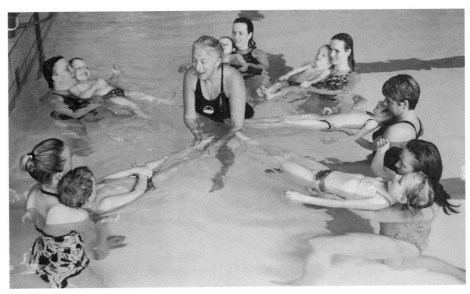

■ FIGURE 14-2 "Now you are going to sleep, all of you." (Photo courtesy of Gudrun Gjesing.)

sition into another and having controlled respiration.)

I continue yelling until all children have placed one hand on "the alarm button" (my head) and they start pressing it into the water (Fig. 14–3). (The goal of this part is to have mobile arms with a stable trunk.) I stay submerged as long as possible. As I emerge, I'm absolutely sure to hear all the children yell, "Let's do it again!" (Fig. 14–4).

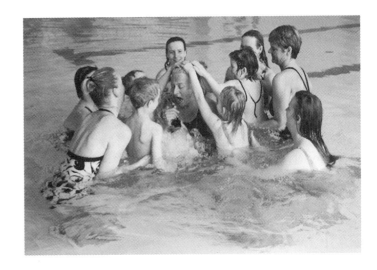

■ FIGURE 14-3 All of the children place one hand on the "alarm button". (Photo courtesy of Gudrun Gjesing.)

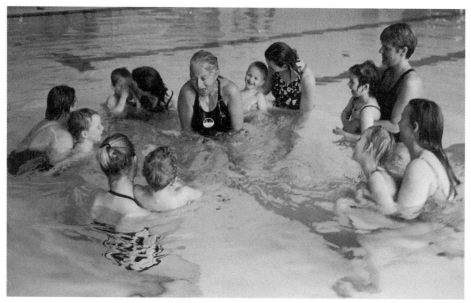

■ FIGURE 14-4 "Let's do it again!" (Photo courtesy of Gudrun Gjesing.)

Hippotherapy

Nancy Lawton-Shirley, OTR

BACKGROUND

The use of horses as a therapeutic medium has been growing in popularity in the United States over the past 20 years. Programs that incorporate intensive therapeutic activities and programming with horses are known as *hippotherapy*. As more programs have been established, the physical and psychosocial benefits of hippotherapy have become recognized in the United States. Many programs have been active in Europe since the early 1960s, and the benefits have been touted since the 1700s (Riede, 1988).

RATIONALE

Hippotherapy combines riding a horse (a highly motivating recreation activity) with simultaneous involvement in a variety of therapeutic activities. Hippotherapy is thought to yield a wide range of benefits, including the development of balance and other postural responses, muscle strength and coordination, ROM, socialization, self-esteem and self-confidence, eye–hand coordination, visual-spatial skill, bilateral coordination, motor planning, and body awareness.

DESCRIPTION

Hippotherapy programs vary widely in physical setup and levels of therapeutic intensity. However, they share some common characteristics. To provide safe, effective instruction, an equestrian instructor who has had training and experience with therapeutic riding facilitates the sessions. Commonly, an occupational or physical therapy practitioner collaborates with the instructor and provides guidance regarding appropriate goals, special adaptations, and program adjustments for each participant.

Horses are selected for their gait patterns, girth, and temperament. These qualities are then matched to the needs of the rider. The horses receive training to attain and maintain a level of responsiveness to clients that is therapeutic. These training sessions include extensive work to accustom the horse to wheelchairs, walkers, unusual behaviors, outbursts of emotion, and other circumstances they might encounter while in the company of persons with disabilities (*Volunteer Manual*, 1999).

The horse walks, trots, or backs up on command as the rider assumes various positions and engages in therapeutic exercises and games. Initially, most riders need adults to lead and control the horses. Thus, many programs incorporate volunteers (called sidewalkers) who walk beside the rider to facilitate participation and ensure safety. As skills improve, the need for this support may diminish. However, riders involved in some therapeutic activities (e.g., assuming four-point kneeling on the back of the horse) likely require continued support. Acquisition of actual riding skills (e.g., reining) varies depending on the developmental level of the individual. In addition, most programs include instructions on safety awareness and care of horses. These foster the rider's independence and sense of responsibility.

RELATIONSHIP TO SENSORY INTEGRATION AND OCCUPATION

The provision of enhanced sensation is inherent to hippotherapy. Furthermore, under certain circumstances (i.e., when the rider is stretching his or her abilities to respond in a more effective way than ever before), involvement and the demand for adaptive behavior also are inherent to hippotherapy. For example, a rider with sensory integrative dysfunction who moves independently into quadruped on the horse's back and remains in that position as the horse moves is likely involved in an activity that reflects the principles of sensory integration theory. When both enhanced sensation and the demand for an adaptive behav-

ior are present, hippotherapy could be viewed as *overlapping with* intervention that reflects the principles of sensory integration.

However, goals addressed and activities used with a particular rider frequently cause hippotherapy to *fall outside the traditional construct of sensory integration*. For example, activities designed to reduce muscle tone and improve passive ROM with a rider who has cerebral palsy fall outside the construct of sensory integration. Similarly, activities designed to maintain muscle strength in a rider with muscular dystrophy would not be considered to be sensory integrative in nature.

Hippotherapy reflects *occupation*. For example, grooming the horse represents a meaningful activity for many riders. For some, hippotherapy provides the opportunity to develop competency in or mastery of a recreational activity or competitive sport. Interacting with the horse may lead to a special bond between animal and rider. Interacting with others involved in the program provides the basis for the development of friendships and opportunities to practice social skills.

POPULATIONS FOR WHOM HIPPOTHERAPY IS APPROPRIATE

Because hippotherapy has potential to facilitate many areas of development, most individuals with special needs can benefit from participation. Hippotherapy has been successfully used with individuals with cerebral palsy, muscular dystrophy, autism, learning disabilities, sensory integrative dysfunction, stroke, traumatic head injury, attention deficit disorder, and attachment disorder. Contraindications for therapeutic riding are advanced hip dislocation, scoliosis over 25 degrees, allergies to horsehair, acute inflammatory conditions of the spine, and atlanto-axial instability (as is often seen in individuals with Down syndrome). Some sources advise against the participation of individuals with myelomeningocele above L_3 (Riede, 1988).

SENSORY INPUT

Riding a horse provides many different kinds of sensory information, including tactile, visual, auditory, vestibular, and proprioceptive. This enhanced information is derived from a number of sources.

For example, grooming and having sustained contact with the horse while riding provide significant tactile input. The movement that accompanies different gaits, sudden starting and stopping, changing direction, and assuming different positions while riding (e.g., prone, supine) provide opportunities to take in enhanced vestibular sensation. Actively changing positions and independently maintaining a position as the horse moves provide intense proprioceptive sensation. Feedback from activated normalized postural movements enhances postural responses. Enhanced sensation facilitates the attainment of a number of different postural and sensorimotor benefits described next.

BENEFITS OF HIPPOTHERAPY

Using a horse as a therapeutic medium is extremely powerful and unique. Many physical and psychosocial benefits that may be generalized to daily life have been associated with participation in hippotherapy

Physical Benefits

One of the remarkable aspects of horseback riding is that the three-dimensional motion caused by the horse's movements is very similar to natural human pelvic movements. As people ride, they respond to the rhythmic movements of the horse's pelvis. Riders experience normal weight shifting, trunk elongation, and mobility (Dertoli, 1998). Riding a horse may be the first experience of these phenomena for riders with significant motor impairments (e.g., cerebral palsy).

Various properties of the gait of the horse lead to different responses from the rider. During steady walking with a horse that has an even stride, riders experience rhythmic movement, which tends to be calming and facilitates visual orientation, attending, and focus. During a trot or fast walk, riders may experience increased proprioceptive and vestibular sensations that facilitate alertness, increased body awareness, trunk stability, postural alignment, balance responses, and midline orientation.

Games and exercises to increase upper extremity function (e.g., ROM, strengthening, midline crossing) and visual orientation and tracking easily can be integrated into the therapeutic session. Reaching for carefully placed objects encourages specific upper extremity movements. Upper extremity positioning, in turn, influences posture. For example, horizontal abduction of the arm increases upper trunk extension. Games that require the rider to focus on various places and events in the arena help to develop visual orientation and tracking and attention to task.

Exercising while seated on a horse facilitates postural responses. The pelvis is held stable by the horse's body, thereby allowing trunk rotation and elongation to occur more easily. Lordotic posture and sacral sitting may be decreased. In fact, improved spinal alignment and mobility are documented as common benefits of hippotherapy (Riede, 1988).

To maintain a seated position on a moving horse, riders must use pelvic, leg, and abdominal muscles, thus strengthening or maintaining strength in these muscles. Actively changing position on the horse (i.e., moving into quadruped, prone, or supine) also facilitates postural responses, midline orientation, weight shifting, motor planning, and attention.

Elongation of and reduced tone in tight muscles can be achieved through the neutral warmth of the horse's body, inhibitory rhythmic movements, and slow stretch provided during riding. Riding draped over the horse in an inverted position may further reduce muscle tone.

The three-dimensional movements of the horse's gait, abdominal activation, and corrected postural alignment resulting from hippotherapy also can enhance circulation and visceral functioning. These benefits have been acknowledged in European literature for centuries (Riede, 1988).

Psychosocial Benefits

Working with and riding a powerful animal intrigues many individuals. Even those who are at first very fearful or gravitationally insecure usually overcome their hesitation as they bond with "their" horse. As they learn to control the horse's movements successfully and the two become a team, riders develop feelings of accomplishment, self-confidence, and mastery.

Some individuals connect more easily with animals than other people. The emotional bond that develops between riders and horses and the comfort that individuals experience from equine companions may result in feelings of belonging and being connected to another living creature. These, in turn, may foster emotional, social, and spiritual development.

Hippotherapy can also open social doors to peers. When the riding experience is provided in a group setting, it provides a common experience on which friendships can be built among peers who share an interest. Team games (e.g., relay races) also can provide the experience of teamwork and collaboration, with which many children who have disabilities have had limited previous experience.

TRAINING RECOMMENDED OR REQUIRED

Hippotherapy programs require the direct involvement and supervision of a trained equestrian instructor, preferably one with training and experience using therapeutic riding techniques. The North American Riding for the Handicapped Association (PO Box 33150, Denver, CO 80233, phone 303-452-1212, 1–800-369 RIDE, fax 303-252-4610, or visit their Website, *www.narha.org*) is a good resource for training.

To be optimally effective, a team of professionals should be involved. Occupational and physical therapy practitioners can be important team members for creating individualized goals and planning programs. Understanding children's social, emotional, and physical needs and ways of optimally facilitating development increases the effectiveness of hippotherapy programs. Because hippotherapy provides intensive sensation, understanding sensory integration theory is especially important. Furthermore, training in neurodevelopmental therapy (NDT) is recommended for understanding the postural components of hippotherapy.

SUMMARY

Hippotherapy is a powerful therapeutic tool that is compatible with both sensory integration and occupation. Horseback riding is motivating and pleasurable and can be a medium for attaining numerous physical and psychosocial benefits. Additionally, hippotherapy can lead to the development of a meaningful recreational interest or hobby.

Oculomotor Control: An Integral Part of Sensory Integration

Mary Kawar, MS, OTR

BACKGROUND

Despite the fact that vision is an integral part of everything occupational therapists do with clients, the oculomotor system has not been viewed as a primary target of intervention using the principles of sensory integration. Because of this, the oculomotor deficits of many clients have "fallen through the cracks." Recognizing the inseparable link between the vestibular system and oculomotor control, Ayres included the postrotary nystagmus test (PRNT) as a part of the assessment of sensory integration function. However, Ayres focused on the vestibular and somatosensory systems and used information derived from the PRNT test primarily as a measure of vestibular function. No other standardized measures of oculomotor control were incorporated into either the Southern California Sensory Integration Tests (SCSIT) or the Sensory Integration and Praxis Tests (SIPT).

Developmental optometrists have specialized in vision training and occupational therapists using sensory integration have specialized in vestibular and somatosensory integration. Although occupational therapists increasingly collaborate with developmental optometrists to incorporate vision screening and therapy into rehabilitation, there are few guidelines for incorporating oculomotor control into assessment and intervention based on the principles of sensory integration. I will attempt to bridge the gap between vision therapy and sensory integration by providing assessment and intervention strategies for integrating posture, bilateral integration, and oculomotor control. Together, I believe these provide a foundation for temporal-spatial orientation in all life tasks.

RATIONALE

Describing the vestibulo-oculo-cervical (VOC) triad, Moore (1994) indicated that dysfunction in any part of the triad disrupts function in the others, resulting in compromised adaptive responses to environmental demands. According to Moore, the vestibular system can be likened to a tripod holding a camera, which maintains the position of the head in order to keep the eyes focused on a target. Furthermore, postrotary and optokinetic nystagmus provide a foundation for volitional saccadic eye movements used for reading and scanning the environment.

Binocular movements are important components of voluntary eye movements (e.g., visual tracking, quick localization). In addition, proprioceptive receptors in the neck help orient the head according to task demands and coordinate movements of the eyes, head, and body. Thus, intervention to improve vestibular and proprioceptive processing should facilitate the development of improved oculomotor control. However, because of its complexity, improved oculomotor control requires specific exercise and activity in addition to activities that provide enhanced vestibular and proprioceptive inputs.

DESCRIPTION

This program consists of assessment and intervention components directed at both the vestibular and oculomotor systems. Each is described below.

Vestibular Testing (Postrotary Nystagmus)

First, test clients in a sitting position, using the PRNT from the SIPT to observe the action of the internal and external rectus muscles in response to stimulation of the horizontal semicircular canals (SSC). Next, rotate the person while he or she is positioned sidelying on a platform swing (head and spine horizontally aligned with the nose rotated 45 degrees toward the floor) to observe the action of the superior and inferior rectus and oblique eye muscles in the vertical plane elicited by stimulation of the superior and inferior SSC. The procedure is done clockwise and counterclockwise while the client lies on the right side and then on the left side at a rate of one revolution per 2 seconds for four or more rotations, depending on the client's tolerance.

Optimally, we see wide excursion, vertical eye movements similar to the typical horizontal PRN eye movements seen after stimulation of the horizontal semicircular canals (in sitting). Be certain that the PRN has stopped before continuing from one rotary procedure to the next. Caution is essential to avoid overloading the system because many clients are particularly sensitive to rotation while in the sidelying position.

When necessary, engage clients in activity that provides heavy proprioceptive input (resistance) to override any adverse vestibular response before proceeding with further rotary testing. When clients can tolerate it, observe PRN through closed eyelids because this eliminates the possibility of ocular fixation to inhibit the PRN response. Clients may close their eyes during and after rotation or may close their eyes from the time that the rotations cease until the PRN has stopped.

Vision Screening

Acuity

The ability to appreciate and interact visually with the environment requires more than visual *acuity,* but acuity is the appropriate starting point for assessment. Tests widely used for vision acuity include the Snellen Chart for individuals age 6 years through adult, the Lea Symbols Test for children age 2.5 to 5 years, and Teller Acuity Cards for children between age 1 and 18 months. Courses and books (e.g., Scheiman, 1997) are readily available for training therapists to screen for acuity.

Oculomotor Control and Visual Efficiency

An occupational therapist can administer many screening tests for *oculomotor control and visual efficiency,* including tests described by Scheiman (1997). Screening for oculomotor control and visual efficiency includes examination of the following functions:

- Binocular vision (eye alignment and sensory fusion)
- Accommodation
- Ocular motility (saccadic fixations and eye pursuits)
- Visual field

Working with a developmental optometrist is another way to learn about screening tools.

Visual Perceptual and Visuomotor Control

In addition to the *visual perceptual and visuomotor* tests included in the SIPT (i.e., Space Visualization, Design Copying, and Figure-Ground Perception), many other useful tests are used frequently by occupational therapists. These include Gardner's Test of Visual Perception Skills (Non-motor; Revised), Gardner's Test of Visual Motor Skills (Revised), Beery's Developmental Test of Visual-Motor Integration (VMI), The Rapid Eye Movement Test, and Gardner's Reversal Frequency Test.

OCULOMOTOR-VESTIBULAR-PROPRIOCEPTIVE INTERVENTION STRATEGIES

Rotary vestibular stimulation in sitting and sidelying (as described previously) is used to reflexively stimulate conjugate eye movements before other intervention. Spinning is essentially a "warm-up" exercise for the active oculomotor work that follows. The number of rotations in each position is determined by each individual's tolerance; initially, some clients can tolerate only one or two rotations in each plane without having an adverse reaction. With their eyes closed, clients concentrate on the reflexive eye movements, noting the ease with which the eyes move horizontally after rotation in sitting and vertically in sidelying.

After completion of the rotations in sitting and sidelying, clockwise and counterclockwise, clients engage in volitional visual tracking exercises that replicate the reflexive, conjugate eye movements. These include looking back and forth several times between two targets placed 16 inches away from the eyes and 6 to 18 inches apart. Targets should be visually compelling and no more than 1 inch in size apart (e.g., two pen lights covered with translucent plastic figures). The occupational therapist changes the relative position of the targets several times so the eyes move in specified directions. In order, these are:

1. Horizontally at eye level
2. Diagonally up to the right and down to the left
3. Diagonally up to the left and down to the right
4. Vertically

Finally, clients follow a moving target two or more times around an infinity pattern that is approximately 24 inches wide by 18 inches high and centered at eye level.

Oculomotor work must be of short duration because the eyes fatigue quickly when visual efficiency is limited. When eyestrain is observed, it is important to do a technique referred to as "palming" (Bates, 1986). Palming involves cupping the palms of each hand over open eyes, thereby creating a seal to occlude the eyes from light exposure. Palming is maintained for approximately 30 seconds; it refreshes the eyes and gives clients the experience of seeing without eyestrain.

After doing localization and tracking exercises, clients engage in whole-body activity with a strong oculomotor component. Linear movements in the prone and supine positions on a scooter board or in a hammock can be very good for working with near–far visual targets that require divergence and convergence of the eyes for depth perception. For example, clients may toss objects into a container as they move past it on a scooter board and then knock a roadblock out of the way. Clients also may pull hand over hand up an inclined rope while prone in a hammock, remove a clothespin clipped at a certain point along the rope, release the rope, and then toss the clothespin in a container while swinging back and forth.

Blow toys (e.g., whistles requiring visual attention and blow darts) also facilitate convergence and divergence. Blow toys (e.g., ball pipe, string pipe) can be adapted with latex tube extenders so convergence on a target can be practiced at various distances from the eyes. These activities can be structured in such a manner that clients are required to monitor the periphery while maintaining central vision on the ball or string pipe. After clients develop a certain level of skill with the pipes, they move through increasingly complex obstacle courses while blowing on the toys. For example, clients can move between, around, and over inflatables, crash mats, and suspended equipment while blowing and catching the ball in the pipe basket or putting a hand in and out of the loop of the string pipe.

Many clients who have learning disabilities also have subtle restrictions to ROM from compromised movement patterns that appear to correlate with eye muscle imbalance. For example, if clients have difficulty converging with the right eye, they may avoid turning the head toward the left so that they do not have to move the right eye medially. Over time, they will lose full ROM of the neck and upper body to the left. Exercises to release these restrictions also seem to free up the VOC triad. Several activities that are particularly effective for developing VOC efficiency and bilateral integration follow.

The Flow (available through Professional Development Products) is a long, soft, bioplastic tube partially filled with water. Clients hold it on each end and move it in many patterns across, over, under, and around the body. For example, an infinity pattern, which extends all the way behind the body on each side in order to look at a visual target behind the individual, is extremely effective for increasing ROM and bilateral integration and for developing highly efficient, coordinated movements of the eyes, head, and extremities around the vertical axis. The Flow comes in six sizes to accommodate preschoolers through adults, and movements can be adapted from very simple to highly complex, depending on the individual.

The Infinity Walk (Sunbeck, 1991) is a method of walking in a large (12+ feet) infinity pattern around two objects (e.g., inner tubes) while maintaining visual fixation on a target that is 6 or more feet away from the inner tubes and aligned with the center point of the infinity pattern. Walking around the infinity pattern requires wide-range head movements in coordination with visual fixation and quick localization of a visual target. The reader is referred to Sunbeck's book for more details.

The trampoline can be extremely useful for developing bilateral integration. For example, clients can alternate jumping jacks with stride jumps or do "twisters" where the feet go one way and the arms the other. The reader is referred to educational kinesiology information (e.g., Dennison & Dennison, 1994) for additional ideas on bilateral integration exercises.

RELATIONSHIP TO SENSORY INTEGRATION AND OCCUPATION

The activities that comprise this oculomotor program use enhanced vestibular and, to a lesser extent, proprioceptive input (from resistance). They also require active involvement. Thus, in many respects, this program represents an *expansion* of intervention based on the principles of sensory integration theory. In fact, many of the activities suggested are typical of those seen in any clinic that uses sensory integration principles.

Two points should be considered because they represent departures from typical sensory integration intervention. First, much of the vestibular input provided by spinning to "warm up" the oculomotor mechanism is applied by a therapist rather than resulting from clients' active movements. Clients' concentrate on the reflexive movements of their eyes before eliciting eye movements volitionally. Second, the oculomotor exercises (i.e., moving between targets and tracking a moving target) may not be highly motivating or meaningful. The latter points to the need for goal-directed intervention. Although clients may find the oculomotor exercises difficult and somewhat tedious, a masterful clinician addressing specific goals can infuse them with meaning. A therapist can point out the relationship between eye movements required in the exercises and those required to meet a goal (e.g., improved reading).

The oculomotor program addresses a performance component important to tasks clients must perform daily (i.e., occupation). Finding one's way, monitoring visual surroundings, succeeding at sports, being at ease in social settings, driving a car, shopping, reading, and copying information are examples of tasks that depend on oculomotor control and the VOC triad. Thus, when carefully planned and implemented, an oculomotor program should improve the client's occupational performance. However, because the link between the oculomotor program and occupation is indirect, therapists should monitor the effect rather than assuming it will happen.

POPULATIONS FOR WHOM THE OCULOMOTOR CONTROL PROGRAM IS APPROPRIATE

The majority of individuals challenged by developmental delays, learning disabilities, attention deficits, traumatic or pre- or perinatal brain injuries have less than optimal oculomotor control. Difficulty separating eye and head movements, tracking moving targets, shifting gaze with accurate saccades, sustaining focus, shifting focus between peripheral and central vision or near and far targets, eye teaming for close work, writing letters and numbers without reversals, and reading without losing one's place are all commonly seen.

In addition, any individual who has a history of recurrent soft tissue swelling caused by ear infections, allergies, sinus infections, or enlarged tonsils and adenoids is at risk for vestibular dysfunction. Because of the relationship between the vestibular and oculomotor systems, these individuals also are at risk for oculomotor deficits. The intervention described here can be adapted to serve clients of all ages who are at risk for oculomotor dysfunction.

TRAINING RECOMMENDED OR REQUIRED

For therapists trained in sensory integration theory to effectively incorporate assessment and intervention designed to improve oculomotor control into practice, further study and training are needed. The materials referenced here provide a good starting point. Continuing education workshops, such as "Full Inclusion: Vision and Hearing in SI Practice" and "From Eye Sight to Insight: Visual/Vestibular Assessment and Treatment sponsored by Professional Development Programs (14524 61st St. Ct. N., Stillwater, MN 55082, 651-439-8865, *www.pdppro.com*), provide excellent opportunities to develop knowledge and skill. Finally, but very importantly, therapists are advised to develop a solid working relationship with a local developmental optometrist.

SUMMARY

Intervention based on the principles of sensory integration can be enriched vastly by:

- Exploring the relation of eye and body movement restrictions
- Enhancing oculomotor control through vestibular and proprioceptive input
- Using reflexive exercises to promote voluntary oculomotor control
- Engaging in activities that require movement of the body through space while shifting visual fixation and that elicit central and peripheral visual processing

Although some of these strategies are already familiar to therapists trained in sensory integration theory, few therapists explicitly address oculomotor development. I have found that vision therapy is much more effective *after* the vestibular and proprioceptive foundation of oculomotor control has been addressed.

Therapeutic Listening: An Overview

Sheila Frick, OTR

BACKGROUND

The early development of the auditory system, its multiple brainstem connections, and its role in spatial perception support its connection with the vestibular, tactile, and proprioceptive systems. Auditory training has been used in Europe since the mid-1900s to address sensory processing disorders. These procedures have become popular in the United States over the past 10 years. Although they are not the only professionals to use these procedures, some occupational therapists incorporate auditory training techniques into intervention based on the principles of sensory integration. Through case studies, a few therapists (Frick & Lawton-Shirley, 1994; Morgan Brown, 1999) have reported promising results.

RATIONALE

The auditory system has numerous ties to the vestibular system. In fact, the two systems are sometimes referred to as one *vestibulo-cochlear system*. The most obvious connection between the auditory and vestibular systems is anatomical. Both share the bony labyrinth of the inner ear and their mechanical receptors operate in very similar fashion. They also share a common cranial nerve and possibly some nerve fibers.

The relationship between the auditory an vestibular systems is manifest in many functional ways. For example, sound localization (auditory) combines with movement (in part, vestibular) to enable the performance of numerous daily life ac-

tivities. Information about sound and movement is integrated at many levels of the CNS, including in brainstem, reticular, and limbic structures. Furthermore, Ayres (1972) described improvements in auditory processing as a result of intervention incorporating enhanced vestibular input.

About the time Ayres was developing sensory integration theory, Tomatis, a French ear, nose, and throat specialist, developed a clinically based approach for clients with listening difficulties. Similar to Ayres, Tomatis believed that the auditory and vestibular systems worked together. Tomatis attributed a number of functions to the combined auditory and vestibular systems, including:

- Integrating information from sound and movement to enable the development of posture, laterality, and language
- Stimulating and balancing the autonomic nervous system

Tomatis emphasized the importance of high-frequency audition for "charging the brain." He developed the first auditory training device, using filtered music that emphasized the higher frequencies of the sound spectrum. Many clinically based auditory training techniques stem from the work of Tomatis (1993) and Berard (1993), his student and colleague.

Berard developed the audiokinetron and a method called auditory integration training (AIT). His method was widely publicized in the United States through *The Sound of a Miracle* (Berard, 1991), in which he described a child with autism who benefited from his approach. Tomatis' ideas about the importance of the high tones were later confirmed and expanded by Steinbach (1997), a German sound engineer. Few individuals can hear above 16,000 Hz (sound waves measured in cycles per second). However, when frequencies between 16,000 and 20,000 Hz are filtered out of music, most listeners notice a difference. Steinbach postulated that the high tones have a powerful impact on the nervous system.

Similar to Tomatis, Steinbach spectrally activated the harmonic range, exaggerating the high overtones. He believed this increased listeners' attention to and awareness of the finer qualities of sound. Steinbach created several different levels of compact discs with varying intensities of spectral activation and filtering.

The techniques of Tomatis and Berard used music modulated and filtered through specialized equipment that tailors sound for each client. The expense of needed equipment and the training required to use it, coupled with the limits placed on intervention by third-party payers, have limited the availability of auditory training techniques. However, because of the work of sound engineers such as Steinbach and Mueller, an American, electronically enhanced music is now available on compact discs (CDs). These provide an affordable alternative to expensive devices. Although similar, they do not replace the Tomatis method or AIT.

DESCRIPTION

In the Therapeutic Listening Program, I use several electronically altered compact discs. These include the lower intensity disc developed by Steinbach and the Electronic Auditory Stimulation Effect (EASE) discs, developed by Mueller. The EASE discs were developed using a form of broad spectrum filtering similar to the modulation Berard used.

Listening times vary, depending on the intensity of the CD and the characteristics of the client for whom a therapeutic listening (TL) program is being implemented. As with all intervention based on the principles of sensory integration, a therapist follows the client's lead. When the listening time is short, clients may sit and listen actively while engaged in respiratory and oral motor play, swinging or playing with tactile materials such as shaving cream or beans. For longer listening times, a client wears headphones and a portable CD player in a belt pack. The child may be very active, jumping on a trampoline, moving through an obstacle course, or playing on a giant air pillow.

Because TL does not involve sophisticated equipment, a prescribed program can be carried out at home, in school, or in a clinic. In schools, trained therapists set up and monitor programs carried out by teachers. Clients require ongoing support from a therapist who is trained in TL.

A typical program may continue for 2 to 6 months. However many clients to find the compact discs useful as part of an ongoing sensory diet (see the Sensory Diet section of this chapter).

RELATIONSHIP TO SENSORY INTEGRATION AND OCCUPATION

Although Ayres (1972) wrote about the relationship between the auditory and vestibular systems, she never directly addressed the use of enhanced auditory input. Thus, when TL is done in the context of activities that require active involvement and adaptive interactions, it represents an *expansion* of intervention based on the principles of sensory integration theory. However, when it is used alone in the absence of any demand for adaptive interaction, it represents pure sensory stimulation and falls *outside* the construct of sensory integration.

TL programs address a performance component important to daily life tasks, including performance in any environment where competing sounds may be present (e.g., school, shopping mall). Thus, when carefully planned and implemented, TL should improve client's occupational performance. However, because the link between TL and occupation is indirect, therapists should monitor the connection rather than assuming it will happen.

POPULATIONS FOR WHOM THERAPEUTIC LISTENING IS APPROPRIATE

Our experience has been primarily with clients ages 2 years and older (throughout the lifespan).

Clients younger than age 2 years may benefit if the program is monitored by a clinician who is experienced in working with very young children and the listening program is modified (e.g., headphone use is not recommended for clients younger than age 2 years).

Clients with many diagnoses (e.g., autistic spectrum disorder, attention deficit disorder, and learning disabilities) have benefited from TL programs. To be a candidate for TL, individuals must demonstrate difficulties with sensory processing. Use of a TL program is contraindicated for clients who have seizures triggered by sound. TL programs should be stopped temporarily when clients have active ear infections.

BENEFITS OF THERAPEUTIC LISTENING

The use of modulated and filtered music in conjunction with intervention based on the principles of sensory integration seems to increase the effectiveness of both. Through sound, we not only influence the auditory system, but we also seem to have a powerful impact on the vestibular system. Clinical experience suggests that TL decreases the time necessary to improve sensory modulation, balance, movement perception, exploration, sense of physical competence, praxis and sequencing, social competence, and language abilities. Children and adults who experience gravitational insecurity often respond very positively to these techniques (Frick & Lawton-Shirley, 1994). In schools, many therapists have reported improvement in children's abilities to attend and in academic performance (Kaliher, 1998).

TRAINING RECOMMENDED OR REQUIRED

Basic training is provided in a workshop entitled Listening with the Whole Body, sponsored by Vital Links Workshops (phone, 919-388-8865). Ingo Steinbach, in conjunction with Samonas International, provides more in-depth training in the Samonas method (phone, 608-278-7075).

The less intense compact discs developed by Steinbach and Mueller are available to therapists who have an understanding of the implications of modulation of sound and its impact on the entire nervous system. The more intense compact discs require training in the use of advanced equipment as well as sound physics. The discs can be purchased through Vital Sounds after participation in an entry-level training course titled "Listening with the Whole Body" (Vital Sounds, 6613 Seybold Rd, Suite D, Madison, Wisconson, 53719, 608-278-9330, *www.vitalsounds.com*).

AN EXAMPLE

At age 2 years, 8 months, Julia was exhibiting decreased sensory registration. She did not seem to perceive sensory information to a degree that she could make sense out of it, integrate the information, or organize it for use. She avoided experiences she did not understand and sought intense sensory experiences apparently to help her register sensation. One of her favorite activities was spinning on a platform swing with side supports. For the most part, the stimulation she sought was relatively passive apparently because she lacked the postural control, strength, and motor coordination to "generate" her own stimulation.

Julia was seen for 3 consecutive days, 2 hours each day. Intervention consisted of TL combined with activities typically associated with sensory integration theory. By the fourth session, she seemed more "energized." She was willing to attempt more motor challenges; her postural control appeared more dynamic; and she began to achieve better stability around her shoulders and hips. She was able to independently jump on a trampoline for the first time.

By the fifth and sixth sessions, she was more active, alert, and expressive. Her verbalizations increased significantly, and she was saying discernible words in conjunction with movement ("down") and in anticipation of movement ("ready, set"). She had used no real words before this intervention.

Julia demonstrated increased trunk rotation and a better understanding of forward and backward space; she began to use vision to direct her movements. By the last session, after a total of 6 hours of intervention, she actively sought multiple opportunities for climbing, jumping, and sliding. She was no longer particularly interested in swinging.

SUMMARY

Ayres pointed out the primacy of auditory input to orientation and spatial localization, critical components of an adaptive response. The use of auditory techniques in a sensory integrative framework appears to increase the efficiency and effect of intervention based on the principles of sensory integration theory.

[Editors' note: The use of TL as described here differs from the more familiar use of the phrase "therapeutic listening" as a counseling term used for effective skills in listening to clients' verbal and nonverbal communication.]

Craniosacral Therapy and Myofascial Release

Nancy Lawton-Shirley, OTR

BACKGROUND AND RATIONALE

Craniosacral therapy (CST) and myofascial release (MFR) are manual techniques that use light touch and, at times, light manual traction to facilitate improved fascial mobility, bony alignment, and physiologic functioning. CST and MFR eliminate tightness in the fascial and craniosacral systems. These techniques affect the functional integrity of the body because the fascial and craniosacral systems interact with each other (Fig. 14–5) and with all other systems of the body. Unless craniosacral and myofascial restrictions are addressed, other interventions addressing improved movement may be less effective or have only temporary impact (Barnes, 1999; Lawton-Shirley, 1988; Upledger & Vredevoogd, 1983).

Craniosacral System

The craniosacral system is a separate physiologic system. The anatomical components are:

- The meningeal membrane
- The bony structures to which the meningeal membranes attach (i.e., cranial bones, C_3, C_2, S_2, coccyx)
- The cerebral spinal fluid
- All structures related to the production, absorption, and containment of the cerebral spinal fluid
- Connective tissue related to the meningeal membrane (Upledger & Vredevoogd, 1983). The craniosacral system provides the protective environment for the brain and spinal cord.

Fascial System

The fascial system is a pervasive three-dimensional head-to-foot web that wraps around every muscle fiber, bone, nerve, and blood vessel. Fascia assists the body with metabolism, fluid and lymphatic flow, cellular elimination, respiration, and protection and support of all organs. Half of all muscular attachments are to fascia; this has tremendous implication for muscle strength and mobility.

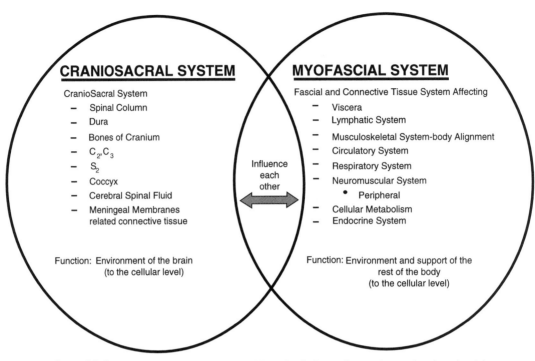

CRANIOSACRAL SYSTEM

CranioSacral System
- — Spinal Column
- — Dura
- — Bones of Cranium
- — C_2, C_3
- — S_2
- — Coccyx
- — Cerebral Spinal Fluid
- — Meningeal Membranes
  related connective tissue

Function: Environment of the brain
(to the cellular level)

Influence
each
other

MYOFASCIAL SYSTEM

Fascial and Connective Tissue System Affecting
- — Viscera
- — Lymphatic System
- — Musculoskeletal System-body Alignment
- — Circulatory System
- — Respiratory System
- — Neuromuscular System
  - • Peripheral
- — Cellular Metabolism
- — Endocrine System

Function: Environment and support of the
rest of the body
(to the cellular level)

■ FIGURE 14-5 Schematic representation of the interaction between the craniosacral and myofascial systems.

DESCRIPTION

CST and MFR involve touch and, at times, gentle manual traction to minimize or eliminate restrictions identified through evaluation. Because they ready the body for optimal response, CST and MFR can be used as preparation for other types of intervention (e.g., sensory integration, NDT, or movement education). They also are easily integrated into tactile and movement activities to help maintain optimal arousal, decrease stress, and facilitate body awareness and postural responses.

RELATIONSHIP TO SENSORY INTEGRATION AND OCCUPATION

Because CST and MFR do not require an adaptive interaction, they are considered to be *outside* sensory integration theory. However, CST and MFR are thought to enhance physical and emotional health, sensory processing, and body alignment and mobility. Thus, these techniques may improve responsiveness to intervention based on the principles of sensory integration theory and

certainly are *complementary* to it (Barnes, 1999; Lawton-Shirley, 1986, 1991; Lawton-Shirley & Wanzek, 1986).

The way in which clients respond to environmental events is influenced by the physical integrity of the body, including the fascial and craniosacral systems. Although CST and MFR do not directly reflect occupation, their indirect contribution to pain-free, effective, and efficient movement and sensorimotor processing may be invaluable. However, because the link between CST and MFR and occupation is indirect, therapists should monitor their connection rather than assuming one will happen.

POPULATIONS FOR WHOM CST AND MFR ARE APPROPRIATE

Because stress can increase tightness in the craniosacral and myofascial systems, most children with physical, emotional, or social challenges may benefit from CST and MFR. Certain conditions seem to place clients at risk for dysfunction in the craniosacral and fascial systems. These include:

- Birth trauma (e.g., C-section, forceps, suction delivery, prolonged labor)
- Traumatic injury (e.g., from car accident or falling)
- Poor postural or joint alignment (e.g., lordosis, scoliosis, neck hyperextension, temporal mandibular joint dysfunction)
- Surgery
- Infection or inflammation (e.g., ear infections, spinal meningitis, chronic respiratory infections)
- Seizure disorders
- Autism
- Attention deficit disorder
- Learning disabilities
- Headaches
- Stress

Identification of clients who would benefit from CST or MFR involves assessment of the fascial and craniosacral system through palpation. Postural analysis also typically is done to identify fascial tightness.

BENEFITS

Arousal and Modulation

CST and MFR facilitate improved autonomic nervous system balance and functioning (Barnes, 1999; Upledger, 1983). Therefore, they indirectly improve the ability to focus and self-regulate. They can help induce a calmer, more organized state as well as clear restrictions that may actually be causing difficulties in arousal, modulation, and self-regulation. These techniques decrease physical and emotional stress and frequently decrease sensory defensive responses.

Improvement in Posture

Postural adaptations to movement and gravity can be restricted by tightness within the fascial system. Because fascia wraps around every fiber, tightness in any area can affect ROM, spontaneous head and trunk righting, rotation, flexion and extension, and fluidity of movement. CST and MFR facilitate bony alignment and mobility (Barnes, 1999; Upledger, 1983). Therefore, freeing the fascial and craniosacral systems from restrictions is vital to postural alignment and fluidity of movement. After restrictions are released, the true status of movement and posture can be

evaluated. These, in turn, result in more appropriate intervention and accelerate responsiveness.

Body Awareness and Neurologic Processes

Proprioceptive receptors are located within connective tissue. Furthermore, the craniosacral system provides the environment for the brain and spinal cord. Thus, connective tissue tightness or craniosacral restrictions potentially interfere with body awareness and perception and neurologic functioning (Lawton-Shirley, 1986, 1991).

Health

Because the craniosacral and fascial systems so profoundly affect all other body systems, they can have an impact on health. Commonly, clients report fewer illnesses (e.g., ear infections, respiratory infections) after administration of these techniques.

Respiration

CST and MFR techniques are effective *before* facilitation of respiration and suck-swallow-breathe synchrony because tightness in the connective tissue supporting the cranium, hyoid, neck, shoulder girdle, rib cage, and pelvis can directly affect these functions. After restrictions are released, the true status of respiration and suck-swallow-breathe synchrony can be assessed and residual difficulties treated with other techniques.

Social and Emotional Development

Because gentle, noninvasive CST and MFR techniques decrease autonomic distress and assist in "rebalancing" the autonomic nervous system (Upledger, 1983), clients have greater capacity for relaxed interaction with family and friends. The physical body stores emotions (Upledger, 1983); by mobilizing the craniosacral and fascial systems, pent-up emotions may be released, thus enhancing emotional health and physical well-being.

Clients who have difficulty meeting challenges presented by everyday life are vulnerable to tremendous stress. Home programs that include CST and MFR techniques can help maintain resilience and eustress within the system. Participation of parents and children in either direct intervention or home program relaxation techniques has a profound affect on healing.

Spiritual Development

Touch applied with respect communicates support for clients' self-healing, interconnectedness, and inner connectedness. Any technique that promotes healing and connectedness potentially promotes spirituality.

TRAINING RECOMMENDED OR REQUIRED

A number of books and chapters (Barnes, 1990, 1999; Boehme, 1991; Manhein & Levitt, 1989; Upledger & Vredevoogd, 1987,1998) address the fundamentals of these approaches. Formal study or

training is necessary to implement these procedures appropriately. Training is available throughout the United States from a variety of sources, including MFR Seminars, 10 South Leopard Road, Suite One, Paoli, PA 19301, and Upledger Institute, 11211 Prosperity Farms Road D325, Palm Beach Gardens, FL 33410-3487; 800-233-5880; *www.upledger.com.*

SUMMARY

CST and MFR can eliminate restrictions that may interfere with development and daily life functioning. Because CST and MFR prepare the body for optimal response, they may enhance the effectiveness of other approaches to intervention. Implementation of occupational or physical therapy *after* CST or MFR is critical for enabling clients to recognize their full benefits.

Environment as a Milieu for Intervention: The Farm

Lois Hickman, MS, OTR, FAOTA

Lynne Harkness, MS, OTR/L

BACKGROUND

Less than 100 years ago, most people in the United States lived on farms or in rural areas in close-knit communities with ample opportunities to be mindful of the natural rhythms inherent to life. Although there are still people living in rural areas, most children in the United States grow up in cities where they may be distant from family,

close-knit communities, and nature. The city environment can have a detrimental effect on growth. As Moore (1996) indicated, "All urban children are at risk to varying degrees. All need access to secure, stimulating outdoor environments where they can discover themselves as individuals and as a community" (p. 75).

Farms involve a way of life for which many people yearn. Awareness of the steady rhythm of the natural world—the seasons and weather, day and night, birth and death, work and play—are fundamental to life on the farm.

Although most therapists do not have access to a working farm, they can use the ideas and principles of the approach described here. Gardens on roofs, in backyards, or in windows can enrich clients' lives and give a stronger sense of connection with the earth and the community. Becoming more "connected" can improve self-awareness, and, in turn, the ability to relate more adeptly with others and in society.

RATIONALE

My (Lois) use of farm-based intervention evolved in stages over several years. I began practicing occupational therapy in hospital and clinical settings with children who had sensory integrative dysfunction. I observed that the children often improved dramatically when they were exposed to natural lighting and other less stressful input and when their families adopted more natural diets. Later, I began to include hippotherapy. Again, I observed that many clients showed dramatic improvement in much less time than they had in more traditional settings. I then began holding intervention sessions on an organic farm and observed many ways in which clients benefited. The farm provided a milieu that promoted responsibility and mindfulness and was a source of natural sensory input and food.

Responsibility for soil, crops, animals, and others promotes growth in children and adults. Through experiences with seeds, plants, and flowers, children can learn language concepts (e.g., light vs. dark, soft vs. hard, rough vs. smooth). They can express their curiosity and awe while watching nature perform its magic (Chamber et al., 1996). Clients can overcome many sensory modulation difficulties by exposure to the predictable, natural experiences provided by animals and "Mother Earth." They also can learn ways to meet physical and intellectual challenges provided by the real-life jobs necessary to daily life on the farm.

DESCRIPTION

We conduct intervention on farms year round, most frequently with children who have sensory integration difficulties. We also conduct a day camp 3 hours a day, 3 days a week for 3 weeks in the summer. Campers' ages range from preschool age through early adolescents.

Two residents live on the farm and work it nearly full time; nearby city dwellers buy annual memberships. In return for their membership fee, they share in the work and the harvest. We conduct intervention sessions during the week when there are fewer people on the farm. The atmosphere is one of openness and acceptance.

Our therapeutic interventions are frequently conducted in partnership with a speech and language pathologist. Clients have the lead in deciding how they want to spend time (e.g., with the animals, dropping sticks in the stream and trying to capture them further downstream, exploring the tree house). Adults model chores and/or activities and invite clients to join. As they become more comfortable, clients become increasingly involved and frequently choose an activity or chore for the day.

Day camp has more planned activities (e.g., games, planting, chores, and lunch). A group consists of seven to 10 children with sensory integration dysfunction or autism. The ratio of campers to therapists is nearly one to one. Children quickly learn the routine. They are always invited and encouraged to try new activities but know that their comfort level for participation will always be respected.

Just as music and story always have been part of the everyday life of "primitive" cultures, intervention on the farm also incorporates music, song, dancing, and storytelling. There are plenty of animals, birds, and nature sounds to emulate. Singing readily contributes to introductions, transitions, describing the steps of a chore, and farewells. Spontaneous songs, sung to a familiar melody but with words that describe what is happening in the moment, become part of the fun and learning.

RELATIONSHIP TO SENSORY INTEGRATION AND OCCUPATION

Individuals with sensory integrative dysfunction may reap many benefits from farm-based intervention. These are addressed, in part, below. Whereas the farm-based intervention is difficult to classify as many of the tasks and activities *overlap* with sensory integration principles, others lie *outside* the realm of sensory integration. Farm-based intervention most directly reflects occupation, a construct much larger than sensory integration. Every aspect of daily life can be addressed in intervention in a farm setting. These include (but are not limited to) activities of daily living, the ability to maintain focus on a task, development of leisure skills and interests, socialization and cooperation, fine and gross motor skills, and tolerance for work and frustration (Mattison, 1992).

POPULATIONS FOR WHOM FARM-BASED INTERVENTION IS APPROPRIATE

Nearly all children and adults, with or without disabilities, can benefit from time spent working and playing on a farm. Intervention goals and strategies are easily tailored to an individual's needs. Although each individual differs, we will discuss some general strategies that reflect common characteristics of several disabling conditions.

By helping to care for farm animals, *children with autism* reach out and relate to other living beings. Some children are drawn first to chickens and later to warmer, "fuzzier" mammals (e.g., rabbits or farm cats). Others are attracted to large, powerful animals (e.g., llamas, horses, or cows), especially if the animals move in slow, nonthreatening ways. By observing the animals to which a child is most drawn, we learn other avenues for relating with that particular child.

Children with learning difficulties, who may find math or reading an almost insurmountable challenge, often enjoy the "real work" of building a nesting box for a mother rabbit. Others, interested in how the farm supports itself, may research the cost of animal feed, seeds, and irrigation water or predict the profit that might be made from farm eggs or produce. For these children, math and reading with a tangible outcome are more engaging than math and reading in the abstract.

Children or adults with sensory modulation disorders get beyond their difficulties when a community goal requires that they confront their fears and aversions. For example, when the goal is to prepare a soil bed for flowers or carrots or brush angora rabbits in order to collect their fur for spinning and weaving, an individual with tac-

tile defensiveness may rise to the challenge. Similarly, an individual with gravitational insecurity may need to climb a ladder to the barn loft to get cartons for gathering eggs or be curious about the tree house. The desire to succeed may provide incentive for overcoming fear of being off the ground.

Individuals who have physical challenges or poor praxis can learn to grade movements by scattering chicken feed gently enough not to startle the chickens or gathering eggs from underneath a hen without disturbing her. They might also learn how to brush rabbits or groom a horse. Individuals with physical challenges can also be invaluable advisors, consulting with the occupational therapy practitioner accessibility issues for everyone. This planning can involve designing trails to various vegetable plots, making greenhouse adaptations, and making animal care possible for ambulatory as well as nonambulatory participants. An individual with a physical disability or an elderly client may gain or regain a sense of self-worth while serving as a consultant or teaching children skills needed to plant, cultivate, or preserve crops or build or repair something needed to keep the farm running smoothly.

BENEFITS

Intervention on an organic farm, with real-life jobs that must be done regularly to keep the land and animals healthy, provides endless opportunities for learning and developing feelings of real accomplishment. Clients benefit in many ways from challenges at various levels and in various areas. Emotionally, there are opportunities to "connect" with farm animals, other clients or campers, staff, and customers. These connections help clients become more aware of their own feelings and presence. Physically, the farm challenges clients' abilities to maneuver around (possibly using a wheelchair or walker), lift, climb, reach, and manage tools. There also are intellectual challenges (e.g., figuring out how much and what kind of food rabbits or chickens need, planning when and how to plant or build). The many textures, noises, and smells of the farm also challenge people who have poor sensory modulation.

Humor and fun are important parts of farm life. Chores offer many humorous situations (e.g., every animal has its own idiosyncrasies) and some frustrations (e.g., gathering the chickens into their coop before a raccoon discovers dinner). The ability to step outside a situation and laugh at oneself can be valuable benefits of such situations when they are handled well by respected adults.

Furthermore, at the same time that individual and farm community goals are being met, the broader community is educated about the benefits of an integrated society. Thus, the benefits of farm-based intervention can be wide reaching.

AN EXAMPLE

Four-year-old Sara was extremely shy and avoided interacting with children and adults other than her family. She had received traditional speech therapy for 2 years, with no change in speech acquisition or ability to relate to others. She attended our farm-based day camp. Child-friendly farm chores were woven into a predictable sequence of activities. Music and singing were used as a way to begin the day, help the children go from one activity to another, and bring closure to therapy sessions. Sara became more engaged and animated every day. By the end of the 3-week camp, she was singing camp songs and talking about her experiences. She maintained the gains she made after camp; Sara continued to respond to the "real life" of the out of doors. Her occupational and speech therapies are now therapeutic horseback riding and farm therapy.

TRAINING RECOMMENDED OR REQUIRED

For information regarding training in horticulture therapy techniques and theory, contact the American Horticultural Therapy Association (AHTA), Center for Horticultural Studies, Attn: Christine Kramer, 909 York St., Denver, CO 80206-3799, e-mail: ahta@ahta.org or *http://www.ahta.org,* phone: (303) 370–8190, fax: (303) 331–5776.

For a Certificate Program: Denver Botanic Gardens Center for Horticultural Studies (AHTA accredited) offers intensive 4- to 5-day courses in a unique format, (9 hours' credit), e-mail info@ahta. org. Another source of information on horticulture therapy is the Virginia Polytechnic Institute and University, Blacksburg, VA, *http://www.hort.vt. edu/human/human.html.*

SUMMARY

When clients are part of a working farm, they are part of a community. The people who work and live on the farm, their friends, and customers who purchase fresh vegetables or eggs all enrich the milieu. Usually, a range of ages and of physical, emotional, and intellectual abilities is represented. Everyone has the opportunity to learn and grow in a natural environment and to attempt tasks that are more threatening in other situations.

Summary and Conclusions

The 10 programs described here represent a sample of the breadth of tools used by occupational therapy practitioners to supplement intervention based on the principles of sensory integration theory. All are alternative or complementary to sensory integration theory; some more closely allied

with it than others. This chapter does not represent an endorsement of any of these programs. Our intent in this chapter is to alert readers to some of the available programs, provide information for learning more about them, and instill in readers an interest in pursuing empirical research in these areas.

References

Wilbarger Approach References

Ayres, A. J. (1972). *Sensory integration and learning disorders.* Los Angeles: Western Psychological Services.

Ayres, A. J. (1979). *Sensory integration and the child.* Los Angeles: Western Psychological Services.

Field, T. M. (1998). Massage therapy effects. *American Psychologist, 53,* 1270–1281.

LeDoux, J. (1996). *The emotional brain: The mysterious underpinnings of emotional life.* New York: Simon & Schuster.

Melzack, R. (1995). Folk medicine and the sensory modulation of pain. In P. D. Wall, & Melzack, R. (Eds.), *Textbook of Pain* (3rd ed., pp. 897–905). New York: Churchill Livingstone.

Oetter, P., Richter, E., & Frick, S. (1995). *MORE: Integrating the mouth with sensory and postural functions* (2nd ed.). Hugo, MN: PDP Press.

Ornstien, R., & Sobel, D. (1987). *The healing brain: Breakthrough discoveries about how the brain keeps us healthy.* New York: Simon & Schuster.

Pert, C. B. (1997). *Molecules of emotion.* New York: Scribner.

Pribram, C. (1991). *Brain and perception: Holonomy and structure in figural processing.* Hillsdale, NJ: Erlbaum.

Wall, P. D., & Melzack, R. (1995). *Textbook of pain* (3rd ed.). New York: Churchill Livingstone.

Wilbarger, P. (1993). *Sensory defensiveness.* Videotape. Hugo, MN: PDP.

Wilbarger, P., & Wilbarger, J. (1991). *Sensory defensiveness in children aged 2–12: An intervention guide for parents and other caregivers.* Denver, CO: Avanti Educational Programs.

Williams, M. S., & Shellenberger, S. (1994). *"How does your engine run?": A leader's guide to the alert program for self-regulation.* Albuquerque, NM: TherapyWorks.

Sensory Diet References

Ayres, A. J. (1972). *Sensory integration and learning disorders.* Los Angeles: Western Psychological Services.

Ayres, A. J. (1979). *Sensory integration and the child.* Los Angeles: Western Psychological Services.

Cermak, S. A., & Daunhauer, L. A. (1997). Sensory processing in the post-institutionalized child. *American Journal of Occupational Therapy, 51,* 500–507.

Field, T. (1995). *Touch in early development.* Hillsdale, NJ: Lawrence Erlbaum.

Field, T. M. (1998). Massage therapy effects. *American Psychologist, 53,* 1270–1281.

Goldberger, L. (1993). Sensory deprivation and overload. In L. Goldberger & S. Breznitz (Eds.), *Handbook of stress: Theoretical and clinical aspects.* New York: Free Press.

Greenough, W. T., & Black, J. E. (1992). Induction of brain structures by experience: Substrates for cognitive development. In M. R. Gunnar & C A. Nelson (Eds.), *Developmental behavioral neuroscience* (Vol. 24, pp. 155–200). Hillsdale, NJ: Lawrence Erlbaum.

Greenough, W. T., Black, J. E., & Wallace, C. S. (1987). Experience and the brain. *Child Development, 58,* 539–559.

Kandel, E. R., Schwartz, J. H., & Jessel, T. M. (Eds.). (1991). *Principles of neural science* (3rd ed.). Norwalk, CT: Appleton & Lange.

Morgan, W. P. (Ed.). (1997). *Physical activity and mental heath. Series in health psychology and behavioral medicine.* Washington, D.C.: Taylor & Francis.

Oetter, P., Richter, E., & Frick, S. (1995). *MORE: Integrating the mouth with sensory and postural functions* (2nd ed.). Hugo, MN: PDP Press.

Ornstien, R., & Sobel, D. (1987). *The healing brain: Breakthrough discoveries about how the brain keeps us healthy.* New York: Simon & Schuster.

Rood, M. (1962). The use of sensory receptors to activate, facilitate and inhibit motor response, autonomic and somatic in developmental sequence. In C. Satterly (Ed.), *Approaches to treatment of patients with neuromuscular dysfunction.* Third International Congress, World Federation of Occupational Therapy. Dubuque, IA: William Brown Group.

Schanberg, S. M., & Field, T. M. (1988). Sensory deprivation stress and supplemental stimulation in the rat pup and preterm human neonate. *Child Development, 58,* 1431–1447.

Sime, W. (1991). Tactile defensiveness: Treatment for developmentally disabled adults. Master's Thesis, Colorado State University, Fort Collins.

Wilbarger, P. (1984). Planning a "sensory diet": Application of sensory processing theory during the first year of life. *Zero to Three, 5,* 7–12.

Wilbarger, P. (1995). The sensory diet: Activity programs based on sensory processing theory. *Sensory Integration Special Interest Section Newsletter.* Rockville, MD: American Occupational Therapy Association, *18(2),* 1–4.

Wilbarger, P., & Wilbarger, J. (1991). *Sensory defensiveness in children aged 2–12: An intervention guide for parents and other caretakers.* Denver, CO: Avanti Educational Programs.

Williams, M. S., & Shellenberger, S. (1994). *"How does your engine run?": A leader's guide to the alert program for self-regulation.* Albuquerque, NM: TherapyWorks.

Zuckerman, M. (1994). *Behavioral expression and biosocial basis of sensation seeking.* Cambridge, UK: Cambridge University.

Alert Program References

Stevens Dominguez, M., Oetter, P., & Westby, C. (1996). *Through shared windows: A training model for the application of the performance competence model*. Albuquerque, NM: University of New Mexico.

Wilbarger, P., & Wilbarger, J. L. (1991). *Sensory defensiveness in children aged 2–12: An intervention guide for parents and other caretakers.* Denver: Avanti Educational Programs.

Williams, M. S., & Shellenberger, S. (1994). *"How does your engine run?": A leader's guide to the alert program for self-regulation.* Albuquerque, NM: TherapyWorks.

Alert Program Recommended Readings

Ayres, A. J. (1979). *SI and the child.* Los Angeles: Western Psychological Services.

Trott, M. C., Laurel, M. K., & Windeck, S. L. (1993). *SenseAbilities: Understanding SI.* Tucson, AZ: Therapy Skill Builders.

Water-Based Intervention References

Association of Swimming Therapy. (1992). *Swimming for people with disabilities* (2nd ed.). London: A. & C. Black.

Campion, M. R. (1985). *Hydrotherapy in paediatrics.* London: Wm. Heinemann Medical Books.

Campion, M. R. (1991). Activity in water: A learning experience. *Interlink, 3,* 12.

Water-Based Intervention Recommended Readings

Gjesing, G. (1997, autumn). Water activities: Purposeful therapy for children with special educational needs. *Newsletter of the National Association of Paediatric Occupational Therapists.* London: Oxford Information.

Gjesing, G. (1998, spring). Water-activities as an OT intervention for children (and adults) with physical and/or mental disabilities. *Newsletter of the Aquatic Therapy Network for Occupational Therapists.* Available from A.T. N., 2424 Hirst Terrace, Havertown, PA 19083–1417.

Lepore, M., William, G. G., & Stevens, S. F. (1998). *Adapted aquatics programming: A professional guide,* Champaign, IL: Human Kinetics.

Hippotherapy References

Dertoli, D. (1988). Effect of therapeutic horseback riding on posture in children with cerebral palsy. *Physical Therapy, 68,* 13–22.

Riede, D. (1988). *Physiotherapy on the horse,* Renton, WA: Delta Society.

Volunteer manual (1999). Galveston: Hope Therapy at Moody Gardens

Oculomotor Control References

Bates, W. H. (1986). *The Bates method for better eyesight without glasses.* New York: Holt.

Dennison, P. E., & Dennison, G. E. (1994). *Brain gym* (Revised; Teachers Edition). Ventura, CA: Edu-Kinesthetics.

Moore, J. C. (1994). The Functional Components of the Nervous System: Part I. *Sensory Integration Quarterly, 22,* 1–7.

Scheiman, M. (1997). *Understanding and managing vision deficits.* Thorofare, NJ: Slack.

Sunbeck, D. (1991). *Infinity walk: Preparing your mind to learn.* Rochester, NY: Infinity.

Therapeutic Listening References

Ayres, A. J. (1972). *Sensory integration and learning disorders.* Los Angeles: Western Psychological Services.

Berard, G. (1991). *The sound of a miracle.* Roxbury, CT: Georgiana Institute, Inc.

Berard, G. (1993). *Hearing equals behavior.* New Canaan, CT: Keats.

Frick, S. M., & Lawton-Shirley, N. (December 1994). Auditory integrative training from a sensory integrative perspective. *Sensory Integration Special Interest Section Newsletter.* Rockville, MD: American Occupational Therapy Association, *17,* 1–3.

Kaliher, M. (1998). Therapeutic listening in an academic setting. Master's thesis, Saint Mary's University, Winona, Minnesota.

Morgan Brown, M. (January, 1999). Auditory integration training and autism: two case studies. *British Journal of Occupational Therapy, 62,* 13–16.

Steinbach, I. (1997). *SAMONAS sound therapy.* Kellinghusen, Germany: Techau Verlag.

Tomatis, A. (1993). *The ear and language.* Norval, Ontario: Moulin.

Therapeutic Listening Recommended Reading

Kandel, E., Jessel, T., & Schwartz, J. (1991). *Principles of neural science.* Norwalk, CT: Appleton & Lange.

Madaule, P. (1993). *When listening comes alive: A guide to effective learning and communication.* Norval, Ontario: Moulin

Craniosacral Therapy and Myofascial Release References

Barnes, J. F. (1999). Myofascial release. In W. I. Hammer (Ed.), *Functional soft tissue examination and treatment by manual methods* (2nd ed.). Gaithersburg, MD: Aspen.

Barnes, J. F. (1990). *Myofascial release: The search for excellence,* Paoli, PA: MFR Seminars.

Boehme, R. (1991). *Myofascial release and its application to neuro-developmental treatment.* Milwaukee: Boehme Workshops.

Lawton-Shirley, N. (June 1986). Overarousal problems: A case report. *Sensory Integration Special Interest Section Newsletter.* Rockville, MD: American Occupational Therapy Association, pp. 2, 3, 7.

Lawton-Shirley, N. (September 1991). Craniosacral/myofascial techniques combined with sensory integration for autistic children. *Sensory Integration Special Interest Section Newsletter.* Rockville, MD: American Occupational Therapy Association, pp. 5–6.

Lawton-Shirley, N., & Wanzek, D. (December 3, 1986). With an eclectic approach: Another piece to the puzzle. *Physical Therapy Forum,* pp. 1–3.

Manheim, C. J., & Levitt, D. K. (1989). *CranioSacral therapy and somato-emotional release: The self-healing body.* Thorofare, NJ: Slack.

Upledger, J. (1983). *CranioSacral therapy.* Seattle: Eastland.

Upledger, J., & Vredevoogd, J. (1983). *Craniosacral therapy.* Chicago: Eastland.

Farm-Based Intervention References

Chambers, N. K., Johansson, S., & Walcavage, D. M. (1996). Classroom? Playground? Garden? Or clinic? *Journal of Therapeutic Horticulture, 8,* 83–87.

Mattison, R. H. (1992). Prescribing health benefits through horticultural activities. In D. Relf (Ed.), *The role of horticulture in human well-being and social development.* Portland, OR: Timber.

Moore, R. C. (1996). Compact nature: The role of playing and learning gardens on children's lives. *Journal of Therapeutic Horticulture, 8,* 75–82.

15

Integrating Sensory Integration with Other Approaches to Intervention

Marie E. Anzalone, ScD, OTR, FAOTA

Elizabeth A. Murray, ScD, OTR, FAOTA

> *Integrating: Forming, coordinating, or blending [parts] into a functioning or unified whole.*
> *Eclectic: Selecting what appears to be best in various [but not necessarily compatible] doctrines, methods, or styles.*
>
> —*Merriam-Webster Dictionary (1989)*

Sensory integration theory is one of many models of practice used for planning and implementing intervention with children; it is particularly helpful for understanding *how* children:

- Modulate responses to the environment
- Acquire new skills
- Approach and interact in novel situations

Sensory integration theory also is an approach to intervention that is focused on remediating underlying central nervous system (CNS) processing rather than providing a structured way to teach new skills. However, the leap from improved processing to improved functioning may be rather large. Because our ultimate goal is to improve children's abilities to engage in occupations and participate fully in social and other roles, sensory integration alone may not be adequate to address all the therapeutic goals for a particular child.

To provide a comprehensive intervention program, other theoretical approaches may need to be integrated with sensory integration theory. This chapter discusses some theories and approaches that may supplement sensory integration and illustrate the use of these approaches in the context of intervention with children who have a range of disabilities.

Integrating theoretical frames of reference requires complex clinical reasoning. The goal of this reasoning is to gain a clearer picture of children's strengths and needs within the context of tasks and roles expected of them and roles they assume. To do this, clinicians must understand the postulates, assumptions, and intervention technology associated with selected theories and approaches and be able to combine them without violating their various premises. To use sensory integration theory in conjunction with other theories and approaches, we need to examine their compatibility and the ways in which each can provide insight into clients' unique needs. A truly integrated approach involves thoughtfully combining theories in the service of meaningful goals.

To illustrate an integrated approach, consider Jill, an 8-year-old girl with a learning disability and sensory integrative dysfunction. Her therapist, Linda, developed several goals that reflect improved sensory integration as the targets for direct intervention. These included improving:

- Modulation of tactile and vestibular input
- Postural and ocular responses
- Body scheme and motor planning

Jill's mother was very committed to improving Jill's underlying sensory integrative abilities. However, she was also very concerned about the fact that Jill was excluded from many of the social activities of her peers because she was unable to ride a bike. This inability influenced Jill's self-esteem as well as her participation in age-appropriate occupations and roles. Bike riding was also very important to Jill, but she was very apprehensive about learning how to ride.

In approaching this clinical problem, Linda decided to integrate developmental and coping theories with sensory integration theory. Linda believed that sensory integrative dysfunction was the underlying reason that Jill was unable to ride a bike, but she also realized that bike riding was a valuable "splinter skill." Linda knew that continuing to work on improved sensory integration would likely improve Jill's underlying dysfunction and ultimately lead to improvement in motor skills, but this process was too slow to meet Jill and her mother's immediate concerns. She recognized that there was no conflict in combining sensory integration procedures with teaching specific skills or in using coping theory to help Jill feel more confident in her ability to take risks. These approaches were compatible.

An important factor contributing to profession-als' judgment about the usefulness of a practice theory is its applicability to the various individuals with whom they commonly intervene. Sensory integration theory cannot be applied to everyone; it has boundaries, and we must be careful not to overstep them. For example, children with Down syndrome often have a cluster of symptoms that suggest deficits in processing of vestibular and proprioceptive sensations and limited praxis. However, these symptoms may be a result of actual abnormalities of brain structure or cognitive limitations rather than a problem in sensory processing. Similarly, young children with muscular dystrophy may display difficulty with balance and low muscle tone, but their problem is with the muscles themselves, not with vestibular processing or sensory integration. Children with cognitive limitations may perform poorly on the Sensory Integration and Praxis Tests (SIPT). Their ideation and motor planning skills reflect limited cognitive ability rather than sensory integrative dysfunction. Sensory integrative dysfunction is not the only explanation for behaviors such as poor balance, low muscle tone, poor motor planning, or even decreased SIPT scores.

Social, environmental, and experiential factors may also result in problems similar to sensory integrative dysfunction. For example, children who have been physically or sexually abused may exhibit behaviors similar to tactile defensiveness. However, their avoidance of touch is not a result of an aversive response to *non-aversive touch,* as in the case of a child with sensory modulation problems. Rather, it is a *learned* response to *extremely aversive touch.* When working with children who have experienced abuse, clinicians must be cognizant of the social and emotional factors that contribute to behavior and not limit intervention to sensory symptoms. Sensory integration may provide a way of understanding these children's behaviors and even working with them, but is must be part of a complex intervention plan that involves other professionals and social service agencies.

Although it may be sometimes appropriate to apply concepts derived from sensory integration theory to children whose disabilities are outside its boundaries, that application will require careful thought and an understanding of the limitations of what can be accomplished. For example, children with cognitive limitations may demonstrate tactile defensiveness. In this situation, a therapist could use sensory integration theory to guide aspects of intervention that relate to decreasing the defensiveness while using a more structured learning or developmental approach to address other goals.

A child with low muscle tone and problems with balance, for whatever reason, may benefit from the varied types of movement activities on suspended equipment that challenge balance and require maintenance of a stable posture. Additionally, because the vestibular system has synaptic connections with extensor muscles (especially of the neck and trunk; see Chapter 2), activities that stimulate the vestibular system may help to facilitate these muscles (Blanche, 1998; Kimball, 1999). Sensory integration procedures have the added benefit of being fun; it is easy to use them to capitalize on children's intrinsic motivation. These properties lead to the kind of repetition, variability of practice, and independent problem solving that are required for motor learning (Gentile, in press). However, when we apply sensory integration theory outside its boundaries, we cannot expect to ameliorate underlying brain damage or musculoskeletal abnormalities.

Often, children's difficulties and needs do not fit neatly into any one approach. There are times when we are unsure whether a client's behaviors are the result of sensory integrative dysfunction, other factors, or both sensory integrative dysfunction and other factors.

Evan is a 6-year-old boy who acquired a mild head injury at age 3 years. Recent testing found him to be below average on tests of praxis and of tactile discrimination. Although we might interpret these findings as indicating that Evan had sensory integrative–based dyspraxia, we also consider that his dyspraxia and poor tactile discrimination may be at least partly the result of his head injury. In this situation, we might wish to use sensory integration procedures for a trial period, carefully monitoring Evan's behavior for improvement in motor planning.

PURPOSE AND SCOPE

This chapter briefly reviews several approaches commonly used by occupational therapy practitioners and discusses their compatibility with sensory integration. Through the use of case studies, the chapter demonstrates how sensory integration theory can be combined with these other approaches for children with a wide variety of disabling conditions.

OTHER APPROACHES TO INTERVENTION

The selected theories or approaches fall roughly into four categories:

1. Developmental
2. Sensorimotor
3. Behavioral or learning
4. Coping theory

Because principles of normal development are incorporated into most direct intervention approaches used with children, including sensory integration, we begin with a discussion of developmental approaches. Sensorimotor approaches are often confused with sensory integration; we discuss three different types of sensorimotor intervention: group or protocol-based sensorimotor interventions, neurodevelopmental intervention (NDT), and sensory stimulation. We then describe behavioral or learning theory, a theory that is compatible with sensory integration in some ways and incompatible in others. We show how behavioral (learning) theory is used both to influence the behavior of a client and to teach specific skills. Finally, we discuss coping theory, a way of influencing emotional and adaptive strategies to manage life experiences despite the presence of sensory integrative dysfunction. We have presented only a flavor of these approaches. Readers who are interested in further information are referred to the references at the end of the chapter.

Developmental Approaches to Intervention

The concept of a developmental approach to intervention is fundamental to the practice of many professions. Unlike sensory integration theory, there is no one clearly delineated developmental intervention theory. Rather, there are many principles of typical and atypical development that are the foundation of developmentally appropriate practice. Although we cannot review all of the theories that contribute to the understanding of human development, there are certain shared premises of most developmental theories that are useful in understanding developmentally based intervention (e.g., Blanche, 1998; Fox et al., 1994; Vygotsky, 1978).

Development is a collection of processes (e.g., motor, cognitive, sensory, and psychosocial) that contributes to maturation across domains of function and in occupational performance (e.g., learning, play, self-care). When using a developmental approach, we frame observations and expectations in terms of clients' chronological or developmental abilities. We would not expect a 2-year-old child to engage in the same type of verbal exchange as a 5-year-old child, and we expect a different level of motor competence in a 6-month-old infant than in a 9- or 12-month infant. Similarly, children's development is expressed differently in terms of play and self-care abilities.

Development in different domains follows a relatively predictable (but not invariable) pattern and has its own markers, or "milestones" (e.g., standing, walking, reach, grasp), that serve to denote achievement. Often we use milestones to gauge an individual's progress and to compare a given child's performance with that of same-aged peers or across domains (e.g., fine motor vs. cognitive). Development across domains and participation in occupational behaviors or roles are both complementary and interdependent. Typically developing children acquire a certain competence in various domains before they can perform a particular occupational behavior. For example, children must develop a certain level of fine motor and visual-motor skill before they can self-feed or engage in manipulative play. Conversely, practice of occupational behaviors fosters the acquisition of skills. As children play or feed themselves, fine motor and cognitive skills may be gained.

Sensory integration theory is, in part, a developmental theory. However, when using a "pure" sensory integrative approach to intervention, we do not explicitly target the acquisition of specific skills because the goal is to improve the underlying capacity to interact with the environment. Nonetheless, we must understand children's developmental capacity in order to engage them in therapeutic activities and interactions. Sensory integration theory helps us understand certain aspects of skill acquisition.

Praxis involves conceptualizing, planning, and executing unfamiliar, purposeful actions (Ayres, 1985). As such, it interacts with the changing developmental competence of young children. An act that requires praxis for the 1-year-old child is already learned and relatively automatic in an 18-month-old child. Praxis enables children to acquire developmental motor skills readily; these become the basis for age-appropriate occupations (Schaaf & Anzalone, in press).

Daniel was a 2-year-old boy who enjoyed walking up and down the scooter board ramp, roaming over, and falling on uneven surfaces in the clinic. His grin and consistent repetition indicated that he enjoyed the postural challenges in combination with the tactile and vestibular and proprioceptive sensations from falling and getting up again. For Daniel, this was a developmentally appropriate sensorimotor activity, and his developing ability afforded him with many opportunities to explore the environment and engage in sensory experiences. When Ariana, his 8-year-old sister, entered the clinic, her behavior was very similar to Daniel's. However, Ariana's behavior was not typical of children her age and reflected poor balance and a limited ability to figure out how to interact with objects in the environment. No doubt, Ariana's difficulties affected many aspects of her development.

Understanding the interactions of developmental processes is an important part of evaluation and intervention. Although developmental processes are thought to proceed in a predictable fashion, there are always variations among individuals, or *inter-individual differences.* Equally important are *intra-individual differences,* or differences within an individual in the pattern and the rates of development of various components (e.g., one child may be advanced in gross motor skills but only average in cognitive or language abilities).

Because development is a process, we are interested in not only what skills a child possesses but also how these skills emerge. Vygotsky (1978) introduced the concept of a "*zone of proximal development*" to describe the process of emerging skills. To understand children's performance, it is necessary to observe what they can accomplish independently as well as with the assistance of a more competent partner. Abilities that can be done with assistance are considered to be in the child's zone of proximal development; they are emerging skills.

Neither Annie nor Diane is able to tie shoes independently. However, if Annie's mother gives Annie minimal verbal cues, Annie is able to tie an acceptable bow. Shoe tying, then, is an emerging skill for Annie; it is in her zone of proximal development. Diane, on the other hand, cannot figure out how to tie no matter what kind of assistance her mother provides. Diane is not yet "ready" to tie her shoes.

The zone of proximal development helps determine the tasks children are ready to learn. Developmentally appropriate goals for intervention should be targeted in the zone of proximal development.

Many developmental theorists view change as occurring in successive stages. A stage is a period of development that possesses distinct characteristics that separate it from other developmental periods. In general, stage theorists believe that children must pass through a stage, learning all of the adaptive behaviors inherent in it, before they can move successfully to other stages. For example, in Piaget's (1952) theory, infants must master the behavioral aspects of the sensorimotor period before they enter the stage of preoperational thought. Although most contemporary researchers (e.g., Adolph, 1997) take a more flexible view, stages provide a means for cataloging development and thinking about the successive steps through which children likely progress.

Most contemporary theorists view development as a transaction between children's biological or genetic endowment (i.e., nature) and the particular human and nonhuman environmental experiences (i.e., nurture) to which they have been exposed (Plomin et al., 1988; Sameroff & Chandler, 1975); heredity and the environment complement each other. Furthermore, the individual and the environment change each other. The goal of intervention is to influence development by engaging children in repeated environmental interactions designed to facilitate change. In the course of the interactions, the environment also changes, providing new challenges for children to master. This developmental premise is at the core of sensory integrative theory; through creating sensory rich experiences in a responsive environment, we foster development (Ayres, 1972; Jacobs et al., in press).

Transactions are also at the core of relationships between children and the social environment (Sameroff & Fiese, 1990). Similar to the transaction between biology and experience, social transactions assume a mutual influence between partners. Just as parents' behaviors influence their children, children's behaviors influence parents. This concept is central to developmentally based interventions. If development occurs within the context of relationships, it is essential to include parents in the formulation of goals and the implementation of intervention.

When Franklin arrived home from work, he took Jamal, his infant son, out of his playpen, sat down with him, and bounced him on his knee. Jamal smiled and giggled. Franklin's behavior obviously has had an effect on his son. Jamal also influenced his father, as seen in Franklin's look of delight and his repeating of the activity. Franklin is likely to try this game again when he wants a smile from Jamal. If Jamal had stiffened and cried when he was bounced, his actions might have had a different effect. In a transaction, both partners have the potential to change the behavior of the other; it is not only the adult who influences the child.

Sensorimotor Approaches

The term *sensorimotor* is used widely to refer to many different approaches to intervention that link sensory input to motor performance. In some of these approaches, sensation plays a narrow, controlled role. For example, Rood described ways in which a specific sensory input (e.g., vibration), presented passively, was expected to produce a specific motor output (i.e., contraction of a muscle) (Horak, 1991). The term *sensorimotor* is also used in a more generic way to refer to a class of intervention theories, including sensory integration, that emphasize the role first described by Piaget (1952) of active, experienced-based learning.

Current theorists writing about perception (Adolph, 1997; Gibson, 1988) and motor control (Gentile, in press; Thelen, 1995) have proposed an action system that reflects the unity of sensory input and motor action to respond to relevant environmental factors (goals). The unity of sensory and motor is reflected in observed behavior and reflects the neural processes underlying the action (Latash & Turvey, 1996). Although preceding their explicit articulation in motor control theory, sensory integration theory was firmly based in both of these sensorimotor premises.

Most sensorimotor intervention approaches are based on Piaget's assumption that children learn about their bodies and their environments through sensorimotor exploration. (For an excellent review of Piagetian theory and its relationship to empirical studies and other theories of cognitive development, see Miller, 1993.) Piaget described a sensorimotor period of development that encompassed the first 2 years of life. During that period, infants develop increasingly purposeful and skilled control over their motor systems and their environments.

Infants learn through their interactions with objects and people. A 12-month-old infant may "experiment" with dropping a toy to see how far it goes, what it sounds like, and how her mother reacts as she throws the toy repeatedly. Repetition and slight modifications of the action are important aspects of these "experiments."

Children learn about their bodies through sensory feedback generated by movement. They develop an expanding repertoire of increasingly complex actions that enable them to learn about causality, space, and objects. This interrelationship between sensory input generated through active engagement with the environment and development of skills and knowledge is the foundation of all sensorimotor approaches. Children learn through doing.

Although sensory integration is a sensorimotor approach, not all sensorimotor approaches to intervention can be called sensory integration. Occupational and physical therapy practitioners and physical educators working with school-aged children frequently use sensorimotor approaches; they also are the basis of many community-based toddler exercise programs. Typically, these intervention programs differ from sensory integration in many ways. One of the most fundamental differences is the fact that although sensory integration is individualized and child directed, most other sensorimotor approaches are therapist directed and are often based on a pre-established curriculum such as the Hawaii Early Learning Profile (Furano et al., 1979).

Sensorimotor approaches are often done with a group of children rather than individually. Because they must meet needs of the whole group, activities are highly structured. Thus, intervention based on a sensorimotor approach often lacks the flexibility and spontaneity characteristic of intervention based on sensory integration theory in which the focus is on client-directed activities tailored to individual needs. Finally, although all sensorimotor programs emphasize the sensory component of active gross motor activities, sensory integration is unique in its use of suspended equipment and graded multisensory input.

John propelled himself through an obstacle course during a sensorimotor group led by his teacher, as well as during an intervention session based on the principles of sensory integration theory, conducted by his occupational therapist. In both situations, he benefited from the vestibular and proprioceptive sensations generated from the activity and learned about the spatial properties of the environment. However, there also were differences in John's experiences in the two situations. During his sensorimotor group, John was one of 10 children going through an obstacle course built by the teacher. He did not receive any individualized assistance, but he was able to do it faster with practice. In contrast, during occupational therapy, John

was involved in selecting the activity as well as in building the obstacle course. While building the course, John developed ideation; experienced enhanced proprioception as he moved the different pieces of equipment; and, most importantly, was involved in a creative and intrinsically motivating activity that resulted from a self-generated goal. His therapist, aware of John's poor antigravity extension, prepared him for the demands of the scooter board before his engagement in the obstacle course by introducing activities that involved enhanced vestibular and proprioceptive sensations.

In programs such as *Movement is Fun* (Young & Kepplinger, 1988) and the *Sensory Motor Handbook* (Bissell et al., 1988), the authors have outlined specific activities and classroom modifications useful for therapists integrating sensorimotor intervention into school programs. Both programs also can help teachers integrate sensorimotor experiences into early childhood programs. We emphasize again that these adult-directed group sensorimotor activities, although frequently beneficial, are not sensory integration.

Neurodevelopmental Intervention

Neurodevelopmental intervention (NDT) is a sensorimotor approach based on both neurologic principles and normal development. NDT is an approach to assessment and intervention of motor performance developed by Berta and Karl Bobath, a physiotherapist and physician, respectively. NDT is used widely with clients who have sustained brain damage (e.g., cerebral palsy or cerebrovascular accidents) (Bobath, 1970; Bobath & Bobath, 1972; Finnie, 1997; Schoen & Anderson, 1999). The primary focus of this approach is to improve the quality of posture and movement through providing experiences of "normal" movement. Components of movement central to NDT include:

- Dynamic interplay between stability and mobility
- Postural tone high enough to sustain movement against gravity but low enough to enable smooth, graded movement
- Dissociation of body parts and movement that is free of synergistic patterns
- Freedom of movement in all three planes (i.e., flexion and extension, lateral flexion and extension, and rotation)

- Appropriate postural control (i.e., righting and equilibrium reactions)

Similar to sensory integration, NDT is concerned with the sensory aspects of movement. Direct intervention involves physically handling the client at key points of control. Handling provides a way of teaching clients to move in as normal and efficient a way as possible. An important tenet of NDT is that normal movement both depends on and results in the generation of normal sensory feedback, which becomes the basis of neuronal models to guide future movement (Bly, 1996; Goodwin, 1999). During intervention, the therapist tries to inhibit abnormal muscle tone and movement patterns and facilitate normal movement. The goal of NDT, as contemporary theorists describe it, is to gradually decrease therapist-controlled handling while increasing the active independent movement of the client who is engaged in functional activities. For more information about intervention and assessment from an NDT perspective, see Schoen and Anderson (1999) or Blanche et al. (1995).

Whereas sensory integration theory emphasizes the ability to take in and integrate sensory information and *plan* movement, NDT focuses on the ability to *execute* movements. Thus, these two approaches differ in focus and in the degree of therapist control. Nonetheless, because of its emphasis, NDT provides a useful way of viewing the disordered postural mechanism and awkward movements of clients who have sensory integrative dysfunction, although their problems generally are milder than those of clients with brain damage.

Eric was an 8-year-old boy with sensory integrative dysfunction whose difficulties included poor postural reactions and mild hypotonia. He tended to move without trunk rotation or diagonal weight shifting. His trunk and pelvis were stiff. As a result, he avoided activities that required dynamic postural alignment. The NDT approach helped his therapist describe and understand Eric's postural difficulties.

Eric's intervention was also influenced by his therapist's knowledge of NDT. However, instead of direct physical handling to facilitate weight shifting and trunk rotation (which would have limited Eric's independent exploration), his therapist created activities that demanded fluid postural adjustments. For example, she suggested a game of "dumper cars." Eric climbed up a mountain of uneven pillows to his "car" (a platform swing). After he was on the swing, he attempted to maintain a quadruped position while the therapist tipped the car from side to side. When ready, Eric pressed an "ejection button" and was dumped into the pillows. In order to get out of the pillows, he had to use trunk rotation, diagonal weight shifts, and antigravity flexion. The therapist manipulated the task demands in order to elicit the desired movement patterns. If Eric had not responded with the desired movements, his therapist might have incorporated some minimal handling.

In a complementary fashion, sensory integration theory can help us in our evaluation of children with cerebral palsy. For example, John, a 4-year-old boy with mild spastic diplegia, had difficulty climbing onto a platform swing. When viewing his problems from an NDT perspective, John's therapist assessed the impact of his spasticity on the quality of his movement. She also observed such things as John's ability to shift weight from one leg to the other and maintain his balance while climbing onto the swing. However, as his therapist viewed the same situation from a sensory integrative perspective, she observed for difficulties with motor planning and signs of gravitational insecurity that limited his engagement in gross motor play. Using both lenses simultaneously added to the richness of her assessment and intervention.

Sensory Stimulation

Although not a theory, *per se,* sensory stimulation is a technique that is frequently confused with sensory integration. When I (Marie E. Anzalone) was a new therapist, Karen, a child with cerebral palsy who was on my caseload at a school for children with physical disabilities had "sensory integration" written into her school schedule. She came to occupational therapy every day as soon as she arrived at school and was swung passively on the platform swing for 10 minutes. This period of stimulation was provided regardless of her state of arousal or her desire for vestibular input. Furthermore, it did not involve any active movement or choice on her part; it was passive sensory stimulation.

Swinging could be beneficial for some children with sensory modulation dysfunction as part of a sensory diet (Wilbarger & Wilbarger, 1991; Williams & Shellenberger, 1996), but only if it was individualized to the particular child's unique needs for graded sensory input. Furthermore, unless it was meaningful to Karen and involved active participation (e.g., Karen swinging herself), it would not be sensory integration.

Because sensory integration and sensory stimulation are not synonymous does not mean that sensory stimulation alone is not therapeutic. For months, Sandra began each intervention session pretending she was a "dusty piece of furniture" and requesting a head-to-toe "dusting" with a furry cloth. After this light touch, she was consistently more active and able to direct her play.

Because enhanced sensation may have an effect on modulation, sensory stimulation techniques also are often used with clients who have sensory modulation dysfunctions. With these techniques, clients may demonstrate increased engagement in or focus on tasks at hand, which are thought to mirror changes in arousal in the CNS. The Wilbarger protocol, described in Chapter 14, involves a program of professionally directed intervention in which parents and other caregivers are taught to provide sensory stimulation in order to alter children's state.

Sensory stimulation can be a useful adjunct to intervention based on the principles of sensory integration. However, state changes occur every rapidly. Thus, passive stimulation must be administered cautiously, especially with clients who are known to have poorly modulated responses to their environment (e.g., premature infants, clients with brain damage). Sensory stimulation can have a strong and cumulative effect on the client's autonomic nervous system. If clients are unable to participate actively, it is essential to *observe their responses carefully*. Some autonomic responses that suggest overarousal include:

- Flushing
- Blanching
- Perspiring
- Nausea
- Yawning
- Changes in sleeping or eating patterns
- Significant changes in activity level

Responses to sensory stimulation may not be immediately apparent. Thus, it is important to let parents and other caregivers know when children have received sensory stimulation so that they can look for signs of sensory overload or sensory disorganization.

Sensory stimulation is always provided most effectively in the context of active engagement in meaningful activity. Active involvement helps to mediate sensation in several ways not available when sensation is passively applied. First, active involvement usually involves proprioception that usually has an organizing effect in conjunction with tactile or vestibular input, which may be more arousing. In addition, the integrative effect of being engaged in an intrinsically motivated, goal-directed activity often increases tolerance for sensation and decreases the chances that clients will become overwhelmed. The Alert program (Williams & Shellenberger, 1996) described in Chapter 14 provides numerous examples of strategies in which enhanced sensation can be attained in the context of meaningful daily life activities.

Behavioral or Learning Theory

Behavioral or learning theory is quite different from the other theories and approaches described here. Behavioral theorists believe that all behaviors except for reflexes are learned. According to Skinner (1968), who had a major impact on the development of this theory "extraordinarily subtle and complex properties of behavior . . . may be traced to subtle and complex features of the contingencies of reinforcement which prevail in environment" (p. 62). Thus, the emphasis in behavioral theory is on the impact of specific aspects of the environment on *observable* behavior.

Behavioral theorists do not concern themselves with anything that cannot be observed directly. Unlike in sensory integration and many other practice theories, proponents of behavioral theory make no assumptions about functions of the CNS and no hypotheses about "changing the brain" through intervention. Behavioral theory, then, is concerned with improving specific behaviors or skills, not with remediating underlying dysfunction. In this way, it is quite different from sensory integration theory. However, many aspects of behavioral theory are useful when designing intervention based in the principles of sensory integration. (For a practical reference on the use of behavioral theory, see Krumboltz & Krumboltz, 1972.)

A basic concept of behavioral theory is that of conditioning. There are two types of conditioning, the first of which is *classical* conditioning. An example of classical conditioning can be seen in Michael, a 3-year-old boy with severe tactile defensiveness, who was particularly sensitive to having his feet touched. Michael was not yet walking, and there was concern that he had some abnormality in the muscles or bones of his feet. During a clinic evaluation, the physician, physical therapist, and occupational therapist each removed Michael's shoes to examine his feet and then put them back on. Michael kicked and screamed each time that his feet were handled. For the next several weeks, he screamed any time he saw his shoes and his mother could not put them on him. Apparently, he had been conditioned to associate his shoes with a particularly upsetting experience. Knowledge of tactile defensiveness, combined with a basic understanding of classical conditioning, helped the occupational therapist explain his behavior to Michael's mother. Although Michael's case is an extreme example, children with sensory modulation dysfunctions sometimes develop associations between an activity and the distress or discomfort they feel from sensory experiences.

The second type of conditioning is *operant* conditioning. The concept of operant conditioning is largely a result of the work of Skinner (1968). Whereas classical conditioning emphasizes the importance of the stimulus to behavior, operant conditioning stresses increasing, maintaining, or decreasing a given behavior. Increasing and maintaining behavior are done through the use of reinforcement, either positive or negative. An object, activity, or other stimulus is said to be reinforcing if it strengthens or increases a behavior. Reinforcers or rewards can be anything from food to a smile. A critical component is that the child performs a behavior in order to receive the reward. We assume by the performance that the reward is something the child desires or enjoys. For example, when given a psychological test, Michael initially refused to try any test items. The psychologist gave Michael a sticker and told him he could earn another one by doing the first test item. Michael then engaged in the test. The stickers seemed to reinforce his test-taking behavior.

When increasing a desired behavior, a reward generally is given on a consistent basis. In order to maintain the behavior, however, the reward is given on an intermittent, or inconsistent, basis. Once Michael was consistently engaging in each test item, the psychologist began giving him a sticker after he had performed several items. The stickers were given randomly so that Michael could not predict when he would receive one. Michael continued to try each test item, suggesting that this intermittent pattern of reinforcement was sufficient to maintain his behavior.

There are times when a client's behavior is inappropriate and we would like to decrease it. One method for decreasing an unwanted behavior is to remove any reinforcement observed to be maintaining this behavior. The process of removing a reinforcer is referred to as *extinction.* Often the unwanted behavior has been inadvertently reinforced by our response to it.

Michael frequently drummed his hands on the table or the chair where he was sitting. The behavior interfered with his ability to engage in fine motor activities, and Susan, his occupational therapist, wanted Michael to stop the drumming. At first, she tried telling him to stop each time, but this did not help. In fact, when she timed his drumming over a few sessions, she found that he was drumming more than ever. Although she had not thought that telling Michael to stop would be reinforcing, it appeared to result in an increase in his drumming. Susan then withdrew this reinforcer and no longer commented on Michael's drumming. At the same time, she engaged him in fine motor activities and gave him stickers as he participated in the activity. In this way, she was *reinforcing a behavior that was not compatible* with the one that she wanted to decrease. The combination of not responding to the undesirable behavior and reinforcing a desired but incompatible behavior was an effective combination.

We may use sensory integration theory to identify reinforcers. For example, the psychologist often used a pat on the head or on the back as a reward during testing. Although this might be reinforcing to some children, Michael had tactile defensiveness. Thus, he probably would not have liked being touched, and touching could have lessened his cooperation.

Punishment is another method of decreasing a behavior. When punishment is used, the behavior is paired with a negative consequence. Although the use of punishment may be effective in decreasing dangerous behaviors (e.g., when clients injure themselves or others), it is not the preferred method in most instances (Krumboltz & Krumboltz, 1972; Landers, 1989). However, we should be aware that with children who have sensory integrative dysfunction, some activities that we might assume would be rewarding actually turn out to be punishment. They could actually result in a decrease in a desired behavior, as in the case of using a pat on the head to reward Michael for engaging in test items.

Another technique often used to decrease unwanted behavior is referred to as *time out*. In time out, a client is removed from a situation so that there is no opportunity to receive reinforcement for any behavior; generally, this involves isolation. However, time out is effective only when the activities from which the client is removed are more rewarding than the time-out process itself. For certain clients, time out actually may be reinforcing because it allows them to sit in a quiet place without being disturbed or having demands placed on them. Consequently, some children misbehave *in order to* be placed in time out.

A technique that bears a superficial resemblance to time out is that of providing children who are easily aroused and who have difficulty modulating sensation with a quiet place away from the activities of the classroom. Some children with sensory modulation dysfunction need to have such opportunities available to them in order to decrease the level of sensation.

Another major component of behavioral theory concerns strategies used to teach specific tasks. We often use these strategies when teaching self-care skills. For example, when a child is unable to perform a task, such as zipping his jacket, we might break that task into a sequence of smaller steps. For zipping a jacket these might be:

1. Holding the two bottom sections of the jacket together and approximating the sides of zipper
2. Hooking the two bottom sections of the zipper together
3. Pulling the zipper tab up with one hand while holding the bottom of the jacket with the other hand

These steps are taught in sequence; when the client becomes proficient at one, the next is added. This process is referred to as *chaining*.

According to behavioral theory, a child will learn a sequenced task most efficiently when a reverse or *backward chaining* method is used. The therapist first does the entire task. Then she performs all but the last step, leaving that step for the client. The therapist completes fewer and fewer steps until the client is doing the whole task independently.

Another technique is called *shaping,* in which a desired behavior is obtained through successive approximations. For example, Timmy was unable to fasten the buttons on his shirt. We began by having him practice on a shirt with larger buttonholes. As Timmy became proficient with larger buttons, we decreased the size of the buttons until they were the same as the ones on his own shirt.

In addition to chaining and shaping, prompts are frequently used to aid in skill acquisition. Prompts can be physical (e.g., placing the child's finger on the zipper tab or helping the child pull the zipper) or verbal (e.g., "pull up the zipper"). Demonstration also can be used as a prompt. To promote the ultimate goal of independence, prompts are *faded,* or slowly removed.

Many aspects of an intervention session conducted according to the principles of sensory integration theory could be reframed from the perspective of behavioral theory. Pieces of equipment are chosen partly because clients enjoy them and will be active participants. Equipment is used to make an activity reinforcing and increase the probability that clients continue to perform it. Sometimes children select activities they cannot perform independently. We modify the activity, providing assistance or prompts as needed so that they can succeed. We may grade the activity until clients are able to perform the one they selected initially. In this way, we shape their performance.

Another situation in which we may use behavioral theory is with a child who has difficulty modulating sensory input. We often introduce sensory stimulation (in the context of the activity) very gradually and provide a great amount of reinforcement for tolerating that stimulation. Sometimes a classical conditioning paradigm is used in conjunction with sensory integration. For example, a child with tactile defensiveness who enjoys movement may roll in a barrel lined with various textures. In this situation, a reinforcing activity (i.e., rolling in a barrel) is paired with an aversive activity (i.e., tactile sensation). When enough of these types of activities are presented over a period of time, the aversive quality of tactile sensation may be lessened.

Although it is possible to use principles derived from behavioral theory to interpret intervention sessions based in sensory integration theory, not all aspects of the two theories are compatible. For example, the teaching of specific skills, rather than improving underlying processes, is characteristic of behavioral theory but not of sensory integration theory. However, there are times when it is essential for a child to learn a specific skill, such as zipping a coat or tying shoelaces. Behavioral theory, which provides a wealth of information on teaching skills, would be an appropriate frame of reference to use for this aspect of an intervention program.

Coping Theory

Coping theory is based on cognitive and behavioral theories. Coping is the process of making adaptations to meet personal needs and respond to the demands of the environment. One of the unique aspects of this theory is that it does not presume pathology. Coping occurs in all of us, and the presence of a disability or delay does not necessarily mean that coping will be problematic. In fact, although there may be a higher incidence of poor or inflexible coping skills in children with disabilities, poor coping is by no means inevitable in children with disabilities. Furthermore, typically developing children are not necessarily good at coping (Williamson & Szczepanski, 1999; Zeitlin & Williamson, 1994).

The coping process is initiated either by internal events (e.g., feelings of anger or sadness) or external events (e.g., the school bell ringing or an unexpected touch) that are filtered through values and beliefs. Determining the meaning of an event is the result of this first step of the coping process. Although cognitive, determination of meaning is not a labeling or problem-solving process; rather, it is a subjective appraisal of the event that can trigger a coping effort if the event is determined to be a threat, harm, or challenge (Garmezy & Rutter, 1983; Lazarus & Folkman, 1984, Williamson & Szczepanski, 1999). Only a "stressful" situation (i.e., one that is potentially harmful or that provides an impetus for change or learning) requires a coping response. Thus, stress is not necessarily negative. One common "stressor" that is a powerful motivator for young children is novelty. Children can attribute threat or challenge to a novel object or event. The action plan will depend on the results of that appraisal.

The second step of the coping process, developing an action plan, is based on available internal and external resources. Internal resources lie in the unique style and capacities each individual brings

to the coping process. Some internal resources are learned and age related (e.g., values or developmental skills); others are innate (e.g., temperament or sensory integrative capacities). External resources are found within the physical and social environments; they are both human (i.e., persons who influence and provide feedback on coping efforts) and material or environmental. Material resources are those things that money can buy (e.g., food, shelter, toys, and medical care). Environmental resources are those conditions of the physical environment that can influence development (e.g., the presence of lead paint, the safety of a play space, or levels of chaos in a classroom).

Internal and external resources combine to determine available coping efforts. A 9-month-old infant, curious about the new carton that has appeared in his living room, brings the developmental skills of creeping and discrete manipulation (internal resources) to his exploration. Whereas a younger child is more limited in internal resources, a 5-year-old child brings many skilled motor and cognitive strategies to the exploration and play.

The action plan is implemented in the third step. Coping efforts can be action oriented (i.e., doing something), affective (i.e., managing emotions associated with the stressor), or cognitive (i.e., learning from the triggering event).

The fourth and final step of the coping process is evaluation of the effectiveness of the strategy. Evaluation can take at least two forms, cognitive (i.e., it worked or did not work) or emotional (i.e., it made the client feel more or less stressed). If the coping effort was successful, it resulted in decreased stress and the coping cycle was complete. If the effort was unsuccessful, a new coping effort may be launched.

Using coping theory along with sensory integrative theory is particularly helpful when thinking about the "big picture" of adaptive behavior and occupation. For example, the presence of a sensory modulation dysfunction, such as tactile defensiveness, can create a situation in which a child interprets an external event (e.g., an affectionate hug) as a threat. That child may possess limited internal resources and, therefore, create an action plan that involves avoidance or aggression (e.g., running away or hitting). Finally, if the action plan resulted in a time out or punishment or created chaos and more sensory stimulation, the child's evaluation of that coping effort may reveal increased stress instead of positive feelings.

Intervention based on coping theory is targeted at three broad categories:

1. Modifying demands
2. Enhancing coping resources
3. Providing contingent feedback
   (Williamson & Szczepanski, 1999; Zeitlin & Williamson, 1994)

When modifying demands, the therapist works to provide a better fit between a client's capacity and the demands of the environment. Some examples are to decrease irrelevant stimuli in a classroom for a child with sensory defensiveness or not to grade handwriting on a history paper for a child with dyspraxia and messy handwriting.

Sensory integration theory provides many different strategies for enhancing coping resources. First, improving sensory integrative functioning helps improve clients' internal resources. Sensory integration theory also provides a rationale for changing external resources so they support optimal action plans.

Coping interventions can be used successfully to enable clients with sensory integrative dysfunction deal with daily life events more successfully. Pat, an adult with a sensory modulation dysfunction, had significant anxiety in social situations because of the demands of social interaction and the increased sensory stimulation (e.g., unexpected touch). Through use of cognitive strategies and an explanation of sensory modulation dysfunction, he was able to understand and reinterpret his discomfort in sensory, rather than emotional, terms (step 1) and then develop and carry out a more adaptive action plan (steps 2 and 3). This resulted in a more positive self-concept (step 4) and greater willingness to engage in social interactions.

A COMPREHENSIVE PLAN: INTEGRATING APPROACHES TO INTERVENTION

We develop intervention procedures to meet explicit goals (see Chapter 9). We consider several factors when setting goals. First, goals and objectives reflect the functional needs of the client. Objectives are statements that address functional behaviors that clients need or want to do in order to meet the challenges of daily life. Second, goals reflect the explicit desires of clients and their families and other caregivers. Motivation is essential to goal achievement and motivation is optimal when goals are meaningful. Third, we must know how a client's disability affects goal attainment. Goals must be not only meaningful but also attainable.

Finally, we phrase goals in terms of change for the client, *not* the therapist. Although Susie may need a splint for her hand, ordering or making a splint is not a goal for *her*. It *may* be a means by which the therapist helps Susie to meet the goal of coloring with a crayon. In short, goals and methods should not be confused.

The choices of intervention approaches and types of service delivery (e.g., direct intervention, consultation) are "driven" by the outcomes desired. Knowledge of boundaries, assumptions, and postulates of each of the approaches is essential to decision making. We also consider clients' strengths and needs and the multiple contexts in which they must function. We then apply intervention thoughtfully and effectively. Because one approach to intervention rarely meets all of a client's needs, we advocate for an eclectic approach. However, *eclectic* does not mean *atheoretical;* rather it means an informed and systematic integration of approaches.

Each of the theories discussed provides insight into intervention and assessment. This discussion is by no means comprehensive, but it does indicate that multiple influences may be contained within a comprehensive intervention plan.

Case Stories

The following case examples illustrate ways in which sensory integration theory can be integrated systematically with other approaches to intervention. Because it is important to understand the implications of specific diagnoses when developing and implementing integrated plans for intervention, we have included clients with diagnoses commonly seen by occupational therapy practitioners. We use these diagnoses not because a diagnosis provides all that needs to be known about any client but because it provides a baseline for expected behavior; the picture is refined as a part of assessment. We open each case with a brief discussion of the application of sensory integration theory to individuals with the diagnosis represented. We begin with a child who has learning disabilities because it was for such children that sensory integration theory was initially developed (Ayres, 1972).

▪ JULIA: COMBINING SENSORY INTEGRATION WITH SENSORIMOTOR AND COPING APPROACHES FOR A CHILD WHO HAS LEARNING DISABILITIES

In IDEA-97 (Individuals with Disabilities Education Act Amendments of 1997), specific learning disability is defined as " . . . a disorder in one or more of the basic psychological processes involved in understanding or in using language, spoken or written, that may manifest itself in an imperfect ability to listen, think, speak, read, write, spell, or do mathematical calculations" (Individuals with Disabilities Education Act of 1997, 1997). A learning disability is not the result of primary visual or hearing loss, motor disability, cognitive limitation, or lack of learning opportunities. Many disorders may occur together with learning disabilities; these include attention deficit disorder with or without hyperactivity (American Psychiatric Association, 1994; DSM IV), motor impairment or clumsiness, and sensory integrative dysfunction.

Learning disabilities may affect much more than an individual's performance at school or at work. They often affect self-esteem, locus of control, socialization, play, vocational choice, and activities of daily living (see Levine, 1987, or Culbertson, 1998, for a comprehensive review). Optimal intervention for clients with learning disabilities involves a comprehensive team of professionals and caregivers, including educators, psychologists, speech and language pathologists, physicians, occupational therapy practitioners, and parents or loved ones. An occupational therapy practitioner's assessment and intervention with clients who have learning disabilities should address not only sensory integrative dysfunction but also any components relevant to educational or psychosocial function within the scope of traditional occupational therapy practice (AOTA, 1999).

Although children with learning disabilities may be seen frequently in practices that specialize in sensory integration, each child presents unique challenges. Julia illustrated the complexity of problems associated with learning disabilities.

Julia was an independent 7-year-old child with a learning disability. She was included in a first-grade classroom but received daily special education help for math and reading. She had been seeing an occupational therapist once a week for direct intervention based on the principles of sensory integration theory.

Julia's learning disabilities were not apparent until she entered kindergarten, when her teacher reported that she had difficulty remaining seated during group activities and was struggling with pre-academic skills (e.g., basic shape and letter recognition, cutting with scissors, drawing). She resisted participating in gross and fine motor activities.

Julia repeated kindergarten but continued to have difficulty with attention and academic readiness. Because of her continued difficulty, she was evaluated by the school psychologist, who found that Julia had average intelligence but performed much better on verbal than nonverbal tasks. This discrepancy between verbal and performance IQ is commonly seen in children with learning disabilities and sensory integration deficits. The psychologist recommended that Julia be evaluated by an occupational therapist to help clarify her problems.

The results of Julia's occupational therapy evaluation revealed sensory integrative–based dyspraxia with particular problems in processing tactile and vestibular and proprioceptive sensations. Interviews with Julia's parents and teachers, as well as classroom observations, revealed that Julia also had tactile defensiveness. She tended to respond to her sensory modulation and praxis problems with either avoidant or rigid, controlling behaviors. Direct intervention was recommended and implemented. General goals for occupational therapy included:

- Improve body scheme to support motor planning
- Improve practic abilities so that Julia would be involved more actively in complex gross and fine motor activities
- Decrease tactile defensiveness, which was thought to be contributing to Julia's difficulty maintaining her attention during group activities
- Increase Julia's flexibility during unstructured activities

Sensory integration was the primary theoretical framework used in Julia's direct intervention. Each session began with tactile and proprioceptive activities. Julia especially enjoyed being in charge of her explorations in the intervention room. She quickly fell into a comfortable routine, with most of her time spent repeating familiar activities (her favorite was a three-part obstacle course). Julia performed this activity successfully but with minimal flexibility and creativity.

Ginny, the occupational therapist, introduced change gradually by modifying the environment. For example, a large ramp would "appear" in the middle of Julia's obstacle course, or a swing that was used every week was no longer available but a similar one, which required more motor planning, took its place.

Initially, modifications triggered refusals and sometimes tantrums. But as Julia developed more trust in Ginny and became more confident in her explorations, Ginny was able to introduce more complex tasks and problem solving into the obstacle courses. Julia also became more involved in the actual building of the course, which added the need for ideation and planning. Moving equipment added proprioceptive sensation, and the fact that the plan was Julia's idea capitalized on her intrinsic motivation.

Julia's initial inflexibility during intervention sessions was characteristic of her behavior at home and school. Her parents described her as controlling and prone to temper tantrums. Similar to many children with sensory integrative dysfunction, Julia was unable to deal with unexpected aspects of social relationships, daily activities, or any demanding motor task. Her coping strategies were ineffective.

Direct intervention based on the principles of sensory integration theory does help children deal more flexibly with sensory and motor challenges, both in the clinic and in daily life. However, Ginny felt that Julia would benefit from direct intervention to improve her coping abilities (e.g., rehearsal, cognitive problem solving) as well.

Eventually, Ginny paired Julia with another child, Morgan; this increased Julia's need for effective coping strategies but also provided considerable support. Julia and Ginny spent some time during intervention explicitly discussing and evaluating Julia's coping efforts and making plans for similar daily life situations. During one session, Julia disagreed with Morgan about how to build an obstacle course. She had difficulty sharing and negotiating. She coped by withdrawing and refusing to try the course after it was built. That session provided an opportunity for specific problem solving and discussion using "STOP," a coping technique (i.e., "*S*top what I am doing, *T*ake a look back to see what has happened, look at my *O*ptions, and *P*lay back a different way of behaving") (Williamson & Szczepanski, 1999, p. 465).

After the problem-solving session, both Julia and Morgan came up with some alternative strategies for their shared task, and the session ended with both feeling better about themselves. Another important part of the intervention plan was consultation with Julia's teacher and parents to ensure carryover of external support for Julia's new coping strategies.

Although Julia was clearly demonstrating progress in her motor planning abilities, she continued to return to familiar activities whenever a new child was in the intervention area or she encountered a difficult challenge. One activity that she returned to frequently was the Pogo Ball, a ball with a Saturn-like ring around it that Julia could stand on and use to bounce herself across the room. Playing with the Pogo Ball is very difficult and requires good balance. In order to succeed at using the Pogo Ball, Julia spent days practicing at home; she was very proud of her accomplishment.

Because Julia's competence on the Pogo Ball was so well learned, it no longer required much praxis; rather, it was a valuable *sensorimotor* experience that provided enhanced proprioception. It represented such an accomplishment, so it also contributed to Julia's self-esteem.

Because of Julia's consistent need to "show off" when other children were around, Ginny believed that Julia would benefit from group sensorimotor activities in which she could improve her skills and demonstrate her accomplishments to her peers. Rather than give up Julia's individual occupational therapy sessions, Ginny referred her to adaptive physical education for an additional group experience. Julia's parents and teacher agreed, recognizing this as an opportunity for Julia to improve both her social and motor skills. Ginny met with the adaptive physical education teacher to provide information about Julia's psychosocial and coping needs.

All aspects of Julia's programming seemed to contribute to her growing self-esteem and improved willingness to try new motor activities. Julia's classroom teacher noticed improvements in Julia's ability to pay attention. She also reported that Julia had befriended another child in the adaptive physical education group. Julia's mother reported that the most significant changes she noticed were Julia's increased willingness to accept help when approaching new challenges and an increased flexibility when dealing with changes in her daily routine.

■ Robbie and David: Combining Sensory Integration with Neurodevelopmental Intervention for Children Who Have Cerebral Palsy

Cerebral palsy is a disorder of movement caused by nonprogressive brain damage. The damage occurs at or soon after birth before development of the brain is completed. The types of motor deficits seen in children with cerebral palsy are variable and range from asymmetry in hand use to complete inability to control movement. Although the most noticeable problem in children with cerebral palsy is motor incoordination, the brain damage may be widespread and result in other associated deficits including language delays, cognitive impairments, or seizure disorders (Dabney et al., 1997; Davis, 1997).

Some children who have cerebral palsy seem to have difficulty performing academic and self-care skills beyond that which can be accounted for by either their motor deficit or cognitive status alone. The specific cause of these functional deficits is unknown; it is likely that there are many. However, these sorts of difficulties are sometimes reminiscent, both in type and in quality, of those seen in children who have sensory integrative–based dyspraxia.

Some children who have cerebral palsy seem to have a fear of movement (i.e., gravitational insecurity) that is out of proportion to their motor deficits (Fisher & Bundy, 1989). Some have also been described as having tactile defensiveness (Blanche et al., 1995; De-

Gangi, 1990). The sensory processing and motor planning deficits seen in individuals with cerebral palsy may be the result of the underlying neurologic lesion. However, the presence of gravitational insecurity and tactile defensiveness suggests that some children may have sensory integrative dysfunction *in addition* to their primary motor deficit. Whether these deficits truly are independent of the cerebral palsy or are a result of brain damage or experiential factors (e.g., avoidance of movement because of poor postural reactions or tactile intolerance because of discomfort with the handling) is not known. However, the symptoms of the dysfunction are sometimes lessened in response to intervention based on the principles of sensory integration theory.

Both Robbie and David were 7-year-old boys with moderate spastic diplegia. Their motor deficits and general developmental levels were about the same, but their functional abilities were quite different. Both were able to walk with crutches; both had the lower extremity spasticity, poor postural reactions, and mildly delayed fine motor abilities typical of diplegia. Intelligence was within normal limits in both boys, and both of them were included in first-grade classrooms.

Both Robbie and David had received occupational and physical therapy services in school since they were quite young. The focus of their intervention had been on improving motor functioning; NDT provided the framework.

Although the boys had many similarities, Robbie was much more successful than David in performing the functional tasks expected of 7-year-old children. In fact, Pam, the boys' occupational therapist, decided to discontinue Robbie's direct intervention. Pam's evaluation revealed that Robbie had no difficulty keeping up in his classroom, at home, or when playing with his many able-bodied friends. His ability to keep up with his friends, despite his obvious physical limitations, constantly amazed observers. Pam continued to provide consultation as needed to Robbie's parents, classroom teacher, and physical therapist.

David, in contrast, had a great deal of difficulty performing the tasks expected of him in school and at home. David's teacher described him as disorganized and distractible. His attention span was limited. David was unable to do many things for which his motor skills were more than adequate. Tasks such as putting on and fastening his jacket, organizing his room, following simple two- to three-step commands, and getting himself ready for school in the morning sometimes seemed insurmountable.

During free play, David tended to watch the other children, initiating interactions only with adults. His play, similar to his schoolwork, was disorganized and lacked spontaneity. He seemed to have difficulty figuring out what to do and did not seem to be aware of his body (i.e., he had a poor body schema). David's poor body schema

is consistent with current research that documents decreased sensory awareness of movement in children with cerebral palsy (e.g., Goodwin, 1999). He spent most of his playtime engaged in a limited repertoire of familiar, solitary activities. Many of these descriptors of David's difficulties are reminiscent of children who have developmental dyspraxia (see Chapter 3).

David also showed evidence of gravitational insecurity. He demonstrated exaggerated fearfulness whenever his balance was challenged in any way, and he disliked having his head out of an upright position (see Chapter 4). His fear of movement during therapy often led to increased postural fixation and spasticity rather than righting and equilibrium reactions. His progress in occupational and physical therapy was slow because of his fear.

Unlike Robbie, David did need ongoing direct occupational therapy. Because of the nature of David's deficits, Pam planned to incorporate sensory integration theory as well as NDT into intervention. Her general goals for intervention were to decrease his gravitational insecurity and improve his motor planning ability. She worked closely with David's physical therapist to inform him of her use of sensory integration and obtain feedback regarding its effectiveness.

In planning intervention, Pam wanted to ensure that David not only increased his tolerance of movement and improved his motor planning but that he also continued to improve the quality of his movements. Therefore, she prepared David using NDT techniques to decrease fixation and abnormal movements and facilitate weight shifting, equilibrium, and fluid movements. Opportunities for enhanced linear vestibular sensation were integrated into intervention very slowly. The first piece of equipment Pam chose was the bolster swing, which ensured good postural alignment (i.e., hip abduction and a wide base of support for sitting) and allowed him to be in control of the duration and speed of movement because his feet were on the floor. The swing provided linear vestibular sensation that was not frightening but instead challenged his righting and equilibrium reactions (see also Fisher & Bundy, 1989). Initially, Pam sat behind David, providing pelvic support, facilitating weight shifting and righting reactions, and grading the postural demands. She was especially aware of David's weak abdominal musculature, so she carefully graded the amount of backward displacement to ensure that he would not lose his balance. Pam's proximity on the swing also decreased David's fear.

As David's fearfulness decreased, Pam introduced more motor planning demands. For example, she placed large cardboard blocks on uneven surfaces throughout the clinic. After David collected them, he used them to build a tower that he knocked over while swinging on the bolster swing. This activity demanded both motor planning and postural adjustments. Initially, Pam needed to facilitate some of David's movements over the uneven surfaces. Gradually, however, David mastered the postural demands, and he needed less handling. Pam began to incorporate into her intervention activities that demanded trunk rotation, controlled movement into flexion and extension, equilibrium reactions, and bilateral coordination.

Close monitoring of David's responses was important to prevent increased tone resulting from overstimulation or increased effort. When tone increased, Pam decreased the demands and incorporated handling, firm touch pressure, and slow rocking to help David organize himself. Sometimes she modified equipment to ensure that David maintained good body positions (e.g., providing lumbar support while his was on the bolster).

David's physical therapist noted changes beginning about 1 month after Pam began using sensory integration. David was much less fearful and stiff and began to move in rotary patterns. In addition, David's mother reported that his ability to organize and perform self-care tasks had improved.

■ CARLOS: COMBINING SENSORY INTEGRATION WITH A DEVELOPMENT APPROACH FOR AN INFANT AT RISK

The number of infants at risk for significant developmental dysfunction is increasing as medical science has begun to keep younger, smaller, and sicker infants alive. The "cost" of these medical advances to a premature infant's developing CNS is, as yet, unknown (Blackburn, 1995; Hack et al., 1995). In addition to the increasing numbers of premature infants who survive, there has also been an increase in the number of full-term infants who have experienced circumstances that may compromise their development (e.g., prenatal drug exposure) (Lester et al., 1995).

Infants whose early histories or whose social or environmental situations have placed them at risk for developmental, learning, or emotional problems are considered to be "high-risk" infants. Although they are at risk, many do not manifest persistent developmental deficits. Nonetheless, a number of sequelae to prematurity and other conditions associated with risk in infancy are commonly described in the experimental literature. A full review of this literature is well beyond the scope of this chapter, but these infants do have some behaviors that are relevant to sensory integration theory (see Hack et al., 1995, for an excellent review).

Als (1986) described the task of early infancy as balancing approach and avoidance responses to the environment. Her description is reminiscent of Ayres's

(1972) concept of organizing sensory input for use. Both involve analysis of environmental demands and the ability to organize a response to them. Both view self-regulation that comes from sensory modulation as a desired response to stimulation.

Some of the behaviors that "preemies" and other high-risk infants exhibit that are consistent with sensory integrative dysfunction include:

- Poorly modulated state behavior
- Slow processing of sensory information
- Disorganized or avoidant exploratory behavior
- Mild motor problems

Many high-risk infants are easily overaroused, do not have effective ways to calm themselves (e.g., sucking or turning away), and have prolonged autonomic effects when overstressed by events or people. Although biological factors account for some of these findings, others likely reflect an interaction between biological and environmental risk factors (e.g., socioeconomic status, parental education, community and cultural values, family support) (Sameroff & Chandler, 1975).

The application of sensory integration theory to high-risk infants presents many unique challenges and opportunities. First, the fragility of infants and young children, coupled with their resiliency and rapid physical maturation, presents an opportunity for developmental neurologic change unmatched in any other stage of life. Second, the dynamic interaction between children's experiences and developmental maturation creates an exceptional opportunity to shape future capabilities. These future capabilities are influenced by the outcomes of sensory integrative functioning: praxis and modulation.

Carlos is, in many ways typical of children born prematurely with some complicating environmental challenges. Carlos was born at 28 weeks of gestation and weighed just over 1000 grams. Severe respiratory disease, which required hospitalization for 125 days, complicated his perinatal course. His home situation was unstable, and his young, single mother had a limited support system and meager financial resources.

Carlos was initially evaluated at 6 months. Because he was born 2 months prematurely, his age was "adjusted" to 4 months. His evaluation revealed hypertonicity with delayed onset of head control and persistent scapular retraction. However, by 7 months' adjusted age, his neurodevelopmental evaluation was normal, and his development was in the low-average range on the Bayley Scales of Infant Development (Bayley, 1993). Carlos' mother, Anita, was given a home program of developmentally appropriate play experiences, but no direct intervention was recommended.

Carlos was next evaluated at 15 months' adjusted age. At that time, he was extremely active and distractible. He had difficulty attending to activities for more than a few seconds. Anita was frustrated in her attempts to manage Carlos' activity and disorganization. She also reported that his sleep patterns were inconsistent and that there were many struggles around bedtime and naptime. Developmental evaluation revealed delays in both mental and motor areas. Carlos did not yet stand or walk. Although his fine motor skills were age appropriate, he did not seem to be interested in manipulating toys. His play consisted of picking up objects, briefly looking, mouthing, and dropping them.

When not sitting on his mother's lap, Carlos spent most of his time in disorganized, nondirected movement, seldom pausing for exploration or manipulation. Additional discussion with Anita and observations of Carlos suggested that he might be gravitationally insecure. Anita reported that Carlos cried whenever she or his grandfather tried to engage him in roughhouse play or tickling. Anita indicated that Carlos seemed afraid when he sat independently on a mattress or other unstable surface.

Anita was dealing with a variety of personal and financial stresses. Consequently, she had particular difficulty dealing with Carlos' disorganized behavior. Although Anita was concerned about Carlos' development, her most immediate need was for assistance in managing his behavior. Leslie, his occupational therapist, and Anita set two general goals for Carlos:

1. Decrease his arousal and increase the organization of his approach to his environment
2. Improve his motor and adaptive skills, especially during play

Because it is not unusual for children who are born prematurely to have difficulty with state regulation, Leslie was not surprised to see this problem in Carlos. She believed, however, that his high level of arousal and decreased organization were contributing to the delays in his development of motor skills. She believed that his overarousal also might contribute to his general sensory defensiveness and gravitational insecurity. Finally, Carlos' disorganized behavior certainly made parenting difficult.

Leslie's intervention with Carlos continued to be based on her understanding of development, but she integrated that understanding with her knowledge of sensory integration. Sensory integration theory helped her teach Anita how and why he became disorganized; it also helped Leslie and Anita to create a better fit between Carlos and his environment. They identified spaces and times that were too stimulating for him at home and in daycare as well as activities and places that were consistently enjoyable and organizing. Carlos needed more calming and organizing sensory inputs, a less distracting environment, and more regularity in his schedule. Deep pressure, calming music, and quiet nesting places were effective for promoting organization. Much intervention with children as young as Car-

los is done effectively by influencing the child's physical and social environments instead of through direct intervention (see Schaaf & Anzalone, in press). Carlos enjoyed being brushed with a surgical scrub brush followed by joint compression, so Leslie taught Anita to do this procedure frequently, particularly before transitions (Wilbarger & Wilbarger, 1991) (see Chapter 14).

Leslie did provide some direct intervention with Carlos, but his mother was always present, and, whenever possible, Anita was the primary person interacting with Carlos. Developmental approaches provided a framework for understanding what was an adaptive behavior for Carlos. Sensory integration theory helped her manage his regulation of arousal and attention and increase his participation in adaptive behaviors.

Leslie wanted to create calming and organizing activities. To do this, she provided proprioceptive input through resistive activities (e.g., pushing a heavy ball to his mother and crawling up a slight incline). Leslie gradually added a vestibular component to the activities when she rode with him on the glider and, finally, introduced the "frog" (see Chapter 11). With children Carlos' age, vestibular input is most often provided through postural challenges rather than through the use of suspended equipment. Children younger than age 2 years can be very easily overstimulated, so swings should be used cautiously, if at all.

As Carlos' arousal decreased to a more optimal level, Leslie and Anita found it easier to engage him in play. Before each session, Leslie reorganized the intervention area to minimize distractions, and she always made sure there was a quiet nesting space (e.g., a barrel or a pile of pillows) that Carlos could go to "cool down" if he was getting too excited. Using toys that Carlos enjoyed, she and his mother used developmental theory and modeling to guide his play, allowing him to set the pace. With this approach, Leslie and Anita saw significant improvement in Carlos' organization and planning of motor activities.

As Carlos became less distractible and more organized, Leslie was able to introduce some structured fine motor activities after the gross motor or sensory integrative activities. Leslie began the manipulative play in a small, quiet area to minimize distractions. She used "responsive" toys, such as the busy box, which require little persistence or skill. Gradually, Carlos became increasingly capable of independent and creative interaction with more complex toys. Eventually, Leslie and Anita introduced form boards and stacking rings into the more distracting environments of the gross motor room and home.

After 6 months of intervention, Anita seemed comfortable managing Carlos' behavior. Carlos, although still highly active, was more directed in his play. His fine motor skills were still slightly delayed, but he was walking and his gross motor and language were developmentally appropriate. Carlos' direct intervention was discontinued, but Leslie continued to consult with Anita monthly to monitor his progress and sensory diet.

■ ADAM: COMBINING SENSORY INTEGRATION WITH BEHAVIORAL THEORY FOR A CHILD WITH MILD COGNITIVE LIMITATIONS

Many children and adults who have cognitive limitations show symptoms suggestive of sensory processing problems (e.g., low muscle tone, defensive reactions to sensory input). In some instances, symptoms *may,* in fact, be a result of sensory integrative deficits. However, we must consider the probability of other causes for these symptoms.

Nonetheless, even when symptoms may also be caused by frank CNS damage or anomaly, incorporating activities based on sensory integration theory into intervention may be appropriate. Sensory integration theory is particularly helpful for addressing sensory defensiveness, gravitational insecurity, and motor planning that seems more impaired than is expected in an individual of that *developmental age.* We always bear in mind, however, that sensory integration theory was developed to explain hypothesized *dysfunction* in the CNS. When there is known suspected brain *damage,* as in many instances of cognitive impairment, the theory may be stretched beyond its boundaries. Certainly, we do not expect to eliminate brain damage or anomaly.

Adam was a 13-year-old boy with mild cognitive limitations of unknown etiology. He had been enrolled in programs for children with special needs since he was 5 years old. Adam was a delightful, interactive young boy who enjoyed the company of both adults and other children. Recent testing indicated that language and academic skills were at the level of a 7- to 9-year-old child. Adam's family recently had moved, and Adam had begun attending a new school. He was referred to Charlotte, the school's occupational therapist, for an assessment to help in planning his program.

Adam's occupational therapy evaluation consisted of interviews with his mother and teacher to obtain information on his daily living skills and behavior, as well as indications of defensive reactions to sensation. Adam was also observed in his classroom. Additionally, Charlotte administered portions of the Bruininks-Oseretsky Test of Motor Proficiency (Bruininks, 1978) and clinical observations of vestibular and proprioceptive sensations.

Charlotte's assessment of Adam revealed several indicators of possible problems with integrating vestibular and proprioceptive sensations. His muscle tone appeared to be low, and he could not assume a prone extension position. His equilibrium reactions were poor for his developmental level, and his performance on the balance subtest of the Bruininks-Oseretksy Test was similar to that of a 5-year-old child. Adam's teacher observed that Adam frequently appeared to be tired. When standing in line, he slouched. When sitting at his desk, he leaned on an elbow, held his head in his hand, or put his head down altogether. Reminders to "sit up straight" didn't seem to help.

Although recognizing that there could be many causes for these difficulties, Charlotte believed that processing of vestibular and proprioceptive sensations was a problem for Adam. Regardless of the underlying cause, Charlotte was concerned that Adam's low muscle tone and poor equilibrium reactions were having an impact on his classroom performance.

Adam also showed evidence of dyspraxia, which seemed to interfere with fine motor tasks. Despite his higher language and academic abilities, Adam's performance on the fine motor portion of the Bruininks-Oseretsky Test was at 4-year-old level. He was unable to figure out how to cut with scissors. His pencil grasp was immature and, although he had learned to write his first name, he had extreme difficulty copying other letters, even those he could name. Although Charlotte expected that Adam's motor planning abilities would be below the norm for his chronological age, she noted that his skills also were well below his cognitive abilities. Further compounding Adam's problem was his sitting posture during these fine motor tasks. He usually leaned on both elbows and sometimes put his head down, making performance far more difficult.

Of even greater concern was the fact that Adam still could not manage fasteners on his clothing. His mother noted that Adam's fingers "don't seem to work quite right" and that it was far easier to assist him with his clothes than to make him struggle with dressing independently. His teacher was concerned because Adam could not manage his clothing in the bathroom. His classroom was in a junior high, and the other boys teased him in the bathroom.

Together with his teacher and mother, Charlotte formulated two general goals for Adam. Their highest priority was for Adam to dress independently, including managing fasteners. Charlotte recognized that Adam's difficulty with this might be caused by dyspraxia, but she also realized that it was imperative for Adam to learn these specific skills as quickly as possible. Part of her therapy program, then, consisted of teaching Adam to zip and button the fasteners on his pants. She used behavioral theory to break the task down into small, sequenced steps. To teach these skills to Adam, Charlotte used a backward chaining procedure; initially, she performed all the steps. Then she left the last step for

Adam to do. As he mastered that step, she added the steps in reverse order until he was able to fasten his pants independently. Charlotte had frequent contact with Adam's mother and teacher so they could carry out the same program. As Adam mastered one specific self-help skill, Charlotte developed a teaching program for another.

The second general goal for Adam was to improve his posture when sitting. Because she believed his low muscle tone and poor proximal stability might be caused by a disorder in processing vestibular and proprioceptive sensations, Charlotte decided to try a program using sensory integration procedures to meet this goal. This portion of direct intervention included activities that emphasized enhanced linear vestibular and proprioceptive sensations incorporated into a variety of activities that required tonic holding against resistance. Charlotte checked with Adam's teacher on a regular basis to see if his posture in the classroom was showing any improvement.

Initially, Charlotte decided to use the sensory integration procedures for the first part of each session and to end with the quieter training activity. In this way, she thought that she would be able to ensure sending Adam back to his classroom quiet and calm. However, within a few weeks, the teacher reported that Adam came back saying he "hated" occupational therapy and that it was boring. Charlotte also noted that although Adam was cooperative for the portion of the session using sensory integration procedures, he was becoming more and more resistant to practicing self-help skills. At times, he refused to get off the equipment or tried to "trick" Charlotte into some other activity.

Realizing that learning to fasten his pants was essential but apparently not very immediately rewarding to Adam, Charlotte turned again to behavioral theory. She began each session with the less appealing task (from Adam's perspective), using the "fun" portion of the session as a reward. Charlotte also made a chart for Adam, which she hung on the wall in the intervention room, so Adam could see the progress he was making on these tasks. With these changes in the sessions, Adam's attitude became much more positive.

As Adam mastered specific self-help skills and his posture began to show improvement, Charlotte discontinued direct intervention. She consulted with the teacher to develop approaches that could be used in the classroom to improve his handwriting; she also suggested that he learn to use the computer for written work. Charlotte helped Adam's adaptive physical education teacher incorporate into his program activities requiring organizing and sequencing of movements. Although she was not intervening directly with Adam, she remained an important member of the team, contributing to the development of his educational goals and objectives and helping his parents and teachers de-

velop strategies that would enable Adam to benefit fully from his educational program.

■ ANDY: COMBINING SENSORY INTEGRATION WITH SENSORY STIMULATION AND BEHAVIORAL THEORY FOR A CHILD WITH AUTISM

Although autism was once thought to be a psychiatric disturbance (e.g., Bettelheim, 1959), it now is associated with neurologic impairment (Waterhouse et al., 1996). Developmental abnormalities of cell structure have been found in both the cerebellum and limbic regions of the brain (Bauman & Kemper, 1985; Kemper & Bauman, 1993), and structural neuroimaging studies have provided support for these findings (Abell et al., 1999; Courschene, 1997).

Research has indicated that a majority of children and adults with autism display unusual responses to sensory input (O'Neill & Jones, 1997), and some authors have suggested that sensory disturbances are a primary deficit underlying autism (Grandin, 1995; Ornitz, 1989; Williams, 1992). Temple Grandin (Grandin, 1995; Grandin & Scariano, 1986), a woman with autism, described herself as overreactive to many sensations, particularly sound, light touch, and movement. However, she craved deep pressure.

The results of a study using the Sensory Profile (Dunn, 1999) suggested that the sensory processing skills in children with autism are different from those of typical children (Kientz & Dunn, 1997). Children with autism tended to be hyperreactive to touch, although their reactions to sounds varied (hyporeactive to some; hyperreactive to others). Additionally, they had increased craving and toleration for rapid movement. Retrospective videotape analysis of children with autism has shown that the appearance of sensory-related symptoms can predate the actual diagnosis by as much as 2 years (Adrien et al., 1993; Williams, 1992). Given the hypothesized role of the limbic system in sensory modulation dysfunctions, it is not surprising that this is one area of the brain in which abnormalities have been found in individuals with autism (see Chapter 4).

Although sensory integrative procedures may be appropriate for those who display problems with sensory modulation, autism is associated with brain abnormalities, not merely with dysfunction. However, sensory integration theory can assist us in addressing the affective reactions to sensory inputs often seen in these clients; it is often mentioned as a worthwhile approach as a part of an overall program (Dalldorf, 1997; Donnelly, 1996).

A great deal of research supports the use of behavioral techniques with children with cognitive limitations and autism. One intervention that has received recent attention is intensive behavioral intervention or discrete trial therapy. Intensive behavioral intervention applies the principles of operant conditioning to learning skills, which are broken into small attainable tasks. This form of intervention, as developed by Lovaas and his associates (Lovaas, 1987, 1993; McEachin et al., 1993) is ideally conducted on a one-to-one basis 30 to 40 hours a week. According to Lovaas and his associates, intervention is most effective if begun by age 3 years. Lovaas (1987) and McEachin et al. (1993) found that children with autism who participated in an intensive behavioral intervention program were later placed in less restrictive school programs and achieved higher IQ scores than did children in a control group.

Certainly, almost any intensive, highly structured intervention would be expected to result in improvement in targeted areas. However, as Mesibov (1993) pointed out, some might jump to the incorrect conclusion that these children have been "cured." He and others have raised concerns that the claims for intensive behavioral intervention are not substantiated by research. For example, no measures have been taken of important skills such as social interaction, conceptual abilities, and social communication, which are important features of autism (Gresham & MacMillan, 1998; Mesibov, 1993).

As Donnelly (1996) points out, although behavioral methods should be a part of most programs for children with autism, the structured training model of Lovaas "does not take into account sensory problems that may underlie the unusual behaviors and communication" (p. 2). Behavioral techniques are only one intervention tool; others include social integration and sensory integration (Donnelly, 1996).

Lovaas and his colleagues have observed that their intervention was not as effective for children for whom autism was not the sole diagnosis. Children with severe cognitive limitations and autistic features showed improvement only in expressive speech (Smith et al., 1997). Children in the original study who were later discovered to have Rett syndrome did not benefit significantly from the program (Smith, Klevstrand, & Lovaas, 1996).

Three-year-old Andy was quite a handful. He seemed to be constantly "on the go," climbing on furniture and counters, pulling things off shelves, and running around aimlessly. He did not seem to hear his parents when they told him to stop and he became very upset, attempting to kick and bite, if either of them tried to restrain him. At first, his parents thought that Andy did not hear them, but it was obvious that he heard other sounds. In fact, he became quite upset when he heard the vacuum cleaner, responding by holding his ears and screaming. The sound of a lawn mower provoked a similar reaction, and often one parent would take him for a ride in the car while the other mowed the lawn.

Andy loved watching television and could repeat several commercials verbatim. But despite his ability to repeat what he heard, he did not use language spontaneously. Andy never asked for a snack or toy. If he did not want to do something, he screamed, but he never said, "No." In fact, he really did not interact with his parents much at all.

One of Andy's favorite activities was going to the playground. He could swing for hours, and his favorite ride was the merry-go-round. Noting his love of spinning, his parents bought him a Sit'n'Spin on which he could spin himself. This activity kept him busy and "out of trouble," for at least part of the day.

In general, toys did not interest Andy. However, he did have a large collection of Matchbox cars that his grandparents had bought him. He kept them on a shelf in his room, periodically taking them down and lining them up. He always lined them up in the same order, and he always placed them back on the shelf in that order. Once when he came into the room after his mother had taken the cars off and was dusting the shelf, he began to scream, evidently distraught that the cars had been moved. From then on, Andy's mother dusted the shelf only when Andy was occupied in another activity.

Mealtime was particularly difficult for Andy and his family. As an infant, he had not been a fussy eater. However, he resisted the transition to solid foods. He did not like food that was either too hot or too cold, and he tolerated only smooth-textured foods.

Getting Andy dressed and undressed also presented problems. He did not like being touched and tried to pull away from his parents when they attempted to dress him. Clothes had to be washed several times before he would wear them.

At their wits' end, Andy's parents turned to their pediatrician. He, in turn, referred Andy to a child neurologist and to his local school system for an evaluation and a program. Andy's evaluation team members found it impossible to use standardized tests. They relied heavily on their own observations as well as on those of Andy's parents. They believed that Andy's greatest problems were his total lack of language use for communication with others and his limited social interactions. In contrast, Andy's gross motor skills and visual-motor skills seemed age appropriate.

Mike, the occupational therapist, noted many indicators of sensory defensiveness, including Andy's resistance to being handled and his food and clothing preferences. His overreaction to noises and craving of movement also suggested that Andy had difficulty modulating sensation.

After reviewing the results of the evaluation and examining Andy, the neurologist diagnosed him as having autism. Andy was enrolled in a special needs program that included occupational therapy services. Mike, who was the occupational therapist for this classroom, was very concerned about the effects that Andy's sensory defensiveness had on Andy and his family. Together with Andy's parents and teacher, Mike formulated a general goal that Andy become more tolerant of being touched and that he become willing to eat a greater variety of foods.

Although Mike used his knowledge of sensory integration theory to help him frame Andy's problems, he was well aware that sensory integration was not the total answer to Andy's difficulties. Given the severity of Andy's problems and his lack of interaction with others, Mike also saw the need to use behavioral principles in direct intervention and when consulting with Andy's parents and teacher.

Mike knew that activities that provided deep pressure might reduce sensory defensiveness and that slow movement and neutral warmth might also be helpful. However, Andy avoided these types of activities, preferring rapid movement. Accordingly, Mike paired activities providing rapid movement with firm touch pressure and neutral warmth. The movement served as a reward for Andy's tolerating other sensory inputs.

Andy enjoyed swinging. A toddler swing with back and side supports was suspended from a hook in the ceiling of the therapy room. The swing was placed so that Andy's feet could not reach the floor; thus, he had to depend on Mike to push him. Mike sat in front of Andy and swung him by pushing on his legs.

Very gradually, over a period of weeks, Mike was able to hold Andy's legs and apply deep touch pressure for a few seconds before pushing him. Mike also placed a blanket in the swing and began to wrap Andy in the blanket as he swung, combining the movement with neutral warmth and deep pressure. In a similar manner, Mike adapted various other movement activities to pair them with tactile sensation.

In addition to intervening directly with Andy, Mike regularly consulted with Andy's teacher and parents. Andy's classroom was small and uncluttered, with only three other students in the room. Andy's teacher was careful not to touch him unexpectedly and watched to make sure the other children did not touch him. Andy seemed particularly fond of a large beanbag chair. By placing heavy pillows on top of him when he was in this chair, the teacher was able to provide him with deep pressure at various times during the day. Andy's tolerance for deep pressure increased over the months, and his teacher thought that he seemed calmer after spending time in the chair.

At Mike's suggestion, Andy's parents dressed him in sweatsuits. Andy seemed to like their softness, and they were easy for his parents to put on and take off. They also bought a beanbag chair for his room and had him sit in it for dressing and undressing. In response to the routine, he became somewhat more tolerant of handling.

Mike began Andy's feeding program by learning from Andy's parents about the foods he liked. Andy tolerated mashed potatoes, strained vegetables, and smooth soups (e.g., tomato), but his favorite foods were strained fruits that were both smooth and sweet. During the next several months, Mike and Andy's teacher and parents worked on increasing Andy's tolerance for textures. They rewarded him for eating a textured food by giving him a spoonful of fruit. They also began mixing lumpy fruits together with the strained fruit, gradually increasing the ratio of lumpy to strained.

By the end of 6 months, Andy was easier to manage at home, although he still was quite active and intolerant of change. He ate a wider variety of foods, and mealtime was not as stressful for Andy or his parents.

In school, Andy now followed the classroom routine. Although he tolerated being handled only for brief periods, his teachers believed he could begin toilet training. More importantly, Andy's parents and teacher reported that they better understood Andy's behaviors. Based on this understanding, which came in part from Mike's simple explanations of sensory integration theory, they developed new and more effective strategies for parenting and teaching Andy.

SUMMARY AND CONCLUSIONS

We have presented an introduction to the ways that sensory integration theory can be combined with other theories and approaches used to meet the needs of children. Evaluation and intervention are *always* based on the *functioning needs* of the client, not on any one theoretical approach. Meeting these needs requires knowledge, flexibility, creativity, collaborative team efforts, and access to a range of intervention approaches and strategies.

References

Abell, F., Krams, M., Ashburner, J., Passingham, R., Friston, K., Frackowiak, R., Happe, F., Frith, C., & Frith, U. (1999). The neuroanatomy of autism: A voxel-based whole brain analysis of structural scans. *NeuroReport, 10,* 1647–1651.

Adolph, K. E. (1997). Learning in the development of infant locomotion. *Monographs of the Society for Research in Child Development. 62,* 1–140.

Adrien, J. L., Lenoir, P., Marineau, J., Perrot, A., Hameury, L., Larmande, C., & Sauvage, D. (1993). Blind ratings of early symptoms of autism based upon family home movies. *Journal of the American Academy of Child and Adolescent Psychiatry, 32,* 617–626.

Als, H. (1986). A synactive model of neonatal behavioral organization: Framework for the assessment of neurobehavioral development in the premature infant and for support of infants and parents in the neonatal intensive care environment. *Physical and Occupational Therapy in Pediatrics, 6,* 3–53.

American Occupational Therapy Association (1999). The guide to occupational therapy practice. *American Journal of Occupational Therapy, 53,* 251–261.

American Psychiatric Association (1994). *Diagnostic and statistical manual of mental disorders* (4th ed.). Washington, DC: Author

Ayres, A. J. (1972). *Sensory integration and learning disorders.* Los Angeles: Western Psychological Services.

Ayres, A. J. (1985). *Developmental dyspraxia and adult onset apraxia.* Torrance, CA: Sensory Integration International.

Ayres, A. J., & Tickle, L. S. (1980). Hyper-responsivity to touch and vestibular stimuli as a predictor of positive response to sensory integration procedures by autistic children. *American Journal of Occupational Therapy, 34,* 375–380.

Bauman, M. L., & Kemper, T. L. (1985). Histoanatomic observations of the brain in early infantile autism. *Neurology, 35,* 866–874.

Bayley, N. (1993). *The Bayley scales of infant development* (2nd ed.). San Antonio, TX: The Psychological Corporation.

Bettelheim, B. (1959). Feral children and autistic children. *American Journal of Sociology, 64,* 455–467.

Bissell, J., Fisher, J., Owens, C., & Polcyn, P. (1988). *Sensory motor handbook: A guide for implementing and modifying activities in the classroom.* Torrance, CA: Sensory Integration International.

Blackburn, S. (1995). Problems of preterm infants after discharge. *Journal of Obstetric, Gynecologic, and Neonatal Nursing, 24,* 49.

Blanche, E. I. (1998). Intervention for motor control and movement organization disorders. In Case-Smith, J. (Ed.), *Pediatric occupational therapy and early intervention* (2nd ed., pp. 255–276). Boston: Butterworth-Heinemann.

Blanche, E. I., Botticelli, T. M., Hallway, M. K. (1995). *Combining neuro-developmental treatment and sensory integration principles: An approach to pediatric therapy.* San Antonio, TX: Therapy Skill Builders.

Bly, L. (September/October 1996). What is the role of sensation in motor learning? What is the role of feedback and feedforward? *NDT Network Newsletter.*

Bobath, B. (1970). *Adult hemiplegia: Evaluation and treatment.* London: William Heinemann Medical Books.

Bobath, K., & Bobath, B. (1972). Cerebral palsy. In P. H. Pearson (Ed.), *Physical therapy services in the developmental disabilities* (pp. 31–186). Springfield, IL: Charles C. Thomas.

Bruininks, R. H. (1978). *Bruininks-Oseretsky Test of Motor Proficiency.* Circle Pines, MN: American Guidance Service.

Courchesne, E. (1997). Brainstem, cerebellar, and limbic neuroanatomical abnormalities in autism. *Current Opinion in Neurobiology, 7,* 269–278.

Culbertson, J. L. (1998). Learning disabilities. In T. H. Ollendick & M. Hersen (Eds.), *Handbook of child psychopathology* (3rd ed., pp. 117–156). New York: Plenum.

Dabney, K. W., Lipton, G. E., & Miller, F. (1997). Cerebral palsy. *Current Opinion in Pediatrics, 9,* 81–88.

Dalldorf, J. S. (Feb 7, 1997). *A pediatric view of the treatment options for the autistic syndrome,* [URL: http://www.unc.edu/depts/teacch/treatmnt.htm] [1999, June 20].

Davis, D. W. (1997). Review of cerebral palsy, Part 1: Description, incidence, and etiology. *Neonatal Network, 16,* 7–12.

De Gangi, G. (1990, March). Perspectives on the integration of neurodevelopment treatment and sensory integrative therapy: Part 2. *NDTA Newsletter,* 1 and 6.

Donnelly, J. A. (1996). The pros and cons of discrete trial training: Is the "Lovaas" behavior modification method appropriate for my student? *ACCESS Express, 4,* 1–2.

Dunn, W. (1999). *Sensory Profile.* San Antonio: Therapy Skill Builders.

Finnie, N. R., (1997). *Handling the young child with cerebral palsy at home* (3rd ed.). Boston: Butterworth & Heineman.

Fisher, A. G., & Bundy, A. C. (1989). Vestibular stimulation in the treatment of postural and related disorders. In O. D. Payton, R. P. DiFabio, S. V. Paris, E. J. Protas, & A. F. VanSant (Eds.), *Manual of physical therapy techniques* (pp. 239–258). New York: Churchill Livingstone.

Fox, L., Hanline, M. F., Vail, C. O., & Galant, K. R. (1994). Developmentally appropriate practice: Applications for young children with disabilities. *Journal of Early Intervention, 18,* 243–257.

Furuno, S., O'Reilly, K. A., Hosaka, C. M., Inatsuka, T. T., Allman, T. L., & Zeisloft, B. (1979). *The Hawaii early learning profile.* Palos Alto, CA: Vort.

Garmezy, N., & Rutter, M. (Eds.) (1983). *Stress, coping, and development in children.* New York: McGraw-Hill.

Gentile, A. M. (2000). Skill acquisition: Action, movement and neuromotor processes. In Carr & Shepard (Eds.), *Movement Science: Foundation for physical therapy in rehabilitation* (2nd ed.). Rockville, MD: Aspen.

Gibson, E. J. (1988). Exploratory behavior in the development of perceiving, acting and the acquiring of knowledge. *Annual Review of Psychology, 39,* 1–41.

Goodwin, A. W. (1999). Sensorimotor coordination in cerebral palsy. *Lancet, 353,* 2090–2091.

Grandin, T. (1995). How people with autism think. In G. B. Mesibov (Ed.), *Learning and cognition in autism. Current issues in autism* (pp. 137–156). New York: Plenum.

Grandin, T., & Scariano, M. M. (1986). *Emergence labeled autistic*. New York: Warner.

Gresham, F. M., & MacMillan, D. L. (1998). Early intervention project: Can its claims be substantiated and its effects replicated? *Journal of Autism and Developmental Disorders, 28,* 5–12.

Hack, M., Klein, N. K., & Taylor, G. (1995). Long-term developmental outcomes of low birth weight infants. *The Future of Children, 5,* 176–196.

Horak, F. B. (1991). Assumptions underlying motor control for neurologic rehabilitation. In M. Lister (Ed.), *Foundation for physical therapy, contemporary management of motor control problems: Proceedings of the II Step Conference* (pp. 11–27). Alexandria, VA: Foundation for Physical Therapy.

Individuals with Disabilities Education Act Amendments of 1997, 40 U.S.C. § 1400 et seq.

Jacobs, S. E., Schneider, M. L., Kraemer, G. W. (in press). Environment, neuroplasticity and attachment: Implications for sensory integration. In E. Blanche, R. C. Schaaf, & S. Smith Roley, (Eds.), *Understanding the nature of sensory integration with diverse populations*. San Antonio, TX: Therapy Skill Builders.

Kemper, T. L., & Bauman, M. L. (1993). The contribution of neuropathologic studies to the understanding of autism. *Neurological Clinics, 11,* 175–187.

Kientz, M. A., & Dunn, W. (1997). A comparison of the performance of children with and without autism on the sensory profile. *American Journal of Occupational Therapy, 51,* 530–537.

Kimball, J. (1999). Sensory integration frame of references: Theoretical base, function/dysfunction continua, and guide to evaluation. In J. Hinojosa & P. Kramer (Eds.), *Frames of reference for pediatric occupational therapy* (2nd ed., pp. 119–168). Philadelphia: Lippincott, Williams & Wilkins.

Krumboltz, J. D., & Krumboltz, H. B. (1972). *Changing children's behavior*. Englewood Cliffs, NJ: Prentice Hall.

Landers, S. (June 1989). Skinner joins aversives debate. *Monitor,* 22–23.

Latash, M. L., & Turvey, M. T. (1996). *Dexterity and its development*. Hillsdale, NY: Erlbaum.

Lazarus, R., & Folkman, S. (1984). *Stress, appraisal, and coping*. New York: Springer.

Lester, B. M., Freier, K. & LaGasse, L. (1995). Prenatal cocaine exposure and child outcome: What do we really know. In M. Lewis & M. Bendersky (Eds.), *Mothers, babies, and cocaine: The role of toxins in development* (pp. 19–40). Hillsdale, NJ: Erlbaum.

Levine, M. D. (1987). *Developmental variation and learning disorders*. Cambridge, MA: Educators Publishing Service.

Lovaas, O. I. (1987). Behavioral treatment and normal educational and intellectual functioning in young autistic children. *Journal of Consulting and Clinical Psychology, 55,* 3–9.

Lovaas, O. I. (1993). The development of a treatment-research project for developmentally disabled and autistic children. *Journal of Applied Behavioral Analysis, 26,* 617–630.

McEachin, J. J., Smith, T., & Lovaas, O. I. (1993). Long-term outcome for children with autism who received early intensive behavioral treatment. *American Journal on Mental Retardation, 97,* 359–372.

Merriam-Webster's collegiate dictionary (9th ed.). (1989). New York: Merriam-Webster.

Mesibov, G. (1993). Treatment outcome is encouraging. *American Journal on Mental Retardation, 97,* 379–380.

Miller, P. H. (1993). *Theories of developmental psychology*. New York: W.H. Freeman and Company.

O'Neill, M., & Jones, R. S. P. (1997). Sensory-perceptual abnormalities in autism: A case for more research? *Journal of Autism and Developmental Disorders, 27,* 283–293.

Ornitz, E. M. (1989). Autism at the interface between sensory processing and information processing. In G. Dawson (Ed.), *Autism: Nature, diagnosis, and treatment* (pp. 174–207). New York: Guilford Press.

Piaget, J. (1952). *The origins of intelligence in children*. New York: W. W. Norton.

Plomin, R., DeFries, J. C., & Fulder, D. W. (1988). *Nature and nurture during infancy and early childhood*. New York: Cambridge University.

Sameroff, A., & Chandler, M. (1975). Reproductive risk and the continuum of caretaker casualty. In F. Horowitz (Ed.), *Review of child development research* (Vol. 4). Chicago: University of Chicago.

Sameroff, A. J., & Fiese, B. H. (1990). Transactional regulation and early intervention. In S. J. Meisels and J. P. Shonkoff (Eds.), *Handbook of early childhood intervention* (pp. 119–149). New York: Cambridge University Press.

Schaaf, R. C., & Anzalone, M. E. (in press). Sensory integration with high risk infants and young children. In S. Smith-Roley, E. Blanche, & R. Schaaf (Eds.), *Understanding the nature of sensory integration with diverse populations*. San Antonio, TX: Therapy Skill Builders.

Schoen, S. A., & Anderson, J. (1999). Neurodevelopmental frame of reference. In J. Hinojosa & P. Kramer (Eds.), *Frames of reference for pediatric occupational therapy* (2nd ed., pp. 83–118). Philadelphia: Lippincott, Williams & Wilkins.

Skinner, B. F. (1968). *The technology of teaching*. New York: Meredith.

Smith, T., Eikeseth, S., Klevstrand, M., & Lovaas, O. I. (1997). Intensive behavioral treatment for preschoolers with severe mental retardations and pervasive developmental disorder. *American Journal on Mental Retardation, 102,* 238–249.

Smith, T., Klevstrand, M., & Lovaas, O. I. (1996). Behavioral treatment of Rett's disorder: Ineffectiveness in three cases. *American Journal on Mental Retardation, 100,* 317–322.

Thelen, E. (1995). Motor development: A new synthesis. *American Psychologist, 50,* 79–95.

Vygotsky, L. S. (1978). *Mind in society: The development of higher psychological processes.* Cambridge, MA: Harvard University.

Waterhouse, L., Fein, D., & Modahl, C. (1996). Neurofunctional mechanisms in autism. *Psychological Review, 103,* 457–489.

Wilbarger, P., & Wilbarger, J. L. (1991). *Sensory defensiveness in children aged 2–12: An intervention guide for parents and other caretakers.* Santa Barbara, CA: Avanti Education Programs.

Williams, D. (1992). *Nobody nowhere.* New York: Avon.

Williams, M. S., & Shellenberger, S. (1996). *"How does your engine run?": A leaders guide to the Alert Program for Self-Regulation.* Albuquerque, NM: TherapyWorks, Inc.

Williamson, G. G., & Szczepanski, M. (1999). Coping frame of reference. In J. Hinojosa & P. Kramer (Eds.), *Frames of reference for pediatric occupational therapy* (2nd ed., pp. 401–430). Philadelphia: Lippincott, Williams & Wilkins.

Young, S. B., & Keplinger, L. (1988). *Movement is fun: A preschool program.* Torrance, CA: Sensory Integration International.

Zeitlin, S., & Williamson, G. G. (1994). *Coping in young children: Early intervention practices to enhance adaptive behavior and resilience,* Baltimore: Paul H. Brookes.

PART III

Focus on Research and Occupation

Advances in Sensory Integration Research

Shelley Mulligan PhD, OTR

Sensory integration theory, which was derived primarily from the fields of medicine, neurology, and child development, attempts to explain relationships among neurologic processes and overt behaviors (Ayres, 1972b). Sensory integration theory aims to increase our understanding of underlying causes of the behavioral difficulties, motor difficulties, and learning problems of some children. As a frame of reference, sensory integration acts as a bridge between theory and clinical practice by providing a set of guidelines for evaluation and intervention. These guidelines are integral tools for promoting research.

Sensory integration has been the subject of more research than any other approach or frame of reference within the field of occupational therapy (Miller & Kinnealey, 1993; Parham & Mailloux, 2001). For many years, it has been one of the most frequently applied frames of reference used by pediatric occupational therapists. Despite this popularity, the research to date has not clearly established professional consensus with respect to the simple question: Is sensory integration intervention effective?

Sensory integration has been criticized, particularly in the educational literature, where its effectiveness has been dismissed by many researchers (e.g., Hoehn & Baumeister, 1994). Scientific legitimacy for this approach has, therefore, not yet been established.

PURPOSE AND SCOPE

The purpose of this chapter is to examine the validity of sensory integration, both as a theory and a frame of reference. To accomplish this task, we review and synthesize the most recent literature (from approximately 1986 to 2000) from both basic and applied methods of scientific inquiry. We also discuss ways in which practitioners who select sensory integration as an intervention approach may apply this research. We conclude by suggesting directions for future research for establishing professional consensus both within and outside occupational therapy regarding the validity of sensory integration theory and its application as an intervention approach.

RESEARCH EXAMINING THE VALIDITY OF SENSORY INTEGRATION

Validation of sensory integration theory involves the integration of information and knowledge from both basic and applied methods of scientific inquiry. Basic research attempts to answer fundamental questions about the nature of behavior. Research questions such as "What is sensory integration?," "What is sensory integrative dysfunction?," and "Why does sensory integration intervention work?" are examples that fall under this category. In addition, basic research examines the many theories upon which sensory integration is derived, including the postulates supporting it.

Applied research is scientific inquiry that directly attempts to solve practical problems. Examples of applied research in the area of sensory integration include studies that examine the effectiveness of sensory integration intervention, studies that aim to develop or evaluate assessment tools measuring sensory integration functions, and case reports that describe the intervention and the functional changes that result from the intervention. Research is about seeking knowledge and developing ways of thinking, organizing, and applying what we know. However, scientific findings and theories are always considered provisional. Regardless of how eloquently a particular theory has been tested, it is always considered tentative—moving closer and closer toward "truth" but never really achieving this end.

Sensory integration theory and its application as a means of evaluating and intervening with children with certain disabilities have continued to evolve since its inception in the early 1960s. This evolution has occurred in response to research findings over time as well as to the practical demands placed on the professionals who practice within this framework. Intervention based on sensory integration theory is very complex, as are the clients best suited for this approach and the theory on which it is based. Therefore, whether a researcher is interested in conducting basic or applied scientific inquiry, complexity provides a significant challenge.

To establish professional consensus regarding the validation of sensory integration theory, evaluation and support for the basic assumptions on which the theory is based are necessary. A clear conceptualization of what sensory integration is, what sensory integrative dysfunction is, and what constitutes sensory integration intervention is crucial. In addition, efficacy studies are necessary to determine whether the intervention is effective, assist in identifying who is most likely to benefit from the intervention, and identify the functional areas affected by the intervention. Finally, efficacy studies must evaluate the intervention in the ways and contexts in which practitioners are applying it in order for the research to be most useful.

We begin by examining research that explores the concept of sensory integration. We emphasize research examining sensory integration intervention as an approach that focuses on remediating underlying etiology or neurologic dysfunction rather than on direct instruction or skill development. We have also included a review of research on central nervous system (CNS) plasticity and hierarchy, two important assumptions supporting sensory integration, and a current model of sensory processing is discussed. Second, we discuss research examining the concept of sensory integrative dysfunction. Third, we present efficacy studies evaluating the outcomes of sensory integration interventions. Finally, we conclude by discussing challenges related to research in the area of sensory integration and include ideas and priorities for furthering our knowledge in this area.

Sensory Integration: A Process Approach

In the educational literature, a *process approach* focuses on remediating underlying neurologic or mental processes believed to be contributing to a child's inability to learn or perform a specific skill as opposed to approaches that directly teach skills. In the late 1960s and 1970s, a number of process approaches, including sensory integration, perceptual-motor (Frostig, 1967; Kephart, 1971), and neurodevelopmental therapy (Bobath, 1980) were popular with practitioners intervening with children with neurologic disorders (e.g., learning disabilities and cerebral palsy). Process approaches are based on the belief that the functioning of specific neurologic systems (i.e., those responsible for sensory processing, motor coordination, and sustaining attention) was required for adequate cognitive development. After the disordered underlying processes were corrected, academic learning could take place normally (Hammill, 1993).

Sensory integration can be viewed as a process approach. Through the provision of enhanced sensory experiences, within the context of meaningful activity, and the production of adaptive responses, CNS functioning improves. This improvement ultimately leads to better performance in any number of functional areas, including behavior, academics, and motor skills (Fisher & Murray, 1991). However, in the mid-1970s and 1980s, researchers (Goodman & Hammill, 1973, 1993; Kavale & Mattson, 1983) conducting efficacy studies evaluating process-oriented interventions in education concluded that these approaches were largely ineffective. Thus, they

16

began to question whether underlying neurologic processes were related to cognitive abilities or academic performance. Eventually, on-task, direct instruction forms of assessment and remediation replaced process approaches. "For the moment, the issue of process training is resolved, and direct instruction has emerged as the model of choice for the remediation of learning disabilities in the United States" (Hammill, 1993, p. 303).

Sensory integration was not tested specifically in these studies, and most of these studies were limited to the examination of process approaches with children with learning disabilities. Nonetheless, the description of sensory integration simply as a process approach has probably contributed to the negative views of some researchers, particularly in the field of education.

Those who accept the effectiveness of intervention based on sensory integration theory believe first that the CNS has the capacity for change or remediation. *Neuroplasticity* is the assumption that the CNS has the capacity for change or is able to modify its structure and function (Lenn, 1991). Second, proponents of sensory integration believe in a certain level of CNS hierarchy because it is assumed that positive change or adaptation of lower (brainstem level) areas may result in improved higher cortical functions, including any number of functional areas and capabilities. Research related to these two basic assumptions on which sensory integration is based is examined below.

Sensory Integration: A Theory Based on Central Nervous System Plasticity and Hierarchical Concepts

There is an abundance of research that supports the concept of neuroplasticity (Bach-y-Rita, 1980; Lenn, 1991; Lund, 1978; McEachen & Shaw, 1996; Stein et al., 1974; Stephenson, 1993; Szekely, 1979). Neuroplasticity is evident throughout development; it involves natural changes in the nervous system that occur during maturation. It also is a reactive process that occurs during the recovery from an injury to the CNS (Schaaf, 1994a). Because the majority of individuals who are treated with sensory integration procedures are children with chronic, developmental conditions (i.e., pervasive developmental disorders, attention deficit hyperactivity disorder, learning disabilities) and because sensory integration theory is not designed to explain adult-

onset deficits (see Chapter 1), research that examines developmental neuroplasticity is most relevant.

Some of the most important factors that promote developmental neuroplasticity are the inner drive to seek, create, challenge, and master the environment (Aoki & Siekevitz, 1988; Parham & Mailloux, 2001), the just-right challenge, and the self-initiation and self-direction to engage in a challenge (Schaaf, 1994a). Inner drive and active involvement in the just-right challenge are fundamental characteristics of intervention based on sensory integration theory (Ayres, 1979) and may be keys to why it works. Therefore, research that examines such factors provides us with helpful guidelines as we continue to seek methods to enhance neuronal organization through sensory integration intervention.

Neuroplasticity takes place through a number of specific neural mechanisms, such as an increase in myelination and synaptic efficiency and in dendritic aborization. Explanations of such mechanisms are beyond the scope of this chapter; however, Schaaf (1994a, 1994b) provided an overview of such mechanisms and how they relate to our understanding of how and why intervention based on sensory integration theory may be effective. Particularly relevant are the ways in which we can enhance neuronal organization and integration through the types of purposeful activities used during intervention.

Although the idea that a more integrated, more efficient CNS results in improved performance in functional skills seems very logical, this issue has been at the core of many debates. Unlike research that supports CNS plasticity (which is very convincing), the connection between improved sensory integration and improved performance in functional skills is less obvious. Both correlational research investigating the relationships between sensory processing and functional skills and research examining brain function as a hierarchical process provide useful information in examining this connection.

Case-Smith (1995) explored relationships among sensorimotor components, fine motor skill, and functional performance in 30 preschool children. The sensorimotor components included two measures of sensory processing. One of these, tactile defensiveness, correlated significantly with measures of fine motor skills. However, the same measure showed only a weak relationship to functional social, play, and self-care skills. Case-Smith concluded that practitioners should not assume that functional skills improve when gains are made in underlying sensorimotor skills. Furthermore, other social, cultural, and environmental factors may be just as important for children to learn, perform, and generalize functional skills. She encouraged practitioners to consider such contexts in their interventions with children.

Sensory integration largely focuses on the remediation of brainstem functions as a way to improve functional skills (Ayres, 1972b). This hierarchical view understands the CNS as having vertically arranged levels that are interdependent yet reflect a trend of ascending control and specialization. This hierarchical approach led Ayres (1972b) to believe that the more primitive or subcortical systems such as the tactile, the vestibular, and the proprioceptive systems provide the foundation for the development of higher-order cortical functions such as academic ability, complex motor skills, and the development of social skills. This relationship is, however, controversial because the indirect correspondence between the stimulus (i.e., improved brainstem functioning) and performance (e.g., motor skill, academic achievement) is, for the most part, unobservable. More importantly, over the past 10 to 20 years, a more popular view of brain function, one that views the brain as a more integrated, holistic system, has emerged (Cohen & Reed, 1996).

Sensory integration theory has evolved to incorporate this view, and today it is consistent with a more holistic view of brain function. Fisher and Murray (1991) described sensory integration theory as being based on a systems view of brain function. In a systems view, rather than viewing sensory integration problems as resulting from specific, dysfunctional primitive sensory systems, such problems are believed to result from a number of interrelated systems that are not functioning optimally. Each part of the system performs a different role. Some are control centers; some fine-tune the instructions from the control center; some carry out instructions; some carry feedback messages. The extent of give and take from each part supports a holistic rather than a strictly hierarchical view.

The amount of literature that describes interventions that apply sensory integration techniques in conjunction with other approaches has increased in recent years. This literature suggests that sensory integrative dysfunction is only one of many problems that contribute to a child's difficulty in performing or learning tasks effectively. Today, intervention based on sensory integration theory is rarely provided in isolation; it is more often combined with other approaches, including the teaching of specific skills (Case-Smith, 1997) and promoting positive play behaviors (see Chapter 15). Intervention activities providing enhanced tactile and vestibular sensations are often used in conjunction with activities that tap higher cortical systems such as those involved in forming the ideas about how to perform motor tasks and with practice of specific functional skills in context (see also Chapter 3).

A more holistic intervention approach does not, however, dispute the emphasis that sensory integration has on the remediation of primitive sensory systems or the importance of healthy sensory integration for performing functional skills. Rather, it has placed this emphasis in context of a more holistic and interactive view of brain function and questions our ability to separate subcortical from higher-cortical functions. Subsequently, the use of other approaches in combination with intervention based on sensory integration theory is encouraged (see also Chapter 1).

Sensory Integration: A Component of Sensory Processing

There has been some confusion related to the use of terminology associated with sensory integration. The inconsistency in the use of this terminology has made interpretation research related to sensory integration rather difficult. The term *sensory integration* has been used to describe a neural process (occurring at the cellular or nervous system level), a behavioral process (observable behaviors that result from these processes), and a frame of reference useful for assessment and intervention. Thus, researchers must differentiate clearly between what they observe in children and what they infer is happening within the nervous system. Miller and Lane (2000) addressed the need to establish a consensus for the use of various terms related to sensory integration, and they provided some clarification for the use of terms, particularly those associated with neurophysiological processes, including peripheral sensory processes and central sensory processes (see also Chapter 4).

Sensory processing is one term that has become popular, and because it is often used interchangeably with *sensory integration,* the differentiation between these two terms requires clarification. Both terms represent theoretical frameworks for explaining the same types of functional deficits and behaviors observed in children. However, sensory processing is a more global, encompassing construct than is sensory integration. *Sensory processing* is the way in which the central and peripheral nervous systems manage incoming sensory information from tactile, vestibular, proprioceptive, visual, auditory, olfactory, and gustatory sensory systems. According to Miller and Lane (2000), the "reception, modulation, integration, and organization of sensory stimuli, including the behavioral responses to the sensory input are all components of sensory processing" (p. 2).

A conceptual model of sensory processing proposed by Dunn (1997) described the relationships among a number of neurobiological factors, including sensory registration (i.e., how one receives incoming sensory information), sensory modulation (i.e., how one regulates incoming sensory information), and habituation and sensitization (i.e., whether the CNS reacts to or ignores incoming sensory information; see Chapter 7). In addition, Dunn attempted to link sensory processing with the ways in which individuals perform daily life activities. Consistent with this more global use of the term *sensory processing,* DeGangi (1991) reported that the sensory processing problems of post-institutionalized children often lead to problems with sensory integration. Therefore, sensory integration should be viewed as only one component of sensory processing. Researchers must make explicit their use of various terms, and consumers of research must attend to the ways in which various terms are used.

RESEARCH EXAMINING SENSORY INTEGRATIVE DYSFUNCTION

Sensory integrative dysfunction is a diagnostic label that is relatively unpopular outside the profession of occupational therapy (Missiuna & Polatajko, 1995), and it is not included in the *Diagnostic and Statistical Manual of Mental Disorders* (*DSM-IV;* American Psychiatric Association, 1994). Rather, sensory integrative dysfunction is often associated with the underlying sensory processing problems characteristic of any number of diagnostic conditions in-

cluded in the *DSM-IV.* The most common *DSM-IV* diagnostic groups that coexist with sensory integrative dysfunction are pervasive developmental disorders (e.g., autism) (Kientz & Dunn, 1997; McIntosh et al., 1999), attention deficit–hyperactivity disorders (Mulligan, 1996), learning disorders (Ayres, 1979), developmental disabilities (Baranek et al., 1997), fragile X syndrome (Miller et al., 1999), and developmental coordination disorder (Missiuna & Polatajko, 1995). Although not all children in these diagnostic groups have sensory integrative dysfunction, many of them have evidence of symptoms associated with it. Based on research to date, it also is not correct to assume causative relationships between sensory integrative dysfunction and these other conditions when they do coexist. The same underlying neurologic deficit may well cause both conditions.

Sensory Integrative Dysfunction and Other Diagnostic Labels

The issue of classification of children has been debated over the years, and the confusion of "labeling" has led to problems both in identifying appropriate children for specific interventions and in selecting subjects for research purposes. A review of four terms: sensory integrative dysfunction, clumsy child syndrome, developmental dyspraxia, and developmental coordination disorder by Missiuna & Polatajko (1995) concluded that these four terms should not be used interchangeably and that clear definitions and characteristic features of each need to identified.

Typically, children are labeled as having sensory integrative dysfunction when they do poorly on tests specifically designed to measure sensory integration (Missiuna & Polatajko, 1995). Such tests, such as the Sensory Integration and Praxis Tests (SIPT; Ayres, 1989), measure the processing of basic sensory systems (i.e., tactile, proprioceptive, vestibular) as well as visual-perceptual and motor planning functions. Specific types of sensory processing deficits are beginning to be identified in children with different diagnostic classifications. This research provides valuable information about the nature of dysfunction characteristic of certain types of children. For example, Mulligan (1996) identified specific patterns of sensory integrative dysfunction in children with attention disorders and Baranek et al. (1997) identified types of sensory defensiveness specific to children and adults with developmental disabilities. Kientz and Dunn (1997) described the sensory processing of children with autism, and Demaio-Feldman (1994) identified somatosensory processing deficiencies of low-birth-weight infants at school age.

The Zero to Three Diagnostic Classification Task Force included a diagnostic classification called multisystem developmental disorders in the Diagnostic Classification of Mental Health and Developmental Disorders of Infancy and Early Childhood (DC 0–3) (as cited by Wieder, 1996). These multisystem disorders are consistent with what has been described as characteristics of sensory integrative dysfunction because they view a variety of functional problems as being secondary to motor planning and underlying sensory processing deficits rather than as primary deficits. The different types of multisystem disorders, however, place more emphasis on sensory modulation (a component of sensory processing) than on sensory integration. For example, the three types of multisystem developmental disorders are a hypersensitive type (type 1), a hyposensitive type (type II), and a motorically disorganized and impulsive type (type III). Research by Miller and colleagues (personal communication, March 15, 2000) is exploring the possibility of sensory modulation disorders as a separate diagnostic entity. This research group has identified and demonstrated types of sensory modulation problems in children with autism and fragile X syndrome, using both traditional measures and neurophysiological measures such as electrodermal responses (McIntosh et al., 1999; Miller et al., 1999).

Types of Sensory Integrative Disorders

Ayres (1972s) believed that many different types of sensory integrative disorders existed and that each was associated with dysfunction in a particular neural substrate. She then developed a typology of sensory integrative dysfunction based on a series of multivariate analyses (Ayres, 1989; see also Chapter 1 and Appendix B). Sensory integrative dysfunction, therefore, has been conceptualized as multidimensional. The identification of different types of sensory integrative dysfunction assists with the understanding of underlying etiology and, more practically, is useful for developing specific intervention for the discrete patterns identified.

Categorical systems for conceptualizing sensory integrative dysfunction, largely based on Ayres' factor analytic work in the 1960s and 1970s, are described by Parham and Mailloux (2001), Fisher and Murray (1991), and Ayres (1989) (see also Chapter 1 and Appendix B). Although there is not perfect consensus on the best way to categorize the patterns of dysfunction, there are recurring themes, and much commonality expressed by all authors.

The exploratory factor analytic studies on which these patterns of dysfunction were based, however, must be interpreted with caution and can be criticized appropriately for limitations in design (Cummins, 1991; Hoehn & Baumeister, 1994; Parham & Mailloux, 2001). Because Ayres was constantly exploring new ideas, she used a different battery of tests in each study. Therefore, none of the studies was a true replication of a preceding one. Furthermore, her samples were heterogeneous and consistently small in number relative to the number of test scores that were analyzed. Terminology used to describe the factors that emerged in these studies was also inconsistent; therefore, comparing results from these studies and drawing conclusions based on their combined contributions are difficult. Nonetheless, the practical implications of these patterns have been very important for our understanding of the nature of the sensory integrative dysfunction seen in children and in interpreting the results of children on the SIPT (Ayres, 1989).

Mulligan (1998) attempted to validate a five-factor model of sensory integrative dysfunction based on the SIPT scores of a large, heterogeneous group of children. The model tested was consistent with current views of patterns of sensory integrative dysfunction and included a bilateral integration and sequencing pattern, a somatopraxis pattern, a visuopraxis pattern, a somatosensory pattern, and a postural-ocular movement pattern. Although the results supported the hypothesized model as reasonable, a number of weaknesses were identified with it that supported further analyses of alternative models. One of the most important findings was the very strong relationship among all of the patterns, suggesting the presence of a higher-order general factor, which initially was termed *generalized practic dysfunction*. (Editors' note: Mulligan later agreed that her higher-order factor may reflect a general inefficiency of CNS functioning, particularly in the areas or systems measured by the SIPT. It might be more appropriate to label this higher-order general factor *general sensory integrative dysfunction.* [Mulligan, personal communication, June 1, 1999].)

In view of this research, rather than purport the existence of separate patterns of dysfunction (related to dysfunction in particular neural substrates), as previous studies have done, Mulligan suggested that specific patterns of dysfunction (based on deficient SIPT scores) should be viewed as extensions of generalized sensory integrative dysfunction (see Chapter 1 for more specifics on Mulligan's factor-analytic study).

The idea of a general factor emphasizes the complexity of our CNS and supports the systems or holistic view of the CNS discussed earlier in this chapter. In examining construct validity of the SIPT, Lai et al. (1996) provided evidence that praxis is a unidimensional construct and that both bilateral integration and sequencing and somatopraxis were a part of this unidimensional construct. Although their study did not examine all patterns of dysfunction believed to comprise sensory integrative dysfunction, these results indicated a shift in thinking regarding the multidimensionality of sensory integrative dysfunction.

Mulligan (1998) also found that the SIPT was not sufficient to detect problems related to postural functioning, supporting Fisher and Bundy (1991), who discussed the importance of using other clinical observations such as examining equilibrium reactions and antigravity postures to determine postural problems (see also Chapter 7). Somatopraxis also did not emerge as a separate pattern (Mulligan, 1998) as it had in previous studies (Ayres, 1966, 1971, 1977; Ayres et al., 1987). A relationship between somatosensory processing and praxis was evident; however, unlike previous models, which identified somatodyspraxia as a separate pattern of dysfunction, the relationship between these two areas was explained by the presence of the general factor (Mulligan, 1998). In view of this new information, Mulligan suggested that therapists be cautious when identifying a child as fitting one of the five specific patterns of dysfunction (based on SIPT scores) previously identified.

In summary, a multitude of diagnostic labels is used to describe children with sensory integrative dysfunction, and care must be taken not to use various terms interchangeably. When conducting research, coexisting diagnoses of study participants need to be identified and reported so that the effects of intervention for different types of dysfunction can be examined and considered in the interpretation of results. Although it appears that the multidimensional view of sensory integrative dysfunction is shifting to a more unified model, a consensus on the best way to conceptualize it has not been reached. Further understanding of how sensory integrative dysfunction relates with other models of sensory processing is necessary.

RESEARCH EVALUATING INTERVENTION BASED ON SENSORY INTEGRATION THEORY

In applied research, the definition of intervention based on sensory integration theory, as an independent variable, has been inconsistent. This is problematic when one attempts to draw conclusions about the efficacy of intervention. Rosenthal and Rosnow (1984) defined an independent variable as an observable or measurable event manipulated by a researcher to determine whether there is any effect on another event (i.e., the dependent variable). Research based on a traditional definition of sensory integrative–based intervention often requires that the independent variable or intervention be administered to every individual in precisely the same manner. Clearly, intervention based on sensory integration theory defies a simple definition.

Integration based on sensory integration theory is complex because the way in which it is administered depends on the individual needs of a client (Ottenbacher, 1991). In addition, the application of intervention as it was conceptualized classically must be distinguished from more current applications that involve the use of indirect, consultative models, and the use of sensory integration principles and activities in combination with those from other frames of reference. Because this distinction is so important, research evaluating each type, "classic" and "nontraditional," will be addressed separately.

Studies of Classic Sensory Integration Intervention

The classic form of sensory integration intervention tends to be practiced more often in private, medically oriented clinics than in educational environments. Such intervention is highly specialized, and it has been recommended that only therapists who have received advanced training administer it. Kimball (1988, 1999) described several characteristics of sensory integration intervention. These can be summarized as follows.

- The goal of the intervention is to facilitate appropriate physical and emotional adaptive responses by improving CNS processing rather than to teach specific skills.
- Intervention activities are individualized and at the upper levels of the client's capacity.
- Intervention is administered by a vigilant practitioner who provides constant feedback.
- Intervention involves purposeful activities that are client directed and result in an adaptive response.
- Intervention activities provide enhanced proprioceptive, vestibular, and tactile sensation.

Although these characteristics provide guidelines for defining the intervention, they are very broad, and there is room for variability within each of them. However, interventions that involve the application of sensory stimulation only, structured group interventions, combined approaches, use of sensory integration in consultative models, or intervention that applies sensory integration principles during the practice of specific functional skills are not considered classic sensory integration intervention. Although all of these approaches are very appropriate for some children, in a research context, care must be taken to differentiate them from classic sensory integration intervention.

In the 1970s and 1980s, many studies were conducted specifically evaluating the effectiveness of sensory integration intervention, with mixed results. Many detailed reviews of this literature are available (Cermak & Henderson, 1989; Hoehn & Baumeister, 1994; Mulligan, 1997; Ottenbacher, 1982; Parham & Mailloux, 2001; Polatajko et al., 1992, Vargas & Camilli, 1999). These early studies demonstrated that sensory integration therapy improved performance in motor, language, and academic areas (Ayres, 1972a, 1972c; Magrun et al., 1981; White, 1979). Ottenbacher (1982) performed a meta-analysis of eight intervention effectiveness studies, which provided support for sensory integration intervention in the remediation of motor, academic, and language functions, with the most improvements noted in the motor area. Specifically in relation to children with learning disabilities, he

reported that "the average learning disabled student receiving sensory integration therapy performed better than 75.2 percent of the learning disabled subjects not receiving therapy" (Ottenbacher, 1982, p. 576).

There have not been many group studies in the past 10 years evaluating the outcomes of sensory integration interventions in comparison with other approaches such as tutoring (Wilson et al., 1992) and perceptual-motor training (Humphries et al., 1992). The more recent studies, however, improved on previous studies in terms of methodological rigor. These studies concluded that sensory integration therapy is not any more effective than these traditional approaches. Polatajko et al. (1992) reviewed seven two- and three-group experimental studies conducted from 1979 to 1992 using sensory integration intervention with samples of children with learning disabilities. They concluded that the results of previous studies do not indicate that sensory integration intervention improves the academic performance of children with learning disabilities more than placebo does. With respect to sensory or motor performance, the results were inconsistent and indicated overall that sensory integration intervention may produce minimal positive effects. However, the generalization of these studies is limited because study subjects included children with learning disabilities only and because the nature and extent of the subjects' sensory integrative dysfunction were often not known. No negative effects of sensory integration interventions were ever reported.

Wilson and Kaplan (1994) conducted a follow-up study of the children who had received either tutoring or sensory integration therapy in their 1992 study. They concluded that the children who received sensory integration intervention performed better on tests of gross motor function than the children who received the tutoring intervention. No significant differences were found on tests that measured reading skills, fine motor skills, visual-motor skills, or behavioral factors. Allen and Donald (1995) conducted a pilot study to determine the effect of occupational therapy intervention (based on sensory integration theory) on five children with documented sensory integrative dysfunction. These case studies revealed that four of the five children receiving the therapy improved in the area of motor performance. The one participant who did not show motor gains was older than the other children (i.e., age 11 years compared with ages 5 to 8 years).

In a meta-analysis of 32 experimental group studies (16 comparing sensory integration intervention with other interventions and 16 comparing sensory integration intervention with no intervention), Vargas and Camilli (1999) expressed three main conclusions. First, when compared with a control situation, the effects of intervention based on sensory integration theory showed positive results in earlier studies but no differences in later studies. Second, effect sizes for measures of motor performance and cognition such as IQ and academic achievement were greater than those for measures of behavior, language, and sensory and perceptual ability. Third, overall intervention based on sensory integration theory was as effective as various alternative intervention approaches.

One way of minimizing or controlling the variation in a complex intervention approach when evaluating it is to reduce the intervention to a small number of standardized and strictly controlled activities. The advantages of doing so are that it allows the researcher to examine the effectiveness of specific components of the intervention while making it easier to operationally define the independent variable. The main disadvantage in doing so is that the resulting intervention approach is probably not very representative of the actual intervention as it is typically practiced, nor of the construct itself.

Reductionistic definitions of sensory integration intervention are common in the literature (Jarus & Gol, 1995; Ottenbacher et al., 1981; Ottenbacher, 1991; Wells & Smith, 1983). Although not specifically defined as sensory integration therapy, De-Gangi et al. (1993) compared a therapist-directed sensory motor intervention approach with a child-directed sensory motor approach. They concluded that the child-directed approach, which is more characteristic of sensory integration, was better than the other approach for the development of fine motor skills but less effective for the improvement of gross motor skills, sensory integration functions, and functional skills. One must take care in interpreting this study because it measures a certain component of sensory integration intervention (i.e., child directed versus therapist directed) and not the intervention itself.

Tickle-Degnen and Coster (1995) examined another component of intervention based on sensory integration theory in the context of intervention sessions. With the use of videotape, they examined a social element, the nature of therapist–child interactions during sensory integration intervention. This social element is one of the most important facets of sensory integration intervention; Ayres emphasized that achieving positive results depends on the involvement of a skilled practitioner who can match both input and adaptive demands to the child's current needs and capacities. Kaplan et al. (1993) also suggested that the bond between a therapist and a child may account for some of the positive perceptions regarding intervention outcomes.

In summary, efficacy research of sensory integration intervention in its "purest" form provides conflicting results. Overall, the results provide little supporting evidence that the intervention is helpful in the remediation of learning or academic difficulties of children. There is some support, however, that it improves sensory processing; improves some behavioral problems in children; and, most clearly, improves gross motor performance in children with learning, behavioral, or motor problems. Results also indicate that intervention based on sensory integration theory is most effective with children who have been specifically identified with sensory integration problems and that the intervention appears most effective with younger children.

Studies of Nontraditional Sensory Integration Intervention

Although the classic approach is still used with some children, intervention based on sensory integration theory is more often modified or used in conjunction with other approaches. For example, practitioners working with children in educational settings have modified the way in which they use sensory integration as a frame of reference to meet the requirements of special education law and to accommodate the specific needs of students. Additionally, they have tried to join the move of educators from process approaches toward more direct instruction models and toward inclusive education (i.e., educating students with special needs in regular classroom environments and within the context of regular classroom activities). For example, the use of consultative services has increased over the past 10 to 15 years (Dunn, 1988; Kemmis & Dunn, 1996) and occupational therapists are applying sensory integration principles to help students to be successful with classroom activities already a part of the typical curriculum (Mulligan, 1997).

There is some empirical evidence supporting the

efficacy of consultative models (Davis & Gavin, 1994; Dunn, 1990; Kemmis & Dunn, 1996), which often include a component of sensory integration theory. For example, Case-Smith (1997) found that one of the most important factors in successful interventions was the practitioner's ability to reframe a child's classroom behaviors using sensory integration theory. Sensory integration was reported to be the primary frame of reference for five of the 13 children examined in her study.

In addition to the increased use of consultation, practitioners often combine sensory integration interventions with other approaches, including the provision of adapted equipment, gross and fine motor skill training, self-care skill training, and parent and teacher support, as part of a child's total intervention program. Few studies however, have examined the effectiveness of sensory integration with other approaches. This is not surprising. As with consultation, it is very difficult to isolate the contributions of the specific components of combined approaches to the ultimate outcomes of the intervention.

A promising study by Case-Smith et al. (1998) demonstrated the effectiveness of school-based occupational therapy services on fine motor skills and other functional outcomes of preschool children with developmental delays. In this study, 44 children with developmental delays and 20 children without delays were pretested with a number of outcome measures at the beginning of the school year and posttested at the end of the school year. The intervention approaches varied depending on the individual needs of each preschooler. The use of activities characteristic of intervention based on sensory integration theory was very common (40.4% of sessions emphasized motor planning and tactile activities; 31.7% emphasized vestibular and proprioceptive activities) as was the use of visuomotor and manipulation activities (81% of sessions). The results of this study supported the use of sensory integration techniques in combination with other approaches for improving fine motor skills, and functional skills of preschoolers with developmental delays.

Operationally defining sensory integration as an independent variable has not become any easier in the past 10 to 15 years. Rather, with the increased use of sensory integration in consultative models and in combination with other approaches, it may very well be more difficult to isolate and define than it was previously. We do, however, have guidelines that can be used (Kimball, 1988, 1999) to help researchers define sensory integration intervention in its classic form (see also Appendix A). Examining components of intervention is also a technique that has been used to further our understanding of the effects of certain qualities of the intervention. Finally, the use of experimental designs that do not attempt to control the intervention, as in the study design used by Case-Smith et al. (1998) and supported by Bower and McLellan (1994), appear to be a useful way to evaluate the effects of complex, multifaceted, and individualized interventions.

DIRECTIONS FOR FURTHER RESEARCH

A number of scholars in the field (e.g., Cermak & Henderson, 1989; Kaplan et al., 1993; Miller & Kinnealey, 1993; Mulligan, 1997; Ottenbacher, 1991; Tickle-Degnen, 1988) have provided direction for future research related to sensory integration theory and intervention. Research questions range from the basic premises on which the theory and hypothesized dysfunction are based to the efficacy of intervention as it is practiced in its varied forms.

For professional consensus to be reached regarding the usefulness of intervention based on sensory integration theory, it must be better defined and conceptualized. Basic research that explores the theoretical bases of sensory integration, including the underlying mechanisms on which it is based, is needed (Tickle-Degnen, 1988). Such research is useful for determining *how and why* intervention works rather than *if* it is effective. Further understanding of the ways in which sensory integration relates to other information processing models, such as those described in the education and psychology literature (see Swanson, 1987) and other sensory processing models (e.g., Dunn, 1997) is also necessary. Such work may someday allow researchers and theorists to converge on a unified paradigm for the study of individuals with sensory integrative dysfunction.

Second, we must better understand the individuals for whom intervention is useful and be better able to describe participants in research samples. Specific tests of sensory integrative dysfunction are recommended to identify individuals appropriate for intervention because only individuals identified as having sensory integrative dysfunction should be used to evaluate intervention based on sensory integration theory. Research examining specific patterns of sensory integrative dysfunction may also be helpful in identifying intervention best suited for certain individuals. Furthermore, coexisting conditions, including other diagnoses and characteristics of participants in studies, should always be reported so the influence of multiple variables can be considered in the interpretation of results.

Third, psychometrically sound tests of sensory integration are necessary for identifying appropriate candidates for intervention as well as for measuring the effects of intervention, supporting research in the area of test development. Mulligan (1998) suggested that a new, shorter test emphasizing the identification of praxis problems and the underlying sensory integration functions that may be contributing to the praxis problems be considered. In addition, further tests of vestibular function and tests that measure sensory modulation need to be developed because it is believed that these are important aspects of sensory integration that have not yet been captured adequately within a standardized tool (Mulligan, 1998). Mulligan also reported that a tool that provides an overall score of sensory integrative dysfunction would be helpful to identify clearly whether dysfunction exists and what the overall severity of the dysfunction is.

The specific goals of intervention based on sensory integration theory and expectations for areas of gain differ for various individuals. Therefore, the dependent measures selected should be consistent with these expectations and be sensitive enough to detect changes. Cermak and Henderson (1989) reported that research is greatly hampered by the lack of good measures of intervention effectiveness (see also Chapter 1). Ways to document both the short- and long-term effects of intervention are needed. In addition to measures evaluating motor, language, academic, and behavioral outcomes, measures of the effects of intervention on occupational performance (e.g., play) and performance components (e.g., attention, organization, and affect) are needed (Cermak & Henderson, 1989). Based on their research examining parental hopes for therapy outcomes, Cohn et al. (2000) discussed the importance of including both child-focused measures (i.e., self-regulation, perceived competence, and social participation) and parent outcomes (i.e., validation of their child's problems and competency in applying strategies to assist their children) when measuring the effectiveness of intervention.

Fourth, the complexity and individualized nature of intervention based on sensory integration theory must be carefully considered when evaluating the effectiveness of the intervention. For traditional experimental designs, sensory integration intervention must be better defined and controlled. Kimball's (1988, 1999) description is useful for identifying the basic and necessary components and characteristics of classic intervention. Specific questions researchers can ask themselves when operationally defining interventions have been outlined by Miller and Kinnealey (1993). For example, researchers must determine how much of the therapy session is child directed and to what degree the sensory input is varied based on the child's responses. Protocols that describe the interventions need to be developed and reviewed by experts in the field, and procedural reliability checks should be implemented to ensure the consistency and accuracy of the application of the protocols. (See also Appendix A for the STEP-SI protocol developed by Miller and her colleagues.)

Reductionistic definitions of intervention based on sensory integration theory, as noted earlier, can also be used to minimize intervention variation and allow the researcher to isolate and examine the effectiveness of specific components of this multifaceted approach. However, care must be taken when generalizing the results of these studies because the sum of the effects of individual components of an intervention do not necessarily add up to the total effects of the intervention.

If interventions are based on a consultative model or are used in combination with other approaches, then all approaches need to be identified, described, and accounted for in the study. It is, however, not always necessary to control the intervention in order to evaluate it. Case-Smith et al. (1998) demonstrated how researchers are able to evaluate therapy services using an experimental design, with the services being individualized and provided in natural contexts. Miller and Kinnealey (1993) cited single subject experimental designs as well as case studies and other qualitative approaches as being particularly relevant when studying the effects of sensory integrative interventions. Rather than masking individual differences and attempting to produce homogeneous groups, these approaches explore the effects of individual differences, allow for individualized intervention, and are useful in determining for whom intervention is most helpful. Regardless of the research method, however, it important for investigators to carefully describe the delivery of the intervention and monitor its implementation throughout the research process.

SUMMARY AND CONCLUSIONS

Sensory integration as a frame of reference has provided a useful framework for assisting occupational therapy practitioners, parents, and teachers in understanding children's behavior in ways that make sense. Despite contradictory empirical evidence regarding the effectiveness of this approach over the years, it has remained very popular. We must not lose sight of the fact that sensory integration has a great deal in common with more global and accepted frames of reference such as developmental approaches and information processing. This commonality with other approaches enhances its credibility and the comfort level of the practitioners who choose to use it. Sensory integration as a frame of reference takes a unique perspective in organizing largely accepted views regarding the way in which the CNS works, what we know about child development, and how one learns and processes sensation.

Developing consensus regarding the validity of sensory integration will require a creative synthesis of past and present empirical efforts. Such efforts require cooperation of a multitude of researchers from various backgrounds and expertise in diverse research methodologies. The science of sensory integration is still in its infancy, and no single research approach has emerged as the methodology of choice in establishing empirical consensus. The absence of a unifying research paradigm is a function of the highly complex subject that sensory integration is. The exploration and application of a multitude of research approaches should be encouraged and is viewed as a positive development.

As concerned, caring professionals, we must believe in the therapeutic merit of what we do. At the same time, we must acknowledge the limitations of the scientific evidence that support the outcomes of the interventions that we strive to achieve with our clients. There is scientific evidence to support the use of intervention based on sensory integration theory for children with sensory processing disorders, and there is scientific evidence to dis-

pute its use. Careful monitoring of the progress of our clients is, therefore, crucial because we must remain accountable. Finally, we must all take some level of responsibility for furthering our knowledge base and our understanding of sensory integration. As a part of this process, we must value research as an integral part of practice.

References

Allen, S., & Donald, M. (1995). The effect of occupational therapy on the motor proficiency of children with motor/learning difficulties: A pilot study. *British Journal of Occupational Therapy, 58,* 385–391.

Aoki, C., & Siekevitz, P. (1988). Plasticity in brain development, *Scientific American, 259,* 56–64.

American Psychiatric Association (1994). *Diagnostic and statistical manual of mental disorders* (4th ed.). Washington, DC: Author.

Ayres, A. J. (1966). Interrelationships among perceptual-motor functions in children. *American Journal of Occupational Therapy, 20,* 335–368.

Ayres, A. J. (1969). Deficits in sensory integration in educationally handicapped children. *Journal of Learning Disabilities, 2,* 160–168.

Ayres, A. J. (1971). Characteristics of types of sensory integrative dysfunction. *American Journal of Occupational Therapy, 25,* 329–334.

Ayres, A. J. (1972a). Types of sensory integrative dysfunction among disabled learners. *American Journal of Occupational Therapy, 26,* 13–18.

Ayres, A. J. (1972b). *Sensory integration and learning disorders.* Los Angeles: Western Psychological Services.

Ayres, A. J. (1972c). Improving academic scores through sensory integration. *Journal of Learning Disabilities, 5,* 338–344.

Ayres, A. J. (1977). Cluster Analysis of measures of sensory integration. *American Journal of Occupational Therapy, 31,* 362–366.

Ayres, A. J. (1979). *Sensory integration and the child.* Los Angeles: Western Psychological Services.

Ayres, A. J. (1989). *Sensory Integration and Praxis Tests.* Los Angeles: Western Psychological Services.

Ayres, A. J., Mailloux, Z., & Wendler, C. L. (1987). Developmental dyspraxia: Is it a unitary function? *Occupational Therapy Journal of Research, 7,* 93–110.

Bach-y-Rita, P. (1980). *Recovery of function: Theoretical considerations for brain injury rehabilitation.* Vienna: Hans Huber Publications.

Baranek, G., Foster, L., & Berkson, G. (1997). Tactile defensivness and stereotyped behaviors. *American Journal of Occupational Therapy, 51,* 91–95.

Bobath, K. (1980). *A neurophysiological basis for the intervention of cerebral palsy.* Philadelphia: J.B. Lippincott Company.

Bower, E., & McLellan, D. L. (1994). Evaluating

therapy in cerebral palsy. *Child Care, Health, and Development, 20,* 409–429.

Case-Smith, J. (1995). The relationships among sensorimotor components, fine motor skills, and functional performance in preschool children. *American Journal of Occupational Therapy, 49,* 645–652.

Case-Smith, J. (1997). Variables related to successful school-based practice. *Occupational Therapy Journal of Research, 17,* 133–153.

Case-Smith, J., Heapy, T., Marr, D., Galvin, B., Koch, V., Good-Ellis, M., & Perez, I. (1998). Fine motor and functional performance outcomes in preschool children. *American Journal of Occupational Therapy, 52,* 788–796.

Cermak, S., & Henderson, A. (1989). The efficacy of sensory integration procedures. *Sensory Integration Quarterly,* Vol. XVII (3), Torrance, CA: Sensory Integration International.

Cohen, H., & Reed, K. (1996). The historical development of neuroscience in physical rehabilitation. *American Journal of Occupational Therapy, 50,* 561–568.

Cohn, E., Tickle-Degnen, & Miller, L., (2000). Parental hopes for therapy outcomes: Children with sensory modulation disorders. *American Journal of Occupational Therapy, 54,* 36–43.

Cummins, R. (1991). Sensory integration and learning disabilities: Ayres' factor analyses reappraised. *Journal of Learning Disabilities, 24,* 160–168.

Davis, P. L., & Gavin, W. J. (1994). Comparison of individual and group/consultation intervention methods for preschool children with developmental delays. *American Journal of Occupational Therapy. 48,* 155–161.

DeGangi, G. (1991). Assessment of sensory, emotional, and attentional problems in regulatory disordered infants. *Infants and Young Children, 3,* 1–8.

DeGangi, G., Wietlisbach, S., Goodin, M., & Scheiner, N. (1993). A comparison of structured sensorimotor therapy and child-centered activity in the intervention of preschool children with sensorimotor problems. *American Journal of Occupational Therapy. 47,* 777–786.

Dematio-Feldman, D. (1994). Somatosensory processing abilities of very low-birth weight infants at school age. *American Journal of Occupational Therapy, 48,* 639–645.

Dunn, W. (1988). Models of occupational therapy service provision in the school system. *American Journal of Occupational Therapy, 42,* 718–723.

Dunn, W. (1990). A comparison of service provision models in school-based occupational therapy services: A pilot study. *Occupational Therapy Journal of Research, 10,* 300–320.

Dunn, W. (1997). The impact of sensory processing abilities on the daily lives of young children and their families: A conceptual model. *Infants and Young Children, 9,* 23–35.

Fisher, A., & Bundy, A. (1991). The interpretation process. In A. Fisher, E. Murray, & A. Bundy (Eds.), *Sensory integration: Theory and practice* (pp. 234–249). Philadelphia: F. A. Davis.

Fisher, A., & Murray, E. A. (1991). Introduction to sensory integration theory. In A. Fisher, E. Murray, & A. Bundy (Eds.), *Sensory integration: Theory and practice* (pp. 3–26). Philadelphia: F. A. Davis.

Frostig, M. (1967). Education of children with learning disabilities. In E. C. Frierson & W. B. Barbe (Eds.), *Educating children with learning disabilities* (pp. 387–398). New York: Appleton-Century-Crofts.

Goodman. L., & Hammill, D. (1973). The effectiveness of the Kephart-Getman training activities. *Focus on Exceptional Children, 40,* 1–9.

Hammill, D. (1993). A brief look at the learning disabilities movement in the United States. *Journal of Learning Disabilities, 26,* 295–310.

Hoehn, T., & Baumeister, A. (1994). A critique of the application of sensory integration therapy to children with learning disabilities. *Journal of Learning Disabilities, 27,* 338–350.

Humphries, T., Wright, M., Snider, L., & McDougall, B. (1992). A comparison of the effectiveness of sensory integration therapy and perceptual-motor training in treating children with learning disabilities. *Journal of Developmental and Behavioral Pediatrics, 13,* 31–40.

Jarus, T., & Gol, D. (1995). The effect of kinesthetic stimulation on the acquisition and retention of gross motor skill by children with and without sensory integration disorders. *Physical and Occupational Therapy in Pediatrics, 14,* 59–73.

Kaplan, B., Polatajko, H., Wilson, B., & Faris, P. (1993). Reexamination of sensory integration intervention: A combination of two efficacy studies. *Journal of Learning Disabilities, 26,* 342–347.

Kavale, K., & Mattson, P. D. (1983). One jumped off of the balance beam: Meta analysis of perceptual motor training. *Journal of Learning Disabilities, 16,* 165–173.

Kemmis, B. L., & Dunn, W. (1996). Collaborative consultation: The efficacy of remedial and compensatory interventions in school contexts. *American Journal of Occupational Therapy, 50,* 709–717.

Kephart, N. C. (1971). *The slow learner in the classroom.* Columbus, OH: Merrill.

Kientz, M., & Dunn, W. (1997). A comparison of the performance of children with and without autism on the sensory profile. *American Journal of Occupational Therapy, 51,* 530–537.

Kimball, J. G. (1988). The issue is integration, not sensory. *American Journal of Mental Retardation, 92,* 435–437.

Kimball, J. G. (1999). Sensory integration frame of reference: Postulates regarding change and application to practice. In P. Kramer & J. Hinojosa (Eds.), *Frames of reference for pediatric occupational therapy* (pp.169–204). Philadelphia: Lippincott Williams & Wilkins.

Lai, J., Fisher, A., Magalhaes, L., & Bundy, A. (1996). Construct validity of the Sensory Integration and Praxis Tests. *The Occupational Therapy Journal of Research, 16,* 75–97.

Lenn, N. J. (1991). Neuroplasticity: The basis for brain development, learning and recovery from injury. *Infants and Young Children, 3,* 39–48.

Lund, R. D. (1978). *Development and plasticity of the brain.* New York: Oxford University Press.

Magrun, W. M., McCue, S., Ottenbacher, K., & Keefe, R. (1981). Effects of vestibular stimulation on the spontaneous use of verbal language in developmentally delayed children. *The American Journal of Occupational Therapy, 35,* 101–104.

McEachen & Shaw (1996). *Brain Research reviews 22,* 51–92

McIntosh, D. N., Miller, L. J., Shyu, V., & Hagerman, R. (1999). Sensory modulation disruption, electrodermal responses, and functional behaviors. *Developmental Medicine and Child Neurology, 41,* 608–615.

Miller, L. J., & Lane, S. (March 2000). Toward a consensus in terminology in sensory integration theory and practice: Part 1: Taxonomy of neurophysiological processes. *Sensory Integration Special Interest Section Quarterly, 23,* 1–4.

Miller, L. J., McIntosh, D. N., McGrath, J., Shyu, V., Lampe, M., Taylor, A. K., Tassone, F., Neitzel, K., Stackhouse, T., & Hagerman, R. (1999). Electrodermal responses to sensory stimuli in individuals with Fragile X syndrome: A preliminary report. *American Journal of Medical Genetics, 83,* 268–279.

Miller, L. J., & Kinnealey, M. (1993). Researching the effectiveness of sensory integration. *Sensory Integration Quarterly,* Vol. XXI(2), Torrance, CA: Sensory Integration International.

Missiuna, C., & Polatajko, H. (1995). Developmental dyspraxia by any other name: Are they all just clumsy children? *American Journal of Occupational Therapy, 49,* 619–627.

Mulligan, S. (1996). An analysis of score patterns of children with attention disorders on the Sensory Integration and Praxis Tests. *American Journal of Occupational Therapy, 50,* 647–654.

Mulligan, S. (1997). Sensory integration: Analyses of patterns of dysfunction and clinical application with children with mild disabilities. Unpublished doctoral dissertation, University of Washington.

Mulligan, S. (1998). Patterns of sensory integrative dysfunction: A confirmatory factor analyses. *American Journal of Occupational Therapy, 52,* 819–828.

Ottenbacher, K. (1982). Sensory integration therapy: Affect or effect? *American Journal of Occupational Therapy, 36,* 571–578.

Ottenbacher, K. (1991). Research in sensory integration: Empirical perceptions and progress. In A. Fisher, E. Murray, & A. Bundy (Eds.), *Sensory integration: Theory and practice* (pp. 387–399). Philadelphia: F.A. Davis.

Ottenbacher, K., Short, M. A., & Watson, P. J. (1981). The effects of a clinically applied program of vestibular stimulation on the neuromotor performance of children with severe developmental delay. *Physical and Occupational Therapy in Pediatrics, 1,* 1–11

Parham, L. D., & Mailloux, Z. (2001). Sensory integration. In J. Case-Smith (Ed.), *Occupational therapy for children* (4th ed., pp. 307–356). St. Louis: Mosby.

Polatajko, H., Kaplan, B., & Wilson, B. (1992). Sensory integration intervention for children with learning disabilities: Its status 20 years later. *Occupational Therapy Journal of Research, 12,* 323–341.

Polatajko, H., Law, M., Miller, J., Schaffer, R., & Mcnab, J. (1991). The effect of a sensory integration program on academic achievement, motor performance, and self-esteem in children identified as learning disabled: Results of a clinical trial. *The Occupational Therapy Journal of Research, 11,* 155–176.

Rosenthal, R., & Rosnow, R. L. (1984). *Essentials of behavioral research: Methods and data analysis.* New York: McGraw-Hill.

Schaaf, R. (1994a). Neuroplasticity and sensory integration: Part 1. *Sensory Integration Quarterly,* XXII(1), 1–5.

Schaaf, R. (1994b). Neuroplasticity and sensory integration: Part 2. *Sensory Integration Quarterly,* XXII(2), 1–7.

Stein, D. G., Rosen, J. J., Butters, N. (1974). *Plasticity and recovery of function in the central nervous system.* New York: Academic.

Stephenson, R. (1993). A review of neuroplasticity: Some implications for physiotherapy in the intervention of lesions of the brain. *Physiotherapy, 79,* 699–704.

Swanson, H. L. (1987). Information processing theory and learning disabilities: A commentary and future perspective. *Journal of Learning Disabilities, 20,* 155–166.

Szekely, G. (1979). Order and plasticity in the nervous system. *Trends in Neuroscience 2,* 245–248.

Tickle-Degnen, L. (1988). Perspectives on the status of sensory integration theory. *American Journal of Occupational Therapy, 42,* 427–433.

Tickle-Degnen, L., & Coster, W. (1995). Therapeutic interaction and the management of challenge during the beginning minutes of sensory integration intervention. *Occupational Therapy Journal of Research, 15,* 122–141.

Varga, S., & Camilli, G. (1999). A meta-analysis of research on sensory integration intervention. *American Journal of Occupational Therapy, 53,* 189–198.

Wells, M. E., & Smith, D. W. (1983). Reduction of self-injurious behavior in mentally retarded persons using sensory integrative techniques. *American Journal of Mental Deficiency, 87,* 664–666.

White, M. (1979). A first grade intervention program for children at risk for reading failure. *Journal of Learning Disabilities, 12,* 26–32.

Wieder, S. (1996). Integrated intervention approaches for young children with mulitsystem developmental disorder. *Infants and Young Children, 8,* 24–24.

Wilson, B., & Kaplan, B. (1994) Follow-up assessment of children receiving sensory integration intervention. *Occupational Therapy Journal of Research, 14,* 244–266.

Wilson, B., Kaplan, B., Fellowes, S., Gruchy, C., & Faris, P. (1992). The efficacy of sensory integration intervention compared to tutoring. *Physical & Occupational Therapy in Pediatrics, 12,* 1–37.

17

Sensory Integration and Occupation

L. Diane Parham, PhD, OTR, FAOTA

> *I guess we can never foresee the path that life will lead us down. To me it is as if people are issued certain tools which they are allowed to use throughout their lives. . . . We have to use them to help ourselves rather than let them weigh us down. I feel that it all comes down to how we use these tools to construct our lives.*
>
> —*Lee & Jackson, 1975, p. 4*

PURPOSE AND SCOPE

The foundational work of A. Jean Ayres has resulted in clinicians, researchers, and families working together to help children who struggle with ordinary sensory and motor challenges that arise at home, in school, and at play. Although the mission to help children with problems has been the most visible theme in sensory integration theory, the link between sensory integration and occupation has been present since the early years of Ayres' work. Over the years, practitioners and families have come to appreciate the need for a deeper understanding of the ways in which the neurologic process of sensory integration affects—and is affected by—participation in the occupations that structure and give meaning to children's lives.

Ayres (1979) defined sensory integration as the "organization of sensation for use" (p. 184). The last two words in that definition, *for use*, are revealing. Unlike neuroscientists, who study neural mechanisms in isolation, Ayres' central concern as an oc-

cupational therapist was with how the nervous system organizes sensory information so that individuals can participate in meaningful and in productive occupations. This concern with occupation permeated Ayres' conceptual framework and intervention programs. Sensory integration–based intervention became a tool for helping children engage in occupations and create rich and meaningful lives.

The purpose of this chapter is to give readers an appreciation of the relationship between sensory integration and occupation and to raise questions that may guide future thinking about this relationship and its applications to real-world problems. The chapter begins with an overview of the concept of occupation, drawing from the occupational science literature. Next, the chapter explores the links between sensory integration and occupation. Finally, the chapter discusses implications for intervention with a focus on the relationship between sensory integration and occupation. I hope that insights into the relationship between sensory integration and occupation will open the door to

413

new strategies to support satisfying and productive lives, not only for children experiencing difficulties but for all individuals.

A BRIEF INTRODUCTION TO OCCUPATIONAL SCIENCE

Throughout this chapter, occupation is discussed from the viewpoint developed within the academic discipline of occupational science in the United States. Occupational science is a discipline that is centrally concerned with the study of occupation, including its form, function, and meaning (Clark et al., 1999; Yerxa et al., 1989). Although the discipline of occupational science emerged out of ideas discussed by many occupational therapists throughout the twentieth century, the establishment of the PhD program in occupational science at the University of Southern California (USC) in 1989 formalized its existence as a legitimate academic discipline (Clark & Larson, 1993; Yerxa, 1993). The study of the discipline is not situated at one particular locale, however. Many scholars working outside of USC have made important contributions to occupational science, including Bundy (1993), Christiansen (1997), Nelson (1988), Trombly (1995), and Wilcock (1998).

Occupational science is not a frame of reference or model of practice; rather, it is an academic discipline that aims to generate knowledge about occupation, so we think of it primarily as a basic rather than applied science (Yerxa et al., 1989). Of course, because most occupational scientists happen to be occupational therapists, scholars within the discipline are often concerned that knowledge gained about occupation will be useful when applied to human problems in living. Nevertheless, research in occupational science per se is not focused on therapeutic issues such as efficacy of intervention. For example, Bundy has conducted research on the relationship between play skills and sensory integration (Bundy, 1989), cross-cultural parental attitudes toward playfulness (Li et al., 1995), and the measurement of playfulness (Bundy, 1997). These studies contribute knowledge about an important type of occupation (i.e., play), but this knowledge does not directly address therapeutic issues such as the effectiveness of intervention. Even so, the knowledge is potentially useful in practice because it can stimulate new ideas for clinical assessment and the design and evaluation of interventions. For example, Morrison and Metzger (2001) described a clinical frame of reference that takes knowledge about play generated in Bundy's research and uses it to guide assessment and intervention for children with developmental problems.

DEFINING OCCUPATION

So what exactly is occupation? The term has been defined a number of ways by occupational scientists and definitions vary somewhat, depending on the particular angle of the author. One of the most widely cited definitions of occupation is "chunks of activity within the ongoing stream of human behavior which are named in the lexicon of the culture, for example, 'fishing' or 'cooking,' or at a more abstract level, 'playing' or 'working'" (Yerxa et al., 1989, p. 5). Most occupational scientists agree that occupation involves intentionality during engagement in an activity and that the person engaged in occupation experiences some degree of meaningfulness or purposefulness. However, the criterion that occupation must always be culturally named is debatable because it can be argued that some people engage in occupations that are intentional and purposeful, yet idiosyncratic, deeply personal in meaning, and not readily named by their culture. This may be true especially for occupations of infants and young children. Because occupations happen in real time and space, temporal and spatial patterns are intrinsic to occupations, as is embeddedness in sociocultural and historical contexts. Occupation is assumed to be related to health, but this assumption is just beginning to be systematically examined (Wilcock, 1998). Furthermore, occupation is usually thought to be involved with adaptation to life challenges, although it may also contribute to maladaptive behavior.

MULTIDIMENSIONALITY OF OCCUPATION

Occupational scientists fairly consistently view occupation as multidimensional, involving physical, biological, cognitive, affective, symbolic, sociocultural, and spiritual aspects that synergistically influence each other. Understanding occupation, therefore, calls for a synthesis of knowledge from many different fields of study, including biology, psychology, sociology, anthropology, theology, and life-span development. Because of this complexity, diverse research methods are often advocated for the study of occupation (Carlson & Clark, 1991; Clark et al., 1991; Parham, 1998).

The multidimensionality of occupation poses an information management challenge. How are we to organize the diverse bodies of knowledge that are relevant to an understanding of occupation? A satisfactory answer to this question has not been reached, but an initial effort to tackle the problem was presented in the form of a graphic model called the USC Model of Human Subsystems that Influence Occupation (Clark et al., 1991) (Fig. 17–1). In this model, six subsystems intrinsic to human beings and essential to the understanding of occupation are depicted. These internal subsystems are interrelated and dynamic processes because they may affect each other. This model acknowledges the environmental challenges and opportunities that influence the person (shown as input); occupation is depicted as behavior produced by the person after integration of processes involving the internal subsystems. Engagement in occupation generates feedback to the person, which further influences internal processing with the subsystems.

This model is a heuristic device for guiding the organization and development of knowledge; we do not intend that it be used as a frame of reference for clinical practice. The six subsystems are not assumed to give a complete picture of all the relevant issues in human engagement in occupation but they do serve as a reminder of the complexity of occupation. Furthermore, scholars at USC have generally found the model to be overly simplistic and limiting when adhered to strictly. Problems that we have encountered include its emphasis on the human's internal characteristics, its downplaying of the complexity and significance of environmental context and of occupation, and the linear sequence of input-processing-output that is depicted. The model was originally designed as a hierarchical, general systems model at a time when the concept of hierarchy was being supplanted by heterarchical, dynamic systems concepts. Today we do not assume that the internal subsystems are subject to hierarchical control, although to some extent they are nested within each other, just as cells of the body are nested within organs or an individual's behavior is nested within the behavior of a group of people. Similarly, we do not consider the internal human subsystems to be clearly demarcated from each other, from the environment, or from the person's occupations in the way that the model implies in its layering of subsystems within a box separating them from contextual influences and from behavior. Nevertheless, the model seems useful as a very rough, general scheme for beginning to think about the multidimensionality of human engagement in occupation, as long as one remembers that it is not literal, comprehensive, or the final word on relevant issues for the study of occupation.

Despite its limitations, this model helps us begin to think about how sensory integration is related to occupation. First, we consider the internal human

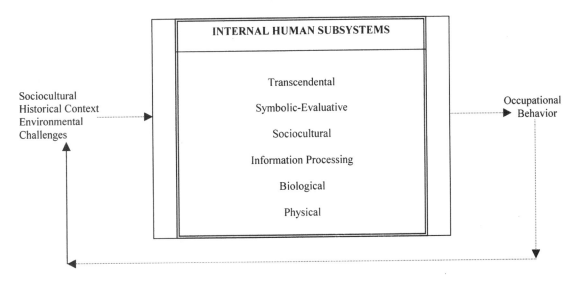

Figure 17–1 The University of Southern California Model of the Human Subsystems That Influence Occupation. (From Clark et al., 1991, with permission.)

subsystems depicted in the model, focusing on issues relevant to sensory integration. (Broader discussion of the model can be found in Clark et al. [1991] and Clark and Larson [1993].) We work our way from the bottom to the top, from the micro to the macro level of analysis. As we work our way up, we see that each subsystem is intertwined with the others. Each incorporates processes from subsystems at a relatively more micro level, but each can also be thought of as having emergent properties (i.e., unique characteristics and processes that are not simply collections of events happening within other subsystems).

Briefly, the *physical subsystem* addresses specific physicochemical processes within the body, such as neural synaptic mechanisms and transmission of sensory information via mechanoreceptors; it deals with micromechanisms within the body. In contrast, the *biological subsystem* deals with biological aspects of occupation that involve the whole organism as a living system rather than with specific micromechanisms within the body (although the living system certainly is dependent on the micromechanisms of the physical subsystem). Here we include the biological drive for mastery (i.e., what Ayres called *inner drive*) and the global sensory integrative processes that allow an individual to experience the physical world as a unified whole rather than fragmented bits of sensory information. Also fitting this subsystem are states of emotion and arousal that reflect the totality of complex neurologic and biochemical events as well as inherited tendencies to use certain behavioral patterns under certain conditions. An example of the latter is temperament, which includes the biological predisposition to react strongly to novel sensory stimuli.

The next subsystem is called *information processing*. Here cognitive operations are addressed in addition to complex conceptual functions used to organize behavior. The concept of praxis as described by Ayres (1989) falls into this subsystem because praxis is thought of as a cognitive function that influences the organization of action. The use of verbal strategies to self-regulate arousal level falls here as well. Again, this subsystem is dependent on the preceding ones. Complex cognitive functions such as praxis are dependent on more rudimentary sensory integrative, perceptual, and behavioral propensities that are biologically rooted and that, in turn, are dependent on specific physicochemical operations within the body.

The three subsystems located in the upper half of the model are less directly related to sensory integrative processes, but they are important in drawing linkages between sensory integration and occupation in its fullest sense. The *sociocultural subsystem* involves the person's understanding of social and cultural expectations regarding occupations, including the times, places, and ways in which they customarily take place in the person's sociocultural milieu. Social experiences shape these expectations and are powerful influences on occupation. However, just as genetic inheritance is a strong influence but does not determine what a person's occupational life will be, sociocultural expectations are not deterministic. The sociocultural subsystem subsumes cognitive information processing because it requires memory, problem solving, planning, and complex processing of subtle social signals, but it goes beyond cognition in addressing occupational patterns that are collectively shared.

The *symbolic-evaluative subsystem* deals with the fact that a person may choose to accept or reject a particular socioculturally entrenched pattern of occupation. This subsystem deals with the individual's assessment of the value of an occupation (Clark et al., 1991) using symbolic systems that may spring from one's idiosyncratic personal history, from sociocultural patterns, or from some combination of the highly personal and the culturally shared. The individual uses symbolic meanings in making choices of which occupations to pursue or to avoid and in prioritizing valued occupations. In the subsystem at the very top of the model, the *transcendental subsystem,* the concern is with the overarching sense of life meaning, purpose, and satisfaction the person experiences as occupations are orchestrated across a lifetime.

LINKING SENSORY INTEGRATION TO OCCUPATION

Now let us focus more specifically on sensory integration and how it articulates with the much broader concept of occupation. We begin this discussion with an imaginary case, using the USC Model of the Human as an Occupational Being (Clark et al., 1991), which was introduced in the preceding section of this chapter. In this case, we focus on how sensory integration relates to the three subsystems at the top of the model, specifically, the sociocultural, symbolic-evaluative, and transcendental subsystems.

Imagine an 8-year-old boy we will call Nick who has sensory integrative difficulties involving hazy tactile discrimination and immature visual perceptual processing. In addition, he has difficulty with the sequencing and timing aspects of praxis. These praxis difficulties make it cumbersome for Nick to manage his body and objects in physical space and in synchrony with time constraints.

With respect to the sociocultural subsystem, Nick is very aware of the general behavioral expectations placed on him by his teacher at school. However, his sensory integrative and praxis problems make it difficult for him to comply with some of these expectations, even though he would like to do so. For example, he knows he is supposed to be able to reach into his desk and find his workbooks and tools (e.g., pencil, eraser, ruler) quickly, but his desk is chaotic, and he seems unable to keep it neat for longer than half a day. His tactile sense is not developed well enough to enable him to find and handle objects quickly and efficiently. He needs to rely on visual inspection to help him find things in his desk, but his visual system is not highly skilled either, so this becomes an arduous task. His somatodyspraxia further interferes with his adeptness in handling classroom materials and tools. His classmates who have well-developed sensory integrative and praxis abilities are able to find and manage their materials quickly and easily, even those who do not have stellar desk organization habits.

Closer observation of Nick may reveal that he actually does not seem aware of some of the finer nuances of his teacher's expectations for her students. Whereas other students figure out that her expectations require that they work out strategies for desk management, Nick does not realize that he needs to do this. This may be at least partially caused by his sensory and praxis difficulties, which have limited his experiences and success with developing effective and sophisticated strategies for organizing and manipulating objects. In Nick's eyes, other kids just magically know how to reach in their desks and immediately find their school materials. His lack of recognition for the need for organizational strategies involving management of his body and physical objects in space and time extends beyond desk management into other realms, such as playground games and sports with peers. Thus, he does not realize the full ramifications of

many social expectations, such as the expectations for team members during a soccer game.

Moving now to the symbolic-evaluative subsystem, Nick's experiences—his successes and failures, pleasures and pains—as he engages in a variety of occupations will influence his future preferences and choices of occupations. He has strong verbal skills and already shows a definite preference for occupations such as reading and telling jokes. He also has an avoidance of sports and games that require skill in sequencing of actions or precision in object manipulation. Of course, not all of his choices will be related to his verbal talents or his sensory integrative difficulties; rather, many will be linked to personally meaningful symbols derived from significant persons, places, things, and events. For example, the flowers that brighten his loving grandmother's backyard give him feelings of joy, security, and contentment. Some day, the pleasant memories of his grandmother's garden may lead him to value the occupation of gardening. This occupation may also become a favorite because he enjoys the sensory experiences of gardening. His sensory integrative characteristics play a role in his occupational choices and may have a lifelong influence on his occupations. In an optimal scenario, he may become a successful attorney if he has supportive family and friends, if he continues to hone his verbal talents, and if he learns to exercise good judgment in deciding when to use verbal strategies to organize tasks and when to delegate. He may experience a great deal of satisfaction and enjoyment while gardening at home. However, it is very unlikely that he will become a professional athlete, and he probably will not choose even to participate regularly in a team sport as a leisure activity.

Clearly, sensory integration is a factor in the formation of Nick's identity, although it most certainly is not the only factor, and it may not even be the most important factor. The formation of his identity is shaped by—and shapes—the occupations in which he engages. Over time, Nick's appraisal of who he is becoming in relation to what he values most in life will affect his overall satisfaction with his life circumstances. This speaks to issues related to the transcendental subsystem. The presence of sensory integrative difficulties definitely does *not* mean that a person is doomed to be unsuccessful or unhappy. But it does present special challenges. Repeated experiences of failure may cumulatively lead to feelings of hopelessness and incompetence, avoidance and fear of challenge, a constricted range of meaningful occupations, and poor life satisfaction. Conversely, if a person's experiences lead to a strong sense of self-efficacy, the challenges posed by sensory integrative difficulties may actually contribute to the forging of self-discipline, determination, hope, character, and, consequently, a rich occupational life with a high degree of life satisfaction.

Does Poor Sensory Integration Cause Occupational Problems?

As we have just seen, sensory integration contributes to what, how, and why a person chooses particular occupations at a particular time in the life cycle. Thus, we think of sensory integration as one of the factors that shapes life outcomes. However, it is one of many potentially powerful factors. I am always reluctant to identify sensory integrative difficulties as *the* cause of a child's problems with daily occupation, or to predict that a child will definitely have future occupational problems because of the presence of sensory integrative difficulties. The complexity and multiplicity of factors that shape lives make it impossible to predict with any precision what the specific life outcomes will be for a particular child who has sensory integrative problems. The developmental process is extremely complex because it is transactional in nature. Biologically based predispositions and environmental influences mutually affect each other through dynamic interchanges, so developmental outcomes are the result of a confluence of a number of factors that change over time as they influence each other (Sameroff & Chandler, 1975). This means that not only is it impossible to predict long-term occupational outcomes for an individual child, but it is usually inappropriate to look back on the life of people who have occupational problems and identify a single, specific cause of their problems.

As an example, consider an infant who is hyperresponsive to tactile, vestibular, and auditory stimuli and has a young, impulsive mother who is very stressed by her low income living situation with limited support from family or friends. The baby recoils when touched by his mother and if environmental sounds become intense (as they often do in the small apartment with thin walls), he screams inconsolably. The infant's defensive behaviors heighten the stress of the mother, who

begins to dread interacting with her infant. She perceives him as a problem baby who does not like her, so she tries to complete infant caregiving activities (e.g., feeding, diapering, and bathing) as quickly as possible in order to be freed to leave him alone in the bedroom to cry and eventually sleep. Her insensitive handling of him aggravates his sensory defensiveness, and consequently he cries more often and more intensely. In a worst-case scenario, the mother may try to cope with this escalating situation by physically neglecting or even abusing the baby.

Four years go by, and we see the baby grow into a preschooler who struggles to engage in play occupations for more than a fleeting time. Not only does he have trouble with solitary play but he also seems unable to play with peers without acting out aggressively and destructively. In the preschool setting, he stands out as a child who is having great difficulty. In this example, what was the original cause of the child's preschool difficulties? His sensory defensiveness or his mother's stress? The mother's impulsive personality or the baby's difficult temperament? Is the cause the mother's lack of access to resources and supports or her lack of knowledge regarding how to engage with the child sensitively during daily routines? All are legitimate causes, because each of these issues affects the others and all of them interact synergistically to shape the child's life. It would be inappropriate to single out one as the sole cause, although some may exert more powerful effects than others.

Even in such an extreme example as this one, the very rocky beginning in the mother–infant relationship will not necessarily doom this infant to future failure. All along the life course, events and experiences arise that shape and guide who the child is becoming. We can imagine a different preschool outcome for the difficult infant in our above example if, for example, we introduce a day care provider into the picture when the baby is a toddler. Let us say this day care provider is gifted at intuiting the toddler's needs and fine tunes the day care environment so that he is not overwhelmed by sensations, he experiences pleasure and mastery in simple sensory-motor activities, and he is cared for by an adult who is nurturing but also sets limits on his behavior in a consistent manner. Furthermore, the day care provider forms a positive relationship with the infant's mother and mentors her in mothering. It is likely that the child's later preschool experiences will not be as negative in this scenario compared with what the situation might have been had he not had the good fortune of an optimal day care experience.

So, in answer to the question, "Does poor sensory integration cause occupational problems?" my answer is, "Yes, but not by itself." Poor sensory integration does not singlehandedly cause difficulties in engaging in occupations; rather, it interacts with talents, physical attributes, environmental opportunities, contexts, past experiences, and a host of other factors, all changing over time and affecting one another, to shape and color the person's occupational life.

Evidence That Sensory Integration Influences Occupation

It is fascinating to contemplate how sensory integration capacities interweave with experiences and environments to shape a person's life. But given the many influences on developmental and life outcomes, how can we be sure that sensory integration really is a significant contributing factor? Is it a critical enough factor that we should pay attention to it when planning intervention for a child?

Currently, most of the evidence that supports the impact of sensory integration abilities on occupation is anecdotal because very little research has specifically examined long-term outcomes for people with sensory integrative problems or talents. However, a few studies exist that provide us with some evidence that sensory integrative characteristics are a potentially critical factor in shaping lives, particularly with respect to occupational concerns. I focus on two studies, one a quantitative study that examined sensory integrative development in relation to children's academic success and the other a qualitative study of an adult whose life history was affected by sensory integrative problems from childhood.

Sensory Integration and Academic Achievement

From an occupational point of view, academic achievement is an outcome of engaging in academic occupations. Reading, writing, and doing mathematics are occupations because they involve doing something that entails intentionality and at least some degree of meaningfulness. These academic occupations contribute to a person's potential for adaptation to changing life circumstances, particularly in highly industrialized societies. When children successfully participate in academic occupations, they acquire literacy skills that will be critical in shaping their occupational lives at work, at home, and in the community.

According to sensory integration theory, children who have poor sensory integrative abilities are at a disadvantage academically, presumably because underlying neural processes make the learning process in an academic setting inefficient or stressful (Ayres, 1972, 1979). Conversely, children with very well-developed sensory integrative abilities should have an advantage in acquiring academic skills. To address the question of whether sensory integration is related to academic achievement, as theory predicts it is, I conducted a 4-year longitudinal study of elementary school children in which I examined the relationship of sensory integration abilities, intelligence, and other characteristics of children (e.g., socioeconomic status) with academic performance in reading and arithmetic (Parham, 1998).

Participants were 32 children with learning disabilities and 35 children who had no known disability. The children were tested initially at ages 6 to 8 years and then retested on the same measures 4 years later at ages 10 to 12 years. To measure sensory integration abilities, I used the Sensory Integration and Praxis Tests (SIPT) (Ayres, 1989). To measure reading and arithmetic achievement, I used the Reading and Arithmetic subtests of the Kaufman Assessment Battery for Children (K-ABC) (Kaufman & Kaufman, 1983). I used the K-ABC Mental Processing Composite score as the measure of intelligence.

Measuring the intelligence of the participating children was an important feature of this study because it allowed me to control for the effects of intelligence when estimating the relationship of sensory integration to academic achievement. Most of the previous research on sensory integration and other perceptual-motor abilities had not controlled for children's intelligence, so any detected effects of sensory integration on academic performance could be explained by the participants' intelligence. In other words, one could argue that children with sensory integration problems score lower on academic achievement measures than children without such problems, not because sensory integration is making an impact, but because children with sensory integration problems have slightly lower intelligence, on average, and it is the intellectual limitation that is having the impact on achievement. So unless I took children's intelligence into consideration, any effect of sensory integration on achievement that I found could be dismissed as an artifact of lower intelligence.

The astute reader may be wondering how I used SIPT scores in this study because the participants at the second wave of data collection were 10 to 12 years old. Raw scores cannot be obtained on most tests of the SIPT, and standard scores require computer scoring using normative data that extend only to age 8 years, 11 months. I dealt with this situation by using the chronological age of the child at the first time of testing for determining standard SIPT scores both the first time it was given and the second time, four years later. For example, if a child was 6 years, 9 months old at the first testing, I used that age to obtain her first set of SIPT standard scores. Then when she was tested 4 years later (at age 10 years, 9 months) I used her original age (6 years, 9 months) to score her second SIPT battery. For all the children in the study, SIPT scores tended to increase quite a bit when tested at the older ages because the child's performance was being compared with the same normative age group as when tested 4 years earlier. This solution worked quite well for the purpose of our study.

The SIPT consists of 17 tests, which brought up another challenge I had to address. How was I going to make sense of statistical results for 17 different measures of sensory integration? The results of the study would be much easier to interpret if I could reduce these 17 scores to just a few. Fortunately, the publisher of the SIPT, Western Psychological Services, provided me with SIPT factor scores that I used in the analyses. The publisher used a statistical formula to condense the 17 SIPT tests into three scores, called *factor scores,* that essentially were composite scores of several factors that had emerged in a factor analytic study of the SIPT (Ayres, 1989). So, instead of having to interpret 17 SIPT scores relative to academic achievement, I ended up with three SIPT scores that I used in the analyses: somatopraxis (which I simply called *praxis*), visuopraxis (which I renamed *visual perception* because this is a more familiar term for most people), and somatosensory (which was primarily determined by the Localization of Tactile Stimuli score). After I received the factor scores for each child at each point in time from the publisher, I proceeded to analyze the data to examine the extent to which

the SIPT factors were related to reading and math achievement concurrently and across the 4-year span of the study.

I used a series of multiple regression models to analyze the data. Results showed that the SIPT factors at ages 6 to 8 years were significant predictors of arithmetic and reading scores 4 years later, at ages 10 to 12 years, even when controlling for intelligence. SIPT scores were very strongly related to math achievement concurrently at ages 6 to 8 years, accounting for 69 percent of the variance in arithmetic scores ($R^2 = 0.69$). In fact, the three SIPT factors together were better predictors of arithmetic achievement at ages 6 to 8 years than was IQ score. Sensory integration, as measured by the praxis and visual perception factors, was even more strongly related to arithmetic achievement 4 years later, with intelligence making a smaller but significant contribution ($R^2 = 0.77$). Sensory integration did not contribute significantly to reading at the younger ages (6 to 8 years) beyond the effects of intelligence and socioeconomic status. However, in predicting reading 4 years later, the praxis and visual perception factors were significant, along with intelligence and socioeconomic status. Across all of the analyses of reading and math, the praxis factor was consistently the most powerful sensory integration factor in predicting academic achievement.

We can conclude that for the children in this study, sensory integration was strongly related to skill development in reading and doing arithmetic and that it contributed something that significantly went beyond the effects of intelligence. Moreover, we have evidence here that is derived from a group of 67 children, with and without disabilities, who were studied over a 4-year period, suggesting that the relationship that we found between sensory integration and academic skill is long lasting and may be characteristic of elementary school children in general. We will have greater confidence that the findings are generalizable to other children if future research replicates these findings.

Because the participants with learning disabilities were not receiving intervention for sensory integration problems, this study does not tell us anything about the effects of intervention. In addition, sensory integration was measured by the SIPT, so our conclusions are drawn in relation to the perceptual, discriminative, and praxis aspects of sensory integration. Because the SIPT does not measure sensory modulation, we cannot tell from this study whether sensory modulation is related to academic skill development.

We also cannot tell from this study why sensory integrative ability appears to contribute to academic skills. We have shown that it is not the same as intelligence, but we still do not know exactly what it reflects that links it to academic achievement. We might hypothesize that children with poor sensory integrative performance experience more stress in school than most children because their basic functions (e.g., postural control, tactile perception, body scheme) are not well developed; therefore, they must exert effort and conscious attention toward these basic functions that should be automatic and effortless by school age. This aspect of the theory has not been tested directly, so we do not yet know if this assumption is correct or if another process is at work. Even if future research verifies this assumption to some extent, it does not explain why sensory integrative performance would be more strongly related to arithmetic than to reading skills, as I found in my study.

My study does not cast light on children as occupational beings while they engage in academic tasks. That is, it does not give us insight into how children individually experience the doing of academic occupations and how sensory integration might influence this. In what ways might academic occupations be meaningful—and in what ways might they not be meaningful—to individual children with different patterns of sensory integrative development? How do the sensory needs of children affect their engagement in academic occupations? What are the temporal and spatial patterns of task organization that children use while engaging in academic occupations, and how are these related to sensory integrative characteristics? How does the orchestration of different activities (e.g., recess, music, art, physical education, academics) throughout the school day affect engagement in academic occupations, and how might the effects vary in relation to the sensory characteristics of children?

Educators and behavioral scientists have grappled for many years with broader questions that dovetail with the interests of occupational scientists. For example, what kinds of academic activities seem to evoke deeper involvement for which children? Are there particular occupational styles of children that fit best with particular strategies for doing academic activities? How does the learning environment affect engagement in academic occupations and the acquisition of academic skills? Of course, experts in other fields have already made very important contributions to these issues (e.g., Armstrong, 1987; Bruner, 1996; Gardner, 1983). I do not presume that occupational science will provide the definitive answers to these complex problems, but an occupational perspective may bring some new insights to the table that could be helpful. Furthermore, a perspective that melds knowledge of occupation with expertise in sensory integration may add a powerful new dimension to understanding children as they engage in academic occupations and acquire academic skills for success and satisfaction in life.

Sensory Integration and Occupations in Adulthood

Now we shift to a different issue that links sensory integration to occupation: the relationship of sensory integration characteristics to occupations across the lifespan. We use another research study to begin this discussion. This study uses a completely different research method than the study discussed in the preceding section.

Fanchiang (1996) examined the life history of a young man who had been diagnosed with sensory integrative dysfunction and received intervention for it as a child. She used a qualitative research design, specifically using narrative analysis with a life history approach. The purposes of this study were dual: to explore long-term outcomes of an adult who had received sensory integrative intervention in childhood and to examine the process of adaptation using occupational interpretations from personal and cultural viewpoints.

The participant, Dale, at age 25 years initiated contact with the clinical site where he had received occupational therapy as a child. At the time that he made this contact, he seemed to be going through a period of reassessing his identity and life goals. Fanchiang (1996), an occupational therapist, recognized the potential for collaborating with him to gain a long-term perspective on adaptation with a learning disability. Dale agreed to participate in hopes that this study would help other people with learning disabilities.

Over a 4-month period, six personal interviews were conducted, each lasting from 3 to 5 hours, as well as four telephone interviews. One year after the initial interview, an additional follow-up interview was conducted. All interviews were audiotaped, transcribed, and then analyzed through a process in which contents were coded, sorted sequentially, and then collapsed to identify themes of life history. A second analysis after the 1-year follow-up interview addressed Dale's occupational metamorphosis during the study.

Analysis of the initial interviews yielded three main themes: one related to Dale's mother's parental strategies, one related to his personal needs for intense sensory experiences ("adrenaline surges" and "hell raising"), and one related to his work experiences and construction of himself as a business deal maker. These themes seemed interrelated. Dale's narratives portrayed his mother as highly invested in channeling her headstrong son's occupations in responsible, constructive directions. In addition to seeking out occupational therapy for his learning disability when he was a child, she structured his life so that he needed to plan and work to earn money for the things he wanted. The work projects and businesses he developed over the years were quite successful for building self-discipline and negotiation skills as well as monetary profits. By the time he reached his mid-twenties, he had a strong sense of himself as a very competent businessman, but he did not experience his work as inspiring, stimulating, or enjoyable.

When contacted for the follow-up interview 1 year after the initial interviews, he was working full time as a massage therapist. Apparently, after the initial interviews had been completed the year before, Dale reassessed his life goals and decided to pursue professional training as a massage therapist. This turned out to be a choice with which he was satisfied; he reported that he felt calm, soothed, and organized when doing this work. In fact, he described himself as being energized by doing massage.

Fanchiang (1996) discussed this case from several angles, drawing attention to how character develops through parental structuring of occupation as well as one's own selection of occupations and how stepping outside of one's habitual routine to take on an alternative viewpoint may be adaptive in making pivotal occupational choices. She also commented that Dale's history suggested a connection between choices of occupations and biological drives.

This last point deserves further comment because it is particularly relevant to sensory integration. Sensory integration is an integral part of the biological makeup of an individual, and individual sensory processing characteristics may give rise to biological drives to seek or even crave certain types of sensations or sensory-motor experiences. Sensory characteristics also can lead to aversions to certain types of experiences that are perceived as stressful and unpleasant. In Fanchiang's study, we do not have any information about the sensory integration diagnosis that was assigned to Dale as a child, but we can infer from his narratives that he probably was a person whose sensory characteristics led him to crave intense sensations. As a teenager, these cravings led him into some potentially maladaptive occupations such as illicit recreational drug use and "hell raising." As he matured, he devoted himself to socially acceptable work as a businessman but apparently felt something was missing from his life, hence his quest to reexamine his identity and his occupational choices. Interestingly, he chose a career in massage therapy, which provided him with frequent doses of strong proprioceptive and tactile stimuli that he experienced as calming.

We can conclude from this study that it is possible for the sensory processing characteristics of an individual to influence occupational choices throughout childhood and into early adulthood and that sensory characteristics may be pivotal in particular life decisions. This is not to say that other factors were not important in this case but simply that sensory aspects played a key role in shaping this person's life. This study does *not* tell us that sensory processing characteristics are central influences in every person's occupational choices, even for every person with sensory integrative problems, nor does it present specific information that is generalizable to a large number of people. Even so, it does provide valuable information because it reveals the potential power of sensory characteristics to shape identity and, consequently, life course. It demonstrates how sensory issues may become a recurrent transformative force that imparts meaning throughout a person's life.

Other research studies reinforce these suggestions that sensory characteristics and experiences may have a strong influence on meaning, identity, and occupational choices across a lifetime for some individuals. For example, Zuckerman (1994), a personality psychologist, developed a theoretical framework around sensation seeking as a lifelong personality trait. Building on a large body of research initiated in the 1960s, Zuckerman (1994) defined sensation seeking as "a trait defined by the seeking of varied, novel, complex, and intense sensations and experiences, and the willingness to take physical, social, legal, and financial risks for the sake of such experience" (p. 27). Perhaps Dale, in Fanchiang's study (1996), represented what Zuckerman called high sensation seekers.

Zuckerman (1994) theorized that within each person's brain, an optimal level of catecholamine system activity is maintained by genetically based characteristics that mediate sensation-seeking or sensation-reducing behaviors. He suggested that high sensation seekers have dopaminergic systems that are genetically predisposed to be strongly active or deregulated (i.e., inconsistently activated), leading to active approach behaviors and pleasure with intense stimulation. This is combined with low tonic levels of norepinephrine, which makes the person easily bored and likely to seek novel stimuli in order to increase arousal. Weak levels of serotonin may contribute to the sensation seeker's reduced inhibition in response to novel or threatening stimuli. Thus, the brains of high sensation seekers may be more accessible to novel or intense stimuli compared with most people. They may be driven to seek novel, varied, or intense stimulation in order to avoid boredom and experience pleasure.

Zuckerman presents evidence from psychophysiological research on electrodermal and heart rate responses to support his hypotheses that high sensation seekers typically have a strong orienting response to an initial stimulus but habituate quickly when it is repeated. This suggests that high sensation seekers are quickly aroused by strong or novel sensations but because they quickly habituate, they often find themselves in a state of stimulus hunger that drives them to seek more novel or strong sensations. Furthermore, Zuckerman presents an impressive body of psychometric and behavioral research that links sensation seeking to choices of occupations and ways of engaging in occupations. For example, evidence indicates that high sensation seeking people tend to enjoy highly stimulating occupations (e.g., skydiving and rock climbing), are likely to choose work that involves a high degree of varied social contact, and usually like foods that are novel (e.g., foreign foods) or stimulating (e.g., spicy or sour foods). Conversely, those who are easily overwhelmed by sensations tend to avoid occupations with high degrees of intense sensory stimuli and high levels of social contact.

Although Zuckerman's theory focuses on the biological aspects of sensation seeking, he does acknowledge that social contexts are also very powerful in influencing a person's behavior. For example, whether a sensation-seeking person becomes a chronic recreational drug abuser or an avid group sports participant may have a great deal to do with social and economic resources and opportunities. Many people with strong drives for intense sensory experiences may develop enough self-awareness to figure out how they can meet their sensory needs in self-regulating ways in order to avoid jeopardizing their health or well being. The case of Dale, who eventually chose to do massage therapy professionally, provided a good example (Fanchiang, 1996). However, many high sensation seekers may need some assistance in gaining insight into their sensory processing characteristics and designing a lifestyle that takes into account sensory needs in order to optimize their health and well being. Creative occupational therapists immediately recognize the therapeutic implications for working with people who are high sensation seekers: help those people redesign their lifestyles so that they provide a lot of novelty and stimulation within safe boundaries, with carefully thought-out risk management. High sensation seekers also could benefit from learning to recognize personal sensory needs so that they can anticipate and manage them before maladaptive urges arise. This is an idea that is the basis for the *Alert Program for Self-Regulation,* which was developed by occupational therapists for application to children with sensory modulation problems (Williams & Shellenberger, 1994).

So far we have discussed sensory seeking (sometimes referred to as *sensory underresponsiveness* or *hyporesponsivity*) in relation to occupational choices across the lifespan. Some research and a great deal of clinical anecdotal evidence also point to the profound effects of sensory overresponding, or defensiveness, the other end of the spectrum from underresponsiveness, on occupational choices throughout life.

Kinnealey et al. (1995) conducted a qualitative study of five adults who had been identified as having sensory defensiveness. Videotaped interviews of these individuals were transcribed and coded in order to identify patterns of sensory experiences and coping strategies that the participants used to deal with situations they perceived as having disturbing sensory qualities. Results revealed examples of how sensory aversions influenced choices of work and leisure occupations and the ways in which activities were done. For example, participants described being unable to tolerate gardening or fishing without gloves, being fearful of playing on playgrounds as a child, avoiding parties, and refusing to go shopping during the holidays because of overwhelming sensations. To cope with their defensiveness, participants described strategies such as avoidance of threatening situations, use of predictability and control by having daily routines and objects arranged in a particular manner, mental preparation for stressful situations, talking oneself through a difficult situation, counteracting defensiveness with sensory experiences that are calming or pleasurable, and confrontation by forcing oneself to go through an aversive experience. These coping strategies seemed to have become engrained into their personalities with age.

The researchers expressed concern that interpersonal relationships and social participation may be profoundly affected by sensory defensiveness. They believed that tactile and vestibular defensiveness (i.e., gravitational insecurity), in particular, had powerful influences on occupational choices and that the coping strategies described by the participants did not diminish their defensiveness over time (although these strategies did help them deal with daily sensory challenges). Intervention suggestions made by these authors included provision of regular tactile and proprioceptive stimulation and a sensory diet that could be incorporated into daily routines. In addition, I wonder if intervention aimed at lifestyle redesign, with an emphasis on gentle sensory enrichment and very gradual, individually tailored sensory challenges to evoke adaptive behavior while maintaining predictability, might result in expanding the occupational repertoire and life satisfaction of individuals with severe sensory defensiveness.

Recently, Dunn (2000) developed an interesting conceptual model that links hypo- as well as hyperresponsive patterns of sensory modulation with neural processes of habituation, sensitization, threshold, and homeostasis (see also Chapter 7). In her model, she identified four main patterns that represent individual differences in nervous system responsiveness: low registration, sensitivity to stimuli, sensation seeking, and sensation avoiding. For each type of pattern, Dunn suggests arranging daily tasks and environments and choosing jobs that maximize the ease with which the person can function in everyday life. For example, for a sensation-

avoiding person who creates rituals in order to make life predictable, Dunn recommended selecting a job with a predictable pattern of activities across the day; identifying the sensory qualities that the person finds comfortable and building them into daily tasks and environments; and preparing for new situations as much as possible (e.g., giving the person information about the new situation in advance). Thus, Dunn's model offers a systematic approach for developing compensatory strategies for individuals with a broad array of sensory characteristics. Her model addresses the various ways that sensory modulation characteristics influence occupation and may be very useful in stimulating ideas for helping individuals build lives that are satisfying and productive.

Throughout this discussion of the impact of sensory integration on occupation throughout life, we have dealt with sensory modulation issues. I am not aware of any studies that examine the long-term effects of sensory discrimination, postural control, or praxis difficulties on occupational choices in adulthood. I suspect that such effects are likely to exist, although they may not be as dramatic as what we see in individuals with modulation issues. Research in these areas would be fascinating. For example, I would expect that children with somatodyspraxia develop specific coping strategies that allow them to compensate for their poor motor planning. I further expect that they make occupational choices in adulthood that minimize motor coordination demands and maximize use of their personal strengths and talents. I wonder to what extent motor planning difficulties interfere with social participation in childhood and adulthood, and if they do interfere, whether it has an impact on their quality of life in the long run. And, of course, because my professional background is in occupational therapy, I wonder whether intervention early in life can alter the long-range life outcomes of individuals with dyspraxia in a positive way.

CAN ENGAGEMENT IN OCCUPATION INFLUENCE SENSORY INTEGRATION?

In thinking about the long-term relationships between sensory integration abilities and occupation, let us revisit the transactional view of development (Sameroff & Chandler, 1975) discussed earlier. In this view, developmental outcomes are not caused solely by characteristics of children or solely by environmental influences but, rather, by transactions between these factors. Therefore, child characteristics change the environment, and environmental influences change child characteristics, in a continual reciprocal cycle as time goes by. In the preceding section, we saw some examples of how sensory characteristics led to environmental changes as individuals sought to cope with or adapt to their sensory-based experiences. For example, Kinnealey et al. (1995) reported that some adults with sensory defensiveness arranged their environments to increase their predictability and personal control in order to minimize aversive responses to sensory experiences. But can environmental qualities and opportunities change the person's sensory integrative characteristics? And furthermore, because occupation involves acting on environmental opportunities, can we say that engagement in occupation leads to changes in a person's sensory integrative abilities and in the neurologic substrates that support these abilities?

A very large body of research provides strong evidence that action on the environment is a powerful force in sculpting brain functions. The past 40 years of animal research on brain development and on the effects of environments on the brain throughout the lifespan have shown that experiences with the environment directly influence brain structure and function. In addition, neurobiological evidence suggests that when a person actively uses particular skills and functions, underlying synaptic mechanisms are strengthened. Conversely, when they are not used, relevant synaptic connections weaken and may be pruned out and replaced by those of competing functions (Chugani, 1994; Diamond & Hopson, 1998; Hubel & Wiesel, 1970; Huttenlocher & de Couten, 1987). Thus, specific types of experience appear to strengthen or weaken specific brain structures and functions. Pert (1997) suggested that engagement in occupations may also alter body chemistry through changes in neuropeptide activity throughout the body.

Building on a lifetime career of studying the effects of environmental enrichment on the brain, neuroscientist Marian Diamond (Diamond & Hopson, 1998) recently summarized current knowledge in this field from nonhuman and human research and made recommendations for enhancing child development using this knowledge. She identified four primary brain-shaping environmental influences:

1. Chemical (e.g., drugs, stress, nutrition)
2. Emotional
3. Educational
4. Vocational (e.g., sports, games, and hobbies)

Thus, academic activities and a variety of types of play activities figure prominently in her formulations for strengthening brain functions through environmental influences. Furthermore, she emphasized children's active involvement and the personal meaningfulness of the activities as important indicators of a potentially brain-shaping experience. In other words, active engagement in occupations is thought to have an effect on underlying brain functions and consequently on relevant skill development.

Most of the human studies on which Diamond based her recommendations focus on visual and auditory capabilities. Compelling evidence indicates that enriched visual-spatial and auditory or language experiences appear to stimulate and strengthen the brain mechanisms that support behavioral competencies using these modalities (e.g., Jacobs et al., 1993; Neville, 1995; Simonds & Scheibel, 1989). Given the existing evidence, it is plausible that particular types of occupational engagement, including participation in sensory integration–based occupational therapy, may result in particular neural changes.

Little is known, however, about specific environmental effects on brain structures or mechanisms that underlie other sensory integrative abilities that are particularly interesting to occupational therapists, such as somatosensory perception and praxis skills or vestibular-proprioceptive processing. Studies of laboratory rats have shown that sensory-motor exploration of enriched environments leads to thicker somatosensory areas in the cerebral cortex, with corresponding luxuriant dendritic branching of neurons in those areas (Diamond et al., 1964).

In an autopsy study of humans, a group of brain researchers examined the relationship between neural synaptic structures and the occupations of subjects. In individuals who held jobs that required a great deal of hand and finger dexterity (e.g., typist), they found bushier dendritic branching in the areas of the cortex that receive somatosensory input from hands and fingers and relatively less dendritic branching in areas that receive input from the trunk (Scheibel et al., 1990). Thus, specific types of experience likely shape the brain mechanisms that support the behavioral competencies being developed. So, although we lack studies of experiential effects on the particular brain structures and functions that underlie specific sensory integrative capabilities, it is reasonable to expect that, in general, when children act on environmental opportunities that challenge their sensory integrative capacities, the supporting brain functions that are involved become better developed. Consequently, the sensory integrative abilities that are being challenged and expressed behaviorally also become better developed.

Of course, this assumption was germane in Ayres' theoretical work on sensory integration. One of the basic ideas proposed by Ayres (1972, 1979) was that adaptive responses are critical in moving sensory integrative development forward. She claimed that when a child organizes an adaptive response to a sensory-motor challenge presented in the environment, the child's brain became better organized to handle the challenge so that, in the future, it will be able to respond more efficiently to similar challenges. Thus, in providing intervention, practitioners should manipulate the environment (including themselves as aspects of the environment) to present challenges at just the right level of novelty or complexity to evoke adaptive responses from the child. These adaptive responses, if they are different or more complex compared with the child's past behavior, were thought to improve the efficiency of the brain's processing of similar information in future environmental transactions. Thus, Ayres' intervention approach rests on the assumption that environmental opportunities, if acted on by the child, are key elements in changing the child's sensory integrative capabilities and, therefore, his or her future environmental interactions.

But is a child who participates in sensory integration–based occupational therapy engaging in occupation? Both the philosophy of treatment and research on the dynamic process of treatment, indicate that the answer to this question is, "Yes."

Researchers from Boston University examined the process of sensory integration–based occupational therapy through microanalysis of videotaped therapist–child interactions (Coster et al., 1995; Dunkerly et al., 1997; Tickle-Degnan & Coster, 1995). The just-right challenge is one of the aspects they focused on in their analyses of naturally occurring therapy sessions. For example, among their many results, they found that the occurrence of events rated as containing a just-right challenge tended to be correlated with therapist variables such as being playful and using equipment and treatment space creatively (Dunkerly et al., 1997). Among the key child variables they identified were engagement in work and play, which are both occupational in nature. They reported that children tended to play before engaging in challenging activities during therapy and that they more often engaged in work when the situation involved a just-right challenge. Other characteristics of children that were correlated with just-right challenges were effort (trying hard), cooperation, seeking assistance, and slight anxiety (Dunkerly et al., 1997).

These researchers' use of the terms *work* and *play* to describe children's involvement during sensory integration–based occupational therapy (Dunkerly et al., 1997) suggests that children are engaged in occupation during this type of intervention. Recall that earlier in this chapter, I stated that occupation involves doing an activity and, furthermore, that it is characterized by intentionality and by some degree of purpose or meaning. These criteria certainly are met for children who participate in sensory integration–based occupational therapy, which emphasizes the active engagement and self-direction of the child (Parham & Mailloux, 2001). So, if Ayres was correct that the intervention she developed brings about changes in the child's neurologic capacity to organize sensory information for use, then engagement in occupation has the potential to change sensory integration mechanisms in the nervous system as well as sensory integrative capabilities that are expressed behaviorally.

Existing intervention effectiveness research on sensory integration does not provide us with evidence that Ayres' hypothesis was correct because direct measures of brain function have not been used in this research, and measures of sensory integrative abilities (e.g., the SIPT) are not generally used as yardsticks for treatment effectiveness. Furthermore, we probably will never have the definitive answer to whether environmental enrichment, including occupational therapy, causes changes in brain function in humans because in order to demonstrate causation, it would be necessary to conduct unethical experimental research entailing controlled manipulation of individuals' environments followed by brain dissection.

However, it is encouraging to note that two

clinical trials found long-term effects of sensory integrative treatment that are consistent with the possibility of brain changes. In these studies, researchers reported maintenance of gains over a 2-year period after cessation of intervention (Grimwood & Rutherford, 1980; Wilson & Kaplan, 1994). One would expect that, if intervention is optimizing brain function and increasing the child's feelings of self-efficacy, then developmental advantages gained in intervention should be self-sustaining (assuming that seriously detrimental changes in environment do not occur) and should not fade when intervention is over. Results of these studies, therefore, are consistent with what we would predict if a change in the biological bases of sensory integration had occurred as a result of intervention in conjunction with self-efficacy. This interpretation must be considered very cautiously, however, not only because the research did not address sensory integrative neural mechanisms but also because alternative explanations could account for the long-term advantages associated with the sensory integration intervention. For example, it could be that the child's newly developed belief in him- or herself as a competent person is the critical ingredient and that underlying neural mechanisms of sensory integration do not change as a result of therapy. Or perhaps the child is developing insight and compensatory strategies through intervention yet underlying neurologic functions responsible for the sensory integration problems are not changing. If future research confirms that sensory integration–based occupational therapy produces long-term developmental advantages, these questions will be important to explore in order to understand why such effects are occurring.

To summarize, we do have some neurobiological evidence that engagement in occupation influences both sensory integrative abilities and the relevant underlying neural structures that are being used. However, our knowledge about this relationship is limited in scope, particularly in relation to the sensory integrative functions with which occupational therapists are most involved. Given the existing evidence, it is plausible that particular types of occupational engagement, including participation in sensory integration–based occupational therapy, may result in particular neural changes. These issues raise important questions in relation to intervention, which is discussed in the next section.

IMPLICATIONS FOR CLINICAL PRACTICE

Although they do not always explicitly mention occupation, the preceding chapters of this volume are full of discussions regarding clinical issues that are relevant to the occupational nature of children and to occupation as a critical ingredient in the dynamic process of sensory integration–based occupational therapy. In this chapter, we have centered on the concept of occupation and its relationship with sensory integration. So far, we have discussed the multidimensional nature of occupation, the evidence that sensory integration influences occupation, and the possibility that occupation influences the behavioral expressions as well as the underlying neural mechanisms of sensory integration. Throughout these discussions, we have adopted a transactional view of development. Now we will consider a few of the implications that these ideas have for clinical practice. What you will see in these sections are my thoughts at the present time, which draw from the current literature on occupation-based practice; however, they may change with ongoing discourse.

Future-Oriented Top-Down Assessment

Because occupational therapy is a practice profession that is centrally concerned with occupation as a key aspect of health and well being, clinicians should place occupation at the front and center of the assessment process. Drawing from the material discussed in this chapter and from current occupational therapy literature, I will offer some suggestions for the occupational therapy assessment process.

Over the past decade, leaders in the profession have recommended that therapists eschew a bottom-up assessment approach and instead embrace a top-down approach (see also Chapter 7). By "bottom-up," we mean that assessment begins with a focus on specific components believed to be affected by the patient's condition, such as strength, coordination, or perceptual skills (Trombly, 1993). An example of a bottom-up assessment strategy is provided by an occupational therapist who administers the SIPT or who tests visual perception or fine motor coordination as the first step in initial assessment of a child who has been referred with a diagnosis of attention deficit disorder. We may think of this approach to assessment as component driven

(Gray, 1998) because concerns with sensory, perceptual, and motor components are driving clinical assessment and subsequent intervention.

In contrast, "top-down" refers to an assessment process that begins with information gathering regarding occupation, specifically, what the person wants and needs to do, the contexts for performing these occupations, and the current strengths and limitations in performing the desired occupations (Coster, 1998; Fisher, 1998; Fisher & Short-DeGraff, 1993). For example, an occupational therapist who uses a top-down strategy with a child diagnosed with attention deficit disorder will initially gather information regarding what the child wants to do and needs to do (according to the child; the parents; and other important people in the child's life, such as teachers), what the contexts are for the child's current occupations (e.g., school, home, community settings), and what the child and others perceive as the current successes and problems the child experiences in doing valued occupations. This initial investigation then leads to decisions regarding whether further assessment of specific tasks or components is warranted, including assessment of performance components such as sensory integrative abilities. Use of a top-down strategy, therefore, puts the assessment of sensory integrative functioning into the broader context of the child's life. This contextualizing of sensory integration assessment is likely to be more helpful and meaningful to the children who are being assessed, as well as to their families.

A potential problem with the top-down assessment approach, as described in the current literature, is that it focuses on problems in occupation only at the time of assessment (Coster, 1998; Fisher, 1998). However, occupational therapists project into the future as they plan the course of therapy with their patients. In fact, based on their qualitative study of occupational therapists engaged in practice, Mattingly and Fleming (1994) claimed that occupational therapists imagine who their patients will become in the future and, furthermore, that they create stories with the patient about what has happened in the past and what will happen in the future as the person's life unfolds. Perhaps occupational therapists should include in their clinical assessments the family and child visions of the future, specifically with respect to

occupations (i.e., what the family and child anticipate that the child will want and need to do in a few years).

The transactional view of development also suggests that assessment should be future oriented. Because development is continually shaped and channeled by transactions between the child and the environment, assessment should be repeated over time. This could take place during the ongoing process of intervention or it could be in the form of intermittent monitoring over time. The purpose of re-assessment is to ensure that the child's occupational development is moving in the desired direction; to detect whether new issues related to the child's occupations have emerged; and to reevaluate intervention or occupational options in order to reformulate the most beneficial plan for helping the child and family, given changes that have occurred. Note that this assessment strategy continues to use a top-down approach, with occupation as the primary reference point, but assessment is not conducted only at one specific point in time. Instead, assessment is ongoing or recurs intermittently as time moves forward.

An implication of bringing a future orientation into clinical assessment is that the prevention of potential problems becomes an issue. When assessment addresses only satisfaction or concerns in relation to the present situation, one's attention is not drawn systematically to information that may signal risk for future problems. A present-only assessment strategy may lead to concluding that a particular child or family will not benefit from intervention because there is no evidence of an occupational problem at the current time, when in fact some assistance or guidance at the present time may be helpful in averting problems that are likely to emerge in the future. If one is consciously imagining the future occupational life of a child by extrapolating from what is known about present occupational patterns and contexts, as well as the current status of performance components, it is more likely that risk factors for later occupational difficulties will be identified and that something will be done to minimize or counteract the risk.

Granted, not much is known about the early risk factors for problems in having a satisfying, productive, and enjoyable work and play life. Additionally, the American health-care and education systems are currently not prepared to designate funding for large-scale preventive programs.

Nevertheless, preventive efforts should be economically advantageous in the long run because prevention should be less expensive than funding intervention, welfare support, or incarceration of people with disturbed or disrupted lives.

Perhaps future research will identify early predictors of occupational problems in childhood, adolescence, and adulthood. We may find that there are times when screening or assessment of occupational components, such as sensory integration, is appropriate for preventive purposes, as when children are screened for vision or hearing problems so that intervention can be introduced before such problems have adverse effects on school performance and other aspects of the child's life. This use of performance components is directed toward ultimately maximizing the child's future occupational life; therefore, we can think of it as a top-down approach in which the top is projected into the future.

Even though research is limited and we must keep in mind the limitations of the existing research, I recommend that occupational therapists incorporate estimations of risk into their assessments by imagining where the child and family might end up in the future if they continue on their current course. In considering how to minimize child and family risk, occupational therapists need to consider all potential resources available that may be helpful to the child or family. For example, we already have evidence that praxis difficulties in early childhood place a child at risk for later academic problems, especially in mathematics (Parham, 1998). Occupational therapists working with young children with dyspraxia may want to share this information with parents and help them identify someone who may be able to give the child additional support for academic skill development before the child experiences repeated failure. Referral to social workers, psychologists, other professionals, family and child care service providers, and community children's programs are other important avenues for connecting families with resources that can help minimize risk.

Consideration of Intervention Options

The multidimensionality of occupation and its enmeshment with environmental contexts suggests that many options for intervention should be considered if clinical assessment indicates that the child is experiencing difficulty engaging in occupations. The occupational therapist's charge is to identify variables that can be altered in order to effect a positive change in the entire system of the child acting in his or her environment (Gray, 1998) and, moreover, to envision how that process of change might unfold over time. Intervention options are then selected and orchestrated to channel the child and family's occupations in a direction that will move them toward achieving the desired occupational goals.

When sensory integrative difficulties contribute to a child's occupational problems, the occupational therapist must consider whether intervention should focus on altering the child's experience or ability to participate in occupations; on changing aspects of the environment to support the child's engagement; or on some combination of these strategies. Would efforts to improve sensory integrative abilities be desirable? If so, would individual occupational therapy be most useful or would it be more helpful to encourage the family to enroll the child in enrichment programs that are available in the community, such as gym classes or swimming? If the child has significant sensory modulation issues, perhaps enrollment in a group such as the *Alert Program* (Williams & Shellenberger, 1994) would be beneficial. If specific motor or social skills are key problems, skill training, either individually or in a group, might be appropriate. Is immediate success in troublesome occupations an urgent need? If so, professional consultation to suggest changes in tasks and activities and their environmental contexts may be the priority. Dunbar (1999) provided a case example that nicely illustrates such an approach to planning intervention. Alternatively, occupational therapists may collaborate with families to redesign their lifestyles so that sensory needs of children are integrated into daily family routines at the same time that parental needs, occupational styles, and values are accommodated.

Consideration of family and child resources, preferences, and occupational styles, as well as community resources, are critical in recommending and discussing intervention options with families. When considering how to be most helpful to a child and family, it is useful to imagine the transactional process of development projecting into the future. Who is this child becoming? Where are the lives of the child and family headed? How might their trajectory be altered if various intervention options are introduced?

Intervention Can Be Both Occupation Centered and Sensory Based

If the decision for intervention involves individual occupational therapy using classical intervention based on the principles of sensory integration theory, this service should be provided in a manner that is occupation centered. Occupation centered means that occupation is both the means and the ends of intervention (Gray, 1998). Classical intervention based on the principles of sensory integration theory uses occupation as means because during intervention, the child is doing highly individualized activities that involve intentionality, imbue some degree of personal control and intrinsic motivation, and are personally meaningful (Parham & Mailloux, 2001). And occupation is the ends of intervention because assessment and intervention processes are centered on the ultimate outcome of improving the child's occupational life, such as play with peers, doing chores at home, and participating successfully in school-based activities. The ideal candidates for this kind of intervention are children whose sensory needs and characteristics are critical aspects of their occupational life in ways that we discussed earlier in this chapter. Furthermore, before recommending this kind of intervention, a therapist should have some indication that exposure to enriched sensory-motor opportunities in the therapeutic environment will lead the child to greater competence and enjoyment of daily occupations. A child is selected as a good candidate for this kind of intervention by the therapist who has used a future-oriented, top-down approach to assessment and has considered multiple options for intervention with family characteristics and resources in mind. Thus, when classical sensory integration treatment is chosen, intervention is simultaneously occupation centered and sensory based.

One question that may arise at this point is whether so-called "passive sensory stimulation" can legitimately be included in occupation-centered intervention. For example, should the Wilbarger protocol (see Chapter 14) be included in occupation-centered intervention, or should it be excluded because it does not involve active, meaningful involvement on the part of the child? What about applying other kinds of tactile, vestibular, or touch-pressure stimuli, such as swinging a child or squeezing the child between pillows in a "mat sandwich?" These activities are often referred to as passive because the child simply receives the stimulation while the therapist does most of the action. However, it is possible that the child may be actively involved in the sensory stimulation activity. In such cases, it may be legitimate to think of the child as engaged in a co-occupation.

In occupational science, the term *co-occupation* refers to an occupation that requires the active involvement of two or more people (Dunlea, 1996; Zemke & Clark, 1996). Caregiving activities are classic examples of co-occupations. At face value, it may appear that a parent is engaged in active occupations when doing caregiving routines (e.g., feeding, bathing, dressing, diapering a child) and that the child passively receives care. However, in occupational science, the active agency of both participants is acknowledged. Infants are active agents when they attend to and respond to the interactive caregiving partner; in such situations, the infant is engaged in a co-occupation even though the parent is in charge and is getting a task accomplished (Dunlea, 1996; Zemke & Clark, 1996).

The concept of co-occupations can be applied to many situations. For example, for many people, a relaxing and very meaningful occupation is receiving a massage. They may plan their time to make sure that this occupation is incorporated into their busy schedules. While receiving a massage, the person may appear on the surface to be simply passively receiving sensory input. We cannot tell from observing a massage whether it is meaningful to the recipient, although we may be able to guess from the way that person behaves before and during the massage whether he or she is actively participating (e.g., by making the massage appointment, showing up on time, and cooperating with the massage protocol of the particular setting). Of course, not all people experience massages as meaningful in a positive way. But for those who do and who incorporate massages into their lifestyle, receiving a massage is a legitimate occupation. Or more precisely put, it is a co-occupation (because another person must be actively involved in giving the massage in order for it to happen).

So, in answer to the question of whether so-called passive stimulation has a place in occupation-centered intervention, I would say "yes," but it depends on whether the recipient experiences the stimulation as a meaningful experience and actively participates in receiving it and whether the therapist is intentionally using it as one aspect of an overall effort to influence the child's occupational life in a positive direction. In some situations, the application of sensory stimulation by the practitioner may truly be a co-occupation in which the child actively cooperates and experiences meaning (e.g., comfort, pleasure, and trust emanating from human contact; the experience of being situated in a body). However, this is not always the case. Application of sensory stimulation when the child is resistive or distressed is not likely to evoke engagement, and it is not likely to impart meaning beyond negative associations with the therapist and the specific sensory input being used.

The issue of personal meaning is critical in evaluating the extent to which a child's activities during sensory integration–based occupational therapy constitute engagement in occupation. An activity cannot be considered to be an occupation unless we have reason to believe that it carries meaning for the person who is doing it (Gray, 1997; Zemke & Clark, 1996). Observation of the person doing the activity does not provide the definitive answer. An activity that appears rote and meaningless to an observer may actually carry important meaning for the doer. Conversely, an activity that seems meaningful to the observer may not actually be meaningful for the person doing it. It is the person's experience of doing that is critical in determining the extent to which occupation is happening, not the structure of the activity itself. As an example, let us consider weightlifting, an activity that is sometimes characterized as rote exercise that very likely has little or no meaning to the client (e.g., Fisher, 1998). For many women and men, lifting weights is a valued occupation that is frequently chosen and is personally meaningful, symbolizing power at the same time that it provides clear feedback regarding physical strength. It would be unfortunate if occupational therapists dismissed the possibility that lifting weights may be a meaningful occupation for a particular client simply because it is sometimes classified as rote exercise. Such classification of specific activities may lead therapists to avoid or embrace a particular activity because it fits or does not fit into a certain category instead of considering its unique meaning for the individual doing it. Many activities that appear to be rote or contrived on the surface may be fully legitimate occupations if the person is personally invested in them and experiences them as meaningful. This is especially true for children, who often choose, create, and enthusiastically engage in occupations that look like fragments of more complex adult activities (e.g., hammering nails into a board or repeatedly moving objects from one place to another).

As a final note, we can consider alternative ways of providing occupation-centered intervention that is also sensory based, aside from the classical intervention based on the principles of sensory integration theory approach. For example, sensory-based occupations may be incorporated into familiar daily routines of children at home and in school; daily routines may be modified taking into consideration the child's sensory characteristics (e.g., see Dunbar, 1999); or new occupations may be introduced into novel nonclinical environments that the child does not ordinarily encounter (e.g., horseback riding). These approaches may be considered sensory based in that they draw heavily from knowledge about the child's sensory functioning for the purpose of immediately boosting the child's success in existing occupational patterns or for the purpose of strengthening the child's sensory vulnerabilities for more competent participation in occupations in the future (see Chapter 14).

SUMMARY AND CONCLUSIONS

From its inception, sensory integration theory has viewed the child as an active agent in the world, whose engagement with the environment affects the development of competence and satisfaction in doing occupations. Within this theory, the neurobiological construct of sensory integration holds an important position as a mediator between the child's physical self and the external world. Because the neural processes and behavioral expressions of sensory integration shape the person's capacity and willingness to act on the environment, sensory integration is relevant to the construction of the self through the doing of occupations.

However, sensory integration is only one of many factors that influences occupation; it interplays with social expectations, physical environments, and personal experiences in shaping an individual's occupational life. We have evidence that sensory integrative characteristics influence the person's competencies in doing various activities, as well as personal choices of occupations and how to perform them, throughout the lifespan. Furthermore, engagement in occupation has the potential to sculpt the neural processes that underlie sensory integrative capabilities. Therefore, we can think of occupation as transformational on many levels, encompassing the biology as well as the personal identity of the individual.

The reciprocal relationship between sensory integration and occupation opens the door to a multitude of intervention possibilities. Because sensory integration affects engagement in occupations, it is one of the many factors that may be considered in assessing the reasons for why a child may be experiencing difficulties with occupations such as participating in home, school, and play activities. One course of action for intervention may be to use knowledge of a child's sensory processing characteristics to modify the tasks, routines, and environments of the child's occupational life in order to maximize the child's success and family satisfaction in the immediate contexts of daily life. Alternatively, engagement in occupations may be used to mold sensory integrative capacities to strengthen the biological foundation for occupations across a longer span of life. This is the intervention approach that is adopted in classical intervention based on the principles of sensory integration theory developed by Ayres, but use of occupations to shape sensory integrative abilities may also be accomplished through community-based activity programs such as swimming and gymnastics classes. Research remains to be done to clarify when particular approaches are most beneficial, for whom, and under which circumstances.

As a concluding thought, I invite readers to consider sensory integration not as simply a neurologic process contained entirely within the individual, but also as a complex process through which the nervous system mediates transactions between individuals and their world. In this view, sensory integration serves as a scaffold for human agency and, therefore, is inextricably linked with occupation.

Acknowledgment

This work was partially supported by the Maternal and Child Health Bureau, Health Resources and Services Administration, Project #5 T81 MC 0008-16.

References

Armstrong, T. (1987). *In their own way*. Los Angeles: Jeremy P. Tarcher.

Ayres, A. J. (1972). *Sensory integration and learning disorders*. Los Angeles: Western Psychological Services.

Ayres, A. J. (1979). *Sensory integration and the child*. Los Angeles: Western Psychological Services.

Ayres, A. J. (1989). *Sensory Integration and Praxis Tests manual*. Los Angeles: Western Psychological Services.

Bruner, J. (1996). *The culture of education*. Cambridge, MA: Harvard University Press.

Bundy, A. C. (1989). A comparison of the play skills of normal boys and boys with sensory integrative dysfunction. *Occupational Therapy Journal of Research, 9*, 84–100.

Bundy, A. C. (1993). Assessment of play and leisure: Delineation of the problem. *American Journal of Occupational Therapy, 47*, 217–222.

Bundy, A. C. (1997). Play and playfulness: What to look for. In L. D. Parham & L. S. Fazio (Eds.), *Play in occupational therapy for children* (pp. 52–66). St. Louis, MO: Mosby.

Carlson, M. E., & Clark, F. A. (1991). The search for useful methodologies in occupational science. *American Journal of Occupational Therapy, 45*, 235–241.

Christiansen, C. H. (1997). Three perspectives on balance in occupation. In R. Zemke & F. Clark (Eds.), *Occupational science: The evolving discipline* (pp. 431–451). Philadelphia: F. A. Davis.

Chugani, H. T. (1994). Development of regional brain glucose metabolism in relation to behavior and plasticity. In G. Dawson & K. W. Fischer (Eds.), *Human behavior and the developing brain*. New York: Guilford Press.

Clark, F., & Larson, E. A. (1993). Developing an academic discipline: The science of occupation. In H. S. Hopkins & H. D. Smith (Eds.), *Willard and Spackman's occupational therapy* (8th ed., pp. 44–57). Philadelphia: J. B. Lippincott.

Clark, F. A., Parham, D., Carlson, M. E., Frank, G., Jackson, J., Pierce, D., Wolf, R. J., & Zemke, R. (1991). Occupational science: Academic innovation in the service of occupational therapy's future. *American Journal of Occupational Therapy, 45*, 300–310.

Clark, F., Wood, W., & Larson, E. A. (1999). Introduction to occupational science. In H. S. Hopkins & H. D. Smith (Eds.), *Willard and Spackman's occupational therapy* (9th ed., pp. 13–21). Philadelphia: J. B. Lippincott.

Coster, W., Tickle-Degnan, L., & Armenta, L. (1995). Therapist-child interaction during sensory integration treatment: Development and testing of a research tool. *Occupational Therapy Journal of Research, 15*, 17–35.

Coster, W. (1998). Occupation-centered assessment of children. *American Journal of Occupational Therapy, 52*, 337–344.

Diamond, M., & Hopson, J. (1998). *Magic trees of the mind*. New York: Penguin Putnam.

Diamond, M., Krech, & Rosenzweig, M. R. (1964). The effects of an enriched environment on the histology of the rat cerebral cortex. *Journal of Comparative Neurology, 123,* 111–120.

Dunbar, S. B. (1999). A child's occupational performance: Considerations of sensory processing and family context. *American Journal of Occupational Therapy, 53,* 231–235.

Dunkerly, E., Tickle-Degnan, L., & Coster, W. J. (1997). Therapist-child interaction in the middle minutes of sensory integration treatment. *American Journal of Occupational Therapy, 51,* 799–805.

Dunlea, A. (1996). An opportunity for co-adaptation: The experience of mothers and their infants who are blind. In R. Zemke & F. Clark (Eds.), *Occupational science: The evolving discipline* (pp. 227–241). Philadelphia: F. A. Davis.

Dunn, W. W. (2000). Habit: What's the brain got to do with it? *Occupational Therapy Journal of Research, 20(suppl I),* 6–20.

Fanchiang, S. C. (1996). The other side of the coin: Growing up with a learning disability. *American Journal of Occupational Therapy, 50,* 277–285.

Fisher, A. G. (1998). Uniting practice and theory in an occupational framework. The 1998 Eleanor Clarke Slagle lecture. *American Journal of Occupational Therapy, 52,* 509–521.

Fisher, A. G., & Short-Degraff, M. (1993). Improving functional assessment in occupational therapy: Recommendations and philosophy for change. *American Journal of Occupational Therapy, 47,* 199–200.

Gardner, H. (1983). *Frames of mind*. New York: Basic Books.

Gray, J. M. (1997). Application of the phenomenological method to the concept of occupation. *Journal of Occupational Science: Australia, 4,* 5–17.

Gray, J. M. (1998). Putting occupation into practice: Occupation as ends, occupation as means. *American Journal of Occupational Therapy, 52,* 354–364.

Grimwood, L. M., & Rutherford, E. M. (1980). Sensory integrative therapy as an intervention procedure with grade one "at risk" readers: A three-year study. *The Exceptional Child, 27,* 52–61.

Hubel, D. H. & Wiesel, T. N. (1970). The period of susceptibility to the physiological effects of unilateral eye closure in kittens. *Journal of Physiology, 206,* 419–436.

Huttenlocher, P. R., & de Couten, C. (1987). The development of synapses in striate cortex of man. *Human Neurobiology, 6,* 1–9.

Jacobs, B., Schall, M., & Scheibel, A. B. (1993). A quantitative dendritic analysis of Wernicke's area in humans. II. Gender, hemispheric, and environmental factors. *Journal of Comparative Neurology, 327,* 97–111.

Kaufman, A. S., & Kaufman, N. L. (1983). *Kaufman Assessment Battery for Children: Interpretive manual*. Circle Pines, MN: American Guidance Service.

Kinnealey, M., Oliver, B., & Wilbarger, P. (1995). A phenomenological study of sensory defensiveness in adults. *American Journal of Occupational Therapy, 49,* 444–451.

Lee, C., & Jackson, R. (1975). *Faking it: A look into the mind of a creative learner*. Portsmouth, NH: Boynton/Cook Publishers.

Li, W., Bundy, A. C., & Beer, D. (1995). Taiwanese parental values toward an American evaluation of playfulness. *Occupational Therapy Journal of Research, 15,* 237–258.

Mattingly, C., & Fleming, M. (1994). *Clinical reasoning: Forms of inquiry in a therapeutic process*. Philadelphia: F. A. Davis.

Morrison, C. D., & Metzger, P. (2001). Play. In J. Case-Smith (Ed.), *Occupational therapy for children* (pp. 528–544). St. Louis, MO: Mosby.

Nelson, D. L. (1988). Occupation: Form and performance. *American Journal of Occupational Therapy, 42,* 633–641.

Neville, H. J. (1995). Developmental specificity in neurocognitive development in humans. In M. S. Gazzaniga (Ed.), *The cognitive neurosciences*. Cambridge, MA: MIT Press.

Parham, L. D. (1998). The relationship of sensory integrative development to achievement in elementary students: Four-year longitudinal patterns. *Occupational Therapy Journal of Research, 18,* 105–127.

Parham, L. D. (1998). What is the proper domain of occupational therapy research? *American Journal of Occupational Therapy, 52,* 485–489.

Parham, L. D., & Mailloux, Z. (2001). Sensory integration. In J. Case-Smith (Ed.), *Occupational therapy for children* (4th ed., pp. 281–329). St. Louis, MO: Mosby.

Pert, C. B. (1997). *Molecules of emotion*. New York: Touchstone.

Sameroff, A. J., & Chandler, M. J. (1975). Reproductive risk and the continuum of caretaking casualty. In F. D. Horowitz, M. Hetherington, S. Scarr-Salapatek, & G. Siegel (Eds.), *Review of child development research* (Vol. 4, pp. 187–244). Chicago: University of Chicago Press.

Scheibel, A., Conrad, T., Perdue, S., Tomiyasu, U., & Wechsler, A. (1990). A quantitative study of dendrite complexity in selected areas of the human cerebral cortex. *Brain and Cognition, 12,* 85–101.

Simonds, R. J., & Scheibel, A. B. (1989). The post-natal development of the motor speech area: A preliminary study. *Brain and Language, 37,* 42–58.

Tickle-Degnan, L., & Coster, W. (1995). Therapeutic interaction and the management of challenge during the beginning minutes of sensory integration treatment. *Occupational Therapy Journal of Research, 15,* 122–141.

Trombly, C. A. (1993). Anticipating the future: Assessment of occupational function. *American Journal of Occupational Therapy, 47,* 253–257.

Trombly, C. A. (1995). Occupation: Purposefulness and meaningfulness as therapeutic mechanisms. 1995 Eleanor Clarke Slagle lecture. *American Journal of Occupational Therapy, 49,* 960–972.

Wilcock, A. A. (1998). *An occupational perspective of health*. Thorofare, NJ: Slack.

Williams, M. S., & Shellenberger, S. (1994). *"How Does Your Engine Run?" Leader's Guide to the Alert Program for Self-Regulation*. Albuquerque, NM: TherapyWorks.

Wilson, B. N., & Kaplan, B. J. (1994). Follow-up assessment of children receiving sensory integration treatment. *Occupational Therapy Journal of Research, 14,* 244–266.

Yerxa, E. J. (1993). Occupational science: A new source of power for participants in occupational therapy. *Journal of Occupational Science (Australia), 1,* 3–10.

Yerxa, E. J., Clark, F., Frank, G., Jackson, J., Parham, D., Pierce, D., Stein, C., & Zemke, R. (1989). An introduction to occupational science, a foundation for occupational therapy in the 21st century. *Occupational Therapy in Health Care, 6,* 1–17.

Zemke, R., & Clark, F. (1996). Co-occupations of mothers and children. In R. Zemke & F. Clark (Eds.), *Occupational science: The evolving discipline* (pp. 213–215). Philadelphia: F. A. Davis.

Zuckerman, M. (1994). *Behavioral expressions and biosocial bases of sensation seeking*. New York: Cambridge University Press.

▪▪ Appendix A

Use of Clinical Reasoning in Occupational Therapy: The STEP-SI Model of Intervention of Sensory Modulation Dysfunction

Lucy J. Miller, PhD, OTR
Julia Wilbarger, MA, MS, OTR
Tracy Stackhouse, OTR
Sharon Trunnell, OTR

Sensory integration is the neurological process that organizes sensation from one's own body and from the environment and makes it possible to use the body effectively within the environment.

—*Ayres, 1989, p. 11*

Occupational therapy using a sensory integration frame of reference is complex and is based on a core set of principles originated by Ayres (1972). Ayres' principles guide the provision of intervention across a broad spectrum of occupational therapy practices worldwide. Although all occupational therapy is individualized, often incorporating a variety of frames of reference, methods, and modalities, detailed principles provide a structure to ensure consistency of application. Kimball (1988) described how "sensory integration intervention is neither predetermined nor fixed, but rather varies from one individual to the next, and changes in response to the individual's responses to therapy" (p. 423).

We, as a profession, must begin to write replicable intervention protocols for effectiveness intervention research. Although these written descriptions can and should be modified by others who use them, using a written manual increases accuracy of application and permits systematic study. Using a reasoning framework described by Mattingly and Fleming (1994) and working in collaboration with members of the occupational therapy sensory inte-

gration team at The Children's Hospital in Denver, Colorado, we embarked on a process to develop a means for ensuring consistency across individualized intervention. This process ultimately resulted in the formation of the STEP-SI clinical reasoning model. The reasoning process, based on Mattingly and Fleming's (1994) seminal work, is briefly synthesized. This Appendix, describes the development and principles of the STEP-SI (Stackhouse et al., 1997) and then details the application of the STEP-SI model to assessment, direct intervention, and home- and community-based intervention. Finally, we illustrate the use of the STEP-SI clinical reasoning model in a direct intervention setting with a case story.

Critical Reasoning in Intervention Based on Sensory Integration Theory

Mattingly and Fleming (1994) completed a detailed study of the ways in which master clinicians make decisions about how to engage in effective intervention. The three types of reasoning they described apply to the framework presented here and elsewhere (Miller & Summers, 2001).

1. *Procedural reasoning:* A highly cognitive approach whereby a practitioner actively considers a child's strengths and difficulties and thinks in advance or retrospectively about specific procedures or activities in which the child might engage to remediate problems.
2. *Interactive reasoning:* An interactive approach that occurs during a session and that assists the practitioner and other caregivers to understand the "whole" child, guiding the ensuing events based on the child's responses; also relates to integrating parents and children's priorities into intervention.
3. *Conditional reasoning:* A complex reasoning process that incorporates interactions, context, and individual clients' responses and needs to achieve quality of life goals. During and after sessions, practitioners use a vast array of information to think about the whole child and family in a social context, including the meaning that the disability has for their client.

Mattingly and Fleming (1994) posited that practitioners use two forms of "knowledge" during intervention. One type, *explicit knowledge,* is information that can be articulated through a conscious reasoning process. The other type, *implicit* or *tacit knowledge,* influences intervention on a moment-to-moment basis. "Tacit knowledge forms the base of all other thoughts and actions that comprise practice" (Mattingly & Fleming, 1994, p. 26). Tacit knowledge is further subdivided into two parts. These are:

1. Background working knowledge (i.e., facts once learned but stored in long-term memory that become part of the wealth of knowledge that the practitioner possesses).
2. Knowledge that is difficult to put into words but uses underlying principles, assumptions, values, judgments and "gut" feelings to guide action. The latter form of tacit knowledge is akin to the "art of therapy" described by Ayres (1972) and further delineated in Chapter 11.

Experts have an implicit understanding of a whole range of minute details of the phenomena that they understand. They recognize small details and nuances and interpret them with impressive speed and accuracy. . . . Therapists . . . can feel small changes in muscle tone . . . or quality of movement . . . and they adjust their own tone of voice or body position almost instantaneously in response to subtle cues indicating the emotional status of the patient (Mattingly & Fleming, 1994, p. 27).

Delineation of the STEP-SI Clinical Reasoning Model

To examine our reasoning process, our team videotaped and later analyzed numerous intervention sessions. We found that our master clinicians used their explicit knowledge to guide their intervention. But more importantly—and certainly much more difficult to describe—these master clinicians used implicit, tacit knowledge *and* an ongoing, interactive reasoning process to decide "in the moment" how to proceed. Ongoing observation, diagnostic assessment, reflection on multiple hypotheses, and *implicit* understanding of the child's needs at the moment guided each individual intervention session.

From these observations, we added several dimensions to the occupational therapy sensory integration principles originated by Ayres (1972) and used by our master clinicians. Analyzing these dimensions, *including (but not limited to) enhanced sensation,* provided a rich basis for enhancing our descriptions of intervention. Eventually, all the components were collapsed into an acronym, STEP-SI (pronounced "Step", "S", "I"), for Sensation, Task, Environment, Predictability, Self-monitoring, and Interaction (Stackhouse & Wilbarger, 1998). The acronym provides a convenient means to discuss the elements of intervention that occur, an important step in promoting our narrative reasoning (Mattingly & Fleming, 1994). The model incorporates elements unique to a master clinician's perspective, specifically a unique understanding of how moment-to-moment and global adaptation to challenges affect our clients. We hope that clarifying the elements and principles of the STEP-SI process will result in development of a replicable and effective intervention protocol useful in future multisite occupational therapy sensory integration intervention efficacy studies.

STEP-SI Clinical Reasoning Model: General Principles

The STEP-SI clinical reasoning model was developed originally for use in treating children with sensory modulation dysfunction (SMD) (Stackhouse et al., 1997). Although it targets children with SMD, the model is also applicable to individuals with other patterns of sensory integration dysfunction. The STEP-SI model is a thinking tool that is intended to facilitate reasoning and communication among parents, occupational therapy practitioners, and other professionals. It provides a structure to organize evaluation and intervention information and to effectively set priorities. Originally conceptualized to assist us to make more effective decisions in the flow of direct intervention, it also assists in training parents, teachers, and other caregivers to construct home and community intervention programs. The model serves to expand a practitioner's conception of intervention beyond the use of enhanced sensory experiences to a more encompassing occupation-based intervention in which sensation plays one key part (see also Chapter 12).

A number of authors have provided good summaries of the principles of intervention based on sensory integration theory (e.g., Ayres, 1972; Fisher et al., 1991; Kimball, 1999; Kinnealey & Miller, 1993; Parham & Mailloux, 2001) (see also Chapter 12). These long-standing principles include:

- Active participation by the client
- Client-directed, intrinsically motivating, and purposeful activities
- Individualized interventions based on the age, developmental status, needs, and responses of the client
- Intervention that provides the "just-right challenge" resulting in an adaptive response (i.e., the task is challenging enough to engage the child yet does not preclude success)
- Use of enhanced sensory experiences in the context of activity
- Focus on improving underlying neurologic processing rather than developing academic or motor splinter skills

Critical to the STEP-SI model is an understanding of Ayres' (1972) traditional principles of intervention such as the adaptive response and the "just-right challenge" (see Chapter 11). Ayres proposed that through the just-right challenge, the level of adaptive response increased, thus facilitating changes in function. We use this core concept to begin the process of STEP-SI clinical reasoning. The practitioner first assesses the child's capacity for adaptation and then *scaffolds* specific challenges to stabilize, broaden, and promote flexibility in the child's range of adaptation. This results in growth toward independent management of behavioral organization.

In the course of intervention, the practitioner manipulates the STEP-SI dimensions to support or challenge the child, developing capacities or skills in identified problem areas. The appropriateness of the child's adaptive response becomes a monitor that guides modification of intervention. Table A–1 elaborates the dimensions of the STEP-SI model.

The four general principles of the STEP-SI model of clinical reasoning are:

- Understand the child's adaptive capacity. Determine the child's state of arousal and ability to attain and maintain appropriate behavioral organization. Attend to the range of arousal and the ability of the child to stay within an optimal range. Be aware of the child's responses to challenges in the day or week and compare the conditions that result in organized versus disorganized responses.
- Examine how each STEP-SI dimension affects the child's state of arousal and ability to attain or maintain appropriate behavioral organization. Determine which aspects of each STEP-SI dimension enable the child to have the best adaptive response and which challenge adaptation.
- Prioritize the use of each STEP-SI dimension to support or challenge clients. Manipulate dimensions of the model to maximize appropriate levels of adaptation and occupational performance.
- Monitor and readjust each STEP-SI dimension based on ongoing assessment of adaptive responses. After optimum adaptive performance is achieved, introduce another just-right challenge by altering some aspect of one or more dimensions of the STEP-SI model. This constant "upping the ante" while scaffolding the child to maintain organization within each new "challenge state" is the key to making the adaptive

■ Table A–1 Dimensions of the STEP-SI Clinical Reasoning Intervention Model

STEP-SI Dimension	Description
S Sensation	Sensory modalities: Tactile, vestibular, proprioception, audition, vision, taste, olfaction, oral input, and respiration
	Qualities of sensation: Duration, intensity, frequency, complexity, and rhythmicity
T Task	Structure, complexity, demand for skill, demand for sustained attention, level of engagement, fun, motivation, and purposefulness (based on standard task analysis)
E Environment	Organization, complexity, perceived comfort and safety, and possibilities for engagement exploration, expansion and self-challenge
P Predictability	Novelty, expectation, structure, routine, transitions, and congruency
	Level of control by child or practitioner and control of events and routines
S Self-monitoring	Moving the child from dependence on external cues and supports to self-directed and internally organized ability to modify own behavior and manage challenges
I Interactions	Interpersonal interaction style, including responses to supportive, nurturing styles versus more challenging, authoritative styles; locus of control (practitioner guided vs. child directed); and demands or expectations for engagement (i.e., passive awareness to active collaboration)

changes suggested by the original intervention theory (Ayres, 1972).

These principles are further delineated below in the context of their use in:

- Assessment
- Specific goals and priorities for intervention
- Direct intervention
- Home and community programs

Using the STEP-SI in Assessment

The STEP-SI model can be used as a structure to organize assessment data. As in any occupational therapy intervention model, the goals of assessment, the parent conference, and the first several intervention sessions are to:

- Build a therapeutic alliance with the child and family members
- Identify the specific challenges that affect the child in daily activities and routines
- Identify child behaviors that affect the family's well being and caregiving capacity

The STEP-SI framework also can assist the practitioner in designing intervention specifically aimed at the events that impact a child's ability to self-regulate. This information, combined with standardized assessment data, assists the practitioner, working in collaboration with families and other caregivers, to establish levels of adaptation in each of the dimension of the STEP-SI model. A comprehensive interview is recommended to initiate this process (for an example, see Miller & Summers, 2001). In addition to reviewing the results of all tests and clinical information gained

through interview, we recommend that the occupational therapy practitioner and parents meet without the child present to formulate specific goals pertinent to improving the quality of life for children and their families (see Cohn et al., 2000; Chapter 9).

During sessions early in the intervention process, the family and occupational therapy practitioner observe and discuss the child's responses to input in each sensory domain and the child's capacity for adaptation in the other dimensions. Initially, we use reasoning to examine how each sensory system serves to support or challenge the child's overall adaptive behavior, using the following guiding questions.

1. How does sensation serve to challenge or support the child?
   - What, if any, sensation (sensory modalities) does the child seek? Avoid?
   - What qualities of each sensation (e.g., intensity, duration) does the child seek? Avoid?
   - How do these seeking and avoiding behaviors enhance or diminish behavioral organization and functional performance?
   - What qualities of sensation enhance or support behavioral organization or functional performance? What qualities of sensation enhance or support challenges in the other dimensions?

2. What kinds of tasks and qualities of tasks serve to challenge or support the child?
   - What qualities of tasks enhance or support behavioral organization or func-

tional performance? What qualities of tasks enhance or support challenges in the other dimensions?

- How does task structure enhance or diminish the child's behavioral organization or functional performance?
- How does task simplicity vs. complexity enhance or diminish the child's behavioral organization or functional performance?

3. What kinds of environments and qualities of the environment serve to challenge or support the child?

- What qualities of the environment enhance or support behavioral organization or functional performance? What qualities of the environment enhance or support challenges in the other dimensions?
- How does the level of stimulation, enrichment, structure, organization, perceived comfort and safety, or possibility for exploration influence the child's ability to adapt in a particular environment?

4. How does predictability serve to challenge or support the child?

- What qualities of predictability enhance or support behavioral organization or functional performance? What qualities of predictability enhance or support challenges in the other dimensions?
- If events that occur are consistent and expected versus surprising and unanticipated, is the child's functioning enhanced or diminished?
- If the child has more or less control over events is his or her functioning enhanced or diminished?

5. How does the child's ability to self-monitor serve to support him or her in challenging situations?

- Can the child recognize how his or her own internal state affects the ability to complete activities or have appropriate adaptive responses?
- What strategies and activities help the child to self-monitor (i.e., modeling, verbal, cue cards, checklist)? What strategies does the child already use?

6. How do interactions challenge or support the child?

- What qualities of interactions enhance or support behavioral organization or functional performance? What qualities of interactions enhance or support challenges in the other dimensions?
- How does the child's performance change with active scaffolding and support compared with more remote and nonintrusive methods of suggesting change? What kinds of social relationships engage the child and intrude on the child?

The above questions, although they are not comprehensive, demonstrate the complexity of the reasoning challenge that faces the occupational therapy practitioners as they strive to find the just-right challenge. Helping parents and teachers understand these complexities is one of our most important jobs—and gifts.

Establishing Specific Goals and Priorities for Intervention

The primary focus of the occupational therapy practitioner is to assist clients to improve their occupational roles and functional performance. Occupational therapy may assist a child by remediating specific sensory or motor dysfunction, but always in the context of occupations, and always focusing on the family's priorities for change. Cohn (2001a, 2001b; Cohn et al., 2000) found that parents of children with SMD valued social participation, self-regulation, self-esteem, and sometimes specific skill areas. Thus, occupational therapy practitioners establish goals before intervention that generally address:

- *Occupational performance:* Activities of daily living, play skills, work and school performance and behaviors, and specific performance components such as fine and gross motor skills
- *Self-regulation:* Adaptability during daily routines; organization during structured and unstructured tasks; sustained concentration and ability to divide attention between two or more focused tasks; task completion; and ability to monitor own behavior in context before it becomes a problem
- *Social participation:* Play with others, cooperation, making and keeping friends
- *Self-esteem:* Positive self-concept and feelings of self-worth.

Significant improvement in the first two goals often facilitates positive social interaction as well as family and peer acceptance. Improvements in occupational performance, such as increased competency in academic and motor (athletic) skills, along with peer and family acceptance lay the groundwork for a positive self-concept (Harter et al., 1998).

A family's priorities for intervention are our guiding beacons when designing intervention. Although we may believe that toilet training is the most important adaptive skill that a 5-year-old client needs to succeed at school, we may find out that in the culture of her particular family, toilet training is not important. Instead, the family may be more concerned about going out in public without worrying if the child is going to fall apart or being able to sleep through the night. Some families' highest priority may be to have one family meal together without someone always having to take the child into the other room. No matter how clear a practitioner may be about what the goals should be, they must always be defined by the priorities of the family.

Case Story for Assessment and Intervention Planning

Now we illustrate the model with a vignette. Jose, a 6-year-old boy in first grade, was from a first-generation American family. Both his parents worked full time and had high expectations for their children, including getting a good education and a high-level professional job. Jose, like his siblings, had above average intelligence. However, Jose had significant problems at school; he often became aggressive with other children or withdrew to a position under the desk. He did not play with other children at recess. He preferred to eat alone, and never ate the school cafeteria food. At school, many children made fun of him, and his teachers worried.

When tested on the Sensory Integration and Praxis Tests (SIPT), Jose demonstrated severe hypersensitivity to touch. In our parent interview, we found that he refused to eat many foods, was extremely sensitive to smells (e.g., refused to enter the kitchen when his mother was cooking certain foods), and became out of control after fast movement experiences (e.g., riding the merry-go-round at the park). We also learned that Jose often

sought strong hugs from his parents, and when he felt overwhelmed, he would squeeze himself into a small space (e.g., under a table or in the back of a closet). He did best when he had a predictable routine, but "fell apart" when the routine was changed or he went somewhere new.

Before his first intervention session, the occupational therapist arranged the environment with several pieces of movement equipment for Jose to explore. First she observed Jose's choices of activities. Jose was curious and explored many movement opportunities. He gravitated toward the glider swing and climbing up a jungle gym. He also loved the small tent with dim lighting. After several minutes, Jose initiated faster movement on the swing and engaged in a tossing game. As the intensity of movement increased, his voice became louder and he began to throw the beanbags randomly, sometimes at the practitioner. After several minutes, Jose dove into the small tent and buried his head under the heavy pillows.

From the assessment and the first few intervention sessions (in reality, an ongoing diagnostic assessment), the occupational therapist learned about Jose's capacity for adaptation. His sensory defensive behaviors were evident; they disrupted his ability to modulate responses to sensation, limited his adaptation to new tasks and environments, and interfered with transitions. Jose was easily overwhelmed and became aroused particularly by stimuli that were intense and nonstructured. His ability to maintain an age-appropriate arousal level after changes in the intensity of stimuli was limited. The occupational therapist discovered that Jose responded positively to deep tactile pressure and proprioception. Other sensory experiences with low intensity and rhythmical quality promoted more adaptive states of arousal. He was bright and capable of excellent focus on challenging academic tasks *if* the environment was nonstimulating. Together, Jose's practitioner and parents reviewed the guiding questions that explore how each dimension of the STEP-SI model served to enhance or disrupt his functioning.

They began by analyzing Jose's responses to qualities of sensation in each sensory domain. They discussed how his extreme tactile, oral, and olfactory sensitivities were minimized by deep pressure and proprioception, slow movement, rhythmical auditory, and low-level visual stimulation. Table A–2 illustrates the outcomes of the reasoning process in which the parents and occupational therapist collaborated.

Next they discussed the other STEP-SI dimensions, again using the guiding questions as a structure. Responses highlighted how Jose's sensory overresponsivity was exacerbated when tasks were unstructured and the environment was cluttered. When overaroused, Jose became aggressive and unable to focus on work at a desk. Neither he nor his parents had "tools" to help him regulate when he became "wired."

To summarize the outcomes of the interview, the occupational therapist and family identified the STEP-SI dimensions that supported more adaptive functioning for Jose.

1. What kinds of tasks and qualities of tasks serve to support Jose?

A task that is cognitively interesting and requires active problem solving or involves an interesting pretend theme will support Jose when he is being challenged in sensory domains or other STEP-SI dimensions.

2. What kinds of environments serve to support Jose?

Environments that are ordered and without clutter, that are consistent each time he sees them, and that offer opportunities for age-appropriate seclusion will allow Jose to handle sensory and STEP-SI challenges.

3. How can we use predictability to expand his abilities in other areas?

Jose will do best when things are consistent, orderly, and scheduled and when he has preparation time for transitions.

4. What kinds of self-monitoring techniques does Jose already use, and what strategies can he learn to remain regulated when challenged?

Jose does not consistently recognize when he is overwhelmed and does not seek out quiet, secluded spaces to become organized. When he does anticipate difficult situations, he refuses to participate, often appearing uncooperative. At other times, he is unable to make overt adaptations, becomes aggressive and "melts down." Jose should be guided to recognize when he is becoming overwhelmed and given some options for appropriate self-monitoring.

5. How are interactions used to support Jose?

Jose prefers situations in which he is allowed to have "distance" from others. Sometimes support from one parent can scaffold him to attempt tasks that are hard for him, but most of the time he resists advice and suggestions from others.

This information is used to plan direct intervention and develop home and community programs. These questions and answers reflect an explicit reasoning process (Table A–3).

Finally, the parents and occupational therapist collaborated on goals for Jose's intervention, which resulted in construction of long-term goals for occupational therapy intervention (Table A–4).

We have found that to gauge success, both families and practitioners benefit from *written goals*. In addition, we bring our *tacit* knowledge to the level of *explicit* knowledge by writing goals as well as charting what we know about each child's sensory systems and other information covered in the STEP-SI dimensions.

■ TABLE A–2   JOSE'S RESPONSES IN EACH SENSORY SYSTEM

Sensory Domains	Jose is Supported by	Jose is Challenged by
Touch	Deep pressure touch	Light or unexpected touch
Movement	Slow, rhythmic, linear movement	Fast, rotary, intermittent, unpredictable movement
Proprioception	Joint input and muscle resistance	None
Vision	Low levels and natural light	Visually distracting environments; bright or fluorescent lights
Vision	Low levels and natural light	Visually distracting environments; bright or fluorescent lights
Auditory	Low, consistent, rhythms and music	High-frequency, loud, intermittent or odd sounds
Olfactory and taste	Sweet smells and tastes	Acrid smells and "yucky" tastes
Oral sensation	Deep pressure and proprioception in mouth	Unexpected textures of food, especially when combined with "yucky" smells or "disgusting" taste"

■ TABLE A–3 **REFLECTIVE QUESTIONS FOR THERAPISTS: ASSESSMENT AND ESTABLISHING GOALS**

What are the child's areas of competency and strength in daily life activities?

Do I understand how the child's strengths can help him or her cope with his problems?

Which STEP-SI dimensions support the child's performance and positive adaptive responses in daily life activities?

Do I understand the family's priorities for the child?

What is the best way to collaborate with the child's parents and share my observations? Do I need to spend more time talking to parents; provide more written materials; or suggest other audio, video, or print resources?

Using the STEP-SI Clinical Reasoning Model in Direct Intervention

To implement the STEP-SI model in direct intervention, an occupational therapy practitioner uses both explicit and tacit reasoning skills. The practitioner carefully considers all the *procedural* information (facts) that he or she has gleaned about the child. Next, the practitioner makes explicit the domains or dimensions of intervention with which he or she will begin intervention (e.g., the equipment to set up before the child arrives and activities that might be needed to increase or decrease the challenge). The general principles of the STEP-SI Model guide the questioning and planning. As the practitioner continues to implement intervention, he or she revisits the STEP-SI guiding questions and the reflective questions above.

First the practitioner works to understand the adaptive capacities of the child. For a child with

■ TABLE A–4 **JOSE'S LONG-TERM GOALS FOR OCCUPATIONAL THERAPY INTERVENTION**

Can successfully manage aggressive tendencies when others invade his "space"

Can successfully engage in social interactions in a stimulating environment, such as the lunchroom or playground

Can stay on task in his classroom and work at a desk

Can increase variety in his diet and eat most meals with his family

Can identify when he is beginning to get overstimulated and use strategies that allow him to stay in the environment or exit in an age-appropriate manner

Can enjoy a variety of movement activities on the play ground, and remain regulated

SMD, the practitioner starts by focusing on how the child responds to sensation and how it affects his or her level of arousal and behavioral organization. The occupational therapy practitioner asks if the child can attain an optimal level of arousal and determines if he or she can maintain this regulated arousal level across various sensory experiences. The optimal level of arousal is the range of activity associated with an individual's most efficient task performance and adaptability, related to central nervous system and autonomic nervous system functions. In Jose's case, we saw that he was overresponsive to sensation and became overaroused and disorganized easily. But children with SMD rarely reach an optimum level of arousal. Some children seem to have behaviors indicating both under- and overarousal, either at different times or in different sensory systems.

From the initial assessment, the practitioner should have a fair idea of the child's adaptive capacities. The practitioner continues to observe the child's behavior and reexamine the child's adaptive capacity and arousal levels during each intervention session.

Second, the practitioner must explicitly understand the supportive and disruptive aspects of each STEP-SI dimension. Furthermore, the occupational therapy practitioner should understand or be developing ideas about how to use each dimension in an intervention session. Each idea the practitioner has about what either supports or disrupts a child should be thought of as a question, and each question tested in an intervention session over the course of several weeks. We conceptualize the first few sessions as an ongoing diagnostic assessment as well as the beginning of intervention.

The third principle is to prioritize which dimensions (and their qualities) will be held constant or used for support and which will be subtly changed. The idea is to choose a single dimension and artfully challenge the child with one aspect of it. After a practitioner understands the child better by testing what challenges and supports the child, the practitioner can balance multiple challenges with multiple supports. The challenge areas are based as much on the practitioner's reasoning as the child's own drive. Following the child's lead is important, and children often gravitate toward a certain activity to challenge themselves while sometimes avoiding areas of challenge. Children also selectively avoid certain challenges. We want to achieve a balance between providing opportunities for child-directed activities and guiding them toward challenges they avoid. Sensation is often a productive dimension to examine first because, by definition, children with SMD have significant disruptions in processing sensation.

The fourth principle, which is key during direct intervention sessions, is to constantly observe the child's adaptive responses with your "critical reasoning" mind actively engaged. Does the child show a positive adaptive response? (e.g., maintaining appropriate arousal, organization, posture, emotional tone, social engagement?) Is the child able to maintain adaptation for increasingly longer time periods? Does the child begin to seek further challenges on his or her own? You can begin to develop an understanding of what works for this particular child. If the child is not demonstrating good adaptation, further supports can be added or challenges reduced. Changes should be subtle. To abandon or radically change an entire activity, especially if the child choses it, often is a mistake. Instead, consider the possibilities for modifying the activity. The acronym *STEP-SI* can provide a reminder of the dimensions that can be changed or adjusted. If a child is demonstrating a good adaptive response, you might want to keep the dimensions constant until the child demonstrates mastery. However, it is important to keep the child moving forward at a just-right rate of challenge. Practitioners must support the child right to the edge of his or her ability to adapt, but not beyond it. The push toward the edge of adaptive ability allows the child to expand his or her adaptive capacities.

The general principles of the STEP-SI model are used dynamically, both within an intervention session and to plan for future sessions. Master clinicians reflect during and after each session regarding the appropriateness of activities, tasks, and the environment. The information gleaned is shared with the family and used to make suggestions for the child at home and in the community. Practitioners must be prepared to explain their *reasoning* to parents. Forcing oneself to articulate the purpose for each intervention activity will improve the practitioner's skills as well as make the rationale for intervention clear to parents.

CASE STORY OF DIRECT INTERVENTION

Now we return to Jose, who has a narrow range of optimal arousal and can easily escalate beyond that range. We have seen how the domains of sen-

sation and the other STEP-SI dimensions either support or disrupt Jose, which allows us to prioritize his intervention. The example below addresses one of Jose's challenges in the dimension of movement sensation. We will explore this one domain as an example of how a practitioner uses reasoning during an intervention session. Jose is challenged by fast or rotary movement, which causes him to become overaroused and disorganized. In his first session, Jose chose to engage in swinging but was not able to maintain adaptation when the movement became faster or rotary. The occupational therapy practitioner, therefore, began the session by asking:

> *How can I best use sensation to support Jose while he tries to maintain a regulated state? What sensory options will support him during movement activities to maintain an optimal arousal range?*

Table A–5 shows how, by writing some initial answers, the occupational therapy practitioner made tacit ideas explicit regarding ways to help Jose, Through this process, she designed the first features to be tested during intervention.

The practitioner should start with one particular supportive domain and then incorporate several ideas from it into the movement activity that she planned for Jose. To find out what is effective, she tests each idea separately and then tests them in various combinations. If too many new features are added at the same time, the overall activity may become too complex. In addition, the practitioner is unable to judge the effect of each feature. Complexity alone adds a dimension of challenge even though all the individual facets may be supportive. *Sometimes less is more.* Table A–6 contains options for using the STEP-SI dimensions to support Jose in upcoming intervention sessions. Before beginning the intervention session, the practitioner has all the sensory equipment and STEP-SI tools nearby that she may use in the session.

INTERVENTION

In the story in this section, the practitioner is referred to as "I" and the child as "he/his." The practitioner's reasoning is italicized.

As a result of the reasoning process summarized in Tables A–5 and A–6, I brought a linear glider into the treatment space so I could manipulate the intensity and rhythmicity of movement Jose experienced. Other movement equipment was available nearby but was not suspended to

■ Table A-5   Example of the Use of the Sensory Domains to Support a Challenge

Options for Support of Challenge in Each Sensory Modality*

Challenge	Tactile	Movement	Proprioception	Auditory	Visual	Oral and Respiratory	Taste and Smell
Poor modulation of fast or rotary movement in a swinging activity	Deep pressure before movement (getting the "warrior" ready for battle) Wrap Jose's extremities or trunk in Ace wraps (as a "shield of armor")	Begin with slow, rhythmic movement (warrior's first exercise) Choose a swing that allows for grading the speed and excursion of movement (ready to ride horse)	Combine movement with muscle resistance such pulling a rope or pushing with arms to move the swing (ready for the lance in battle) Weight the swing to provide more resistance to the movement (strong arms to wrestle the enemy to the ground)	Reduced extraneous sound (the hush before the battle) Slow, rhythmic music** (getting ready for the troops to move all together)	Establish a point of focus or target (focus on other side's troops) Dim lights (ready for a dawn attack)	Provide things for Jose to put in his mouth to bite, chew, suck, or blow*** (to keep the troops quiet until the leader raises the battle call)	Try different taste qualities for things in his mouth such as sweet, sour, salty or bitter (things he can sucked on during battle to give him special powers) Avoid wearing perfumes, hairspray, and so on**

*These suggestions should occur in the context of a comprehensive intervention plan for addressing Jose's sensory defensiveness (e.g., a sensory diet and the Wilbarger approach to treating sensory defensiveness; see Chapter 14).
**Specific sound therapy programs have been developed (see Frick's section in Chapter 14).
***See Oetter et al., 1993.

▪ TABLE A–6	EXAMPLE OF THE USE OF *STEP-SI* DIMENSIONS TO SUPPORT A CHALLENGING ACTIVITY				
Task	**Environment**	**Predictability**	**Self-Monitoring**	**Interaction**
Use structured targeting activities and tasks that emphasize a cognitive challenge (e.g., shooting arrows at a target during swinging to practice for battle)	Low levels of background noise and light; structured and neat Provide only a few interesting options for activities (e.g., clear the battlefield so the great warrior can focus)	Set up a routine for beginning and ending sessions with taking off shoes Start with a familiar activity from the previous session Give Jose control through choices (e.g., warriors must have a ritual they follow)	Provide a hideout space Give Jose verbal feedback regarding when he is able to stay calm and when he is getting overwhelmed (e.g., use hideout when the battle "gets too rough")	Use a nurturing, low demand and a calm and steady voice (e.g., you are the battle coach and you don't want the other side to hear you)

keep the environment more organized visually. A variety of activity options were available but out of sight. I had decided to try the "warrior in King Arthur's army" as a fantasy theme to make our sessions more playful. These were built into each step but are not explained in detail here.

I began with Jose with our previously established, predictable routine of removing and storing his shoes. Before entering the "King Arthur's campground," Jose was talking rapidly and incessantly about a TV program he had seen. He seemed overaroused. We entered the gym, and Jose immediately approached the familiar linear glider swing and then stood on it. He tried to move the swing forward and backward, but he was unsteady and disorganized in his movement. Quickly, Jose began acting silly and making quick, repetitious, and ineffective attempts to get the swing going.

I need to get his state more organized right away. How can I slow him down and get better postural responses? . . . Maybe I should try intensifying the deep pressure and proprioceptive input to get his movement more organized?

I got a weighted vest (armor) and helped him put it on (*use of sensation*).

How can I help him control the speed, rhythmicity, and direction of movement?

I decided to get on the swing with him so that I could guide the glider's movement (*use of sensation*). I realized that Jose's poor postural control was exacerbating the problem.

How can I get him to sit down to improve his postural control? . . . Maybe a task that engages his attention will help him achieve a more organized state?

I asked his mother if she would build a huge tower of blocks in the center of our battleground

for practice with the lance, near one end of the swing (*use of task*). Jose then began to swing more rhythmically, pretending he was swinging a lance at the enemy. He became intent on knocking down the tower. He gradually stopped talking, and the volume of his voice volume lowered to a normal range (*manipulation of sensation and task*).

This might quickly get too easy and boring. What can I do to increase the challenge so that it is just right for Jose without adding so much challenge that he cannot succeed?

After twice using his "lance" to knock down the tower his mother built, I guided him to stand up and continue without me on the swing. As Jose started to stand, I could see that he was beginning to lose his balance. He started talking loudly, and then he jumped off the swing and tried to bang the tower with the glider swing!

Too much challenge . . . now what should I do?

With firm, steady pressure on his shoulders (*use of sensation*), I physically guided him back to the swing. Then I sat behind him and stabilized his pelvis while he pushed and pulled on the rope to activate the swing (*use of deep touch pressure, postural support, and rhythmical movement*) until his movements become smooth and symmetrical. He focused on the activity and began having fun. He laughed and said, "I can do this! Better watch out, Enemies!" He slowly began to incorporate more adaptive postural organization.

I know that I've got to keep this session moving forward . . . keep it fun but just a little more challenging from moment to moment.

I asked Jose's mother to put cotton balls (spies) on top of the tower, at the level of Jose's eyes. Giving Jose a straw, I said, "Can you eliminate the enemy spies [blow the cotton balls] off the lookout tower?" He playfully engaged in the task of moving the glider swing back and forth, while blowing the enemy spies off the "lookout tower." *(We have subtly manipulated the task for more challenge, and the sensory input has assisted him to stay organized.)* I modeled for Jose's mother, giving reinforcing verbal feedback to Jose, using my "steady and calm voice" *(manipulation of interaction).* Soon Jose's mother took over giving positive reinforcement. Jose was demonstrating an adaptive response, with increased postural organization, purposeful engagement in the task, and persistence.

Where do I go from here?

I wanted to challenge him to maintain this regulated state with more movement. I asked his mother, "What can we do to make it just a little harder for him?" She suggested that we move the tower back gradually (enemy forces slowly withdrawing from Jose's powerful onslaught) to allow the movement to increase, as Jose continued blowing. We tried this. After several minutes, Jose was still able to focus on this activity and was playful. However, I soon realized, by Jose's waning interest in the activity, that he was going to need another subtle shift, a new challenge, but along the same lines, not a big change in activity.

Jose gets especially overaroused by rotary movement, yet he is really focusing here. I wonder if I can use the focus of the task and the fact that the swinging and blowing is happening in a predictable manner to begin rotary movement?

I decided to shift the movement of the swing so that it offered a circular pattern (looking for other enemy spies that were out there in other directions).

What can I do to help him stay focused during this transition while I switch the glider to a different hook that allows rotary movement?

Intuitively, I began conversing with Jose *(using interaction).* I asked him to help me carry the heavy glider (cannon) *(using sensation)* and talked about how strong he is in fighting the enemy. We talked more about how he could help his mother by carrying heavy things for her at home.

During this conversation, Jose got off the glider swing, removed his weighted vest, and conversed appropriately. I encouraged Jose to get on the rotary swing in prone while I placed sequential picture cards of a battle scene in a circle on the floor beneath the swing *(using a challenging task to increase demand for cognitive concentration).* "Jose, see if you can pick up the pictures *in order* as you swing," I said. Jose propelled himself around to explore the pictures *(using rotary movement sensation)* and began collecting them in sequence.

I see that he is doing pretty well, but I sense that he is about to go out of an appropriate arousal level, and so I decide to ask him to tell me the story of the pictures as he picks them up (using interaction and manipulating the task).

He calmed as he verbalized the story about the warriors and their battle shown in the pictures. In addition, the proprioceptive input he received through his extensor muscles in the prone position and by pushing with his upper extremities, the visual scanning and focus, and the challenge of the cognitive task supported him to stay organized. These supports helped grade the speed and intensity of his rotary movement. When all the cards were picked up, he immediately began spinning faster and faster.

Should I let him experiment a little, or should I introduce another task?

I decided to allow him to explore the rotary movement briefly, encouraging intermittent direction change. In the meantime, I explained to his mother the behaviors I look for as specific signs that he is still maintaining a regulated state of arousal rather than escalating out of control. However, I knew this activity had the potential to get Jose overaroused.

What should I add to this now? I'm feeling just a little "stuck" here. I want him to experience the rotary movement, but I don't want him to escalate. Well, if he is to maintain this level of organization, perhaps I should add some heavy work patterns.

I then guided Jose to throw weighted "cannon balls" into a bucket as he went swinging by *(use of proprioception).* He stayed with this activity for 5 minutes as I varied the targets *(use of novel task)* and increased the weight of the balls *(use of proprioception).* Our session was nearing a close. Realizing that warning Jose about the coming up transition out of the intervention session would help him be regulated through the transition, I said, "We've almost won the battle! Only 10 more minutes . . . 6 more minutes . . . 3 more minutes" *(use of predictability).* And then I said, "What should we do to finish up this battle for the last 3 minutes, Jose?" He decided to swing freely forward and backward, "planning his attack for the next battle" while gently tossing some balls (giving verbal instructions to his soldiers and to his mother). I put a slow, quiet tape in the tape recorder and let him play catch and plan his next attack plan with his mother for a couple of minutes. Then I said, "Now its time to clean up," which we did together at the end of each session (*use of predictability*). Today Jose was able to voluntarily stop throwing the ball and help clean up. He also put on his shoes while maintaining an organized state. Jose seemed much more regulated than when he came into the session.

As I walked out Jose and his mother, we discussed how what happened today in our session could translate to home during the week. I explained the kinds of sensory input we have used (proprioceptive, linear, and then rotary movement) and the adaptive and nonadaptive responses that we observed. I reminded her of the STEP-SI acronym and described how this sessions used Sensation, Task, Predictability and Interaction to calm Jose as he began to escalate out of an appropriate range. Because Jose's mother had seen him play with movement while remaining organized and the effects of specific interactions with him, she understood exactly what I meant. She said that she would go to the playground a couple of times that week with the whole family after dinner. Jose could try out the merry-go-round, and his mother would monitor his activity level and excitability. She would guide him to intersperse play on the merry-go-round with climbing and digging activities. And, the next week was Jose's father's turn, so his father would then fill me in on how the playground time went.

Where will I direct the intervention next week? Should I continue with the "battle theme" or suggest another one? What happens if I set up the environment with more challenging movement equipment in the beginning? Can Jose verbalize to me how his "engine" is speeding up? Can he choose between several options for calming himself if I have them out and ready? What would happen if I made the environment more challenging (i.e., more distracting)? Is Jose ready to bring a sibling into his session so we can work on maintaining a good state of arousal while being challenged to remain socially engaged in play with a stimulating movement activity as preparation for success with peers on the playground at school . . . or maybe I should wait a few more weeks for that one . . . (Table A–7).

The STEP-SI clinical reasoning model is a "decision tree" analysis that is automatic and ongoing, directing the practitioner's choice of intervention during each direct session. Decisions are made in the moment by master clinicians based on knowledge gained during years of experience and

---

▪ TABLE A–7   REFLECTIVE QUESTIONS FOR THERAPISTS AFTER A DIRECT INTERVENTION SESSION

What important things happened in this intervention session?
How did the child respond? What was the adaptive response? Did the child or therapist find the just-right challenge? Was any of the session child directed? Was the child purposeful and intrinsically motivated?
What worked to provide support and appropriate challenges? How did you know what worked? Why did it work?
What didn't work to provide support and appropriate challenges? How did you know it didn't work? Why didn't it work? Did the child's overall adaptive capacity change as a result of this intervention session?
What will you do next time? What would you do the same or different from this session?
What questions do you have for the next intervention session?

---

responses from many young clients who have become their "professors." The more explicit the occupational therapy practitioner's understanding of the child's competencies and needs, the better prepared he or she is for each session. This takes time, of course, time that is precious to everyone. However, with experience, many of the options are integrated into the practitioner's tacit knowledge and become a part of an ongoing reasoning process. However, to practitioners new to this way of thinking, the process may seem overwhelming. Take the time to ask and answer questions about the child's responses as you conduct each session, and you will find that you have the information you need to decide how the intervention should proceed (Table A–8).

Using the STEP-SI to Develop Home and Community Programs

Next practitioners bring their reasoning skills to the development of home programs. What the practitioner has learned in direct intervention about the child's adaptive capacities and how to support the child during real-life challenges is then translated into the child's daily routine. The home or community program should provide family members and other caregivers with the following:

- An education about the meaning of the child's behavior
- Concrete and reasonable solutions to everyday challenges
- Tools to solve problems on their own

■ TABLE A–8 **REFLECTIVE QUESTIONS FOR THERAPISTS AFTER SEVERAL WEEKS OR MONTHS OF DIRECT INTERVENTION**

Do the parents seem comfortable with me and the direction of intervention? Am I communicating adequately with the family?

Do the parents understand the meaning of their child's behavior from a sensory integration frame of reference?

Do they understand the rationale behind intervention and home program suggestions?

Have I tried to counteract problems in sensory domains using strategies based in the dimension of the STEP-SI model?

What can I do to better meet the needs of the child as well as of family members?

Education for caretakers, suggestions for activities, and adaptations for the home should be established immediately after assessment.

Providing education to families and other caretakers about the nature of their child's strengths and problems is a critical feature of occupational therapy. As parents begin to understand their child's responses to the world, tensions often begin to ease and more positive interactions are established. Parents and caregivers can refocus on developing new solutions to the child's behaviors.

The practitioner and parent together build a home program to support the child in mastering challenging situations. The practitioner reviews the child's daily routine with parents, identifies problem areas, and develops a plan to support child through the challenge. An example for Jose is provided in Tables A–9 and A–10.

The charts constructed for Jose are examples of how social participation, self-regulation, self-esteem, and daily living tasks are addressed for a small part of the day for one child. This approach includes using specific dimensions of the STEP-SI model to address a specific problem at home, at school, and in the community.

These recommendations require multiple levels of reasoning on the part of the practitioner, who must give equal consideration to the family's priorities and the child's needs. Any plan

---

■ TABLE A–9 **JOSE'S HOME PROGRAM**

Activity	This Is Easy Because	This Is Difficult Because	Suggestions to Support
Waking up in the morning	It is not easy, but it is assisted by a loving and understanding family	Jose is very sluggish in the morning and can't seem to alert himself	Use sensation to support appropriate levels of alertness in Jose Have a morning wake-up routine with a song to sing while jumping on the mini trampoline
Getting dressed	Once clothes are decided on, his ability to dress himself is excellent	Jose has trouble choosing what to wear and seems overwhelmed by possibilities	Modify the task to support Jose to make clothing choices Use Garanimals Limit choices to a few known favorite clothes
Eating breakfast	His feeding skills are good; the only struggle is what to eat	Jose is a very picky eater and will only eat smooth vanilla yogurt or dry cereal for breakfast	Use sensation to support the task of eating Use oral pressure 10 minutes before meals Have Jose "drink" yogurt with a straw and then offer him a new food choice
Completing daily care activities (e.g., brushing teeth)	This is not easy, but it is helped by a behavioral chart with stickers that he uses	Jose is extremely sensitive to tactile stimulation in his mouth	Use sensation to support the task of tooth brushing Use oral pressure 10 minutes before meals and tooth brushing
Leaving for school	This is not easy, but it is supported by his siblings' leaving at the same time and understanding that he needs to be able to leave with them	Transitions are always a battleground Jose tantrums and refuses to leave the house	Combine sensation and predictability to support Jose through a transition Develop a "stomp-march" routine for transitions and use in conjunction with a picture schedule

■ TABLE A–10 JOSE'S COMMUNITY PROGRAM			
Activity	**This Is Easy Because**	**This Is Difficult Because**	**Suggestions**
Participating in circle time at school	Jose is very smart and quick to respond to all cognitive tasks as long as no one is too close to him	Teachers report that Jose will not sit near the other children	Use sensation to support by engaging in a deep pressure or proprioceptive task before circle or modify the environment by giving him "special" mat next to an adult or quiet child who won't touch him
Transitioning to lunch	This is not easy, but his teacher and all other classroom personnel are aware of his problem related to regulation and are willing to assist him by putting him at the end or beginning of line, giving him warnings, and so on	Jose hates to change from one place to another	Support with modification to the environment by allowing him to stay in the classroom with a buddy at lunch Support with preparatory sensation such as wall push-ups
Playing on the playground	This is not easy, but playground personnel are aware and willing to help him	Jose has difficulty with unexpected touch and dislikes recess very much	Support play by altering the playground task (challenge) Show him games he can play with one other child or a small group Encourage self-monitoring (e.g., when his engine gets too fast, its time to go try a pull-up or get into a small space on the climbing structure)
Going to Cub Scouts	This is not easy, but the Cub master is open to trying to learn about Jose so that Jose can participate	Jose has difficulty if the activities are not well supervised He can be terrified if he doesn't know what is coming up next	Support Jose by reinforcing the Cub master's positive interactions Support with increased predictability by asking the Cub master to start each meeting by listing what is going to happen that day or by making a daily chart
Going to Tae Kwon Do	This is not easy, but Jose is extremely motivated to be like the other children and to participate	Jose has a hard time keeping focus when other children are around	This activity intrinsically incorporates sensation that is supporting his ability to be part of a community group

must be sensitive to the beliefs, resources, and limitations of the family. Sometimes small alterations can make a huge difference (e.g., as soon as Jose wakes up, he is immediately urged to jump on a mini trampoline in his bedroom). This facilitates his ability to alert and self-regulate in the mornings. However, sometimes what seems like a "small alteration" to a practitioner can feel overwhelming to a parent (e.g., "How do you expect me to lay out all his clothes the night before? I'm so tired I can barely drag myself to bed!"). All matters related to the child's functioning in the home must be handled with cultural competence, maturity, and flexibility.

An equally important feature of the home or community program is providing education to help the family and the child learn critical reasoning skills. We may provide parents with education about the principles of sensory integration and teach them to use the STEP-SI dimensions as a guide to their own reasoning process. We point out how each intervention idea addresses a supportive feature of one of the dimensions of the STEP-SI model. We model problem solving by constructing options for helping a specific goal using the STEP-SI dimensions.

In addition to his parents developing tools for problem solving, Jose must also understand his own behavior and how to regulate it. Expanding Jose's capacities for self-monitoring is an essential feature. Modeling for the parent is essential, and specific programs such as the Alert Program may also be useful (Williams & Shellenberger, 1994; see also Chapter 14).

Probably the most important feature of successful critical reasoning is self-reflection. Questions such as those in Table A–11 may assist practitioners as they begin to use the principles outlined in this chapter.

Summary and Conclusions

Occupational therapy administered with a sensory integrative frame of reference is complex; it may seem like play when it really is work for both the practitioner and child. Effective intervention requires balancing multiple dimensions and principles. Because each program is individualized, not only in its overall focus but also "in the moment" based on the responses of the child, no concrete protocol or sequence of activities can be prescribed. Therapists must rely on tacit reasoning, which develops after explicit knowledge is obtained about the principles of intervention. While retaining individuality, for intervention research purposes, occupational therapy must be described in a manner that

it is replicable and so that fidelity to an intervention model can be guaranteed and that model tested empirically. The framework laid out in this chapter is designed to guide practitioners' critical reasoning by articulating the principles that guide intervention. The STEP-SI clinical reasoning model is a "thinking tool" for understanding how to apply and adjust multiple dimensions in the course of intervention. We have discussed this reasoning process for a child with severe movement sensitivity and an overall difficulty with sensory modulation. A similar thinking process is engaged for the other patterns of sensory integration dysfunction.

"Just as the continued production of research results in constantly changing neurological concepts, so also will this theory need to undergo frequent revision" (Ayres, 1972, p. ix).

Acknowledgments

We would like to acknowledge the important contributions made by each member of the Sensory Integration Team at The Children's Hospital of Denver during the duration of this project, including Julie Butler, Becky Greer, Corene Jack, Patty Kenyon, Nicki Pine, Robin Seger, Clare Summers, and Lisa Waterford. In addition, the careful edit and review by Barbara Hanft resulted in a much more coherent manuscript. The ongoing mentorship of Dr. Marshall Haith was the guiding influence that highlighted the need for this initial manuscript, which we will build on with feedback

---

■□ TABLE A–11   **REFLECTIVE QUESTIONS FOR THERAPISTS**

Have I developed the home program address the family and child's key issues and goals?

Is my program easy for the parents able to carry out at home? Does it fit the family's values and resources? Does it flow with the family's schedule?

Have I explained the STEP-SI model well enough that parents can automatically use it to assist their child at home and make adaptations as needed?

Have I given the parent and child a "toolbox" of ideas that they can use in everyday situations to assist the child?

Have I adequately addressed the child's social participation at home or community? What problems does he still have participating with his parents, siblings or peers in activities? Are there additional special family or social activities that I can recommend?

Have I adequately addressed the child's self-regulation at home or community? Have I given the parents and teachers tools to help the child begin to recognize when he is losing control? Do they understand how and when to use the tools? Am I helping the child recognize when he is beginning to become dysregulated? Are there any additional strategies I could add to the child's daily intervention?

Have I adequately addressed the child's self-esteem issues at home or in the community? Is the child able to verbalize what his or her sensory modulation dysfunction is and how it affects him or her? Does the child realize that the problem is not his or her "fault" but is caused by how his or her brain was when he or she was born? How does the child feel about the problems? What can I do to address affective issues for the child related to the dysfunction?

Have I adequately addressed the child's occupational performance needs? Is the child able to participate adequately in self-care and assist in household chores? Can the child adequately care for his or her belongings at home or at school? Does the child have an appropriate range of play skills and activity? Is the child adequately participating in school-related tasks?

from the professional community. Finally, this work could not have been completed without funding from the Wallace Research Foundation and a career award to the first author from the National Institutes of Health, National Center for Medical Research and Rehabilitation. The administrative support of Dr. Dennis Matthews, Chairman of the Department of Rehabilitation and Brian Burne, Director of Occupational Therapy at The Children's Hospital in Denver is also gratefully acknowledged.

References

Ayres, A. J. (1972). *Sensory integration and learning disorders*. Los Angeles: Western Psychological Services.

Ayres, A. J. (1989). *Sensory Integration and Praxis Tests*. Los Angeles: Western Psychological Services.

Cohn, E., Miller, L. J., & Tickle-Degnen, L. (2000). Parental hopes for therapy outcomes: Children with sensory modulation disorders. *American Journal of Occupational Therapy, 54,* 36–43.

Cohn, E. S. (2001a). Parent perspectives of occupational therapy using a sensory integration approach. *American Journal of Occupational Therapy, 55,* 285–294.

Cohn, E. S. (2001b). From waiting to relating: Parents' experiences in the waiting room of an occupational therapy clinic. *American Journal of Occupational Therapy, 55,* 168–175.

Fisher, A. G., Murray, E. A., & Bundy, A. C. (1991). *Sensory integration: Theory and practice.* Philadelphia: F. A. Davis.

Harter, S., Waters, P., & Whitesell, N. R. (1998). Relational self-worth: Differences in perceived worth as a person across interpersonal contexts among adolescents. *Child Development, 69,* 756–766.

Kimball, J. G. (1988). Hypothesis for prediction of stimulant drug effectiveness utilizing sensory integrative diagnostic methods. *Journal of the American Osteopathic Association, 88,* 757–762.

Kimball, J. G. (1999). Sensory integration frame of reference. In P. Kramer & J. Hinojosa (Eds.), *Frames of reference for pediatric occupational therapy* (2nd ed.). Baltimore: Lippincott, Williams & Wilkins.

Kinnealey, M., & Miller, L. J. (1993). Sensory integration/learning disabilities. In H. L. Hopkins & H. D. Smith (Eds.), *Willard & Spackman's occupational therapy* (8th ed., pp. 474–489). Philadelphia: J.B. Lippincott.

Mattingly, C., & Fleming, M. H. (1994). *Clinical reasoning: Forms of inquiry in a therapeutic practice.* Philadelphia: F.A. Davis.

Miller, L. J., & Summers, C. (2001). Clinical applications in sensory modulation disruptions: Assessment and intervention considerations. In S. Roley, R. Schaaf, & E. Blanche (Eds.), *Sensory integration and developmental disabilities* (pp. 249–276). San Antonio, TX: Therapy Skill Builders.

Oetter, P., Richter, E. W., & Frick, S. M. (1993). *M.O.R.E. integrating the mouth with sensory and postural function.* Hugo, MN: PDP Press.

Parham, L. D., & Mailloux, Z. (2001). Sensory integration. In J. Case-Smith (Ed.), *Occupational therapy for children* (4th ed., pp. 329–381). St. Louis: Mosby.

Stackhouse, T., & Wilbarger, J. L. (1998). Treating sensory modulation disorders: A clinical reasoning tool. Paper presented at the American Occupational Therapy Association 1998 Annual Conference and Exposition, Baltimore, MD.

Stackhouse, T. M., Trunnell, S. L., & Wilbarger, J. L. (1997). *Treating sensory modulation disorders: The STEP-SI: A tool for effective clinical reasoning.* Denver: The Children's Hospital.

Williams, M. S., & Shellenberger, S. (1994). *"How does your engine run"?: A leader's guide to the alert program for self-regulation.* Albuquerque: TherapyWorks.

Appendix B
Sensory Integration and Praxis Tests

A. Jean Ayres, PhD, OTR, FAOTA
Diana B. Marr, PhD

> *Tests yield numbers and numbers can do things that words or ideas cannot do. In occupational and physical therapy, measurement is central to differential diagnosis, gain or loss assessment, information across fields. It is difficult to accomplish any of the goals without some form of measurement.*
>
> —Ayres, 1989a, p. xi

[Editors' note: This appendix reflects the contributions of A. Jean Ayres and Diana Marr to Fisher et al. (1991). It has been revised to include more recent research addressing validity of the SIPT and to make the terminology parallel with that in the rest of the book.]

This section describes the nature, purpose, development, standardization, validity, reliability, and psychometric basis for the interpretation of the Sensory Integration and Praxis Tests (SIPT) (Ayres, 1989b). This integrated battery of tests was designed to contribute to the clinical understanding of children age 4 through 8 years with mild to moderate learning or motor difficulties. The tests that make up the SIPT are based on a neurobiological model that primarily addresses relationships among tactile processing; vestibular and proprioceptive processing; practic ability; and form and space, visual-motor, and constructional ability, all of which are considered essential to person–environment interaction and the organization of behavior.

Description of the Tests

Each of the 17 tests in the SIPT is individually administered; the entire battery generally can be completed in approximately an hour and a half. The tests are computer scored, which ensures precise scoring and allows for complex statistical comparisons between the tested child's pattern of SIPT scores and the typical score patterns observed in six different cluster groups.

The tests included in the SIPT are of the performance type. None of the SIPT requires verbal responses, and only one is strongly (and intentionally) dependent on auditory-language comprehension. The SIPT can be categorized into four overlapping groups, which are measures of:

1. Tactile and vestibular-proprioceptive sensory processing
2. Form and space perception and visuomotor coordination
3. Practic ability
4. Bilateral integration and sequencing (BIS)

The SIPT are intended primarily for the detection, description, and explanation of a cluster of symptoms interfering with daily life function rather than the detection of changes in sensory integrative functioning occurring from intervention. Most investigations of the psychometric properties of the SIPT have been conducted based on that assumption. However, in a pilot study, Kimball (1990) investigated the use of the SIPT for measuring change after intervention. She evaluated nineteen 6- to 8-year-old boys using an experimental version of the SIPT both before and after 6 months of intervention. Kimball grouped the SIPT into four categories and found statistically significant changes in three of the four groupings (all except form and space). Furthermore, the diagnostic categories for 17 of 19 of the boys changed from pretest to posttest. Thus, Kimball concluded that, unlike the Southern California Sensory Integration Tests (SC-SIT), the SIPT *may* prove to be sensitive measures of change. Kimball's conclusions are highly preliminary and need to be replicated. Thus, they should be viewed with caution.

Tactile, Vestibular, and Proprioceptive Sensory Processing Tests: Kinesthesia, Finger Identification, Graphesthesia, Localization of Tactile Stimuli, Postrotary Nystagmus, and Standing and Walking Balance

These six tests assess integration and interpretation of body sensation. The tactile tests and Kinesthesia (KIN) together make up the somatosensory tests. All five somatosensory tests are administered with vision occluded.

In the Finger Identification (FI) test, children point to the finger (or fingers) touched by the examiner. The Graphesthesia (GRA) test requires children to draw the same designs on the back of a hand that the examiner drew there. In the Localization of Tactile Stimuli (LTS) test, children touch the spot on a hand or arm that was touched by the examiner.

Kinesthesia (KIN), Postrotary Nystagmus (PRN), and Standing and Walking Balance (SWB) evaluate certain aspects of CNS processing of vestibular or proprioceptive sensory input. Kinesthesia measures conscious perception of position and movement of the arms and hands with vision occluded. Postrotary Nystagmus is identical in design (but not in normative data) to the Southern California Postrotary Nystagmus Test (SCPNT) (Ayres, 1975). In administration of the Postrotary Nystagmus test, the examiner records the duration of the oculomotor reflex after body rotation. Both atypically high (prolonged) and atypically low (depressed) scores are considered abnormal. Static and dynamic balance with eyes open and closed are evaluated in the SWB test. Balance is included in the SIPT because of its strong dependence on integration of vestibular and proprioceptive sensation.

Form and Space Perception and Visual-Motor Coordination Tests: Space Visualization, Figure-Ground Perception, Manual Form Perception, Motor Accuracy, Design Copying, and Constructional Praxis

Space Visualization (SV) assesses visual space perception and the ability to mentally manipulate objects in two-dimensional space. In this test, children decide which of two blocks fits into a hole in a form board. Because motor performance is not required and does not enter into scoring, the test is one of visual perception rather than a visual motor test. Although children are not required to put the blocks into the form board, most do so, providing information about their hand preference and tendency to use the contralateral versus ipsilateral hand in extracorporeal space. Scores derived from these observations are discussed below with the tests of BIS.

Figure-Ground Perception (FG) requires visual separation of a foreground line drawing from a rival background. This is a motor-free test. To eliminate contamination of a strictly visual perception score by motor or practic function, children indicate the answer to each test item by merely pointing to one of six multiple choice response figures. The decision time for each item is recorded, and a time score, separate from the accuracy score, is obtained.

Manual Form Perception (MFP) evaluates the haptic or stereognostic sense through identification of a plastic form held in the hand. In part 1 of this test, children point to an equivalent visual stimulus of the form; in part 2, they use the other hand to identify an equivalent form.

Visual motor coordination is assessed by the Motor Accuracy (MAc) test. In this test, children draw a red line over a heavy, curved, printed black line; the score is based on the extent of error. Separate scores for preferred and nonpreferred hands enable comparison of performance of the two hands.

In addition to these four tests of visual and haptic perception and visual-motor coordination, two tests, Design Copying (DC) and Constructional Praxis (CPr), described later in this chapter, assess construction and include elements of form and space perception. Design Copying also assesses an element of visual motor coordination. [Editors' note: Based on the results of factor and cluster analyses, Ayres (1989b) labeled this group of tests, which tended to be related to one another, tests of visuopraxis. The term *visuopraxis* reflected the common conceptual component between visual perception and motor planning. Visuopraxis does not refer to the *motor* manifestations of a practic deficit. Because of the confusion that arises from its use, we believe the term *visuopraxis* should be avoided and the test scores broken down into the following elements: form and space perception, visual construction, and visuomotor coordination.]

Praxis Tests: Design Copying, Constructional Praxis, Postural Praxis, Praxis on Verbal Command, Sequencing Praxis, and Oral Praxis

Practic skill is appraised in six behavioral domains. Two of these primarily assess visual construction rather than praxis. Design Copying (DC) evaluates the ability to conceptualize, plan, and execute two-dimensional designs. In part 1, children duplicate a design superimposed on a dot grid. In part 2, they copy the design in a designated blank space. All designs are scored for spatial accuracy; some also are scored for atypical drawing approaches such as segmentations, reversals, inversions, and extension of the drawings beyond their designated boundaries (see Ayres, 1989b for more detail).

Constructional Praxis (CPr) uses a block-building task to assess skill in relating objects to each other spatially. Block structures are scored for various errors in block placement, including rotation, reversal, mislocation, and omission.

The major tests of praxis include Postural Praxis (PPr), Praxis on Verbal Command (PrVC), Sequencing Praxis (SPr), and Oral Praxis (OPr). Postural Praxis evaluates aptitude in planning and assuming unusual body postures demonstrated by the examiner. Hand and arm postures are most frequently used, but head, trunk, and finger positions are critical on some of the items. Although Postural Praxis requires visual interpretation of each demonstrated position, no visual memory of that position is required. Praxis on Verbal Command taps the ability to assume a number of different positions based on an examiner's verbal command. Sequencing Praxis evaluates competency in perceiving, remembering, and executing a demonstrated sequence of unilateral and bilateral hand and finger positions. In the Oral Praxis test, the child imitates the examiner's movements of the tongue, lips, cheeks, or jaw. Most items consist of a sequence of movements. [Editors' note: Because the examiner demonstrates each item, both Sequencing Praxis and Oral Praxis involve visual interpretation and visual memory.]

Bilateral Integration and Sequencing Tests: Oral Praxis, Sequencing Praxis, Graphesthesia, Standing and Walking Balance, Bilateral Motor Coordination, Space Visualization Contralateral Use, and Space Visualization Preferred Hand Use

Through a series of factor and cluster analyses of SIPT scores, five tests in the SIPT were found to be related to BIS. Four of these tests, Oral Praxis, Sequencing Praxis, Graphesthesia, Standing and Walking Balance, were described above. The fifth test is Bilateral Motor Coordination (BMC). Bilateral Motor Coordination requires imitation of smoothly executed movements of hands and feet demonstrated by the examiner. Reciprocal interactions of the right and left extremities are stressed to assess integration of the two sides of the body.

Two additional scores related to BIS, the Space Visualization Contralateral Use (SVCU) score and the Space Visualization Preferred Hand Use (PHU) score, are derived from the observation of the hand used to pick up the block to be placed in the form board. The Space Visualization Contralateral Use score, a test of crossing the midline, is based on the proportion of responses in which the child crosses the midline of the body with the hand to select a block from contralateral space. The PHU score, a measure of hand preference, is based on the proportion of items on which children use their preferred hand during the Space Visualization test. The preferred hand is defined as the hand the child uses for writing.

Test Development and Standardization

The SIPT evolved over several decades. Initially, a number of clinical procedures commonly used to assess agnosia and apraxia in individuals with adult-onset brain damage were redesigned for use with children with minimal brain dysfunction or learning disabilities. Through statistical analyses,

Ayres (1965, 1969) selected the procedures that provided the most useful clinical information, showed the highest factor loadings, and showed the strongest capacity to discriminate between children with and without dysfunction. First appearing as several individual tests, they were later published in combined form as the SCSIT (Ayres, 1972a; 1980) and as the SCPNT (Ayres, 1975).

The Postrotary Nystagmus test and 12 of the tests in the SCSIT were retained or revised for the SIPT. Decisions as to which of the SCSIT to revise and include in the SIPT were based on:

- The results of a number of factor analyses (Ayres, 1966, 1972b, 1977; Silberzahn, 1975)
- The ability of the tests to contribute to the understanding of children's problems
- The results of a survey of the faculty of Sensory Integration International

In addition, four new praxis tests were developed for the SIPT. In developing new tests and revising tests from the SCSIT, the selection of items was based on extensive field testing, several pilot studies evaluating each item's capacity to distinguish between children with and without dysfunction, and interrater and test-retest reliability.

The SIPT were standardized on a nationwide sample of approximately 2000 children. The children in the normative sample were chosen to be as representative as possible of children from age 4 years, 0 month to age 8 years, 11 months living in the United States. A modified random sampling procedure was used, stratified to reflect the population characteristics from the 1980 U.S. Census. The number of children tested in each region was based on the number of children between the ages of 4 and 14 years reported in the census data. The ethnic composition of the normative sample and the percentage of urban vs. rural children in each region were based on census figures. Because sensory integration principles were used throughout Canada, a number of Canadian children were also included in the standardization sample. Table B–1 shows the geographic distribution of children in the normative sample.

The normative data analyses were conducted in three stages. These included:

1. Preliminary analyses, which examined age- and gender-related differences in performance and determined the appropriate scoring and stopping rules for the tests

2. Computation of means and standard deviations, which included the examination of developmental trends and the normality of the score distribution for each of the 17 tests

3. Determination of the extent to which each of the various tests discriminated between children with and without dysfunction

Preliminary analyses indicated significant gender differences on all of the tests except Manual Form Perception and Postrotary Nystagmus. Therefore, separate norms were developed for boys and girls. There also were significant age effects on all tests except Postrotary Nystagmus. The developmental curves for the tests indicated that the optimal age groupings for the normative data should cover 4-month intervals for children younger than age 6 years and 6-month intervals for children age 6 years and older. Therefore, separate norms were developed for boys and girls in each of 12 age groups. For each of these groups, SIPT scores generally fit a normal distribution curve. Means and standard deviations were computed for each normative subgroup so that each child's score can be reported as an index of the degree to which the child's performance differs from the average performance of children of the same age and gender.

Ayres wanted to be able to discontinue testing when children seemed unable to complete any more items. Because many items are administered in order of increasing difficulty, it was possible to determine appropriate stopping rules for eight of the 17 tests. Stopping rules were added only for those tests in which predictive validity was not significantly lowered by a stopping rule and only when the differences were negligible between the scores with and without the stopping rule.

Most of the individual tests yielded several subscores (e.g., time and accuracy). For both theoretical and pragmatic reasons, it seemed likely that children in different diagnostic groups might exhibit different speed-accuracy tradeoffs in test performance. Thus, time-adjusted accuracy scores were important on a number of tests. Optimal statistical weights for time and accuracy were identified to discriminate between children with and without dysfunction, within and across the 12 age groups.

Validity of the SIPT

Validity is the ability to draw meaningful inferences from test scores to meet an intended purpose.

TABLE B-1 Normative Sample by Age, Sex, and Geographic Region

		Geographic Region																					
Age Group		New England		Mid Atlantic		South Atlantic		East No. Central		East So. Central		West No. Central		West So. Central		Mountain		Pacific		Canada		Total
(yr/mo)		m	f	m	f	m	f	m	f	m	f	m	f	m	f	m	f	m	f	m	f	
4/0–4/3		3	2	3	2	2	3	7	5	1	1	2	3	1	1	1	2	4	0	0	1	44
4/4–4/7		7	3	3	5	5	6	10	9	6	3	6	5	4	6	2	3	3	7	3	3	99
4/8–4/11		3	5	7	7	7	4	9	7	4	2	4	8	5	4	1	1	9	9	4	4	104
5/0–5/3		4	6	8	5	6	3	13	17	3	5	2	6	8	7	2	1	6	3	3	0	108
5/4–5/7		2	6	10	6	16	9	14	17	9	3	6	3	11	12	4	4	7	6	9	3	157
5/8–5/11		3	3	10	13	16	17	14	20	9	10	5	6	10	9	8	6	7	7	7	4	184
6/0–6/5		4	3	14	15	21	23	28	24	11	10	8	10	10	14	13	14	12	11	6	8	259
6/6–6/11		2	2	9	11	22	21	19	18	10	9	6	12	10	11	9	7	10	12	9	7	216
7/0–7/5		2	2	14	12	17	14	18	19	8	5	11	14	12	12	6	9	10	8	10	9	212
7/6–7/11		1	4	13	13	15	16	20	25	6	6	8	8	10	12	8	12	12	11	7	9	216
8/0–8/5		3	2	12	11	14	15	14	20	9	9	10	9	13	6	9	7	6	8	1	1	191
8/6–8/11		4	5	11	15	22	17	19	25	11	6	5	7	12	8	10	4	6	7	7	6	207
		38	43	114	115	163	148	185	206	87	69	73	91	106	102	73	70	92	89	72	61	1997
TOTAL		81		229		311		391		156		164		208		143		181		133		1997

We address two types of validity-related evidence: construct-related and criterion-related evidence. To ensure that validity estimates would not be inflated by age and gender differences, all analyses were conducted using standard scores.

Construct-Related Validity

Identification of relevant sensory integrative processes and the organization of related behavioral parameters into meaningful theoretical constructs have been accomplished through factor and cluster analyses. Factor analysis is a statistical technique that identifies groups of test scores that are correlated. For example, we expect that form and space tests define a factor; if a child has a low score on one, it is likely that he or she will have low scores on all of them (see Chapter 1). Cluster analysis is a statistical technique that is conceptually similar to factor analysis. However, cluster analysis is used to identify groups of children who demonstrate similar test score patterns on a battery of tests.

Data from the SIPT, the SCSIT, and related clinical observations have been included in these analyses. As a part of the interpretation of the factor or cluster analyses, the researcher names the resulting factors or clusters.

EARLY FACTOR ANALYSES

An early factor analysis of the scores of one hundred 6- and 7-year-old children on a number of perceptual-motor measures revealed four factors (Ayres, 1965). Ayres labeled these:

- Developmental dyspraxia with major loadings for tactile and motor planning tests
- Form and space perception deficit, best represented by tests of visual and haptic form and space perception, and kinesthesia
- Bilateral integration deficit, with highest loadings for right–left discrimination, crossing the midline, and bilateral motor coordination
- Tactile defensiveness, characterized by tactile defensiveness, distractibility, and poor tactile perception

Similar factors did not emerge from scores on the same measures in a group of 50 age- and gender-matched typically developing children.

In a subsequent study of 4- to 8-year-old children, a somatomotor factor linked tactile perception and kinesthesia with motor planning in a group of 92 children (including some with dysfunction), but not in a group of 164 children with typical early development (Ayres, 1966). A Q technique factor analysis (Ayres, 1969) of 64 observations for each of 36 learning disabled children (mean age = 97.7 months; standard deviation [SD], 11.3 months) expanded the identifying markers of the score pattern earlier referred to as bilateral integration deficit. In this analysis, clinically observed postural and ocular responses were statistically associated with the bilateral integration measures.

The tactile, proprioceptive, and visual perception tests tended to share variance in a 1972 factor analysis of scores of 148 children with learning disabilities (mean age = 92.6 months; SD = 12.0 months) on measures of sensory integration, psycholinguistic ability, academic achievement, intelligence, and postural and ocular responses. Motor planning, hyperactivity, and tactile defensiveness were closely associated. Psycholinguistic and intelligence test scores were significantly correlated (Ayres, 1972b).

The close association between praxis and tactile perception was also demonstrated in a later analysis, in which postural and ocular functions again shared variance. Auditory-language abilities loaded on a single separate factor in that analysis (Ayres, 1977).

A study by Ayres et al. (1987) addressed the issue of whether there are different types of dyspraxia. Scores on the SCSIT; several auditory-language tests; postural and ocular observations; a block-building test; and early forms of the SIPT Praxis on Verbal Command, Oral Praxis, and Sequencing Praxis tests were analyzed for 182 children known or suspected to have dysfunction (mean age = 78 months; SD = 17.4 months). Praxis on Verbal Command, Oral Praxis, Sequencing Praxis, block building, and all of the SCSIT except Bilateral Motor Coordination loaded on one major factor reflecting praxis. Other scores that did not load on this factor included Postrotary Nystagmus, prone extension, supine flexion, and Space Visualization Contralateral Use. The auditory-language tests identified the second factor, on which Praxis on Verbal Command and Sequencing Praxis also had loadings above 0.30. The ability to integrate the two sides of the body in a series of sequential movements was reflected in a third factor with major loadings for Bilateral Motor Coordination, Oral Praxis, and Sequencing Praxis.

Ayres et al. (1987) concluded that the data neither supported the existence of a unitary dyspraxia function nor different types of dyspraxia. Rather, the data supported the idea of a general practic function with different practic skills defined by behavioral tasks. The data also supported the idea of a common conceptual component to praxis and visual perception. Throughout all of these pre-SIPT studies, there was a tendency for auditory-language measures to be less closely associated with sensations from the body than were measures of perception and sensory integration.

In summary, the results of factor-analytic studies conducted by Ayres, supported the presence of the following constructs:

- Tactile-kinesthesia linked with poor praxis (somatopraxis)
- Form and space perception
- Postural-ocular scores linked with bilateral integration (defined by Bilateral Motor Coordination, right–left discrimination, and crossing the midline of the body)
- Tactile defensiveness (tactile defensiveness is a construct not measured by the SIPT)

Finally, some of the factor-analytic studies suggested the presence of a more "generalized" construct of poor sensory processing (vestibular-proprioceptive and tactile), praxis, bilateral integration, form of space, and academic achievement.

Factor Analyses of the SIPT

Ayres conducted a number of factor analyses of SIPT scores, which further clarified the nature of the constructs evaluated by the SIPT. In this discussion, only factor loadings greater than or equal to 0.35 are reported.

SIPT Normative Sample

A four-factor solution of a principal components analysis of the SIPT normative sample categorized the tests as those that were primarily visuopractic and those that were primarily somatopractic.

The term *somatopraxis* was derived from findings of a close association between somatosensory (tactile-proprioceptive) processing and motor planning. The use of the term *visuopraxis* originated in the earlier recognition of a common conceptual link between praxis and visual perception (Ayres et al., 1987). Highest loading tests on the visuopraxis factor were, in decreasing order of magnitude, Con-

structional Praxis, Space Visualization, Design Copying, Manual Form Perception, Figure-Ground Perception, and Praxis on Verbal Command. Highest loading somatopraxis tests were (in decreasing order of magnitude) Oral Praxis, Bilateral Motor Coordination, Graphesthesia, Postural Praxis, Sequencing Praxis, Standing and Walking Balance, and Finger Identification. The third factor to emerge was a vestibular-somatosensory processing factor. Tests with the highest loadings on the vestibular-somatosensory factor were Postrotary Nystagmus and three somatosensory tests (i.e., Kinesthesia, Finger Identification, and Localization of Tactile Stimuli). The fourth factor was a Kinesthesia-Motor Accuracy doublet. This factor also had a negative loading on Postural Praxis.

Children With Dysfunction

A principal components analysis of the SIPT scores of 125 children with learning or sensory integrative deficits (mean age = 7.27 years; SD = 0.97 years) showed a differentiation of sensory integrative problems into five different categories or patterns. The results of this analysis are shown in Table B–2.

The first factor to emerge, representing the greatest proportion of the SIPT's variance, was a BIS factor. The tests representing this factor were Sequencing Praxis, Bilateral Motor Coordination, Graphesthesia, Standing and Walking Balance, Oral Praxis, and Manual Form Perception.

On the second factor, Postrotary Nystagmus had a large positive loading, and Praxis on Verbal Command had the largest negative loading. This relationship suggested that problems in translating verbal directions into body postures are apt to be associated with prolonged postrotary nystagmus. The relationship is consistent with a previous factor analysis (Ayres, 1977) in which the SCPNT had a substantial negative loading on an auditory-language factor. Figure-Ground also had a negative loading on this factor.

Factor 3, somatosensory processing with oral praxis, linked Localization of Tactile Stimuli, Kinesthesia, and Oral Praxis. Factor 4, visuopraxis, was best represented by the form and space perception tests and by the visual construction tests (Design Copying and Constructional Praxis). Factor 5, somatopraxis, was identified by high loading for three praxis tests (Postural Praxis, Constructional Praxis, and Oral Praxis) and one tactile test (Graphesthesia).

■ TABLE B–2 FACTOR ANALYSIS OF SIPT SCORES OF 125 CHILDREN WITH LEARNING OF SENSORY INTEGRATIVE DEFICITS

	FACTOR 1	FACTOR 2	FACTOR 3	FACTOR 4	FACTOR 5
	Bilateral Integration & Sequencing	*Praxis on Verbal Command*	*Somatosensory Processing & Oral Praxis*	*Visuopraxis*	*Somatopraxis*
Space Visualization [SV]	−.08	−.11	−.08	.64	.30
Figure-Ground Perception [FG]	.20	−.36	.05	.54	−.02
Manual Form Perception [MFP]	.38	−.10	.12	.20	.17
Kinesthesia [KIN]	.24	.13	.74	.02	−.14
Finger Identification [F]	.24	.31	−.07	.37	.30
Graphesthesia [GRA]	.57	.09	−.03	−.04	.42
Localization of Tactile Stimuli [LTS]	−.27	−.11	.83	.04	.09
Praxis on Verbal Command [PrVC]	.32	−.59	.14	.06	.14
Design Copying [DC]	.18	.00	.06	.67	.06
Constructional Praxis [CPr]	.07	−.07	.10	.38	.54
Postural Praxis [PPr]	−.07	−.03	−.02	.07	.89
Oral Praxis [OPr]	.40	.00	.37	−.22	.51
Sequencing Praxis [SPr]	.78	.04	−.02	.04	.08
Bilateral Motor Coordination [BMC]	.69	−.31	−.04	.07	−.10
Standing and Walking Balance [SWB]	.54	.15	.16	.26	−.07
Motor Accuracy [MAc]	−.03	.20	.09	.78	−.11
Postrotary Nystagmus [PRN]	.06	.76	.04	.07	.01
Factor Correlations: 2	−.08				
3	−.26	.04			
4	−.37	.00	.18		
5	−.34	.08	.16	.31	

CHILDREN WITH AND WITHOUT DYSFUNCTION

Scores of a combined sample of 176 typically developing children and 117 children with learning or sensory integrative deficits (mean age = 7.3 years; SD = 1.0 year) were examined in an additional principal components analysis. The first factor to emerge was primarily a somatopraxis or BIS factor, with highest loadings for Oral Praxis, Graphesthsia, Bilateral Motor Coordination, Sequencing Praxis, and Standing and Walking Balance, in that order. Praxis on Verbal Command loaded moderately on this factor, as did Postural Praxis.

The second factor was identified as a visuopraxis factor, with highest loadings for Space Visualization, Figure-Ground Perception, Design Copying, Motor Accuracy, and Constructional Praxis. The third factor, vestibular functioning, was defined by a high loading for Postrotary Nystagmus. Finally, the fourth factor, somatosensory processing, was identified with highest loadings for Localization of Tactile Stimuli and Kinesthesia.

In summary, these factor analyses resulted in the identification of four factors: visuopraxis (form and space, visual construction, and visual motor coordination), somatopraxis, BIS, and praxis on verbal command, associated with pro-

longed postrotary nystagmus. Vestibular and somatosensory processing factors emerged in several analyses, perhaps suggesting an underlying deficit in sensory processing. [Editors' note: Ayres gave various labels to these sensory processing factors.]

CLUSTER ANALYSES OF THE SIPT

Using the same sample of 117 children with dysfunction and 176 typically developing children described previously, cluster analysis was used to identify distinct groups of children who could be characterized by different score profiles on the SIPT. Children with and without dysfunction were included in the sample in order to ensure that obtained clusters would differentiate between them. The analysis used Ward's method of clustering, which generally produces the most accurate results for the type of data obtained from the SIPT (see, for example, Lorr, 1983).

Cluster solutions were generated to extract from two to 10 clusters; a six-cluster solution seemed to be the most appropriate based on both statistical and clinical criteria. Solutions with more than six clusters tended to split the children into very small groups, some of which had only two or three members; solutions with fewer than six clusters combined groups that theoretically and clinically could be delineated. The six-cluster solution identified groups that Ayres labeled as follows:

- Low Average BIS
- Generalized Sensory Integrative Dysfunction
- Visuo- and Somatodyspraxia
- Low Average Sensory Integration and Praxis
- Dyspraxia on Verbal Command
- High Average Sensory Integration and Praxis

The means and standard deviations for each group on all of the 17 major SIPT scores are shown in Table B–3. The plotted scores are the cluster group mean scores, which are also listed in Table B–3.

Approximately 19 percent of the children in the sample were identified as belonging to the Low Average BIS cluster group. This group scored close to the mean on most of the SIPT, but with somewhat lower scores on the five tests that are associated with BIS (i.e., Oral Praxis, Graphesthesia, Standing and Walking Balance, Sequencing Praxis, and Bilateral Motor Coordination). Children in this group also had lower scores on the Postural Praxis test. However, because low scores on the Postural Praxis test did not emerge in the factor analyses, this score was thought to be less important.

Approximately 12 percent of the children in the sample were identified as belonging to the Generalized Sensory Integrative Dysfunction cluster group. They tended to score substantially below the mean on all of the SIPT; however, their Localization of Tactile Stimuli and Postrotary Nystagmus mean scores were in the average range. Another 12 percent of the children were identified as members of the Visuo- and Somatodyspraxia cluster group. Children in the Visuo- and Somatodyspraxia cluster group also tended to score below the mean on all of the SIPT, but their scores were not nearly as low as those of the Generalized Sensory Integrative Dysfunction cluster group.

Approximately 24 percent of the total sample belonged to the Low Average Sensory Integration and Praxis cluster group. This group's SIPT scores tended to fall just below the mean, with the lowest scores (still within average limits) on Postural Praxis, Finger Identification, Sequencing Praxis, Design Copying, and Localization of Tactile Stimuli.

The Dyspraxia on Verbal Command cluster group included approximately 10 percent of the total sample. This group's profile of scores was distinguished by very low scores on Praxis on Verbal Command and the highest mean Postrotary Nystagmus score; other scores were in the average or low average range. This group also had low scores on Bilateral Motor Coordination, Sequencing Praxis, Standing and Walking Balance, Design Copying, and Oral Praxis.

Finally, 24 percent of the children in the sample

■ TABLE B–3   SIPT MEANS AND STANDARD DEVIATIONS FOR THE SIX CLUSTER GROUPS

Test	GROUP 1 Low Average BIS Mean	SD	GROUP 2 Generalized SI Dysfunction Mean	SD	GROUP 3 Visuo- and Somato- dyspraxia Mean	SD	GROUP 4 Low Average SI & Praxis Mean	SD	GROUP 5 Dyspraxia on Verbal Command Mean	SD	GROUP 6 High Average SI & Praxis Mean	SD
Space Visualization [SV]	−.03	.67	−1.36	.79	−.90	.80	−.32	1.03	−.48	.87	.54	.60
Figure-Ground Perception [FG]	.03	1.02	−1.35	1.04	−.60	.70	−.30	1.08	−.81	.76	.60	.89
Manual Form Perception [MFP]	−.13	.87	−1.60	.97	−.65	1.04	−.09	1.17	−.57	.72	.36	.85
Kinesthesia [KIN]	−.34	.96	−1.60	1.50	−1.20	1.21	.14	.74	−.78	1.20	.14	.96
Finger Identification [FI]	.01	.93	−1.40	.97	−1.02	1.12	−.51	1.01	−.41	.67	.43	.77
Graphesthesia [GRA]	−.81	.93	−2.13	.88	−1.01	.91	−.08	.93	−.72	.80	.42	.86
Loc. of Tactile Stimuli [LTS]	−.24	1.04	−.66	1.31	−.41	.92	−.43	1.14	−.12	1.09	.61	.81
Praxis on Verbal Command [PrVC]	.18	.66	−2.41	.84	−.15	.68	−.08	.93	−2.38	.76	.56	.49
Design Copying [DC]	−.02	.74	−2.11	.62	−1.61	.81	−.43	.96	−1.07	1.00	.74	.74
Constructional Praxis [CPr]	.16	.69	−1.58	1.05	−.88	.71	.07	.62	−.53	.58	.53	.64
Postural Praxis [PPr]	−.52	.95	−2.14	.93	−.98	1.13	−.55	.93	−.76	.88	.53	.90
Oral Praxis [OPr]	−.94	.99	−2.20	.72	−.47	.89	.13	.77	−1.04	.83	.24	.86
Sequencing Praxis [SPr]	−.66	.90	−2.06	.74	−1.21	.84	−.42	.66	−1.44	.97	.41	1.03
Bilateral Motor Coord. [BMC]	−.46	.79	−1.46	.72	−1.11	.94	−.24	1.07	−1.56	.59	.47	.99
Standing/Walking Balance [SWB]	−.77	.79	−2.28	.63	−1.28	.94	.12	.77	−1.17	.85	−.49	1.05
Motor Accuracy [MAc]	−.17	.65	−1.03	.48	−.98	.39	−.19	.73	−.70	.45	.21	.83
Postrotary Nystagmus [PRN]	−.36	.88	−.48	.84	−.63	.78	.11	.78	.47	.84	.09	.71

belonged to the High Average Sensory Integration and Praxis cluster group. This group tended to score above the mean on all of the SIPT.

Table B–4 shows the representation of typically developing children, children with learning disabilities, and children with sensory integrative deficits in each of the six cluster groups. As expected, most of the typically developing children had score profiles that matched either the high average or two low average cluster groups. In fact, 88 percent of the typically developing children fell into one of these three groups (37 percent matched the High Average Sensory Integration and Praxis cluster; 30 percent matched the Low Average Sensory Integration and Praxis cluster; and 21 percent matched the Low Average BIS cluster).

In contrast, only 3 percent of the children with learning disabilities or sensory integrative dysfunction matched the High Average Sensory Integration and Praxis cluster, and 29 percent matched either the Low Average BIS cluster or the Low Average Sensory Integration and Praxis cluster. The remaining 68 percent of the children with learning disabilities or sensory integrative dysfunction matched one of the three dysfunctional cluster groups, and more than 27 percent matched the Generalized Sensory Integration Dysfunction cluster. Factor analysis of the data from children with dysfunction revealed that the Low Average BIS cluster group may be composed of two groups of children, one group that is normal on the BIS factor and another group that is made up of children with dysfunction.

CONFIRMATORY FACTOR ANALYTIC STUDIES

More recently, in an effort to confirm the factors most commonly identified by Ayres and address the criticism of small sample sizes in Ayres' work

(Cummins, 1991), Mulligan (1998) conducted the largest study to date of SIPT data. She used confirmatory factor analysis with data from more than 10,000 children, about 1000 of whom had learning disabilities. Based on Ayres' work, Mulligan hypothesized that sensory integration dysfunction had a five-factor structure consisting of BIS, postural ocular movements, somatosensory processing, somatopraxis, and visuopraxis. She did not consider sensory modulation because the SIPT do not provide evidence of this or praxis on verbal command because it is thought to reflect left hemisphere rather than sensory integrative functioning.

Although Mulligan found a reasonable fit to the data using the five-factor model, she also found numerous weaknesses, including low factor loadings and strong correlations among factors. Thus, Mulligan conducted exploratory factor analyses in an attempt to identify the most parsimonious solution with the best fit of the data.

Mulligan generated two solutions, each of which appeared to reflect the data better than the model drawn from Ayres' work. In the first, she identified a first-order four-factor model; she labeled the four factors *visuoperceptual, bilateral integration, somatosensory,* and *praxis.* However, because these factors were highly correlated, she also identified a second-order, four-factor model in which a higher order factor she labeled generalized *practic dysfunction* emerged; the four first-order factors remained very similar. [Editors' note: Mulligan later indicated that generalized practic dysfunction might be more accurately labeled *generalized sensory integrative dysfunction.*]

Using the second-order, four-factor model, Mulligan again conducted confirmatory factor analyses using both the original data set and a data subset of children with learning disabilities. Her results with both groups were similar to those of the exploratory

---

■ TABLE B–4 **REPRESENTATION OF NORMAL, LEARNING-DISABLED, AND SI DEFICIENT CHILDREN IN THE SIX SIPT CLUSTER GROUPS**

	GROUP 1	GROUP 2	GROUP 3	GROUP 4	GROUP 5	GROUP 6	
	Low Average BIS	*Generalized SI Dysfunction*	*Visuo- and Somato-dyspraxia*	*Low Average SI & Praxis*	*Dyspraxia on Verbal Command*	*High Average SI & Praxis*	*TOTAL*
Normal Children	36	2	13	54	6	65	176
Learning-Disabled	11	28	13	13	21	3	89
SI Dysfunctional	8	4	9	4	2	1	28
TOTAL	55	34	35	71	29	69	293

factor analysis. Thus, she concluded that the latter model represented the best of the three models of sensory integration. This model is presented in Figure 1–7.

Mulligan discussed a number of interesting points. First, no pattern related to postural ocular movement emerged. This is likely because of the absence of sufficient measures on the SIPT to discriminate such a function. These results confirmed earlier suggestions made by Fisher and Bundy (1991) regarding the need to include clinical observations of postural functions in the assessment of sensory integration.

Second, Mulligan found no evidence of a somatopraxis factor. This result was surprising because Ayres repeatedly found associations between praxis and somatosensory measures. Mulligan concluded that children with poor scores on both tactile and praxis measures would be described most accurately as "having generalized practic dysfunction with weaknesses in the areas of praxis and somatosensory processing" (Mulligan, 1998, p. 825). [Editor's note: We believe it is *always* best to describe both the practic problem and its apparent underlying basis in *any* report of sensory integrative functioning.]

Finally, Mulligan discussed the possibility of a shorter test to measure sensory integration. She found that PRN, KIN, SWB, and MAc failed to support any patterns. In addition, she believed that eliminating some of the visual perceptual tests would make testing more efficient. Because of its poor test-reliability, FG seems a likely candidate for elimination.

Mulligan's study represents the largest study to data of SIPT patterns. Thus, her results must be considered carefully. However, as she used the same sample for both exploratory and confirmatory factor analysis, her work also must be viewed with caution until it is replicated. Clearly, further research is needed.

Criterion-Related Validity

Because the tests in the SIPT are intended for the detection, description, and explanation of current developmental irregularities rather than for the prediction of criterion scores at a later time, criterion-related evidence is primarily concurrent in nature. Co-occurrence, of course, is not to be confused with causation. Although some work has been done comparing the whole SIPT—or categories within

it—with assessments thought to reflect the same (convergent validity) or different constructs (divergent validity), there are generally few tests of sensory integration and praxis against which to compare the SIPT. Thus, inferences about the meaning of a given test profile in the current life of a child are generally collected through testing children with known, different, and previously determined diagnoses. In this respect, prior research using the SCSIT and SCPNT with various populations contributes to an evolving ability to derive accurate inferences from SIPT scores.

Comparison of Diagnostic Groups

Means and standard deviations, calculated during SIPT development for children in nine diagnostic groups are shown in Table B–5. The mean scores of all nine groups combined were below average on the SIPT. Scores of some, but not all groups, show recognizable patterns.

Learning Disability

For 195 children with learning disabilities (mean age = 7.3 years; SD = 1.0 years), scores on all tests in the SIPT tended to be below average. The lowest scores were on five of the six praxis tests and on Graphesthesia and Standing and Walking Balance. By definition, children with learning disabilities have IQs within normal limits. Thus, the high incidence of sensory integrative dysfunction among this group supported the idea that intelligence and sensory integration are relatively distinct constructs.

Sensory Integrative Dysfunction

A group of 36 children with sensory integrative dysfunction (mean age, 6.9 years; SD = 1.1 years) tended to score in the low average range on most of the tests but had considerably lower scores than average on Graphesthesia, Postural Praxis, Sequencing Praxis, and Standing and Walking Balance. This pattern may reflect a selective factor in the referral and acceptance of children for intervention. As in the learning disabled group, fairly large standard deviations on some of the tests indicated considerable heterogeneity. Different patterns of scores may have been obscured by the computation of mean scores across a fairly heterogeneous group of children.

Reading Disorders

The mean SIPT scores of 60 children with reading disorders (mean age = 7.1 years; SD = 0.9

■ Table B-5 SIPT Means and Standard Deviations for Different Diagnostic Groups

Test	Learning Disabled (n = 195)		Brain Injured (n = 10)		Mental Retardation (n = 28)		SI Dysfunction (n = 36)		SpinaBifida (n = 21)		Reading Disorder (n = 60)		Language Disorder (n = 28)		Cerebral Palsy (n = 10)		Attention Deficit Hyperactivity Disorder (n = 309)	
	Mean	SD	Mean	SD	Mean	SD	Mean	SD	Mean	SD	Mean	SD	Mean	SD	Mean	SD	Mean	SD
V	-0.71	.85	-1.03	1.01	-1.51	.97	-0.67	1.04	-0.74	.63	-0.52	.92	-0.75	1.15	-0.85	.37	-0.89	0.96
FG	-0.75	1.07	-1.31	1.29	-1.73	1.68	-0.29	1.05	-1.00	0.86	-0.92	0.79	-0.81	1.16	-0.68	.88	-0.46	1.10
MFP	-1.02	1.23	-1.90	1.30	-2.79	0.32	-0.46	0.99	-1.90	1.25	-0.99	1.10	-1.17	1.14	-0.65	.21	-1.61	1.40
KIN	-1.09	1.36	-1.69	1.59	-2.73	0.55	-0.60	1.08	-1.10	1.30	-1.30	1.02	-1.01	1.48	-0.60	1.5	-1.73	1.64
FI	-1.02	1.03	-0.80	1.01	-1.90	0.89	-0.73	1.05	-0.53	1.06	-1.02	1.02	-1.04	1.00	-1.60	1.2	-1.36	1.42
GRA	-1.37	1.14	-1.57	1.15	-2.42	0.69	-1.09	1.06	-1.90	0.69	-0.63	1.18	-1.17	1.01	-1.28	1.4	-0.81	1.13
LTS	-0.65	1.20	-1.18	1.09	-1.63	1.77	-0.61	1.20	-1.30	1.12	-0.33	1.07	-0.86	1.04	-1.80	.94	-1.15	1.98
PrVC	-1.40	1.36	-1.58	1.50	-3.00	0.00	-0.49	1.25	-0.99	1.24	-1.01	1.32	-1.74	1.38	-0.63	1.5	-0.73	1.34
DC	-1.60	1.12	-1.43	1.35	-3.00	0.00	-0.86	1.05	-2.00	1.13	-1.24	1.27	-1.33	1.11	-2.33	.99	-0.61	1.39
CPr	-0.91	.95	-0.83	1.02	-2.17	0.53	-0.46	0.95	-1.10	1.09	-0.60	0.88	-0.78	0.93	-1.00	.95	-0.60	1.36
PPr	-1.44	1.13	-2.28	1.00	-2.74	0.61	-1.05	1.33	-1.50	0.83	-1.42	1.01	-0.92	1.08	-1.73	1.0	-1.09	1.20
OPr	-1.37	1.17	-2.34	.88	-2.67	0.66	-0.77	1.23	-2.00	0.79	-0.70	1.10	-1.30	0.99	-1.58	2.4	-1.23	1.45
SPr	-1.48	.98	-1.56	1.11	-2.36	0.74	-1.17	0.8?	-1.10	1.00	-0.78	0.83	-1.36	0.84	-0.93	.76	-0.78	1.62
BMC	-1.15	.99	-1.68	.91	-1.85	0.49	-0.71	1.16	-1.10	0.81	-0.58	0.92	-1.47	0.54	-1.23	.86	-1.23	1.77
SWB	-1.58	1.11	-2.17	1.17	-2.87	0.31	-1.46	.98	-2.90	0.11	-0.61	1.01	-1.31	1.00	-2.73	.32	-0.68	1.27
MAc	-1.04	1.02	-1.97	.97	-2.44	0.83	-0.89	1.00	-1.20	1.16	-0.47	0.86	-0.67	1.00	-1.98	.83	-1.21	1.25
PRN	-0.12	1.22	1.09	1.46	-1.04	1.44	-0.84	1.00	N/A	N/A	-0.21	0.80	-0.05	0.77	.19	.31	-0.46	1.91

years) fell largely in the low average range, but scores were considerably lower than average on Postural Praxis, Kinesthesia, and Design Copying. The mean scores for this group generally fell somewhere between those of children with learning disabilities and children with sensory integrative dysfunction. The group with reading disorders differed more from these two groups on Standing and Walking Balance than on any of the other tests, suggesting that the children in this group had better vestibular and proprioceptive processing.

LANGUAGE DISORDER

The SIPT means and standard deviations of 28 children with language disorders (mean age = 6.6 years; SD = 1.6 years) indicated some impairment in the areas tested. More than half the scores were considerably below average, and the score pattern was a fairly good approximation of the profile for the Dyspraxia on Verbal Command cluster group. This suggests that children matching this cluster group profile may have left hemisphere rather than sensory integrative deficits.

ATTENTION DEFICIT HYPERACTIVITY DISORDER

Mulligan (1996) investigated potential differences in SIPT scores between children with (n = 309) and without (n = 309) evidence of attention deficit hyperactivity disorder. The mean scores for Postural Praxis, Praxis on Verbal Command, Oral Praxis, Kinesthesia, and Graphesthesia all were less than -1.0, suggesting that praxis may be an area of difficulty for many children with attention deficits. Multivariate Analysis of Variance (MANOVA) procedures revealed highly significant differences on four individual tests: Design Copying, Space Visualization, Postrotary Nystagmus, and Standing and Walking Balance. Furthermore, discriminant analysis revealed that, when considered together, Space Visualization, Constructional Praxis, Manual Form Perception, Design Copying, Postrotary Nystagmus, and Standing and Walking Balance significantly predicted group membership. Mulligan discussed a possible contribution of the vestibular system to attention deficits (because 46 percent also had depressed nystagmus) and the difficulty the children had settling in to testing.

The remaining four groups have identified central nervous system abnormalities or damage associated with obvious sensory, neuromotor, or cognitive impairments. If we administer the SIPT to children with known sensory, neuromotor, or cognitive impairments and can show that expected test scores are low, we can use this evidence to support the hypothesis that the SIPT are tests of neurobehavioral functioning. *However, this does not mean that the low scores on these tests obtained by these children necessarily reflect sensory integrative dysfunction.*

COGNITIVE IMPAIRMENTS

Scores for a sample of 28 children with cognitive impairments (mean age = 7.1 years; SD = 1.3) were consistently low. This may suggest that many of the SIPT have a cognitive component. However, it also is likely that the same neural conditions that lead to cognitive impairments also influence SIPT scores. The groups' highest mean score (excluding Postrotary Nystagmus) was slightly below the seventh percentile on Space Visualization (i.e., approximately -1.5). The mean scores on all six praxis tests were below the third percentile (i.e., < -2.0). Their low tactile, vestibular, and proprioceptive scores may reflect cortical abnormalities rather than poor sensory integrative functioning per se.

SPINA BIFIDA

The scores of 21 children with spina bifida (mean age = 7.5 years; SD = 0.9 years) were below average on all of the SIPT. Excluding scores on Standing and Walking Balance, for neuromotor rather than sensory integration-related reasons, the lowest scores (i.e., Oral Praxis, Bilateral Motor Coordination, Sequencing Praxis, and Graphesthesia) suggested that children with spina bifida have visual motor as well as gross motor (including bilateral) deficits. However, this does *not* suggest that children with spina bifida have sensory integrative dysfunction. Visual perception tasks with little demand for motor planning (i.e., Space Visualization, Figure-Ground Perception) were easier for these children than were visual perception tasks that require motor planning (i.e., Design Copying, Constructional Praxis).

TRAUMATIC BRAIN INJURY

Mean scores of six boys and four girls who had sustained traumatic brain injuries (mean age = 7.6 years; SD = 0.8 years) were generally low to very low. The standard deviations tended to be fairly high, suggesting rather large differences among these children. Nevertheless, some general patterns were evident. The Postrotary Nystagmus score, which was unusually prolonged, was consistent with the belief that brain injury may decrease the inhibition on the vestibulo-ocular reflex. In addition, the pattern of scores indicated that their sensory processing abilities and neuromotor status at the time of testing was poor. Their generally low scores should be interpreted with caution because the sample size was small and performance may be impaired by primary sensory and neuromotor deficits.

CEREBRAL PALSY

For the sample of 10 children with cerebral palsy (mean age = 6.1 years; SD = 1.4 years), the majority of scores were quite low. The scores on all tests with a motor component likely were depressed by the cerebral palsy. This group as a whole had trouble on tests of somatopraxis, visual perception, visual-motor coordination, and constructional abilities but, in this instance, the depressed scores may stem from the same cause as in those with cerebral palsy. Poor tactile perception also may be associated with brain damage. The possibility that some scores were lowered by the neuromotor deficits was supported by relative strengths in form and space perception tasks that do not involve motor execution and in following the verbal instructions of Praxis on Verbal Command.

COMPARISON OF THE SIPT WITH OTHER TESTS

Another approach to the evaluation of test validity is to correlate test scores on alternate measures, of which some are presumed to assess similar abilities (i.e., convergent validity) and others are presumed to assess different abilities (i.e., divergent validity). The pattern of correlations is then examined to determine whether or not the obtained results are consistent with theory.

Ayres administered both the SIPT and the Kaufman Assessment Battery for Children (K-ABC) (Kaufman & Kaufman, 1983) to a combined sample of typically developing children, children with learning disabilities, and children with sensory integrative disorders. The K-ABC is a standardized intelligence test that also is used to screen for level of achievement. Correlations of the subscales on the SIPT and the K-ABC are shown in Table B–6. As expected, SIPT measures of sequential processing (e.g., Sequencing Praxis and Bilateral Motor Coordination) have higher correlations with the K-ABC Sequential Processing scale than the Simultaneous Processing scale in the control group. Furthermore,

the SIPT tests that should require little or no sequential processing (i.e., Finger Identification, Localization of Tactile Stimuli, and Postrotary Nystagmus) generally show the lowest correlations with the K-ABC Sequential Processing scale.

In general, whereas the more basic tactile tests in the SIPT show the lowest correlations with the K-ABC scales, the complex praxis tests generally have the highest correlations. The processes common to both the K-ABC and the SIPT praxis tests are probably of a complex cognitive nature. As shown in Table B–6, the overall pattern of correlations was similar for children with and without dysfunction, although the magnitude of the correlations differed somewhat across the two subsamples.

Cermak and Murray (1991) investigated construct validity of Design Copying and Constructional Praxis using two procedures. They examined differences in scores between children with and without learning disabilities and correlated DC and CPr with four other constructional measures (Primary Visual Motor Test, Developmental Test of Visual-Motor Integration [VMI], Block Design subtest of the Wechsler Intelligence Scale for Children-Revised, and the Rey-Osterreith Complex Figure Test). Cermak and Murray found statistically significant differences between the groups and strong correlations among most of the measures with children who had learning disabilities. However, only two correlations were statistically significant for the control group. They interpreted their results as lending support to the construct validity of DC and CPr, especially in children with learning disabilities.

Because many of the tests in the SIPT are revisions of tests from the SCSIT (Ayres, 1972a; 1980), correlations between these tests and other relevant measures may provide some additional evidence for the validity of the SIPT. For example, parts of Luria-Nebraska Neuropsychological Battery, Children's Revision (Golden et al., 1980) assess parameters that are similar to those assessed by the SCSIT. Both tests were designed to evaluate neurological dysfunction. Kinnealey (1989) administered the tactile-kinesthetic sections of both tests to thirty 8-year-old typically developing children and thirty 8-year-old children with learning disabilities and obtained a correlation of 0.73 ($p < 0.001$) between the total scores. The total tactile score for the SCSIT was a sum of the z scores for each of the somatosensory tests; the t score for the tactile section of the Luria was used as the total score for that

SIPT Test	Arithmetic	Riddles	Decoding	Understanding	Sequential Processing	Simultaneous Processing	Mental Proc. Composite	Achievement
Results for a Group of Normal (n = 47) Children								
Space Visualization [SV]	.24*	.41*	.21	-.20	.17	.20	.23	-.02
Figure-Ground Perception [FG]	.12	.46*	.26*	.19	.28*	.15	.25*	.05
Manual Form Perception [MFP]	.04	-.01	-.07	-.23	.30*	.15	.26*	-.13
Kinesthesia [KIN]	.20	.28*	.36*	-.27*	.22	.03	.19	.27*
Finger Identification [FI]	.09	.07	-.09	-.35*	-.16	.19	.01	-.06
Graphesthesia [GRA]	.01	-.09	-.02	.00	-.06	-.14	-.15	.16
Loc. of Tactile Stimuli [LTS]	.11	.03	.10	.04	.03	.08	.15	.11
Praxis on Verbal Command [PrVC]	.14	.22	.10	-.03	.21	.18	.28*	.24*
Design Copying [DC]	.21	.29*	.43*	.24*	.20	.15	.25*	.17
Constructional Praxis [CPr]	.11	.14	.15	-.06	.22	.29*	.36*	-.10
Postural Praxis [PPr]	.16	.15	.14	.12	.28*	.02	.19	.14
Oral Praxis [OPr]	.00	.33*	-.04	.14	.06	.13	.19	-.05
Sequencing Praxis [SPr]	.23	.16	.45*	.10	.46*	.38*	.46*	.17
Bilateral Motor Coord. [BMC]	.34*	.20	.45*	.53*	.31*	.20	.32*	.06
Standing/Walking Balance [SWB]	.21	.16	.18	.23	.15	-.01	.07	.38*
Motor Accuracy [MAc]	-.16	.23	.21	.28*	.05	-.03	.12	.02
Postrotary Nystagmus [PRN]	-.08	-.21	-.02	.41*	.04	-.26*	-.19	.16
Results for a Group of Learning-Disabled (n = 35) Children								
Space Visualization [SV]	.13	-.21	.15	-.06	.27	.28*	.33*	.02
Figure-Ground Perception [FG]	.41*	.40*	.33*	.12	.30*	.45*	.48*	.47*
Manual Form Perception [MFP]	.30*	.22	-.10	-.23	.15	.57*	.51*	.05
Kinesthesia [KIN]	.45*	.07	.13	.02	.36*	.41*	.47*	.22
Finger Identification [FI]	-.30*	-.41*	-.12	.03	-.17	-.12	-.21	-.32
Graphesthesia [GRA]	.21	-.21	.18	.00	.32*	.27	.36*	.11
Loc. of Tactile Stimuli [LTS]	.07	.17	.02	.27	.09	.09	.03	.06
Praxis on Verbal Command [PrVC]	.41*	.55*	.11	.26	.44*	.31*	.47*	.41*
Design Copying [DC]	.51*	.14	.27	.22	.17	.49*	.45*	.37*
Constructional Praxis [CPr]	.59*	.10	.11	.03	.26	.44*	.44*	.24
Postural Praxis [PPr]	.41*	.07	.08	.00	.25	.46*	.47*	.13
Oral Praxis [OPr]	.40*	.14	.23	.18	.45*	.55*	.63*	.29*
Sequencing Praxis [SPr]	.49*	-.08	.47*	.48*	.47*	.15	.37*	.40*
Bilateral Motor Coord. [BMC]	.24	-.00	.38*	.32*	.29*	.14	.24	.32*
Standing/Walking Balance [SWB]	.50*	.34*	-.03	.09	.36*	.34*	.44*	.21
Motor Accuracy [MAc]	.28*	.07	.22	.35*	-.01	.20	.14	.24
Postrotary Nystagmus [PRN]	.04	-.14	-.15	-.16	-.12	.19	.08	-.13

continued on following page

467

■ TABLE B-6 PEARSON PRODUCT-MOMENT CORRELATIONS BETWEEN SIPT SCORES AND STANDARDIZED K-ABC SCORES (CONTINUED)

SIPT Test	Arithmetic	Riddles	Decoding	Understanding	K-ABC Scale Sequential Processing	Simultaneous Processing	Mental Proc. Composite	Achievement
Results for a Combined Group of Normal (n = 47), Learning-Disabled (n = 35), and SI Disordered (n = 9) Children								
Space Visualization [SV]	.47*	.41*	.43*	.12	.43*	.43*	.50*	.19*
Figure-Ground Perception [FG]	.54*	.61*	.50*	.30*	.55*	.50*	.53*	.26*
Manual Form Perception [MFP]	.56*	.49*	.37*	.15	.54*	.61*	.59*	.15
Kinesthesia [KIN]	.67*	.54*	.54*	.36*	.59*	.55*	.58*	.36*
Finger Identification [FI]	.33*	.27*	.28*	.02	.22*	.32*	.24*	.12
Graphesthesia [GRA]	.55*	.36*	.50*	.28*	.51*	.44*	.43*	.31*
Loc. of Tactile Stimuli [LTS]	.39*	.27*	.32*	.10	.30*	.29*	.27*	.21*
Praxis on Verbal Command [PrVC]	.68*	.68*	.53*	.41*	.63*	.60*	.65*	.24*
Design Copying [DC]	.73*	.60*	.64*	.46*	.57*	.66*	.66*	.34*
Constructional Praxis [CPr]	.70*	.56*	.53*	.30*	.57*	.66*	.68*	.24*
Postural Praxis [PPr]	.57*	.46*	.44*	.30*	.55*	.50*	.52*	.28*
Oral Praxis [OPr]	.60*	.57*	.51*	.39*	.59*	.60*	.61*	.24*
Sequencing Praxis [SPr]	.66*	.46*	.65*	.45*	.67*	.59*	.63*	.33*
Bilateral Motor Coord. [BMC]	.56*	.45*	.59*	.54*	.56*	.48*	.51*	.26*
Standing/Walking Balance [SWB]	.68*	.59*	.48*	.42*	.58*	.53*	.54*	.44*
Motor Accuracy [MAc]	.62*	.59*	.61*	.49*	.52*	.58*	.51*	.29*
Postrotary Nystagmus [PRN]	.04	.05	.08	.16	.12	.03*	.08	.14

*p<

test. In a comparable study of the motor tests of the Luria and the SCSIT, Su and Yerxa (1984) obtained a correlation of 0.83 ($p < 0.001$) between total scores on the two tests with thirty 8-year-old children who had been referred for evaluation of or intervention for sensory integrative dysfunction.

Although the Bruininks-Oseretsky Test of Motor Proficiency (Bruininks, 1978) is a test of motor skill rather than sensory integration, it does contain a number of tests that require practic ability. Ziviani et al. (1982) administered both the SCSIT and the Bruininks-Oseretsky to 32 boys. They obtained significant correlations between the Bruininks-Oseretsky Fine Motor Scale and 13 of the SCSIT. Fewer of the SCSIT correlated significantly with the Bruininks-Oseretsky Gross Motor Scale. However, the overall pattern of correlations suggested that the two tests share a common practic-postural domain.

Scores on the Bender-Gestalt Test (Bender, 1938) predicted a SCSIT space perception composite score ($r = 0.65$, $p < 0.01$) in a group of children (mean age = 84.8 months; SD = 12.8 months) with suspected sensory integrative dysfunction (Kimball, 1977). The Bender-Gestalt did not correlate significantly with tests of posture and bilateral integration.

Evidence Supporting Individual Test Validity

Although SIPT profiles are usually interpreted as a whole or as an overall pattern that can be related to SIPT cluster groups, inferences sometimes must be drawn from the relationships among a smaller number of scores. To explore the meaning of these relationships, Ayres generated a number of correlation and factor analyses among the tests in the SIPT. These analyses can be found in the manual for the SIPT (Ayres, 1989b).

Taking a different approach to construct validity, Lai et al. (1996) used Rasch analysis to determine that each of the five SIPT praxis tests measures a single unidimensional construct. However, when they combined all the items from the five tests into one 117-item test, the items continued to identify a single practic function. Based on the latter results, they concluded that a unitary practic component underlies both BIS and that a shorter test could potentially provide all the essential diagnostic information attained through the SIPT.

RELIABILITY

Interrater reliability indicates the extent to which children's test scores agree when their performance is evaluated by different examiners. Most tests have some margin for human error. Examiners may differ in the accuracy and precision with which they measure the time it takes children to perform a task or the leniency with which they evaluate accuracy. A high interrater reliability coefficient is an indication that children's scores will be very similar when their performance is evaluated by different examiners. Test–retest reliability indicates the extent to which test scores for individuals are consistent across time. Insofar as the constructs assessed by the SIPT are assumed to be fairly stable over time, a good measure of these constructs should have fairly high test–retest reliability. The reliability statistics for the SIPT are summarized in Table B–7.

To evaluate interrater reliability, the SIPT were administered to 63 children from 5 years, 0 months to 8 years, 11 months (50 boys, 13 girls; mean age = 7.26 years; SD= 1.04 years). This sample included 19 children with diagnosed reading disorders, 41 children with other learning disabilities, and three children with spina bifida. Eight examiners participated in the interrater reliability study, and each child's performance on the SIPT was evaluated by two different examiners. All of the reliability coefficients were very high, ranging from 0.94 to 0.99.

These reliability coefficients, summarized in Table B–7, indicate that different examiners should be able to obtain similar results from the SIPT. However, all of the examiners in the interrater reliability study had completed a comprehensive test administration course. Interrater reliabilities probably would be considerably lower among untrained examiners.

Test–retest reliability of the SIPT was evaluated in a sample of 41 children with dysfunction (24 boys, 17 girls; mean age = 6.5 years; SD = 1.3 years) and 10 typically developing children (4 boys, 6 girls; mean age = 6.8 years; SD = 1.4 years). Children were tested twice at intervals of 1 to 2 weeks. To ensure that reliability coefficients would not be inflated by age differences, all coefficients were computed using standard scores. Test–retest reliability coefficients are shown in Table B–7.

As a group, the praxis tests had the highest test–retest reliability, but reliability for all but four of the other tests was acceptable; these included

TABLE B-7 SIPT Reliability Statistics

Interrater Reliability

	r	(n)
SPACE VISUALIZATION [SV] Time-Adjusted Accuracy	.99	(63)
FIGURE-GROUND PERCEPTION [FG] Accuracy	.99	(58)
MANUAL FORM PERCEPTION [MFP] Total Accuracy	.99	(47)
KINESTHESIA [KIN] Total Accuracy	.99	(60)
FINGER IDENTIFICATION [FI] Total Accuracy	.95	(62)
GRAPHESTHESIA [GRA] Total Accuracy	.96	(54)
LOCALIZATION OF TACTILE STIMULI [LTS] Total Accuracy	.99	(59)
PRAXIS ON VERBAL COMMAND [PrVC] Total Accuracy	.98	(62)
DESIGN COPYING [DC] Total Accuracy	.97	(58)
CONSTRUCTIONAL PRAXIS [CPr] Total Accuracy	.98	(63)
POSTURAL PRAXIS [PPr] Total Accuracy	.96	(62)
ORAL PRAXIS [OPr] Total Accuracy	.94	(63)
SEQUENCING PRAXIS [SPr] Total Accuracy	.99	(51)
BILATERAL MOTOR COORDINATION [BMC] Total Accuracy	.96	(48)
STANDING AND WALKING BALANCE [SWB] Total Score	.99	(60)
MOTOR ACCURACY [MAc] Weighted Total Accuracy	.99	(62)
POSTROTARY NYSTAGMUS [PRN] Average Nystagmus	.98	(56)

Test-Retest Reliability

	Combined Sample Test Mean	Test SD	Retest Mean	Retest SD	r	(n)	Learning-Disabled Sample Test Mean	Test SD	Retest Mean	Retest SD	r	(n)
SPACE VISUALIZATION [SV] Time-Adjusted Accuracy	-.42	0.93	-.25	1.17	.69	(49)	-.58	.87	-.48	1.11	.62	(39)
FIGURE-GROUND PERCEPTION [FG] Total Accuracy	-.67	1.24	-.28	1.02	+.56	(47)	-.90	1.23	-.41	1.02	+.54	(38)
MANUAL FORM PERCEPTION [MFP] Total Accuracy	-.99	1.10	-.34	1.24	+.70	(31)	-1.07	1.14	-.43	1.25	+.69	(26)
KINESTHESIA [KIN] Total Accuracy	-.94	1.31	-.55	1.19	+.50	(46)	-1.29	1.19	-.76	1.15	+.33	(37)
FINGER IDENTIFICATION [FI] Total Accuracy	-.52	1.33	-.62	1.28	.74	(46)	-.67	1.33	-.76	1.27	.75	(38)
GRAPHESTHESIA [GRA] Total Accuracy	-.28	1.37	-.21	1.37	.74	(42)	-.60	1.37	-.55	1.31	.72	(32)
LOCALIZATION OF TACTILE STIMULI [LTS] Total Accuracy	-.42	1.08	-.29	1.24	.53	(47)	-.65	1.02	-.54	1.16	.54	(37)
PRAXIS ON VERBAL COMMAND [PrVC] Total Accuracy	-.87	1.34	-.61	1.43	+.86	(48)	-1.17	1.31	-.91	1.44	+.88	(38)
DESIGN COPYING [DC] Total Accuracy	-.47	1.45	-.08	1.60	+.93	(36)	-.68	1.50	-.36	1.64	+.94	(27)
CONSTRUCTIONAL PRAXIS [CPr] Total Accuracy	-.39	1.12	-.42	1.10	.70	(51)	-.54	1.17	-.56	1.09	.67	(41)
POSTURAL PRAXIS [PPr] Total Accuracy	-.52	1.30	-.12	1.46	+.86	(49)	-.65	1.37	-.30	1.50	+.88	(39)
ORAL PRAXIS [OPr] Total Accuracy	-.47	1.53	-.25	1.43	+.90	(49)	-.76	1.50	-.52	1.41	+.89	(39)
SEQUENCING PRAXIS [SPr] Total Accuracy	-.77	1.16	-.55	1.22	+.84	(47)	-1.03	1.10	-.74	1.23	+.84	(38)
BILATERAL MOTOR COORDINATION [BMC] Total Accuracy	-.74	1.07	-.52	1.14	+.82	(45)	-1.08	.82	-.76	1.08	+.77	(36)
STANDING AND WALKING BALANCE [SWB] Total Score	-1.50	1.42	-1.68	1.33	.86	(48)	-1.88	1.32	-2.06	1.19	.80	(38)
MOTOR ACCURACY [MAc] Weighted Total Accuracy	-.44	1.20	-.43	1.20	.84	(45)	-.59	1.27	-.53	1.29	.84	(35)
POSTROTARY NYSTAGMUS [PRN] Average Nystagmus	.03	.77	.11	.67	.48	(39)	-.03	.87	.12	.72	.47	(29)

+Indicates significant practice effects on retest ($p < .05$).

Postrotary Nystagmus, two of the somatosensory tests (Kinesthesia and Localization of Tactile Stimuli), and one form and space test (Figure-Ground Perception). Test–retest reliabilities for Kinesthesia and Localization of Tactile Stimuli are quite similar to those reported for the SCSIT version of these tests (Ayres, 1980). The reliability of the SIPT Figure-Ground Perception test is slightly higher than the reported reliability of the SCSIT version.

The test–retest reliability coefficient of 0.49 for Postrotary Nystagmus is considerably lower than coefficients previously obtained with typically developing children for the SCPNT. Ayres (1975) reported a 2-week reliability coefficient of 0.83 with 42 typically developing children. Kimball (1981) obtained a coefficient of 0.80 with 63 typically developing children (ages 5 through 9 years) after more than 2 years. Punwar (1982) reported a 0.82 coefficient after 2 weeks with a sample of 56 typically developing children, age 3 through 10 years. And Dutton (1985) reviewed the published SCPNT reliability data and found that reliability coefficients ranged from 0.79 to 0.81 for typically developing 4- to 11-year-old children. Although these studies suggest that the Postrotary Nystagmus Test may be more reliable than is suggested by the 0.49 reliability coefficient, they had considerably smaller sample sizes than the SIPT standardization sample, so their results must be viewed with caution.

Interpretation of SIPT Results

The SIPT were designed for children with mild to moderate difficulties with learning and behavior. SIPT results should never be used as the sole source of information when making diagnostic judgments. In addition, practitioners should have knowledge of:

- Presenting problems, including, when possible, formal testing related to occupational and role performance
- Relevant history
- The child's intellectual capacity, language development, and academic achievement
- Any pertinent psychological and medical diagnoses
- Clinical observations of posture, defensiveness to sensation, and gravitational security

The SIPT scores should be interpreted in light of all of these additional sources of information.

Interpretation of Full and Partial Profiles

The computer-generated SIPT Test Report provides comprehensive information about performance on each test. In addition, the Test Report compares a child's overall pattern of scores with patterns that characterize the six different diagnostic clusters described below.

DEFICIT IN BILATERAL INTEGRATION AND SEQUENCING

The scores of this cluster group present a relatively clear picture of BIS deficit. Although their mean scores were all within average range, Ayres found that this group showed the prototypic pattern of deficit in the BIS function. They tended to score in the low average range on Oral Praxis, Standing and Walking Balance, Sequencing Praxis, Bilateral Motor Coordination, Graphesthesia, and Postural Praxis. In contrast, they tended to score in the average to high average range on Figure-Ground Perception, Finger Identification, Praxis on Verbal Command, Design Copying, and Constructional Praxis. Contrast between scores on the BIS tests, when they fall below the normal range, and the rest of the tests, is an important criterion in diagnosis.

In general, a diagnosis of BIS deficit should be made only when there are no other conditions that would account for the child's performance (e.g., low tactile scores associated with somatodyspraxia or low Praxis on Verbal Command scores and prolonged nystagmus). BIS deficits are generally associated with poor vestibular and proprioceptive processing characterized by postural dysfunction. However, postural dysfunction cannot be diagnosed reliably with the SIPT alone; clinical observations of neuromotor performance are required.

VISUO- AND SOMATODYSPRAXIA

Members of this group scored lowest on Design Copying, Standing and Walking Balance, Sequencing Praxis, Kinesthesia, Bilateral Motor Coordination, Postural Praxis, Motor Accuracy, Graphesthesia, and Finger Identification, in that order. They generally scored highest on Praxis on Verbal Command. This group has the lowest Postrotary Nystagmus score of the six groups. Whereas both somatopraxis scores and scores reflecting visual perception, visuomotor coordination, and construction were low for children in this cluster, children likened to this cluster on the

SIPT Test Report may demonstrate low scores only in somatopraxis or only in the form and space, visuomotor and constructional grouping (sometimes called *visuopraxis*).

Dyspraxia on Verbal Command

Ayres found this type of dysfunction was the most discrete and least variable in its manifestation. The major identifying feature was the contrast between a very low Praxis on Verbal Command score and a relatively high Postrotary Nystagmus score. This group also had low scores on Design Copying, Oral Praxis, Sequencing Praxis, Bilateral Motor Coordination, and Standing and Walking Balance. Equally important in characterizing the dyspraxia on verbal command profile were average to low-average scores on the rest of the tests, which include the somatosensory, the visual form and space, and the visuopraxis tests. Dyspraxia on verbal command is believed to be associated with cortical, rather than sensory integrative, dysfunction.

Generalized Sensory Integrative Dysfunction

This group tended to score far below average on all of the SIPT. Generalized dysfunction is characterized by consistently low performance rather than by any discrete pattern. Careful analysis of scores of children in this group suggested that they were better identified as having severe deficits in somatopraxis; BIS; or form and space, visuomotor, and construction.

Low Average Sensory Integration and Praxis

This group was also characterized by its general level of performance rather than by any distinguishing pattern of scores. Children in this group tend to fall in the low average range on most tests.

High Average Sensory Integration and Praxis

Ayres found that members of this group were also distinguished by their general performance and not by any pattern of scores. They tended to fall in the average to high average range on most of tests.

Partial Patterns

Study of a large number of factor analyses (Ayres, unpublished data) revealed natural linkages among tests. These partial patterns also appeared on some of the children's profiles. In one analysis,

Postrotary Nystagmus shared variance with Design Copying, Constructional Praxis, Space Visualization, Finger Identification, Motor Accuracy, Manual Form Perception, and Figure-Ground Perception. The pattern suggested inefficient vestibular processing and may be associated with poor form and space perception.

Another analysis showed strong relationships among Space Visualization, Figure-Ground Perception, Design Copying, Motor Accuracy, and Constructional Praxis. Two or more of these tests could identify a visual form and space perception deficit, with or without dyspraxia. The term *construction deficit* could be used when Design Copying and Constructional Praxis scores are low. The term *visual motor coordination deficit* could be used when Motor Accuracy and Design Copying scores are low, and *poor visual form and space perception* could be used when Space Visualization and Figure-Ground scores are low.

Postural Praxis and Oral Praxis appeared essentially as a doublet in several analyses, indicating a likely linkage. In a number of analyses, the somatosensory tests correlated with each other and independent of praxis, suggesting a sensory integrative deficit without dyspraxia. In other analyses, Postrotary Nystagmus correlated with the somatosensory tests, suggesting a vestibular and somatosensory processing deficit.

Readers interested in additional information concerning the interpretation of individual tests are referred to the SIPT manual (Ayres, 1989b). Interpretation is always based on clusters of test scores that, when considered together, can be interpreted in a meaningful manner. Some of the SIPT tests have limited reliability when considered in isolation; therefore, when several scores assessing the same construct are low, diagnosis can be made with more confidence.

Finally, diagnostic judgments never should be made without evidence regarding the child's current performance at home and in school; relevant history; other available test scores; and clinical observations of postural responses, sensory defensiveness, and gravitational security. The art of interpretation of the SIPT is discussed in Chapter 8.

Validity of Individual SIPT

Sensory Processing Tests

Kinesthesia correlated most consistently with Sequencing Praxis, Standing and Walking Balance,

Constructional Praxis, Design Copying, Motor Accuracy, and Oral Praxis, suggesting a possible proprioceptive link among these tasks. In factor analyses, Kinesthesia loaded highest on (and helped to identify) somatosensory processing factors.

Finger Identification correlated most strongly with Graphesthesia and with visuo- and somatopraxis tests and had the lowest correlations with Praxis on Verbal Command. In factor analyses, Finger Identification loaded most strongly on somatopraxis and somatosensory processing factors; visuopraxis factors; and factors reflecting positive correlations between Postrotary Nystagmus and somatosensory processing.

Graphesthesia correlated most strongly with tests that identified the BIS function, but it also correlated substantially with Postural Praxis and with the visual construction tests. In factor analyses, Graphesthesia loaded consistently and strongly on BIS factors and on somatopraxis factors. These loadings possibly point to the sensitivity of Graphesthesia to deficits in complex tactile processing and in translating complex stimuli into planned bilateral action sequences.

Localization of Tactile Stimuli correlated most strongly with Kinesthesia, Bilateral Motor Coordination, and Oral Praxis. In factor analyses, Localization of Tactile Stimuli loaded strongly on somatosensory processing factors. A considerable link between Localization of Tactile Stimuli and Oral Praxis was also demonstrated in one of the three factor analyses. The data reaffirmed the close relationship between tactile processing and certain practic abilities.

Correlations between Postrotary Nystagmus and other SIPT were fairly weak. In a sample of 125 children with sensory integrative deficits, Postrotary Nystagmus had a significant negative correlation with Praxis on Verbal Command. In a combined sample of 117 children with learning disabilities or sensory integrative deficits and 176 matched children from the normative sample, Postrotary Nystagmus had significant, but low, positive correlations with Finger Identification, Motor Accuracy, and Graphesthesia.

Standing and Walking Balance correlated significantly with many of the other tests in the SIPT, suggesting that some process needed for body balance may also contribute to performance on the other tests in the SIPT. The strongest associations were with the BIS function, proprioception, and visual construction. The most likely basis for these relationships was the degree of integration of sensation from the vestibular and proprioceptive systems. Analyses suggested that Standing and Walking Balance was more apt to be low when duration of postrotary nystagmus was prolonged than when it was depressed but that relationship was not invariable. In fact, Standing and Walking Balance performance, as well as the other tests of BIS, were apt to be depressed in each of the domains of sensory integrative dysfunction, suggesting a vulnerability of body balance to dysfunction. However, when a BIS deficit is associated with prolonged postrotary nystagmus, the problem is thought to be due to cortical dysfunction.

Form and Space and Visual Motor Tests

The adjusted Space Visualization score correlated best with Design Copying, Constructional Praxis, and Motor Accuracy. Space Visualization loaded well on a factor Ayres labeled visuopraxis, suggesting a strong visual space perception component.

The Figure-Ground Perception accuracy score loaded consistently on visuo-praxis factors. Of the 17 tests in the SIPT, Figure-Ground Perception is the least related to somatosensory processing. Figure-Ground performance was sometimes associated with the same conditions that contributed to prolonged postrotary nystagmus.

Manual Form Perception loaded primarily with the form and space, visuomotor, and constructional tests, indicating a haptic form perception component with a strong visualization component. The test also showed some linkage to somatosensory processing and BIS.

Motor Accuracy (preferred and nonpreferred hand scores) correlated most strongly with Design Copying, Sequencing Praxis, Space Visualization, Oral Praxis, Bilateral Motor Coordination, Constructional Praxis, and Standing and Walking Balance, suggesting that visuomotor coordination may be linked with form and space perception, BIS, and visual construction. In the normative sample, both preferred and nonpreferred hand scores correlated significantly with almost all other SIPT scores and subscores, indicating that the test taps a fundamental sensorimotor process related to most of the SIPT. This may indicate that poor visuomotor coordination is an endproduct of sensory integrative dysfunction. In factor analyses, Motor Accuracy loaded most strongly and consistently on visuopraxis factors.

Praxis Tests

The Praxis on Verbal Command accuracy score was the major identifying test of the Praxis on Verbal Command factor and the dyspraxia on verbal command cluster group. In both instances, low Praxis on Verbal Command scores were associated with abnormally increased Postrotary Nystagmus scores. Praxis on Verbal Command also correlated with Design Copying, Constructional Praxis, and Postural Praxis. In addition, there were substantial correlations with Bilateral Motor Coordination, Sequencing Praxis, Standing and Walking Balance, and Oral Praxis. These latter correlations do not necessarily stem from the same condition that is central to the BIS function—that is, when Postrotary Nystagmus scores are high and Praxis on Verbal Command scores are low, low scores on the tests of BIS are presumed to be caused by cortical dysfunction.

Of all the SIPT, Design Copying appears to be one of the best indicators of construction ability, especially in two-dimensional space; it correlated most highly with Constructional Praxis, Space Visualization, Motor Accuracy, and Sequencing Praxis. In the factor analyses, Design Copying accuracy held one of the highest loadings on the factor it helped to identify as visuopraxis (form and space, visuomotor, and construction) and on the function it helped to identify as visuo- and somatopraxis. All the Design Copying atypical approach parameters consistently loaded on praxis factors.

Constructional Praxis correlated positively and significantly with all other tests in the SIPT except Postrotary Nystagmus. Highest correlations were with Design Copying, Postural Praxis, and Sequencing Praxis. Constructional Praxis loaded most strongly on the visuopraxis (form and space, visuomotor, and construction) and somatopraxis factors. Overall, the data suggested that three-dimensional construction involves more than visual space perception and that Constructional Praxis assesses a basic visual and somatopraxis skill.

Postural Praxis correlated positively with most of the other SIPT, indicating high representation of praxis element in these tests. Correlations with Oral Praxis, Sequencing Praxis, Graphesthesia, Design Copying, and Constructional Praxis were particularly strong. Postural Praxis loaded substantially on somatopraxis factors.

Oral Praxis correlations and factor loadings demonstrated three major links with Oral Praxis performance: somatosensory, BIS, and motor planning ability. Oral Praxis loaded strongly on somatopraxis factors and on BIS factors.

Sequencing Praxis was most highly correlated with tests that defined the BIS function, with the form and space, visuomotor, and constructional tests, and with the somatopraxis tests. The correlations suggested that Sequencing Praxis evaluates a central practic ability that subserves most aspects of praxis under evaluation by the SIPT. Sequencing praxis consistently carried high loadings on the BIS factor in numerous factor analyses.

Bilateral Integration and Sequencing Tests

Bilateral Motor Coordination correlated most strongly and positively with other tests that identify the BIS function, especially with Sequencing Praxis, Oral Praxis, and Graphesthesia. Bilateral Motor Coordination also correlated with the visual motor coordination tests (i.e., Motor Accuracy and Design Copying). Finally, Bilateral Motor Coordination had a positive association with Praxis on Verbal Command.

The Space Visualization Contralateral Use score effectively discriminated between 49 children with dysfunction and 49 typically developing children ($p < 0.05$). In a group of 1750 normal children, Space Visualization Contralateral Use scores correlated significantly with the majority of the other SIPT scores. The highest correlations were with the arm and feet items of Bilateral Motor Coordination. The positive association between Space Visualization Contralateral Use and Bilateral Motor Coordination also emerged in factor analyses, emphasizing the bilateral integration aspect of Space Visualization Contralateral Use. The data also linked low Space Visualization Contralateral Use scores to right–left and reversal drawing approaches in Design Copying and poor somatosensory processing. These correlations supported the interpretation of Space Visualization Contralateral Use as a reflection of integration of the two body sides.

Children with dysfunction tend to have lower Preferred Hand Use scores, indicating that they exhibit less strong hand preference than typically developing children. In children both with and without dysfunction, boys exhibited weaker hand preference than girls. Correlations between Preferred Hand Use and Space Visualization Contralateral Use ranged from 0.47 to 0.52 ($p < 0.001$).

Additional data supported associations between hand preference and integration of the two body sides, right–left reversals, visual motor coordination, and duration of postrotary nystagmus. These associations were not necessarily strong and could easily be overshadowed by other linkages in children with dysfunction.

The high correlation of the Bilateral Motor Coordination arm items with the Space Visualization Contralateral Use score emphasized their common reflection of integration of two body sides. In factor analyses, Bilateral Motor Coordination loaded strongly on the somatopraxis factors and helped identify the BIS factors. In some factor analyses, Bilateral Motor Control and Postural Praxis loaded strongly on the same factor, suggesting that Bilateral Motor Coordination may depend, in part, on a more general practic ability.

References

Ayres, A. J. (1965). Patterns of perceptual-motor dysfunction in children: A factor analytic study. *Perceptual and Motor Skills, 20,* 335–368.

Ayres, A. J. (1966). Interrelation among perceptual-motor functions in children. *American Journal of Occupational Therapy, 20,* 68–71.

Ayres, A. J. (1969). Relation between Gesell developmental quotients and later perceptual-motor performance. *American Journal of Occupational Therapy, 23,* 11–17.

Ayres, A. J. (1972a). *Southern California Sensory Integration Tests manual.* Los Angeles: Western Psychological Services.

Ayres, A. J. (1972b). Types of sensory integrative dysfunction among disabled learners. *American Journal of Occupational Therapy, 26,* 13–18.

Ayres, A. J. (1975). *Southern California Postrotary Nystagmus Test manual.* Los Angeles: Western Psychological Services.

Ayres, A. J. (1977). Cluster analyses of measures of sensory integration. *American Journal of Occupational Therapy, 31,* 362–366.

Ayres, A. J. (1980). *Southern California Sensory Integration Tests manual: Revised 1980.* Los Angeles: Western Psychological Services.

Ayres, A. J. (1989a). Forward. In L. J. Miller (Ed.), Developing norm-referenced standardized tests [special issue]. *Physical and Occupational Therapy in Pediatrics, 9,* 1.

Ayres, A. J. (1989b). *Sensory Integration and Praxis Tests manual.* Los Angeles: Western Psychological Services.

Ayres, A. J., Mailloux, Z., & Wendler, C. L. (1987).

Developmental dyspraxia: Is it a unitary function? *Occupational Therapy Journal of Research, 7,* 93–110.

Bender, L. (1938). *A visuo-motor gestalt test and its clinical use (Research Monograph No. 3).* New York: American Orthopsychiatric Association.

Bruininks, R. H. (1978). *Bruininks-Oseretsky Test of Motor Proficiency manual.* Circle Pines, MN: American Guidance Services.

Cermak, S. A., & Murray, E. A. (1991). The validity of the constructional subtests of the Sensory Integration and Praxis Tests. *American Journal of Occupational Therapy, 45,* 539–543.

Cummins, R. (1991). Sensory integration and learning disabilities: Ayres' factor analyses.

Dutton, R. E. (1985). Reliability and clinical significance of the Southern California Postrotary Nystagmus Test. *Physical & Occupational Therapy in Pediatrics, 5,* 57–67.

Fisher, A. G, & Bundy, A. C. (1991). Sensory integration. In H. Forssberg & H. Hirschfeld (Eds.), *Movement disorders in children* (pp. 16–20). New York: Karger.

Golden, C. J., Hemmeke, T. A., & Purisch, A. D. (1980). *The Luria-Nebraska Neuropsychological Battery.* Los Angeles: Western Psychological Services.

Kaufman, A. S., & Kaufman, N. L. (1983). *Kaufman Assessment Battery for Children.* Circle Pines, MN: American Guidance Service.

Kimball, J. G. (1977). The Southern California Sensory Integration Tests (Ayres) and the Bender Gestalt: A creative study. *American Journal of Occupational Therapy, 31,* 294–299.

Kimball, J. C. (1981). Normative comparison of the Southern California Postrotary Nystagmus Test: Los Angeles vs. Syracuse data. *American Journal of Occupational Therapy, 35,* 21–25.

Kimball, J. G. (1990). Using the Sensory Integration and Praxis Tests to measure change: A pilot study. *American Journal of Occupational Therapy, 44,* 603–608.

Kinnealey, M. (1989). Tactile functions in learning-disabled and normal children: Reliability and validity considerations. *Occupational Therapy Journal of Research, 9,* 3–15.

Lai, J. S., Fisher, A. G., Magalhaes, L. C., & Bundy, A. C. (1996). Construct validity of the Sensory Integration and Praxis Tests. *Occupational Therapy Journal of Research, 16,* 75–97.

Lorr, M. (1983). *Cluster analysis for social scientists.* San Francisco: Jossey-Bass.

Mulligan, S. (1996). An analysis of score patterns of children with attention disorders on the Sensory Integration and Praxis tests. *American Journal of Occupational Therapy, 50,* 647–654.

Mulligan, S. (1998). Patterns of SI dysfunction: A confirmatory factor analysis. *American Journal of Occupational Therapy, 52,* 819–828.

Punwar, A. (1982). Expanded normative data: Southern California Postrotary Nystagmus Test. *American Journal of Occupational Therapy, 36,* 183–187.

Silberzahn, M. (1975). Sensory integrative function in

a child guidance population. *American Journal of Occupational Therapy, 29,* 28–34.

Su, R. V., & Yerxa, E. J. (1984). Comparison of the motor tests of SCSIT and the L-NNBC. *Occupational Therapy Journal of Research, 4,* 96–107.

Ziviani, J., Poulsen, A., & O'Brien, A. (1982). Correlation of the Bruininks-Oseretsky Test of Motor Proficiency with the Southern California Sensory Integration Tests. *American Journal of Occupational Therapy, 36,* 519–523.

■■ Glossary

Adaptive Interaction: Interactions between an individual and the environment in which the individual meets the demands of the task. Ayres emphasized the need for a client's actions to be just a little better than they had ever been before. Adaptive interactions give rise to production and outcome feedback.

Angular Movement: Circular movement or movement that, if continued, would culminate in a circle.

Aversive Response (Intolerance) to Movement: A type of sensory modulation dysfunction characterized by autonomic nervous system reactions to movements that most individuals would consider non-noxious; thought to be the result of poor processing of vestibular information.

Bilateral Integration and Sequencing Deficits: A relatively high-level sensory-integrative-based dyspraxia characterized by poor bilateral coordination and difficulty with projected action sequences; thought to have its basis in poor processing of vestibular and proprioception information

Body Schema: An unconscious mechanism underlying spatial motor coordination that provides the central nervous system with information about the relationship of the body and its parts to environmental space.

Central Auditory Nervous System: That portion of the auditory mechanism that receives, transmits, and analyzes sound stimuli detected by the peripheral hearing mechanism. It includes a specialized series of nerve fibers and neural pathways in the brainstem and the brain.

Central Auditory Processing: The process whereby auditory signals are converted into meaningful messages after they have been detected by the peripheral hearing mechanism. This phenomenon is particularly important for the understanding of speech signals. Failure to process auditory speech information accurately results in a breakdown in the communication process.

Central Auditory Processing Disorder: A disorder that occurs when the central auditory nervous system fails to efficiently process important speech stimuli. Adults and children with this type of disorder have difficulty processing auditory information in environments where even minimal ambient noise is present.

Clinical Observations: A fairly standard group of tests commonly used to supplement standardized testing of sensory integration especially in the area of posture; these tests generally lack normative data.

Cluster Analysis: A set of statistical procedures that can determine typologies by grouping subjects according to similar characteristics.

Constructional Ability: The ability to perform the sequences of movement involved in producing two- or three-dimensional representations as in drawing or assembling tasks. Construction has a strong spatial component since accurately reproducing a two-dimensional or three-dimensional design requires grasping the spatial relationships among the parts of a design.

Contralateral Ear: Literally, ear on the other side. Refers to acoustic stimuli that are present in the ear opposite to the ear being tested.

Decibel: A unit of measurement for expressing differences in power of acoustic stimuli.

Depth Perception: The visual system converts a two-dimensional retinal image into three dimensions based on the unconscious integration of visual information with head and eye movement. We experience depth through cues provided by motion parallax, optical expansion, stereoscopic vision, and linear perspective. The perception of depth is as direct as the perception of color.

Diadokokinesia: Rapidly alternating movements; when testing for sensory integrative dysfunction, we generally evaluate diadokokinesis of the forearms.

Dichotic: The simultaneous presentation of different stimuli to the two ears; this can be in the form of different consonant-vowel-consonant, words, or sentences.

Dynamic Balance: Balance in the context of voluntary movement.

Dyspraxia: A developmental condition in which

the ability to plan unfamiliar motor tasks is impaired.

Enhanced Sensation: More than that typically derived from daily life activity.

Factor Analysis: Examination of a set of data by looking at how variables are correlated; creates categories, or factors, that are statistically related

Feedback: Information arising from the response itself (i.e., production feedback) or from changes that occur in the environment as a result of the response (outcome feedback)

Feedback-Dependent Actions: Relatively easy tasks in which actors can adjust their movements in response to feedback obtained from the body. Generally occur when neither the actor nor the target is moving rapidly or very far.

Feedforward: Signals sent ahead of a movement to prepare for an upcoming motor command or to ready the system for the receipt of some kind of feedback information.

Feedforward-Dependent Actions: Relatively difficult tasks that are anticipatory in nature; they must occur before any feedback can be gathered. Generally occur when the actor, the target, or both are moving rapidly or great distances.

Grasp Phase of Reaching: In preparation for grasp, the hand begins to shape to accommodate the size of the object and the forearm rotates to position the hand to match the orientation of the object.

Gravitational Insecurity: A type of sensory modulation dysfunction thought to result from poor processing of vestibular and proprioceptive sensation; manifested as fear of moving, being out of the upright, or having one's feet off the ground which is out of proportion to any danger and also to any postural deficits the individual has.

Hearing Level: The number of decibels above an accepted average normal threshold for acoustic signals. For example, 10 dB HL refers to a level 10 decibels above the average reference for normal for a specific acoustic signal.

Ideation: Conceptualizing an action; knowing what to do.

Ipsilateral Ear: Literally, ear on the same side. Refers to more than one acoustic stimulus presented to the same ear. For example, when speech stimuli are presented to the right ear along with a competing speech-band noise spectrum.

Linear Movement: Movement occurring in a straight plane.

Learning Disability: A disorder of presumed neurological origin that results in difficulty with one or more of the processes involved in perceiving, understanding, using language, or doing mathematical calculations. It is not the result of primary visual or hearing loss, motor handicap, cognitive limitations, or lack of learning opportunities.

Neurodevelopmental Treatment: A sensorimotor approach to assessment and intervention of motor performance developed by Berta and Karl Bobath that is based on both neurological principles and normal development.

Neuromodulation: The balancing of excitatory and inhibitory inputs, and adapting to environmental changes.

Object Vision ("What" System): Neural processing attuned to the features of objects that enable us to identify and remember them.

Object-Focused Spatial Abilities: Skills tapped by many formal assessments including several of the performance subtests of the WISC (e.g., Block Design, Object Recognition) that involve recognition of the spatial relationships of objects to each other irrespective of their relationship to the individual.

Optic flow (Optic Array): The pattern of visual stimulation on the retina, including the visual stream across the retina, which occurs with every movement of the eyes, head, or body. Optic flow is a major source of information for the perception of depth, distance and movement.

Perception of Motion: Motion of (a) the self relative to a stable surround, (b) objects relative to the surround, (c) the surround relative to self, and the relative motion of moving objects.

Peripheral Hearing Mechanism: Classically referred to as the ear; a system that is separated into four main sections: (1) outer ear, (2) middle ear, (3) inner ear, and the (4) eighth cranial nerve. The peripheral hearing mechanism is typically tested using traditional hearing techniques to determine level of hearing, discrimination of speech in quiet, and possible site-of-lesion status.

Pre-rotary Nystagmus: Nystagmus taking place during angular movement of the head. The nystagmic eye movements are tied to the movement of endolymph in the canals, and they begin with the onset of movement. As movement continues at a steady pace, the endolymph catches up with the movement of the head, the cupula regains an upright position, and input to the CNS returns to baseline.

Post-rotary nystagmus: Involuntary rhythmic movements of the eye following short (~20 second duration) rotation. It consists of rapid movements of the eyes in one direction followed by a slow movement in the opposite direction. In post-rotary nystagmus the fast component is in direction opposite that of the spin.

Postural Dysfunction: Outward manifestation of vestibular proprioceptive processing deficits; characterized by difficulty with proximal stability, low extensor muscle tone, poor prone extension, poor neck flexion against gravity, and often, poor equilibrium.

Praxis on Verbal Command: A type of practic dysfunction identified by scores on two SIPT tests: low scores (<-1.0) on Praxis on Verbal Command and high scores ($>+1.0$) on Postrotary Nystagmus; not a sensory-integrative-based dyspraxia; thought to stem from higher level dysfunction.

Primary Functions of Human Vision: The guidance of motor actions and the visual identification of the objects in our environment. Different neural networks at subcortical and cortical levels mediate these two functions. Spatial vision is felt to be more related to the processing of vision in the parietal lobe and object vision to processing in the temporal lobe.

Projected Action Sequence: A series of actions driven forward by prediction. The action sequence is derived from an internal model of the world (based on previous experience).

Proprioception: Sensations derived from movement (i.e., speed, rate, sequencing, timing, and force) and joint position. Derived from stimulation to muscle and, to a lesser extent, joint receptors, especially from resistance to movement

Pure Tone Average: The average of an individual's air conduction pure tone thresholds at 500 Hz, 1000 Hz, and 2000 Hz for each ear.

Reach: Movement of the hand to a desired location. Reach is coded for direction and distance in relationship to the body schema; the object's location in relation to a person is important for the action.

Responsiveness: Behavioral manifestation of sensory modulation.

Scaffolding: A process in which a therapist or other caregiver adjusts and controls task elements that are just beyond a child's skills allowing the child to focus on elements that are within his or her abilities and to achieve success in completing the task.

Sensation Level: The number of decibels, above or greater than, a threshold for a particular sound stimulus at which a signal is presented.

Sensorimotor Approaches: The application of specific sensory stimulation through handling or direct stimulation with the purpose of eliciting a desired motor response.

Sensory Defensiveness: Fight or flight reaction to sensation that most others would consider non-noxious.

Sensory Detection: First step of sensory processing within the central nervous system.

Sensory Integration: The neurological process that organizes sensation from one's own body and from the environment and makes it possible to use the body effectively within the environment; the entire sequence of central nervous system events from reception to the display of an adaptive environmental interaction.

Sensory Integration and Praxis Tests (SIPT): A battery of 17 tests designed to evaluate several aspects of praxis as well as some aspects of somatosensory and visual discrimination and postural control in children 4 through 8 years of age with mild to moderate learning or motor difficulties. Their primary use is to contribute to understanding a child's difficulties and planning intervention.

Sensory-Integrative-Based Dyspraxia: Developmental difficulty with planning unfamiliar movements resulting from poor body scheme, which is based in turn on poor processing of sensation, especially vestibular, proprioceptive, and tactile. Generally, we speak of two types: deficits in bilateral integration and sequencing and somatodyspraxia.

Sensory-Integrative-Based Therapy: A program of intervention involving meaningful therapeutic activities characterized by enhanced sensation, especially tactile, vestibular, and proprioceptive, active participation, and adaptive interaction.

Sensory Integrative Dysfunction: Difficulty with CNS processing of sensation, especially vestibular, tactile, or proprioceptive, which is manifested as poor praxis, poor modulation, or both.

Sensory Modulation: The ability to regulate and organize reactions to sensory input in a graded and adaptive manner (behavioral).The balancing of excitatory and inhibitory inputs, and adapting to environmental changes (neurophysiological).

Sensory Modulation Dysfunction: A pattern of dysfunction of sensory integration in which a person under- or over-responds to sensory input from the body or environment. There are several types: gravitational insecurity, aversive response to movement; sensory defensiveness, under-responsiveness.

Sensory Processing: Functions related to sensation occurring in the central nervous system; includes reception, modulation, integration, and organization of sensory stimuli; also includes the behavioral responses to sensory input.

Sensory Registration: Noticing sensory stimuli in the environment.

Sensory Stimulation: A treatment technique that involves the application of direct sensory stimulation with the purpose of eliciting a generalized behavioral response, such as increased attention or calming.

Sensory Synthesis: The process of combining sensation between or within a sensory system.

Signal-to-Noise Ratio: The ratio of noise to the primary signal. For example, a signal-to-noise ratio of +6 dB refers to a primary signal presented 6 dB higher or more intense than the noise stimulus.

Somatodyspraxia: A relatively severe form of sensory-integrative-based dyspraxia characterized by difficulty with both easy (feedback-dependent) and more difficult (feedforward-dependent) motor tasks; thought to be based in poor processing of tactile and likely vestibular and proprioceptive sensations

Spatial Cognition: Higher-order visual spatial abilities involving the ability to recognize and remember the relationships between features within an object or design, between two or more objects, or between oneself and objects

Spatial Constancy: Neurophysiological mechanism that ensures stable vision while the eyes are moving. Spatial constancy depends upon the central registration of eye, head, and body movements coordinated with the central registration of the changes in the retinal pattern caused by those movements. It is a critical mechanism of the human visual system and the foundation of motor and perceptual functions in the physical world.

Spatial Vision ("Where" System): Neural processing which determines the locations and positions of objects, both relative to ourselves and to other objects. It processes the features of objects that are needed for actions.

Speech Recognition (Discrimination): A test score reflecting the percentage of correctly identified items on a standardized word-discrimination test.

Tactile: Sensation derived from stimulation to the skin.

Tactile Defensiveness: A subset of sensory defensiveness; a fight or flight reaction to touch that most others would consider non-noxious.

Tactile Discrimination Deficits: Impaired ability to recognize the spatiotemporal characteristics of touch generally identified through tactile tests on the Sensory Integration and Praxis Tests

Threshold: The level at which signals (stimuli) are barely perceptible. With regard to auditory stimuli, the threshold is determined to be the level at which the individual is able to detect its presence 50 percent of the time.

Topographical Orientation (Wayfinding): Ability to go from place to place in familiar surroundings without getting lost and to learn how to find the way in new environments.

Vestibular: Sensation derived from stimulation to the vestibular mechanism in the inner ear that occurs through movement and position of the head; contributes to posture and the maintenance of a stable visual field.

Zone of Proximal Development: The distance between children's independent performance and their performance under adult guidance or in collaboration with more capable peers.

■■ Index

Page numbers followed by an "f" indicate figures; page numbers followed by a "t" indicate tables.